Atlas of Mammography

THIRD EDITION

ELLEN SHAW de PAREDES, MD, FACR

Founder and Director
Ellen Shaw de Paredes Institute for Women's Imaging
Glen Allen, Virginia

Clinical Professor of Radiology
University of Virginia
School of Medicine
Charlottesville, Virginia

Clinical Professor of Medicine
Virginia Commonwealth University
Richmond, Virginia

Wolters Kluwer | Lippincott Williams & Wilkins
Health
Philadelphia · Baltimore · New York · London
Buenos Aires · Hong Kong · Sydney · Tokyo

Acquisitions Editor: Lisa McAllister
Managing Editor: Kerry Barrett
Developmental Editor: Leanne McMillan
Marketing Manager: Angela Panetta
Project Manager: Nicole Walz
Manufacturing Coordinator: Ben Rivera
Design Coordinator: Stephen Druding
Cover Designer: Cathleen Elliott
Production Services: Aptara, Inc.
Printer: Maple Press—York

Printed in the United States of America

Library of Congress Cataloging-in-Publication Data

de Paredes, Ellen Shaw.
   Atlas of mammography / Ellen Shaw de Paredes.—3rd ed.
     p. ; cm.
   Rev. ed. of: Atlas of film-screen mammography.   2nd ed. c1992.
   Includes bibliographical references and index.
   ISBN-13: 978-0-7817-6433-9
   ISBN-10: 0-7817-6433-5
   1. Breast—Cancer—Diagnosis—Atlases. 2. Breast—Radiography—Atlases.
 I. de Paredes, Ellen Shaw. Atlas of film-screen mammography. II. Title.
   [DNLM: 1. Breast Neoplasms—radiography—Atlases. 2. Mammography—Atlases.
   WP 17 D278a 2007]
   RC280.B8D38 2007
   616.99'44907572—dc22

2006037826

To Victor, for his tremendous encouragement, support, advice, and dedication.

and

To my parents, George and Julia Shaw, who inspired me to achieve my goals.

I am forever grateful.

CONTENTS

"The heights by great men reached and kept
Were not attained by sudden flight
But they, while their companions slept
Were toiling upward in the night"
                                    —Longfellow

Mammography is a well established technique that has been proven to reduce the death rate for breast cancer in screened populations of women. Since the last edition of this book, major changes have occurred in breast imaging. Mammography has been well established and is utilized as a screening and diagnostic tool. Breast ultrasound and MRI are also used frequently in the evaluation of abnormalities. Breast interventional procedures are more varied and serve to diagnose breast lesions. Digital mammography has been developed, approved by the Food and Drug Administration and is utilized in the United States and abroad. The Mammography Quality Standards Act was passed by Congress and implemented, and is an important mechanism for standardizing and improving the quality of mammography services. The training of radiologists in breast imaging is now a well established component of radiology residency programs. Even with improved techniques, tools and training, the challenge for the radiologist remains to identify breast cancer when it is small and curable.

The focus of this book is to present via mammographic images, the patterns of normal and abnormal breasts so that radiologists may be better equipped to identify breast cancers. *The Atlas of Mammography* serves as a primary training tool as well as a reference source when one is faced with a diagnostic dilemma. The book is organized based on a pattern-recognition format, thereby facilitating its use as a reference source.

Chapters on anatomy, techniques and positioning and an approach to mammographic analysis are once again included as well as a series of chapters on masses, calcifications, dilated ducts, the edema pattern and asymmetries. The male breast, the axilla, the post surgical and augmented breast are covered as well as a series of chapters on breast interventions and the roles of ultrasound and MRI. New chapters in this book are those on asymmetries and distortions, the augmented breast, galactography, needle localization, percutaneous breast biopsy, ultrasound and MRI. In each chapter, comprehensive differential diagnoses are presented with cases demonstrating the various entities.

Images were acquired on Siemens analog and full field digital units. All mammographic images are presented with the patient's left to the reader's left. I prefer to read film screen images in this orientation so that the surface glare from the non emulsion side of the film is reduced.

There are many individuals I wish to thank for their contributions to this book. First, my technologists, Diane Loudermilk, Chrystal Sullivan, Robyn Ost, Deborah Smith, and Lanea Bare are responsible for the excellent radiography that served as the source material for this book. Dr. Ami Trivedi was instrumental in case collection and organization. Image production and graphics were carefully prepared by Whitney Shank and who was assisted by Mariel Santos. The photographs were prepared by Carlos Chavez. The editorial assistance provided by my mother, Julia Shaw was invaluable. The pathology images were provided by Dr. Michael Kornstein to whom I am most thankful. Some of the unusual cases were provided by former fellows including Drs. Neeti Goel, Thomas Poulton, Thomas Langer, Deanna Lane, Patricia Abbitt, and Lindsay Cheng.

I gratefully thank my secretary, Ms. Louise Logan who tirelessly worked on the manuscript preparation, giving attention to all the details. I also thank Kerry Barrett at Lippincott Williams & Wilkins for her editorial assistance.

The Ellen Shaw de Paredes Research Foundation provided support through a grant for book production and preparation of materials, and I am most grateful for the unwavering support of the Board.

Several individuals who are extremely important to me helped to guide my career into the subspecialty of breast imaging, a field that has so much meaning and importance in improving patients' lives. My parents, George and Julia Shaw, encouraged me to be a physician and taught me the value of education and the importance of self discipline. My selection of the field of radiology was suggested by my husband, Dr. Victor Paredes, who encouraged me to write the first Atlas and has been incredibly supportive and encouraging of this endeavor. I thank Dr. Theodore Keats, who was the first radiology chair under whom I worked, and who directed me into breast imaging, giving me the opportunity to develop the section at the University of Virginia.

As I write this preface, I reflect on the many nights that I sat up late until the early morning hours, working on the book. As life has become busier with clinical work, the effort to produce this book has been far greater than that for the earlier editions. This effort was energized by the kind support and constant encouragement of my husband, the loyalty of my dear dog Sam, who warmed my feet as I wrote every word, and the powerful self discipline that my mother has taught me. But most importantly so many of my former residents and fellows have taught me how much their training in mammography and their knowledge has changed their own patients' lives. I hope that this work will provide the reader with greater insight into the complexities of mammography.

Ellen Shaw de Paredes, M.D.

PREFACE to the FIRST EDITION

"People see only what they are prepared to see."
(Ralph Waldo Emerson, Journals, 1863)

The early detection of breast cancer depends primarily on mammography. With the increasing emphasis on screening mammography by organizations such as the American Cancer Society, there is rapidly expanding utilization of mammography services, and there is a concomitant need for increased training of radiologists and radiology residents.

High-quality images are absolutely necessary for the detection of subtle abnormalities. There are tremendous differences in patterns of the breast parenchyma among women. Although the number of diseases that affect the breast is not vast, the perception and analysis of an abnormality can make mammography seem difficult.

The purpose of this book is to present through images the various manifestations of breast diseases, so that the reader may use it not only as a reference source, but also as a tool for developing pattern recognition skills in mammography. The book will be useful to practicing radiologists or to radiology residents in the process of learning mammography.

Each chapter is introduced with a brief review of the various processes that are manifested as a specific pattern, and is followed by a series of radiographs demonstrating the lesions. Correlation of clinical findings, mammographic findings, and histologic diagnosis is made. In some cases, not only mammography but also ultrasound images and histopathologic sections are correlated.

The initial sections discuss the anatomy and physiology of the breast, the proper techniques for performing film-screen mammography, and the analysis of a mammogram. The body of the text deals with chapters divided by patterns—well-defined masses, ill-defined masses, calcifications, prominent ducts, and thickened skin. The remainder of the text covers the axilla, the male breast, and interventional procedures in mammography.

The recent technical trends are towards film-screen mammography. This book covers only film-screen techniques, and all images are film radiographs. The images were produced almost entirely at the University of Virginia on either an Elscint Mam-II unit, which does not utilize a grid, or newer Siemens Mammomat B and the Mammomat-2 units with grids. The higher contrast and improved image quality on the radiographs from the equipment with grids are apparent on the reproductions. Film-screen systems that have been utilized are Kodak Ortho M film and Min-R screens and Kodak T-Mat M film with Min-R Fast screens.

I wish to acknowledge the fine work of my dedicated technologists. Deborah Smith, Diane Loudermilk, Mary Owens, Bonnie Mallan, Marie Bickers, Theresa Breeden, and Lisa Elgin, who are responsible for the radiographs. My special thanks go to Deborah Smith for assisting in writing the section on patient positioning. Manuscript preparation was carried out by Joy Bottomly and Patsie Cutright. Esther Spears, Catherine Payne, Kim Nash, Adair Crawford, Susan Bywaters, Tracy Bowles, and Lisa Crickenberger assisted in the collection of cases and other production work. The line drawings were produced by Craig Harding, and the reproductions of radiographs were done by Ursula Bunch, Connie Gardner, and Patricia Pugh of the Biomedical Communications Division. I wish to thank Dr. Sana Tabbarah for her assistance with the pathology slides and descriptions. My postresidency fellows, Drs. Patricia Abbitt and Thomas Langer, have assisted greatly with clinical work, leaving me time to work on this project. My appreciation also goes to other physicians who have sent me interesting cases: Drs. Luisa Marsteller, George Oliff, Jay Levine, Alexander Girevendulis, A.C. Wagner, Bernard Savage, M.C. Wilhelm, Melvin Vinik, and James Lynde. Lastly, I wish to thank my husband, Dr. Victor Paredes, for his assistance with the production and editing of the book. Without their help, this work would not have been possible.

Ellen Shaw de Paredes, M.D.

FOREWORD from the SECOND EDITION

Although many years of effort have been spent in improving surgical and radiotherapeutic techniques, the mortality rate from breast cancer remains appalling. It is commonly conceded that early detection is the best means of reducing this mortality. Fortunately, mammography has finally evolved as a means of achieving this purpose. At last we have an opportunity to improve significantly the cure rate for patients with breast cancer.

Mammography today is far different from what it was when I became involved with it more than 25 years ago. Progress has resulted from the dedicated efforts of the pioneers in this field, such as Egan and Wolfe and their associates. Today, this progress continues with further improvement in image quality, techniques for localizing lesions, and biopsy procedures. These advances have led to greatly improved detection rates. They have also made it necessary for the radiologist constantly to modify his or her patterns of practice and to become a perennial student in the field.

Dr. Ellen Shaw de Paredes has been tireless in the pursuit of excellence in her mammographic program at the University of Virginia. Her work exemplifies the enlightened state of modern mammography. This book reflects her clinical experience and contains a wealth of teaching axioms gleaned from working with many residents, fellows, and surgical colleagues. Her new edition includes additional case material to amplify her teaching points. Also included are discussions of interventional procedures and a valuable chapter on the postoperative breast. These additions should further enhance the scope of this valuable work.

Theodore E. Keats, M.D.
Professor and Chairman
Department of Radiology
University of Virginia School of Medicine
Charlottesville, Virginia

Anatomy of the Breast

The breast or mammary gland is a modified sweat gland that has the specific function of milk production. An understanding of the basic anatomy, physiology, and histology is important in the interpretation of mammography. With an understanding of the normal breast, one is better able to correlate radiologic-pathologic entities.

DEVELOPMENT

The development of the breast begins in the fifth-week embryo with the formation of the primitive milk streak from axilla to groin. The band develops into the mammary ridge in the thoracic area and regresses elsewhere.

If there is incomplete regression or dispersion of the milk streak, there is accessory mammary tissue present in the adult, which occurs in 2% to 6% of women (1). Accessory breast tissue, particularly in the axillary area, that is separate from the bulk of the parenchyma may be identified on mammography in these women (2) (Fig. 1.1). The orientation of the milk streak is slightly lateral to the nipple above the nipple line and medial to the nipple below the nipple line. Therefore, patients with accessory breasts, accessory parenchyma, or accessory nipples are found to have these in the axillary region or just medial to the nipple in the inferior aspect of the breast or upper abdominal wall (Figs. 1.2, 1.3). In women with accessory breast tissue, changes occur cyclically and with pregnancy and lactation, as they do within the breasts themselves. Therefore, these patients may note that areas of accessory breast tissue may enlarge with pregnancy and may produce milk when the patient is lactating if there is a duct orifice or nipple present.

At 7 to 8 weeks of embryologic development, there is an invagination into the mesenchyma of the chest wall. Mesenchymal cells differentiate into the smooth muscle of the nipple and areola (1,3). At 16 weeks, epithelial buds develop and branch. Between 20 and 32 weeks, placental sex hormones entering the fetal circulation induce canalization of the epithelial buds to form the mammary ducts.

At 32 to 40 weeks, differentiation of the parenchyma occurs, with the formation of the lobules (3,4).

The mammary gland mass increases by fourfold, and the nipple-areolar complex develops (1). Developmental anomalies include polymastia (accessory breasts along the milk streak), polythelia (accessory nipples), hypoplasia of the breast (Fig. 1.4), amastia (absence of the breast), and amazia (absence of breast parenchyma) (Fig. 1.5) (1). Systemic or iatrogenic influences in childhood may be related to breast hypoplasia or amazia. Iatrogenic causes of amazia include excision of the breast bud during biopsy of the prepubertal breast and the use of radiation therapy to the chest wall during childhood (1) (Fig. 1.6).

During puberty in girls, the release of follicle-stimulating hormone and luteinizing hormone by the pituitary causes release of estrogens by the ovary. Hormonal stimulation induces growth and maturation of the breasts. In early adolescence, the estrogen synthesis by the ovary predominates over progesterone synthesis. The physiologic effect of estrogen on the developing breast is to stimulate longitudinal ductal growth and the formation of terminal ductule buds (1). Periductal connective tissue and fat deposition increase (1), accounting for increase in size and density of the breasts.

STRUCTURE

The adult breast is composed of three basic structures: the skin, the subcutaneous fat, and the breast tissue, which includes the parenchyma and the stroma. Beneath the breast is the pectoralis major muscle, which is also imaged during mammography. The breast parenchyma is enveloped by deep and superficial fascial layers; Cooper's ligaments, the fibrous strands that support the breasts, traverse the parenchyma and attach to the fascial layers. The parenchyma is divided into 15 to 20 segments, with each drained by a lactiferous duct (Fig. 1.7). The lactiferous ducts converge beneath the nipple, with about 5 to 10 major ducts draining into the nipple. Each duct drains a lobe composed of 20 to 40 lobules (Fig. 1.8).

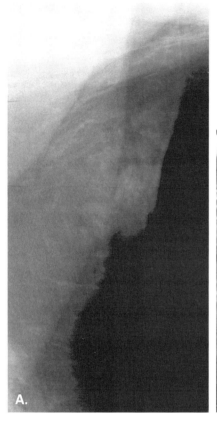

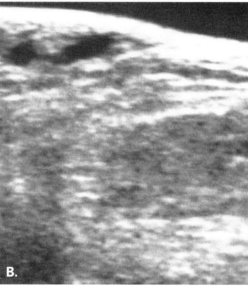

Figure 1.1

HISTORY: A 30-year-old woman in the 32nd week of pregnancy, presenting with an enlarging axillary mass.

MAMMOGRAPHY: Right axillary (A) view shows a prominent ductal and glandular pattern in the area of the mass in the axilla. On ultrasound (B), dilated ducts are noted in the subcutaneous area. The findings are consistent with accessory breast tissue that is enlarging secondary to the pregnancy.

IMPRESSION: Accessory breast in the axilla, with changes related to pregnancy.

The microanatomy of the breast was described by Parks in 1959 (4). Each lobule is 1 to 2 mm in diameter and contains a complex system of tiny ducts (the ductules), which terminate in blind endings. The ductules can respond to hormonal stimulation of pregnancy by proliferation and formation of alveoli (3). Two types of stroma are present: the perilobular connective tissue, which contains collagen and fat, and the intralobular connective tissue, which does not contain fat (4).

Wellings et al. (5) further classified the microstructure of the normal breast into the terminal duct lobular unit (TDLU) (Fig 1.9). Small branches of the lactiferous ducts lead into terminal ducts that drain a single lobule. The terminal duct is composed of the extralobular segment and the intralobular segment. The lobule is composed of the intralobular terminal duct and the blindly ending ductules (5). The ductules are lined by a single layer of epithelial cells and a flattened peripheral layer of myoepithelial cells (5). A loose fibrous connective tissue stroma supports the ductules of the lobule.

The TDLU is a hormone-sensitive gland varying from 1 to 8 mm in diameter in the nonpregnant state and having the potential of milk production (6). The lobules normally regress at menopause, leaving blunt terminal ducts; however, in women older than 55 years with

breast cancer, Jensen et al. (6) found the TDLUs remain well developed.

The work of Wellings et al. (5) has suggested that the TDLU is a basic histopathologic unit of breast from which many benign and malignant lesions arise. Fibroadenomas, sclerosing adenosis, apocrine cysts, lobular hyperplasia, and lobular carcinoma in situ are thought to develop in the lobule itself; ductal hyperplasia and ductal carcinoma in situ develop in the TDLU. Solitary intraductal papillomas, epithelial hyperplasia of the larger ducts, and duct ectasia occur in the main lactiferous ducts (4). Correlative studies between radiographic and histologic appearances of the breast parenchyma suggest that small nodular densities on mammography represent lesions of the terminal duct lobular units and that linear densities are due to periductal and perilobular fibrosis (7).

BLOOD SUPPLY AND LYMPHATIC DRAINAGE

The primary arterial supply to the breast is from the perforating branches of the internal mammary and lateral

(text continues on page 5)

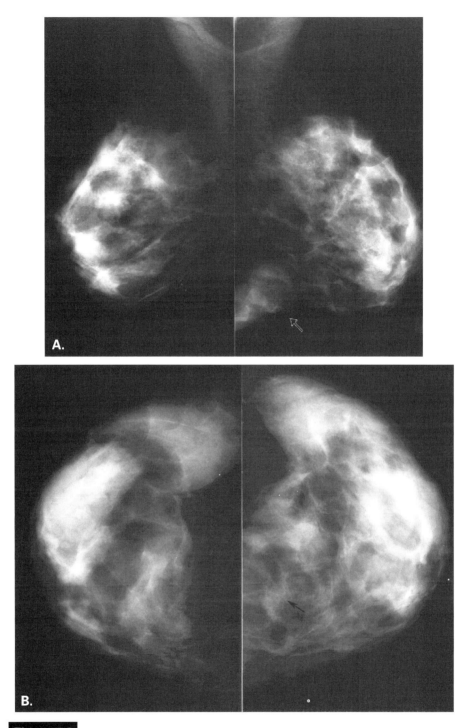

Figure 1.2

HISTORY: A 50-year-old woman with fullness in the right breast inferiorly.

MAMMOGRAPHY: Bilateral MLO (**A**) and CC (**B**) views show heterogeneously dense breasts. In the right breast at 6 o'clock is a prominent focal area of asymmetric breast tissue (**arrow**). Ultrasound showed no focal abnormality. No mass was palpable on clinical examination of this area.

IMPRESSION: Focal asymmetric breast tissue consistent with accessory breast.

NOTE: Accessory breast tissue is typically located laterally above the nipple line and medially below the nipple line.

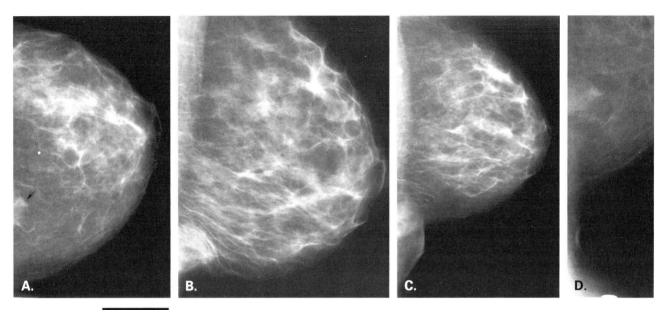

Figure 1.3

HISTORY: A 55-year-old woman with slight fullness of the inferior aspect of the right breast.

MAMMOGRAPHY: Right CC **(A)** and MLO **(B)** views show a focal rounded asymmetry in the inferior aspect of the right breast, located slightly medially **(arrow)**. On a ML **(C)** view of the lower aspect of the breast, the very inferior location of the asymmetry in the inframammary area is noted. On the cleavage view **(D)**, the rounded aspect of the asymmetry is seen.

IMPRESSION: Accessory breast tissue.

NOTE: Accessory breast tissue below the nipple line is located slightly medially, because it develops from the primitive milk streak.

Figure 1.4

HISTORY: A 26-year-old gravida 0, para 0 woman with a history of ectodermal dysplasia. She had bilateral breast implants placed during adolescence because of the lack of breast development.

MAMMOGRAPHY: Bilateral MLO views. There are bilateral breast implants present. There is some dense glandular tissue in the subareolar area on the left side, but there are only rudimentary ducts on the right **(arrow)**. The appearance on the right is similar to a normal male breast or a preadolescent female breast. In the condition of ectodermal dysplasia, there is a lack of normal development of epithelial structures such as nails, teeth, skin, hair, and sweat glands. Because the breast is a modified sweat gland and is derived from epithelium, the development of the breast can be impaired in this condition.

IMPRESSION: Maldevelopment of the breast secondary to ectodermal dysplasia.

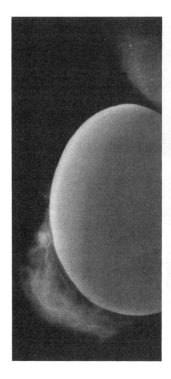
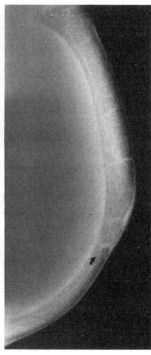

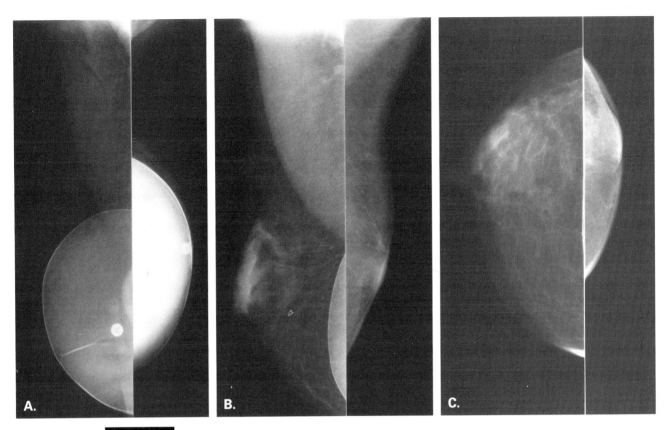

Figure 1.5

HISTORY: Screening mammogram in a patient who is status post augmentation mammoplasty that was performed for marked asymmetry of breast size.

MAMMOGRAPHY: Bilateral MLO (**A**) and MLO implant displaced (**B**) views show that prepectoral saline implants are present. On the displaced views (**B**), the left pectoralis major muscle is present, but no similar structure is seen on the right. There is marked disparity of breast size, with the right breast being smaller and less glandular than the left, also confirmed on the CC implant displaced (**C**) views.

IMPRESSION: Mammary hypoplasia secondary to Poland's syndrome.

NOTE: Poland's syndrome is lack of development of the pectoralis major muscle.

thoracic arteries. Minor contributions to the blood come from the branches of the thoracoacromial, subscapular, and thoracodorsal arteries (1). Venous drainage is primarily via branches of the internal mammary, intercostal, and axillary veins. If there is obstruction of the subclavian vein, collateral drainage produces dilated, tortuous vascular structures, easily visible on mammography (Fig. 1.10).

Lymphatic drainage is via the superficial plexus to the deep plexus to the axillary and internal mammary lymph nodes. The low axillary nodes are often visible on mammography, as are small intramammary nodes. It is unusual to identify on mammography intramammary nodes in a location other than the superficial region of the middle- to upper-outer quadrant of the breast.

MUSCULATURE

The breast lays over the musculature of the chest wall: the pectoralis major and minor muscles. The pectoralis major muscle has its origins at the anterior medial surface of the clavicle, the sternum, and the aponeurosis of the external oblique muscle and its insertion on the proximal humerus. The pectoralis major muscle, therefore, lies obliquely over the chest wall. This angle of obliquity varies with the body type of the individual. A parameter for a well-positioned mediolateral oblique (MLO) mammographic view is that the pectoralis major muscle is visible from the axilla down to the level of the nipple. Before positioning the patient for the MLO view, the

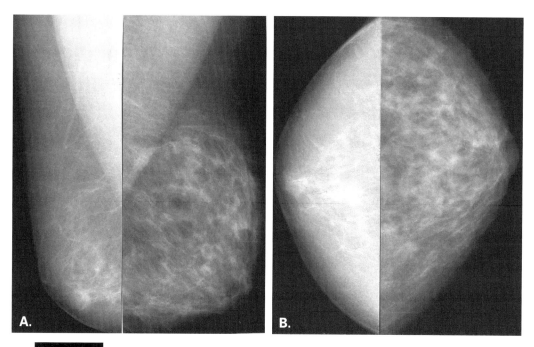

A.   B.

Figure 1.6

HISTORY: A 49-year-old gravida 2, para 2 woman with a history of a plasma cell tumor of the left lung, treated with pneumonectomy and radiation therapy at age 4 years. The left breast has been significantly smaller than the right since development. The patient has no history of breast surgery.

MAMMOGRAPHY: Bilateral MLO **(A)** and CC **(B)** views. Marked asymmetry in the appearance of the breasts is seen. The left breast is significantly smaller, and there is a paucity of glandular tissue in comparison with the right. This striking lack of glandular development is presumably related to the lack of development of the breast bud, either from atrophy secondary to the radiation therapy or from surgery in the left midchest area, which may have involved incidental removal of part of the breast bud.

IMPRESSION: Hypoplasia of the left breast, presumably of iatrogenic origin.

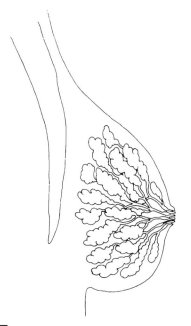

Figure 1.7

Gross anatomy of the normal breast.

technologist must determine the angle of obliquity of the pectoralis major muscle. She then angles the mammographic receptor and compression device into this position. She is thereby able to compress the breast along the plane of the pectoralis muscle and to include more breast tissue. The pectoralis major muscle may be seen on the craniocaudal (CC) view in about one fourth to one third patients. Often, the muscle is seen as an area of density along the posterior aspect of the breast. Occasionally, the medial aspect of the muscle at the sternal border is prominent and can appear masslike on the CC view only.

An inconstant muscle that may be present unilaterally or bilaterally is the sternalis muscle. This is a muscle band that runs vertically, parallel to the sternum. The sternalis muscle occurs in 3% to 5% of individuals and is more frequently observed in women. When present, the sternalis may be visible on mammography as a triangular or rounded density on the CC view only, and it is located at the medial, posterior edge of the breast (Figs. 1.11–1.14). It is not evident on the MLO or mediolateral (ML) views, and ultrasound is normal. If in doubt, a

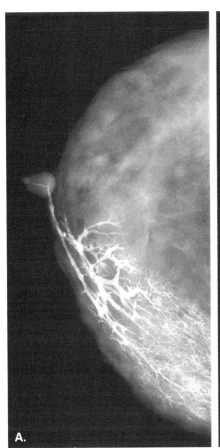
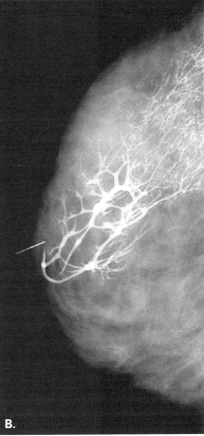

A.   B.

Figure 1.8

HISTORY: Patient presenting with a left serous nipple discharge.

GALACTOGRAM: Left CC (**A**) and ML (**B**) views show filling of the parenchymal system in the upper-inner quadrant via the cannulated duct. The normal ductal structures are seen, ramifying back into smaller ductal elements and eventually filling the rounded lobules.

IMPRESSION: Normal ductal anatomy.

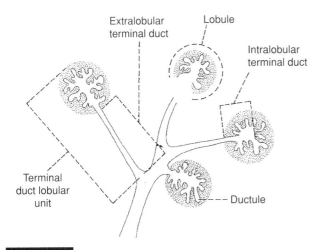

Figure 1.9

Classification of the microstructure of the breast (from Wellings SR, Jensen HM, Marcum RG. An atlas of subgross pathology of the human breast with special reference to precancerous lesions. *J Natl Cancer Inst* 1975;55:231–273 .)

computed tomography (CT) scan can be performed and will demonstrate the sternalis muscle clearly.

LIFE CYCLE

At birth and in childhood, only rudimentary ducts are present (Fig. 1.15). At puberty, growth and elongation of ducts occur, and buds of the future lobules form at the end of the ducts (4,8). Periductal collagen is deposited, and mammographically the breast appears very dense and homogeneous. In the adult, in response to progesterone, the second stage of glandular development occurs, namely, the formation of the lobules (8) (Fig. 1.16).

With pregnancy, changes in the parenchyma occur to make milk secretion possible (8). There is marked increase in numbers of lobules and an increase in their size and complexity (4) (Fig. 1.17). In the second and third trimesters of pregnancy, the terminal ductules expand into the secreting alveoli (4). Prolactin, in the presence of insulin, growth hormone, and cortisol, changes the epithelial cells of the alveoli into a secretory state (1). With

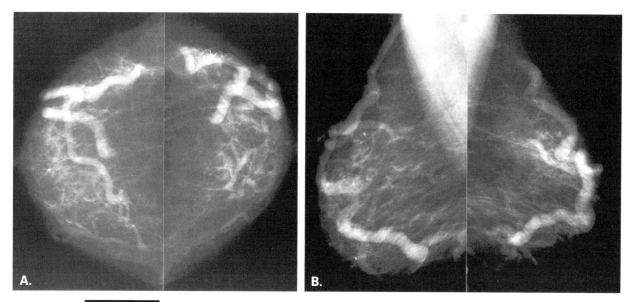

Figure 1.10

HISTORY: A 71-year-old woman with a history of diabetes, chronic renal failure, pulmonary embolism, and thrombophilia.

MAMMOGRAPHY: Bilateral CC **(A)** and MLO **(B)** views show circuitous vascular structures extending into the axillary regions. These are enlarged venous collaterals, likely secondary to the history of pulmonary embolism and a clot in the superior vena cava.

IMPRESSION: Enlarged venous collaterals.

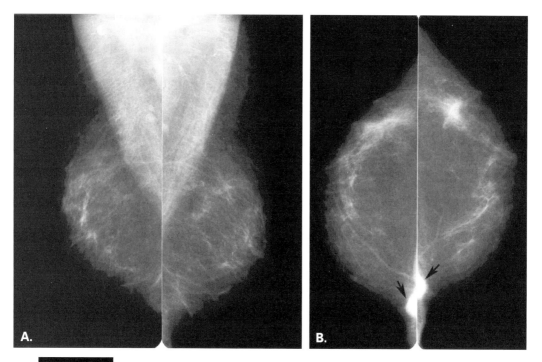

Figure 1.11

HISTORY: A 51-year-old women for screening mammography.

MAMMOGRAPHY: Bilateral MLO **(A)** and CC **(B)** views show scattered fibroglandular densities. There are bilateral dense ovoid masslike densities located far medially at the chest wall **(arrows)**. The obtuse angle at the chest wall is typical of a muscular structure.

IMPRESSION: Sternalis muscle.

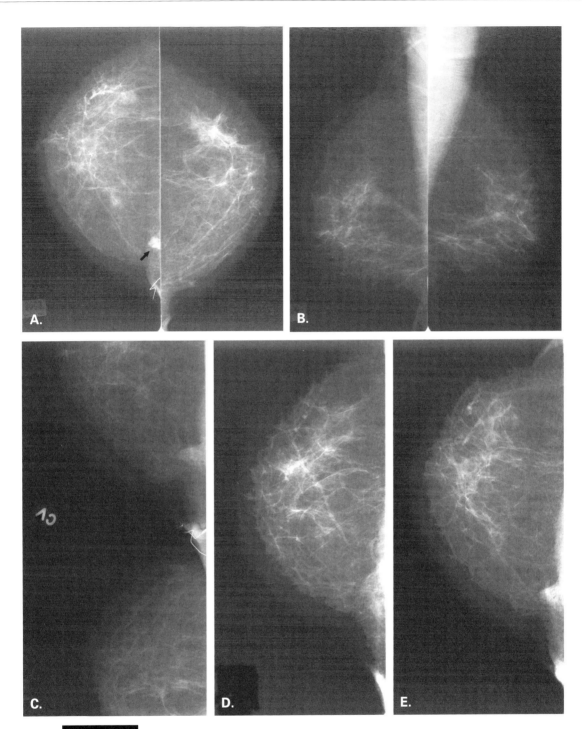

Figure 1.12

HISTORY: Screening mammogram.

MAMMOGRAPHY: Bilateral CC views **(A)** show a focal masslike density in the far medial posterior aspect of the left breast **(arrow)**. The normal pectoralis major muscle extends obliquely down the chest wall on the MLO view **(B)**, however, the focal density is not seen. The masslike density is evident on the cleavage view **(C)**. On the rolled CC lateral **(D)** and medial **(E)** views, the density changes shape and appears more obtuse at the chest wall.

IMPRESSION: Sternalis muscle.

the onset of lactation, the alveoli become maximally dilated, and milk production occurs. On mammography (Figs. 1.18 and 1.19), the lactating breast usually appears extremely dense, and dilated ducts may be seen. However, in a study of 18 women who were pregnant or lactating, Swinford et al. (9) found that these patients did not always have dense breasts. In this study, all seven lactating women had heterogeneously dense or extensively dense breasts, yet in 4 of 6 women, the density had not increased from the prepartum mammogram. After lactation ceases, the hypertrophied lobules shrink and may disappear. The breasts of parous women tend to appear more fatty and radiolucent than those of nulliparous women.

With menopause, there is further involution of the parenchyma. The terminal lobules disappear, and the small ducts eventually atrophy. The main ducts are not greatly affected (4) (Fig. 1.20). The postmenopausal breast appears more radiolucent (10,11), and only minimal glandular elements are generally seen (Fig. 1.21). However, in some patients who have marked fibrocystic changes premenopausally or who are nulliparous, persistent dense parenchyma may be seen postmenopausally (Fig. 1.22).

The effects of endogenous hormones related to the menstrual cycle have been observed on the histologic appearance of the normal breast (12). During the first half of the menstrual cycle, the effect of estrogen is to stimulate breast epithelial proliferation. In the second half of the cycle, after ovulation, progesterone causes ductal dilatation and differentiation of the ductular epithelial cells into secretory cells. In the 3 to 4 days before menses, edema and enhanced ductular acinar proliferation occur (1,12,13). Mammography at this time is more difficult

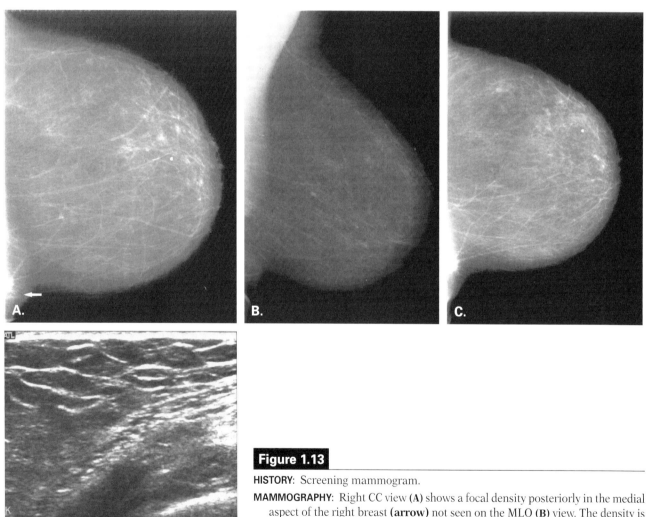

Figure 1.13

HISTORY: Screening mammogram.

MAMMOGRAPHY: Right CC view **(A)** shows a focal density posteriorly in the medial aspect of the right breast **(arrow)** not seen on the MLO **(B)** view. The density is more triangular in appearance on the exaggerated CC medial **(C)** view; no abnormality was found on ultrasound **(D)**. The location and appearance of this structure are characteristic of a normal variant, the sternalis muscle.

IMPRESSION: Sternalis muscle.

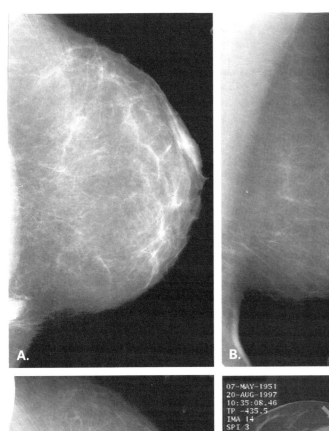

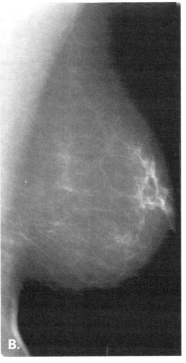

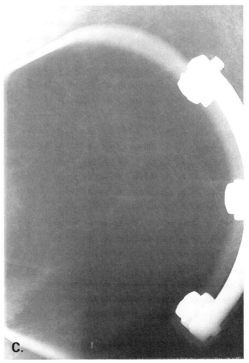

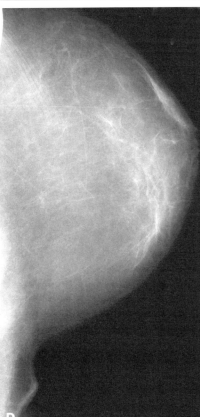

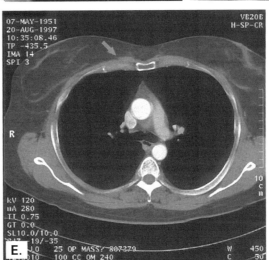

Figure 1.14

HISTORY: A 46-year-old patient referred for needle localization of a right breast mass.

MAMMOGRAPHY: Right CC view **(A)** shows an oval masslike density located at the chest wall, far posteriorly **(arrow)**. The lesion was not seen on the MLO view **(B)**, however, it persisted on the spot-compression CC **(C)** view. On the rolled medial CC view **(D)**, the area changes shape considerably, becoming more obtuse with the chest wall. Ultrasound was performed of the entire medial aspect of the breast and was negative. On CT **(E)**, the asymmetry of the parasternal musculature is seen **(arrow)**. There is an accessory muscle on the right consistent with sternalis muscle and corresponding to the mammographic finding.

IMPRESSION: Right sternalis muscle.

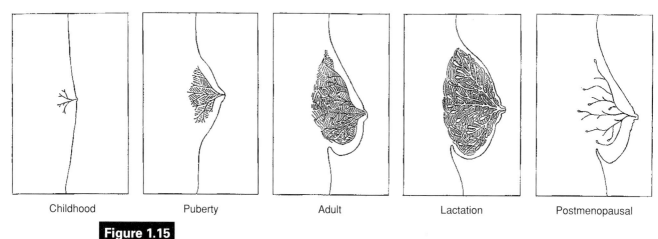

Childhood   Puberty   Adult   Lactation   Postmenopausal

Figure 1.15

Changes that the normal breast undergoes during the life cycle.

because the breasts are tender and may appear more dense. In a study of women aged 40 to 49 years, who were not on exogenous hormones, White et al. (14) found that breast parenchyma is less radiographically dense in the follicular rather than the luteal phase of the menstrual cycle. Postmenstrually, the edema is reduced, and secretory activity of the epithelium regresses (1,12).

Exogenous hormones may also have an effect on the mammographic appearance of the breast (Fig. 1.23). An increase in mammography density has been observed in 10% to 73% of women on combined therapy with estrogen and progesterone (15–24). Marugg et al. (19) found that 31% of patients treated with combination hormone replacement therapy (HRT) had an increase in fibroglandular tissue compared with 8.7% of women treated with estrogens alone, and this difference was statistically significant. Laya et al. (20) found that the increase in density was more pronounced in women with a lower baseline

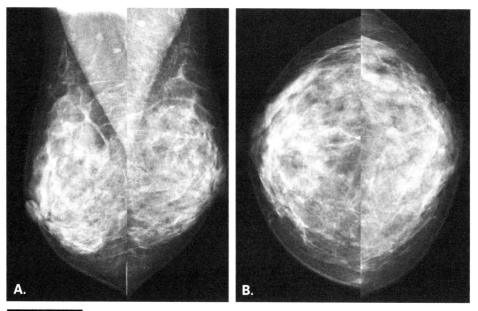

Figure 1.16

HISTORY: A 32-year-old gravida 2, para 2 woman with a positive family history of breast cancer, for screening mammography.

MAMMOGRAPHY: Bilateral MLO **(A)** and CL **(B)** views show diffusely dense breast tissue with no focal abnormalities. This parenchymal pattern is often seen in young patients, and the density is related to parenchymal and stromal elements.

IMPRESSION: Normal breast, young patient.

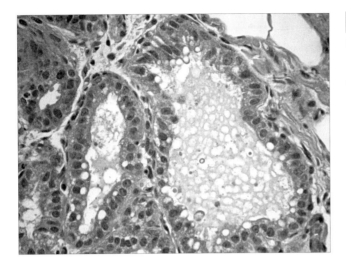

Figure 1.17

HISTOPATHOLOGY: High power section of a lactating breast: the lobules are distended and filled with an eosinophilic material; secretory vacuoles are noted in the cells lining the glands.

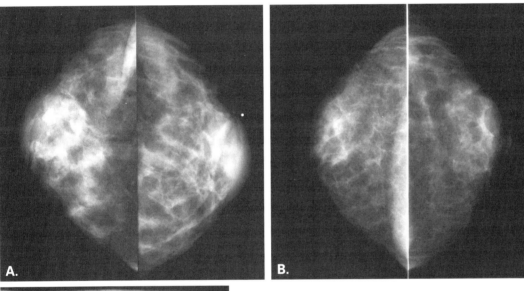

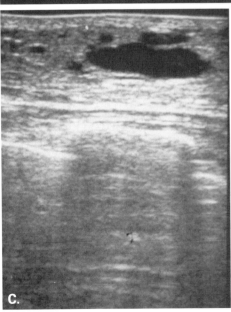

Figure 1.18

HISTORY: A 32-year-old lactating woman, with a family history of premenopausal breast cancer in the grandmother, presents with a palpable right subareolar mass.

MAMMOGRAPHY: Bilateral CC (A) views show marked increase in density bilaterally with ductal dilatation. Comparison with a prior study (B) shows the parenchymal changes related to lactation. Ultrasound of the subareolar area (C) shows fluid-filled dilated ducts.

IMPRESSION: Lactational changes, dilated ducts.

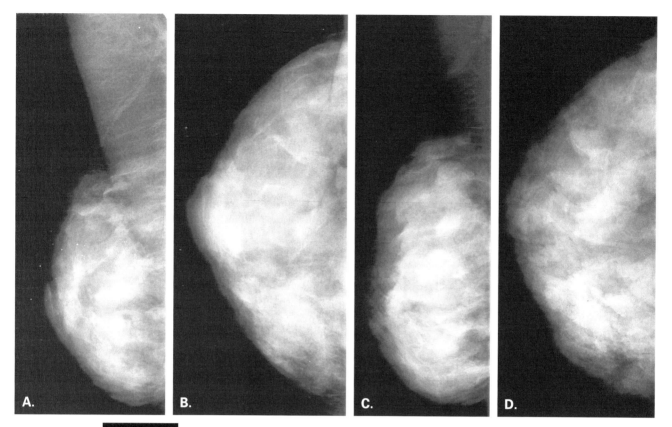

Figure 1.19

HISTORY: Screening mammograms 1 year apart in a 37-year-old patient at high risk for breast cancer. At the time of the second study, the patient was lactating.

MAMMOGRAPHY: Initial left MLO **(A)** and CC **(B)** views show heterogeneously dense parenchyma. On the subsequent postpartum study **(C, D)**, when the patient was lactating, there was marked overall increase in density and size of the breast. These changes were bilateral and are consistent with the normal lactating breast.

IMPRESSION: Normal changes in the lactating breast.

parenchymal density. In the Women's Health Initiative randomized trial, McTiernan et al. (25) found that the mean mammographic percent density increased by 6.0% at year 1 in women placed on combined HRT versus decreasing by 0.9% in women not on hormones. Rutter et al. (26) found that the relative risk of an increase in breast density was 2.57 in women who initiated HRT; after discontinuation of HRT, the relative risk of a density decrease was 1.81. Therefore, the breast density changes associated with HRT are dynamic, increasing with initiation and decreasing with discontinuation.

Stomper et al. (16) found changes related to hormonal influences in 24% of women placed on estrogen; these changes included diffuse increase in density (14%), multifocal areas of asymmetry (4%), and cyst formation (6%). Trapido et al. (27) found an increased risk of benign breast disease (both fibroadenomas and fibrocystic disease) in women on estrogen replacement therapy in comparison with a control group. The risk of benign breast disease

was greater with increasing years of use of estrogen and was also higher in women with bilateral oophorectomy than in other postmenopausal women (27).

Another systemic effect on the breast, weight loss, may produce a striking change in the mammogram. The loss of body fat is accompanied by a loss of fat in the breasts, and the density of the parenchyma may appear much greater on mammography. Similarly, weight gain may cause the breasts to appear less radiographically dense because of increased fat deposition.

Danazol is sometimes used in the treatment of severe fibrocystic and cystic disease of the breast. The effect of danazol on the breast is to decrease pain and tenderness. The density of the breast also may decrease on the mammogram, allowing better visualization of the parenchyma (28). Tobiassen et al. (29) found that a significant decrease in the amount of glandular tissue on mammography was present in women treated with danazol for fibrocystic changes. The mammographic visualization of cysts

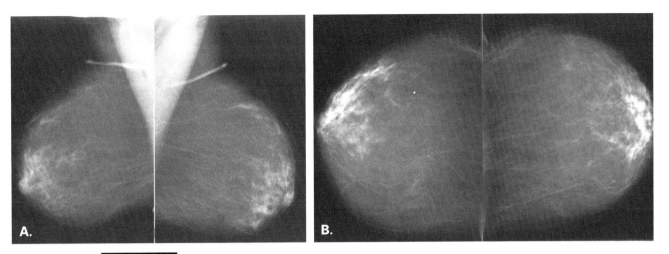

Figure 1.20

HISTORY: A 62-year-old woman for screening.

MAMMOGRAPHY: Bilateral MLO (**A**) and CC (**B**) views show scattered fibroglandular densities. There are prominent tubular densities in both subareolar areas, radiating back from the nipple.

IMPRESSION: Bilateral duct ectasia.

NOTE: Because the ducts are evident as discrete tubular structures, and because of their diameter, duct ectasia is present.

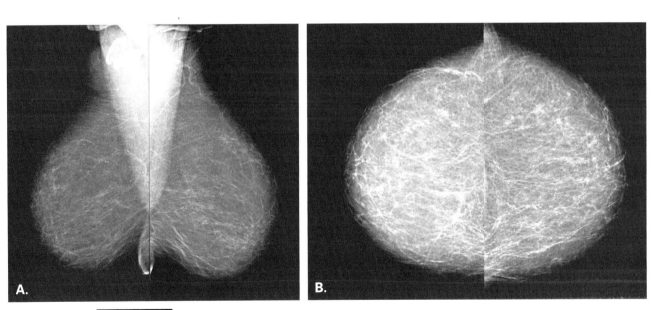

Figure 1.21

HISTORY: A 66-year-old para 0 woman for screening mammography.

MAMMOGRAPHY: Bilateral MLO (**A**) and CC (**B**) views show the breasts to be fatty replaced. These findings are the typical mammographic findings in a postmenopausal patient without a history of fibrocystic changes.

IMPRESSION: Normal postmenopausal breasts.

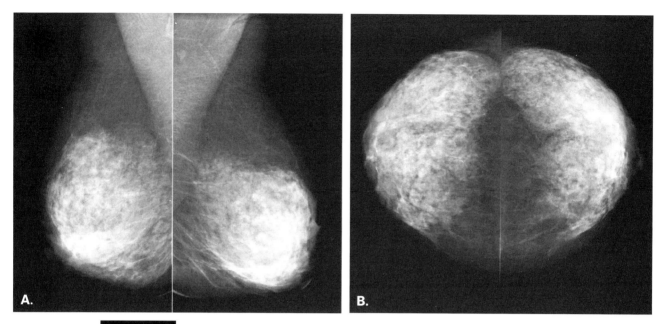

Figure 1.22

HISTORY: A 62-year-old gravida 2, para 2 patient for screening mammography. The patient was not taking hormone replacement therapy. She had a history of fibrocystic breasts.

MAMMOGRAPHY: Bilateral MLO (**A**) and CC (**B**) views show heterogeneously dense symmetrical-appearing breasts. Although the patient was not on hormones, the parenchyma is dense for the age of the patient. These findings often reflect diffuse fibrocystic changes.

IMPRESSION: Dense breasts in a postmenopausal patient.

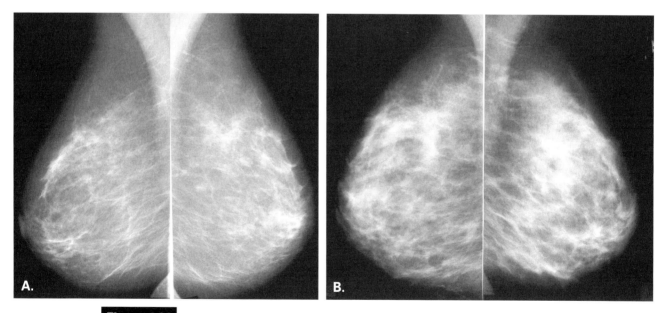

Figure 1.23

HISTORY: Screening mammograms a year apart in a postmenopausal patient who was placed on hormone replacement therapy in the interval.

MAMMOGRAPHY: Initial bilateral MLO (**A**) views show scattered fibroglandular densities. One year later (**B**), there is marked overall increase in parenchymal density bilaterally, consistent with changes related to hormone replacement therapy.

IMPRESSION: Effect of hormone replacement therapy on mammography.

increased initially because of the marked regression in the obscuring glandular tissue, but thereafter, a decrease in the size and number of cysts occurred.

A decrease in breast density has been described in premenopausal women who take calcium and vitamin D supplements. Berube et al. (30) found that a total daily intake of 400 IU vitamin D and 1,000 mg calcium was associated with an 8.5% lower mean breast density in premenopausal women. A similar effect was not observed in postmenopausal women.

The effect of tamoxifen on glandular density has been studied in several small series. Konez et al. (31) found that the majority of patients on tamoxifen therapy had no change in parenchymal density on mammography. Tiersten et al. (32) found that breast density was inversely related to age and postmenopausal status, but that there was no correlation between breast density and tamoxifen use. However, Chow et al. (33), in a study of 28 high-risk women on tamoxifen, did find a decrease in mammographic density as quantitated on digitized images.

By keeping in mind the normal structure of the breast—both macroscopically and microscopically—and the effects on the breast of the hormonal changes during the life cycle, one can be better prepared to interpret the normal and the abnormal mammogram.

REFERENCES

1. Osborne M. Breast development and anatomy. In: Harris JR, et al. *Breast Disease*. Philadelphia: JB Lippincott, 1987;1–14.
2. Adler DD, Rebner M, Pennes DR. Accessory breast tissue in the axilla: mammography appearance. *Radiology* 1987;163: 709–711.
3. Hughes ESR. The development of the mammary gland. *Ann R Coll Surg Engl* 1950;6:99–105.
4. Parks AG. The micro-anatomy of the breast. *Ann R Coll Surg Engl* 1959;25:235–251.
5. Wellings SR, Jensen HM, Marcum RG. An atlas of subgross pathology of the human breast with special reference to precancerous lesions. *J Natl Cancer Inst* 1975;55:231–273.
6. Jensen HM. On the origin and progression of human breast cancer. *Am J Obstet Gynecol* 1986;154:1280–1284.
7. Wellings SR, Wolfe JN. Correlation studies of the histological and radiographic appearance of the breast parenchyma. *Radiology* 1978;129:299–306.
8. Netter F. The reproductive system. In: Oppenheimer E, ed. *The CIBA Collection of Medical Illustrations*. Summit, NJ: CIBA, 1965:2.
9. Swinford AE, Adler DD, Garver KA. Mammographic appearance of the breasts during pregnancy and lactation: false assumptions. *Acad Radiol* 1998;5(7):567–572.
10. Fewins HE, Whitehouse GH, Leinster SJ. Changes in breast parenchymal patterns with increasing age. *Breast Dis* 1990;3: 145–151.
11. Boyd N, Martin L, Stone J, et al. A longitudinal study of the effects of menopause on mammographic features. *Cancer Epidemiol Biomarkers Prev* 2002;11(10 Pt 1):1048–1053.
12. Vogel PM, Georgiade NG, Fetter BF, et al. The correlation of histologic changes in the human breast with the menstrual cycle. *Am J Pathol* 1981;104:23–34.
13. Fanger H, Ree HJ. Cyclic changes of human mammary gland epithelium in relation to the menstrual cycle: an ultrastructural study. *Cancer* 1974;34:574–585.
14. White E, Velentgas P, Mandelson MT, et al. Variation in mammographic breast density by time in menstrual cycle among women aged 40–49 years. *J Natl Cancer Inst* 1998;90(12): 875–876.
15. Pock DR, Lowman RM. Estrogen and the postmenopausal breast. *JAMA* 1978;240:1733–1735.
16. Stomper PC, Vanvoorhis BJ, Ravnikar VA, et al. Mammographic changes associated with postmenopausal hormone replacement therapy: a longitudinal study. *Radiology* 1990; 174:487–490.
17. Marchesoni D, Driul L, Ianni A, et al. Postmenopausal hormone therapy and mammographic breast density. *Maturitas* 2006;53(1):59–64.
18. Conner P, Svane G, Azavedo E, et al. Mammographic breast density, hormones, and growth factors during continuous combined hormone therapy. *Fertil Steril* 2004;81(6):1617–1623.
19. Marugg RC, van der Mooren MJ, Hendriks JH, et al. Mammographic changes in postmenopausal women on hormonal replacement therapy. *Eur Radiol* 1997;7(5):749–755.
20. Laya MB, Larson EB, Taplin SH, et al. Effect of estrogen replacement therapy on the specificity and sensitivity of screening mammography. *J Natl Cancer Inst* 1996;88(10):627–628.
21. Jackson VP, San Martin JA, Secrest RJ, et al. Comparison of the effect of raloxifene and continuous-combined hormone therapy on mammographic breast density and breast tenderness in postmenopausal women. *Am J Obstet Gynecol* 2003;188(2): 389–394.
22. Persson I, Thurfjell E, Holmberg L. Effect of estrogen and estrogen-progestin replacement regimens on mammographic breast parenchymal density. *J Clin Oncol* 1997;15(1):3201–3207.
23. Berkowitz JE, Gatewood OMB, Goldblum LE, et al. Hormonal replacement therapy: mammographic manifestations. *Radiology* 1990;174:199–201.
24. McNicholas MMJ, Heneghan JP, Milner MH, et al. Pain and increased mammographic density in women receiving hormone replacement therapy: a prospective study. *AJR Am J Roentgenol* 1994;163:311–315.
25. McTiernan A, Martin CF, Peck JD, et al. Estrogen-plus-progestin use and mammographic density in postmenopausal women: women's health initiative randomized trial. *J Natl Cancer Inst* 2005;97(18):1366–1376.
26. Rutter CM, Mandelson MT, Laya MB, et al. Changes in breast density associated with initiation, discontinuation, and continuing use of hormone replacement therapy. *JAMA* 2001;285(14):1839–1840.
27. Trapido EJ, Brinton LA, Schairer C, et al. Estrogen replacement therapy and benign breast disease. *J Natl Cancer Inst* 1984;73:1101–1105.
28. Ouimet-Olivia D, Van Campenhut J, Hebert G, et al. Effect of danazol on the radiographic density of breast parenchyma. *J Can Assoc Radiol* 1981;32:159–161.
29. Tobiassen T, Rasmussen T, Doberl A, et al. Danazol treatment of severely symptomatic fibrocystic breast disease and long-term follow-up: the Hjorring project. *Acta Obstet Gynecol Scand* 1984;123(Suppl):159–176.
30. Berube S, Diorio C, Masse B, et al. Vitamin D and calcium intakes from food or supplements and mammographic breast density. *Cancer Epidemiol Biomarkers Prev* 2005;14(7): 1653–1659.
31. Konez O, Goval M, Reaven RE. Can tamoxifen cause a significant mammographic density change in breast parenchyma? *Clin Imaging* 2001;25(5):303–308.
32. Tiersten A, Ng YY, Pile-Spellman E, et al. Relationship between mammographic breast density and tamoxifen in women with breast cancer. *Breast J* 2004;10(4):313–317.
33. Chow CK, Venzon D, Jones EC, et al. Effect of tamoxifen on mammographic density. *Cancer Epidemiol Biomarkers Prev* 2000;9(9):917–921.

Techniques and Positioning in Mammography

During the past three decades, there has been significant improvement in the equipment and image-recording systems for mammography. In addition to providing better images, these developments have resulted in a significant reduction in radiation dose. Mammography has evolved from more dedicated equipment and industrial film, through xeromammography, dedicated film-screen mammography, and now to full-field digital mammography (Fig. 2.1). With the importance of an emphasis on mammography in the role of early detection of breast cancer, it is of utmost importance that meticulous techniques be used. Factors that affect the image quality include equipment, image-recording system, processing, compression of the breast, and the technologist's skill in positioning the patient. Adherence to strict quality assurance guidelines is critical in mammography to maintain optimum image quality (1,2). The Mammography Quality Standards Act (MQSA) (3) was passed in 1992 and regulates mammography facilities in the United States. The entire mammography process is addressed through MQSA, but importantly, the quality of images is carefully evaluated.

The interpretation skills of the radiologist are limited by a suboptimal image. A poor-quality mammogram or poor positioning can account for many of the cancers missed by mammography (4,5), and technical errors should not be overlooked or accepted. For the radiologist to detect subtle signs of malignancy, high-quality images are a must. The emphasis of this book is on interpretation and pattern recognition, but it is important to review briefly the technical factors that affect the mammographic image.

EQUIPMENT

Only dedicated units should be used for film-screen mammography. Dedicated units are those with special focal spots, target and filter materials, low kilovoltage, and compression devices designed to optimize the mammographic image at low radiation doses. Under no circumstances can nondedicated equipment produce images of similar quality to those performed with dedicated units.

There are three types of target materials used for mammography: molybdenum, rhodium, and tungsten. With molybdenum targets, 0.3-mm molybdenum filtration is used; the molybdenum targets are particularly well suited for mammography because of the low kiloelectron volt x-rays produced. The characteristic peaks for molybdenum are 17.9 and 19.5 keV, which provide high-contrast images for breasts of average thickness.

When the 0.3-mm molybdenum filter is used, the photons at energies greater than 20 keV are suppressed, and a larger number of low-energy photons are used in recording the images (6). The kilovolt peak (kVp) setting for molybdenum targets is generally at 25-28 kVp (6).

Alternative target/filter combinations for mammography include molybdenum/rhodium, rhodium/rhodium, and tungsten/rhodium. With tungsten targets, a beryllium window and minimal aluminum filtration are recommended. In comparison with a molybdenum target, even at low kVp settings, the tungsten target produces more high-energy photons, and the subject contrast is, therefore, lower (Fig. 2.2). Generally, settings of 22–26 kVp should be used for tungsten targets (A) (6–8). For most patients, a molybdenum target and a 0.06-mm molybdenum filter is automatically in place at low kVp settings; to penetrate thick dense breasts, the 0.05-mm rhodium filter is used at higher kVp settings (2).

Resolution is affected by the recording system's unsharpness, geometric unsharpness, and motion (9). The size of the focal spot of the tube is of particular importance in mammography because of the high resolution required for this work. To reduce geometric blurring, the focal spot

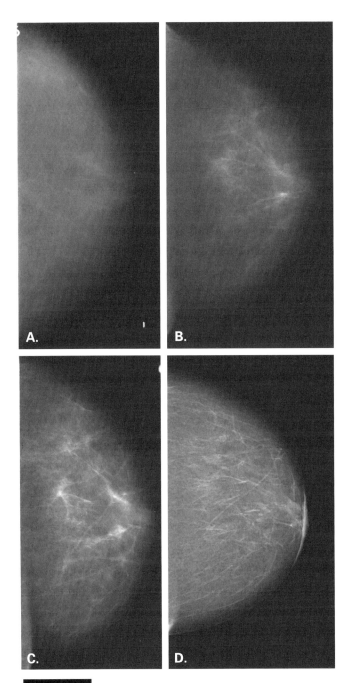

Figure 2.1

HISTORY: Series of screening mammograms over 22 years.

MAMMOGRAPHY: Right CC view in 1985 (**A**), 1987 (**B**), 1996 (**C**), and 2006 (**D**) performed with the following equipment and techniques: **A:** Dedicated unit with a tungsten target, aluminum filter, and no grid. **B:** Dedicated unit with molybdenum target and filter and a grid. **C:** Dedicated unit with molybdenum target/filter, grid, and a newer film-screen combination with extended processing showing contrast improvement. **D:** Full-field digital unit with a tungsten/rhodium target/filter and a selenium detector showing excellent contrast and visibility of structures.

size and the distance between the breast and image receptor should be kept as small as possible, and the object-to-focal-spot distance should be maximized (10). The size of the focal spot becomes even more important in magnification mammography (6), where it is generally recommended that the measured focal-spot size be no greater than 0.3 mm (11) and preferably in the range of 0.1 to 0.2 mm (12,13).

The use of grids in mammography improves image quality by reducing scatter, thus increasing contrast; there is a concomitant increase in radiation dose to the patient (14). Grids are of particular advantage in imaging the more dense, thick breast, in which more scattered radiation is present (15). However, because of the improvement in image quality with a grid, all routine mammography is performed with a grid. Mammography units have reciprocating grids with a ratio of approximately 5:1 (6). The grids used in mammography are thinner than conventional grids and contain carbon fiber interspace material for lower absorption. Typical reciprocating grids are composed of 16-μm lead strips separated by 300-μm carbon-fiber resin interspaces (7). The increase in the radiation dose with a grid is about two times that of a nongrid film, but this may be compensated for by using faster screen-film combinations. Grids are not utilized for magnification mammography because of the increased dose and length of exposure.

Dedicated mammography units should be equipped with a firm radiolucent compression device that forms a 90-degree angle with the chest wall. No rounded or curved edge compression devices should be used because the posterior aspect of the breast will not be adequately visualized (16). Proper compression of the breasts during mammography is extremely important in terms of producing an image of satisfactory diagnostic quality. Compression of the breasts is a very important factor in reducing scatter radiation, which degrades the image. With compression, there is spreading of the tissues apart, and small lesions are more easily identified within the parenchyma. The immobilization of the breasts decreases motion blurring, and the location of structures in the breast closer to the film receptor decreases geometric blurring. There is less variation in the density of the areas of breast with compression to a uniform thickness from nipple to chest wall. Importantly, the radiation dose to the breast is decreased with compression (7).

IMAGE RECORDING SYSTEM

It is important that a film-screen system specifically designed for analog mammography be utilized in order to

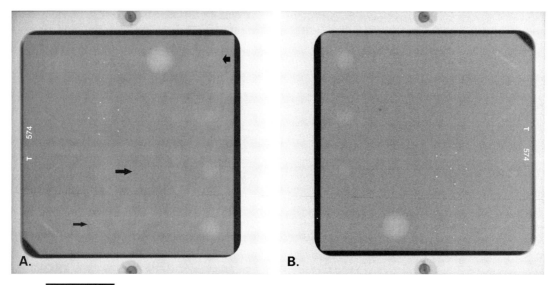

Figure 2.2

Digital images of the American College of Radiology Accreditation phantom demonstrating the effect of target/filter combination on contrast. **A** was obtained using molybdenum/molybdenum target filter at 28 kVp and 97 mAs. **B** was obtained using tungsten/rhodium target/filter at 28 kVp and 83 mAs. The contrast is higher on the Mo/Mo image **(A)**, and more objects are clearly visible **(arrows)**.

obtain the proper diagnostic quality of the images. With dedicated units and the common use of grids and magnification techniques, it is also important that the film-screen combination chosen have the lowest radiation dose while the quality of the images is maintained. Single-emulsion film is recommended for contact mammography because of the image degradation secondary to crossover in double-emulsion systems. In 1972, DuPont introduced the LoDose screen-film systems, which was followed by the DuPont LoDose 2 system. Kodak introduced the MinR system in 1976 and OM film in 1980. Since then, numerous film-screen combinations have been designed specifically for mammography. Some of these films have been specifically developed to be used in either standard 90-second or the extended 3-minute processors. The screens used for most routine mammography are single-back screens. The film and screen are in intimate contact, with the emulsion in contact with the top of the screen (17). Mammographic film-screen combinations have a much higher resolution than that of conventional radiography systems (2). Kimme-Smith et al. (17) found that the screens are of primary importance for good resolution, whereas contrast is affected more by type of film and processing (2,17).

Cassettes specifically designed for mammography are most commonly used, but polyethylene envelopes that are vacuum sealed have also been used. The cassette and its screen should be dusted daily to maintain proper quality control and to reduce dust artifacts. Weekly, wet cleaning of the screen is necessary to optimize image quality in reducing artifacts.

Quality control of film processing is of great importance in mammography. It is important to follow the manufacturer's recommendation for film processing in terms of the chemicals used, replenishment rate, development time and temperature. Using a temperature that is lower than that recommended by the manufacturer for mammography causes a loss in film speed and contrast (2), thereby necessitating a higher dose to produce films of satisfactory optical density (18). Many facilities have used extended-cycle processing for single-emulsion films (2,19,20). With extended-cycle processing, the film spends more time in the developer, thereby increasing the total processing time to 3 minutes. It is important that the processor be dedicated to mammography if extended-cycle processing is used. A reduction in radiation dose by 30% (2,19) and an increase (19) in contrast of 11% were found when Kodak OM1-SO177 film was tested in 3-minute rather than 90-second processing. Kimme-Smith et al. (21) found that extended cycle processing increased noise and decreased dose, but diagnostic capabilities were not compromised. More recently, newer films and screens have been developed that provide the higher contrast and lower dose afforded by extended cycle processing, yet the processing time for these films is 90 seconds.

IMAGE CONTRAST

Contrast is dependent on subject contrast (radiation quality and kVp), film contrast, film processing (darkroom, chemistry, development time and temperature), and scattered radiation (compression, grid) (22). There are a number of factors in the darkroom that affect radiographic contrast. The film should be processed according to the manufacturer's recommendations. The purity of the chemistry, the replenishment rate of the chemicals, and the temperature all affect the contrast. The time for processing also affects contrast significantly. Extended cycle processing has been used for mammography to increase the contrast of the images.

Another major effect on contrast is scattered radiation. The use of grids in mammography reduces scatter and increases contrast. The grid attenuates the primary radiation, though, and the dose is increased about twofold (23).

RADIATION DOSE

The parenchyma of the breast, not the skin, is the area that is of greater concern regarding exposure. Therefore, the absorbed glandular dose, not the skin entrance dose, is the more important measurement (6). For a 5-cm-thick average breast, the mean absorbed dose using OM film at 28 kVp with a molybdenum target is approximately 0.05 rad (6). Factors that affect radiation dose include breast-tissue composition and thickness, x-ray tube target materials, filtration, kVp, grid use, film-screen combination, and processing (2). With the development of dedicated mammography equipment and the improvement in

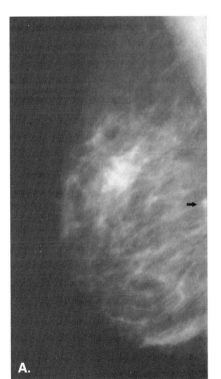
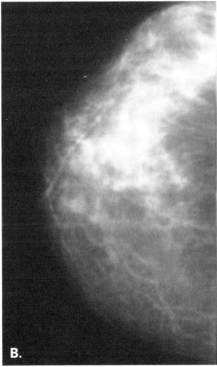
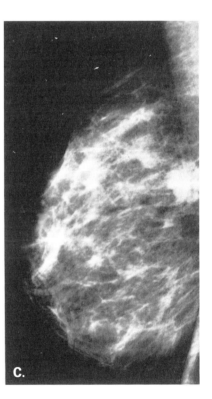

Figure 2.3

HISTORY: A 50-year-old woman with a lump deep in the left breast.

MAMMOGRAPHY: Left ML **(A)**, CC **(B)**, and MLO **(C)** views. No abnormalities are seen on the CC view, but on the ML view a questionable density **(arrow)** is seen positively. However, on the MLO view, there is a high-density nodular mass deep in the breast near the chest wall. This emphasizes the importance of performing the MLO view routinely in order to visualize the posterior aspects of the breast adequately.

IMPRESSION: Carcinoma.

HISTOPATHOLOGY: Infiltrating ductal carcinoma.

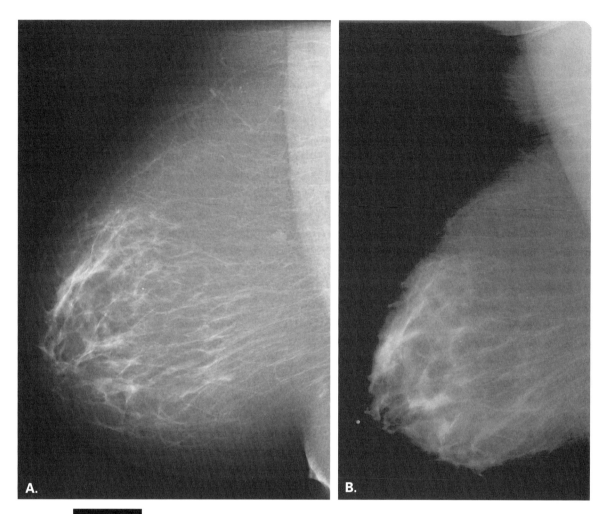

Figure 2.4

HISTORY: Screening mammogram with prior films for comparison on a difficult-to-position patient because of her size.

MAMMOGRAPHY: Current left MLO **(A)** view performed with a full-field digital unit shows the breast to be well positioned, especially for the large size. The pectoralis major muscle is visualized down to the level of the nipple. There is however, some overlap of the upper abdomen at the inframammary fold. A normal lymph node is noted in the axillary tail. Comparison with the prior study **(B)** shows that significantly more breast tissue has been included on the current study. The muscle, the node, and several centimeters of posterior breast tissue are visible on the well-positioned MLO versus the prior study.

IMPRESSION: Normal left mammogram with better positioning on the current MLO view.

film-screen systems, there has been a tremendous decrease in the radiation dose from mammography over the last decades.

DIGITAL MAMMOGRAPHY

Because of the resolution requirements for mammography, the technical developments to achieve full-field imaging have been challenging. Yet, full-field digital mammography has been developed and tested, and is clinically available. Other than the diagnostic improvements with digital compared with analog or film-screen mammography, as shown in the Digital Mammographic Imaging Screening Trial (DMIST) (24), there are distinct technical improvements as well.

With film-screen mammography, the various functions related to imaging are accomplished on a piece of film:

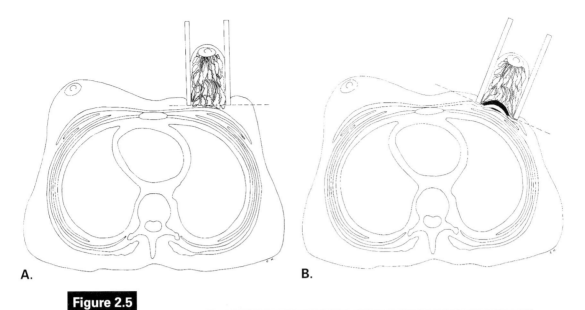

A.   B.

Figure 2.5

Cross sections through the thorax show that the axillary tail of the breast may not be included on a ML projection **(A)**, but on the MLO projection **(B)**, the axillary tail and pectoralis major muscle are imaged.

image acquisition, interpretation, and storage. With digital mammography, these three functions are separated, and each is optimized. The large dynamic range and improved contrast overcome some of the limitations of film-screen mammography. The dynamic range of digital mammography is approximately 1,600:1 versus 100:1 for film (25). The digital mammogram is particularly helpful because of increased contrast resolution in dense breast tissue.

The spatial resolution of digital mammography is less than that of film, with the current units having a resolution of 50- to 100-μm pixel size. The line pair resolution of film mammography translates to an approximate pixel size of 25 μm. However, because of the other favorable factors with digital imaging, fine detail observation is not compromised (26).

Digital detector development has included several different technologies. An early unit was composed of multiple small detectors (charge-coupled devices) stitched together to create a larger detector. Another technology is slot scanning, in which a long narrow CCD is scanned along with the x-ray beam over the breast. The GE unit was the first unit approved by the Food and Drug Administration and has a flat panel detector composed an amorphous silicone photodiode array with a spatial resolution of 100 μm. More recently, Siemens and Hologic have developed and received approval for units that are based on direct digital image capture on an amorphous selenium plate.

Simultaneous development of computerized radiography has occurred for mammography. Photostimulable phosphor plates are exposed to x-rays and develop a latent image. The plates are scanned by a laser beam, and the images are printed onto film. Like digital mammography, the phosphor plates offer a higher dynamic range than film mammography (26).

Digital images may be interpreted as hard copy or soft copy. With hard-copy interpretation, the images are laser printed onto film. Soft-copy interpretation involves interpretation at a high-resolution workstation. Because of the amount of information in one image, the images are not displayed at full resolution on a 2 K × 2 K workstation. The images are enlarged to full resolution and panned to see the entire breast, or the magnification tool is used. A distinct advantage of interpretation at the workstation is that the image may be postprocessed. Window leveling, zoom, and magnification are all useful tools to improve observations and analysis.

Another important advantage of digital imaging is improved archiving of the images. Instead of a large film room and the challenges of maintaining it, digital images are archived in a PACS (picture archiving and communication system) or in a local and remote server. Because of the communication aspects of digital imaging, telemammography is possible and allows for remote interpretation.

(text continues on page 26)

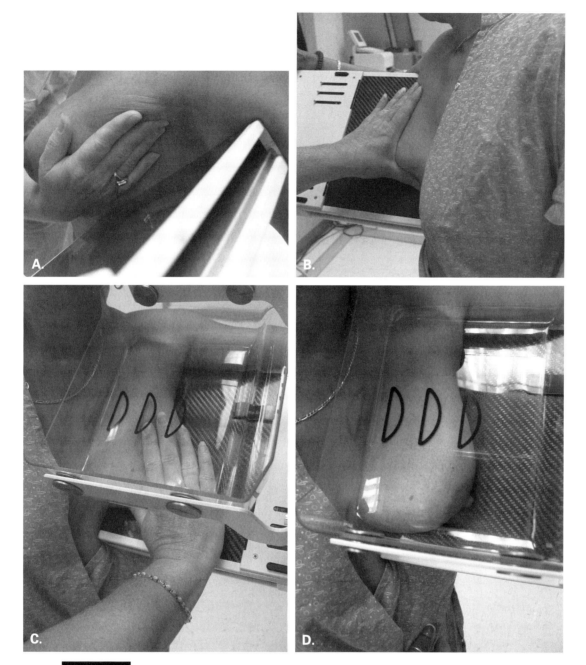

Figure 2.6

Steps in positioning the patient for the MLO view. **A:** The technologist determines the angle of the obliquity of the pectoralis major muscle by lifting the breast medially and turning the image receptor to this angle. **B:** The Bucky is turned to the angle of obliquity of the pectoralis major muscle (35 to 60 degrees). The breast is placed over the Bucky with the arm draped behind the receptor. The technologist maintains the breast in a up-and-out position as she moves the compression device into position. **C:** The inframammary fold is open, and the breast is elevated as the compression is applied. **D:** Final position shows the entire breast and low axilla in the field of view.

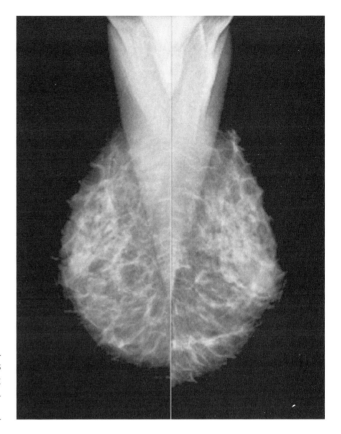

Figure 2.7

Well-positioned MLO views show the pectoralis major muscles bulging forward and visualized as a triangle with the apex at the level of the nipple. The nipple is elevated, and the inframammary fold region is open; the breast is well compressed.

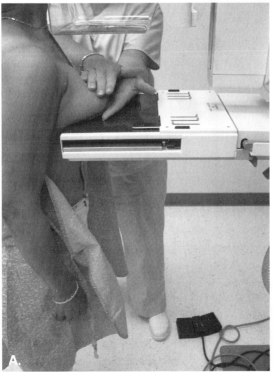
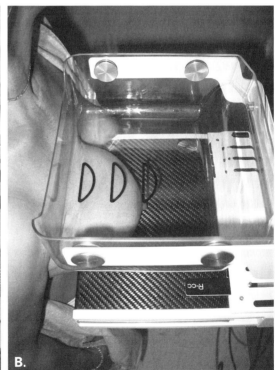

Figure 2.8

Positioning the patient for the CC view. **(A)** The technologist is using both hands to pull the breast forward over the receptor, and the receptor has been elevated to the elevated inframammary fold position. **(B)** On final positioning, the breast is pulled straight forward, and the medial aspect of the opposite breast is draped over the receptor.

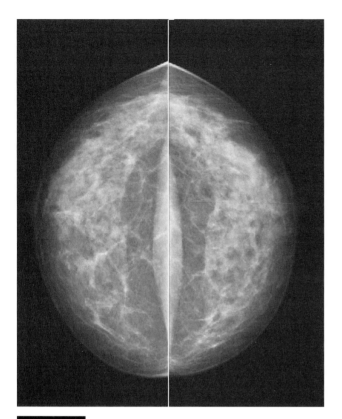

Figure 2.9

Well-positioned CC views show the breasts positioned straight forward and not rotated. The pectoralis major muscles are seen bilaterally. The nipple is in profile, and the breast is well compressed.

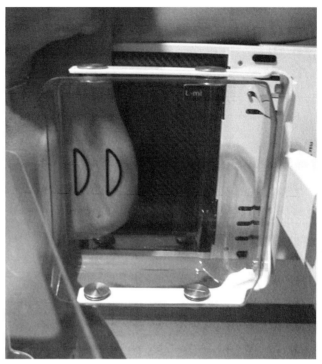

Figure 2.10

ML. Positioning the patient for the ML view. The breast is compressed from the medial aspect, and the degree of obliquity is 90 degrees. The axillary tail is not as included in the field of view as it is on the MLO view.

POSITIONING

Most authors agree that two views should be performed for routine mammography (27,28). The craniocaudal (CC) view and the mediolateral oblique (MLO) view (29) are recommended as standard projections. Before the determination of the MLO projection, the views for mammography were a CC and a mediolateral (ML). With the advent of MLO positioning, more posterior tissue could be included in the field of view (Fig. 2.3). Additional views may be necessary to evaluate specific areas within the breast (30–32), and the techniques for positioning the patient for these various views are described in this chapter. For all views, it is of utmost importance that the breast be compressed properly.

Mediolateral Oblique View

When the patient is positioned properly, the MLO view will demonstrate the pectoralis major muscle and the entire breast, including the inferior portion and the axillary tail, on one film (Fig. 2.4). The concept of the MLO view is that the breast is compressed at the same angle of obliquity as the pectoralis major muscle transverses the chest wall. In compressing the muscle in this plane, the technologist is more able to pull the muscle forward over the cassette; therefore, the posterior breast tissue is also pulled forward (Fig. 2.5). The pectoralis major muscle has a triangular shape, with the apex at the level of the nipple. In general, the parenchyma should not extend to the posterior edge of the image on the MLO view. Instead, the parenchyma should be separated from the chest wall edge of the image by the retroglandular fat (33).

The MLO view is performed by angling the receptor and compression device, 45 to 60 degrees in a caudal direction from the vertical position. The level of angulation is determined by the orientation of the pectoralis major muscle on the chest wall. The technologist determines this angle by visualizing the edge of the patient's

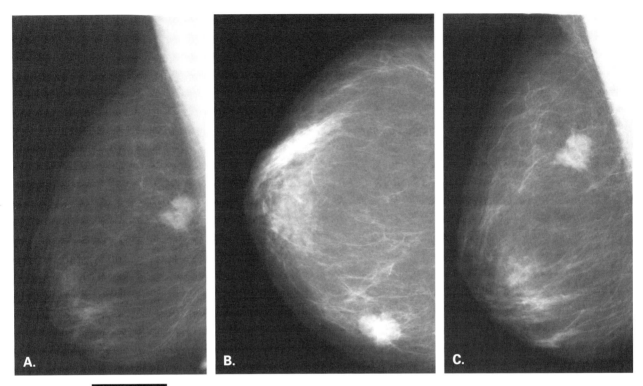

Figure 2.11

HISTORY: A 39-year-old woman with a palpable mass left breast.

MAMMOGRAPHY: Left MLO **(A)** and CC **(B)** views show a lobular, high-density mass with indistinct margins. On the ML **(C)** view, the lesion appears to be located higher than on the MLO, confirming a medial location.

IMPRESSION: Highly suspicious for carcinoma.

HISTOPATHOLOGY: Medullary carcinoma.

NOTE: Lesions that are in the medial aspect of the breast will appear higher on the ML than on the MLO view.

pectoralis major muscle in the anterior axillary line, and she moves the equipment to this angle. The degree of obliquity depends on the patient's body habitus; a thin patient needs a steeper oblique; a heavy, short patient may be examined with a lesser degree of obliquity. The patient stands with the ipsilateral arm elevated to no more than 90 degrees over the receptor. The receptor is placed behind the breast, high into the axilla, and the patient may gently hold the cassette holder or handle.

The positioning of the breast is improved when the technologist uses the natural breast mobility in positioning. The lateral and inferior aspects of the breast are more naturally mobile than are the medial and superior aspects (34). Therefore, in positioning the patient for the MLO view, the lateral aspect of the breast and the pectoralis

major muscle are displaced medially and anteriorly and then positioned over the image receptor. When properly positioned, the MLO view includes nearly all of the breast tissue (34) (Figs. 2.6 and 2.7).

In this position, the pectoralis major muscle can be most easily pulled forward from the chest wall, enabling greater visualization of the posterior aspects of the breast. The patient should not be allowed to tense the arm, because this will also tighten the pectoral muscle and prevent the breast from being pulled forward easily. All aspects of the lateral side of the beast and the axilla should be in contact with the cassette; if the opposite breast is in the radiographic field, the patient should press it up and against the chest wall. If this is not done, the opposite nipple can project into the radiographic field, simulating a nodule (35). The breast is pulled for-

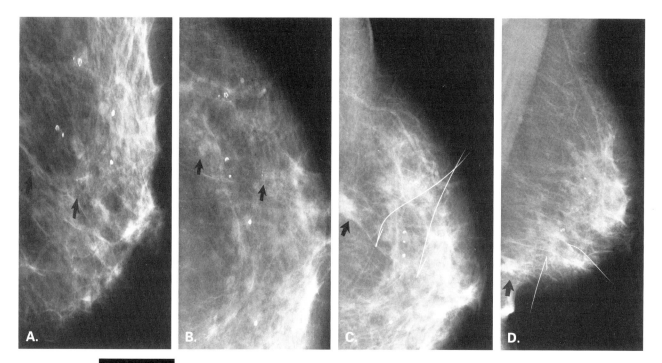

Figure 2.12

HISTORY: A 56-year-old woman with a history of multiple benign breast biopsies, presenting now with nystagmus and neurologic findings suggesting a paraneoplastic syndrome. An outside mammogram had been interpreted as nonsuspicious for a primary breast cancer.

MAMMOGRAPHY: Enlarged right MLO **(A)** and magnification (2X) CC **(B)** views and right XCCL **(C)** and ML **(D)** views from a needle localization. The breast is moderately dense. There are two clusters **(arrows)** of microcalcifications, irregular in contour and separated by approximately 2 cm in the right lower outer quadrant **(A and B)**. These calcifications were considered highly suspicious for malignancy, and needle localizations were performed before excisional biopsy. The XCCL **(C)** and ML **(D)** views from the needle localization **(C and D)** show a spiculated 8-mm mass **(arrow)** deep in the lower outer quadrant near the chest wall.

HISTOPATHOLOGY: Infiltrating ductal with multicentric intraductal carcinoma.

NOTE: The ML view may demonstrate a lesion near the chest wall in the inferior aspect of the breast better than the routine MLO view. In this case, the demonstration of the mass was serendipitous, because the final films for the localization included a standard ML view, on which the lesion was seen.

ward and up as the compression device is applied. In doing so, the inframammary fold is open, and the posterior and inferior aspect of the breast is visualized. Vigorous compression must be applied without allowing the breast to sag on the cassette.

Craniocaudal View

The CC view is a standard transverse view of the breast. The CC complements the MLO view by visualizing the far medial and posterior aspects of the breast. The CC view includes most of the parenchyma except for the far lateral and posterior regions of the breast. On the CC view, the central and subareolar areas are well compressed and well depicted.

In considering the natural mobility of the breast, the inferior aspect is elevated during the positioning of the CC view. With this maneuver, the superior and posterior tissue are included in the field of view and are better visualized. The patient stands facing the mammographic unit with the head turned away from the breast being examined. The patient should lean slightly forward, and the technologist places one hand under the breast, elevating it. The image receptor is placed at the level of the

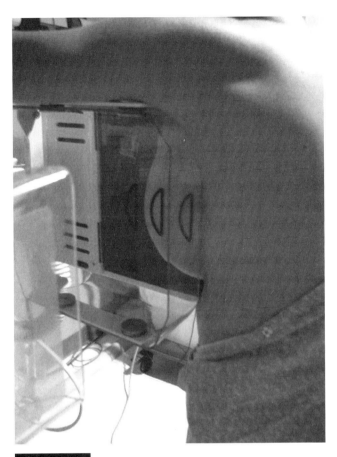

Figure 2.13

Positioning of the patient for the left LM view. This is a 90-degree lateral view in which the compression plate is placed on the lateral side of the breast. The x-ray beam is directed from the lateral to medial direction. The medial aspect of the breast is closest to the receptor, thereby optimizing imaging of medial structures.

elevated intramammary fold. The breast is pulled forward over the cassette with both hands. Skin folds and wrinkles should be smoothed out; rotating the shoulder slightly back helps to smooth out the skin folds at the anterior axillary line. The nipple should be in profile if at all possible. The medial aspect of the opposite breast is draped over the edge of the receptor (Fig. 2.8). The films are marked in the axillary region, and firm compression is applied to the breast.

On a well-positioned CC view, the distance from the edge of the film at the chest wall to the nipple should be no more than 1 cm greater or less than the distance measured from the nipple to the anterior border of the pectoralis major muscle on the MLO (the posterior nipple line [PNL] measurement) (34). In a study of 1,586 CC mammograms,

Bassett et al. (36) found that in 79% of cases, the measurement of the PNL on the CC view was within 1 cm of the PNL on the MLO view. The authors (36) also found that the pectoralis major muscle was seen on 32% of the CC views (Fig. 2.9).

Occasionally, a lesion is seen only on the CC view and not on the MLO view. A rolled CC view can be obtained by sliding the superior aspect of the breast medially or laterally and the inferior aspect of the breast in the opposite direction (31). If the "lesion" persists, the direction of its movement relative to its position on the standard CC view indicates its relative vertical position in the breast.

Supplementary Views

In addition to the routine CC and MLO views, supplementary views may be used in the evaluation of a mammographic or palpable abnormality. A tailored examination with views selected to evaluate the potential abnormality is a diagnostic mammogram. The purpose of the additional views is multifactorial: to determine if a potential lesion is real, to evaluate its position in the breast, to evaluate its characteristics, and sometimes to search for other occult lesions. These additional views include the reverse obliques (lateral-medial oblique, superoinferior oblique), 90-degree lateral views (ML, lateral medial), exaggerated CC views (lateral, medial), rolled CC views, cleavage view, off-angle obliques, spot compression, magnification, axillary tail and axillary views, tangential views, and implant displaced views.

True Lateral (90-Degree) Views

The ML view may not demonstrate the posterior and axillary portion of the breast in entirety; therefore, the MLO view is recommended instead for the routine examination (29). The ML view, however, is essential in localizing a lesion and may also be of help in differentiating a true lesion from superimposition of glandular tissue. With the cassette placed against the lateral aspect of the breast and compression applied from the medial direction, the ML view is a true sagittal view (Fig. 2.10). The ML view may also be extremely useful in demonstrating a lesion located high in the upper inner quadrant, an area sometimes not included on the MLO view, or a lesion deep near the chest wall in the inferomedial or inferolateral aspect of the breast. The ML view can be used to locate a lesion demonstrated on an MLO view but not seen on a CC view. A lesion that is lower in position on the ML view than on the MLO view is located laterally; a lesion that is higher in position on the ML view than on the MLO view is located medially (Figs. 2.11 and 2.12).

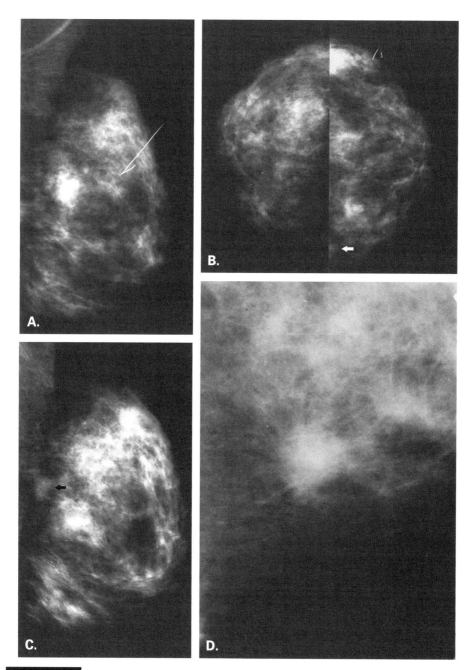

Figure 2.14

HISTORY: Screening mammogram on a patient with a history of multiple cysts and fibrocystic changes.

MAMMOGRAPHY: Right MLO **(A)** and bilateral CC **(B)** views show the breasts to be heterogeneously dense. There is an indistinct mass seen at the posteromedial aspect of the right breast on the CC view only **(arrow)**. Because of the position of the lesion, a lateromedial LM view **(C)** was obtained to try to locate the lesion on the sagittal plane and to place it closer to the image receptor. The mass is visible on the LM view superiorly **(arrow)** and is also visible on the spot CC **(D)** view.

IMPRESSION: Dense indistinct mass located at 2 o'clock posteriorly on the right breast, demonstrated on the LM view.

HISTOPATHOLOGY: Invasive ductal carcinoma.

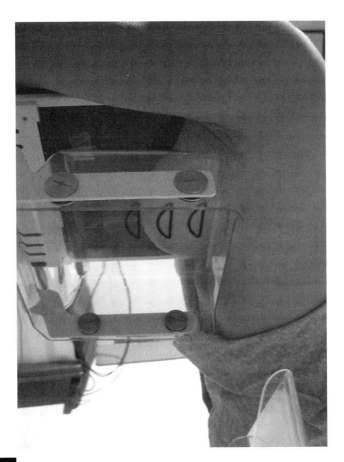

Figure 2.15

Positioning for the LMO view shows the breast compressed from the lateroinferior to the medio-
    superior direction. The angulation is usually the same degree of obliquity as is used for the
    MLO view.

Lateral Medial

The lateral medial (LM) view is also a 90-degree lateral
view; however, in this case the breast is compressed from
the lateral aspect. The x-ray beam is directed from the lateral to the medial direction. This view places the medial
aspect of the breast closest to the receptor, which is particularly useful for improving the visibility of lesions that
are located medially (Figs. 2.13 and 2.14).

Lateromedial Oblique

The advantage of performing the lateromedial oblique
(LMO) view is to image lesions located far medioposteriorly that are seen on the CC view only or to image palpable lesions in the inner quadrant that are not seen on
mammography. To position the patient for this view, the
tube and cassette holder are tilted 45 to 60 degrees
toward the contralateral breast (Fig. 2.15). The medial
aspect of the breast to be examined is placed against the
cassette holder, and the ipsilateral arm rests over the
receptor. The breast is elevated so that it does not droop,
and compression is applied from the lateral direction.
This view is also used for patients who are very kyphotic
or in patients with a pacemaker or a port located in the
upper inner quadrant. The view may also be helpful to
demonstrate lesions located medially and not seen on the
MLO (Fig. 2.16).

The superoinferior oblique (SIO) view, like the LMO, is
used for kyphotic patients or those with pacemakers and
central lines. The view is an oblique projection, but
instead of the x-ray beam being directed medially to laterally, it is in a superolateral to inferomedial direction.
The compression plate is placed against the lateral and

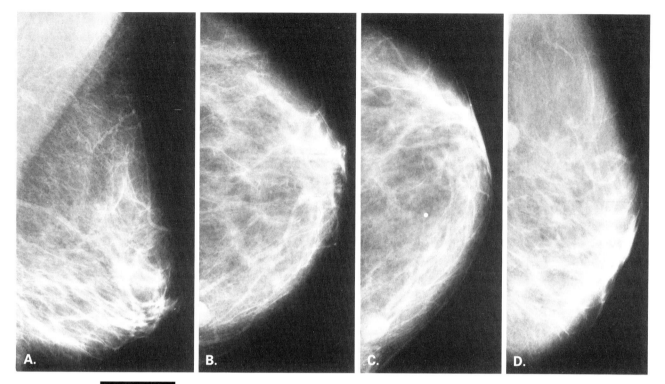

Figure 2.16

HISTORY: A 44-year-old gravida 3, para 2, abortus 1 woman with no palpable findings, for screening.

MAMMOGRAPHY: Right MLO **(A)**, CC **(B)**, XCCM **(C)**, and LMO **(D)** views. Although on the routine MLO view **(A)** no abnormality is seen, the edge of a well-circumscribed mass **(arrow)** is present far medioposteriorly on the CC view **(B)**. An XCCM view **(C)** demonstrates the lesion more clearly. To identify the exact position of the mass, the LMO view **(D)** was performed and showed the mass to be in the upper inner quadrant.

HISTOPATHOLOGY: Fibroadenoma.

NOTE: The LMO is particularly useful for demonstrating lesions located medially, near the chest wall.

superior area, and the breast is compressed from this direction (Fig. 2.17).

Exaggerated Craniocaudal Views

The tissue in the extreme lateroposterior or medioposterior aspects of the breast may not be visualized in entirety on the routine CC view. When a lesion is found on the routine MLO view deep in the breast and is not seen on the CC view, an exaggerated lateral or medial CC (XCCL or XCCM) view will be of help in defining the location of the abnormalities. For the XCCL view, the lateral aspect of the breast is placed forward on the cassette in the CC position (Fig. 2.18). For the axillary tail of the breast to be in good contact with the film, the patient must lean backward slightly, keeping the ipsilateral arm extended over the top of the cassette. For the XCCM view (Fig. 2.19), the patient is rotated anteriorly, extending her chest forward, with the far medioposterior aspect of the breast being imaged. If the lesion is located high in the upper inner quadrant, it may be necessary to elevate the cassette holder and compress the uppermost aspect of the breast.

The exaggerated views are used to determine the location in two projections of a lesion seen only on the MLO posteriorly. The XCCL is performed first because more parenchyma and more lesions, especially cancers, are located in the upper outer quadrant than elsewhere (Figs. 2.20–2.23).

If a lesion is located at the chest wall on the MLO and not seen on the XCCL, it is presumably located medially. In this case, the XCCM view is performed to extend the

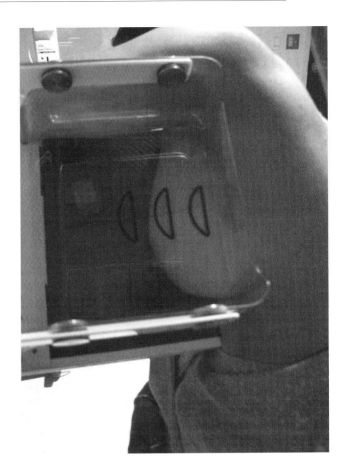

Figure 2.17

Positioning the patient for the SIO view. The degree of obliquity is the same as for the MLO view, but the breast is compressed from the lateral side. The direction of the beam is from the superolateral to inferomedial direction. This is used for kyphotic patients and those with pacemakers.

field of view posteriorly at the medial side of the breast (Fig. 2.24).

In addition to the XCCM, the cleavage view is performed for possible medial and posterior lesions (Fig. 2.25). For the cleavage view, both breasts are placed over the image receptor with the cleavage in the center of the field. Usually a manual technique, rather than phototiming is used, because the photocell is not covered completely by breast tissue.

For lesions that are seen only on the MLO and not demonstrated on the ML or CC, step obliques or off-angle obliques can be most helpful. The concept is that the angle of obliquity is changed about 10 degrees more than and less than the obliquity the MLO. If the lesion is visible on these additional obliques, it is real. The displacement of the lesion on the additional views also is used to locate it. Lesions that are located in the lateral aspect of the breast appear lower on the higher angle of obliquity (approaching the 90-degree lateral) (Fig. 2.26).

Spot Compression

Most mammographic units have a smaller compression paddle that can be used for spot compression. The area of concern, identified on the standard view, is spot compressed, with the surrounding normal tissue pushed away by the compression device (Fig. 2.27). The technologist must estimate the location of the lesion in the breast from the initial images, and care must be taken to be certain that the area of concern is included in the spot field. Spot compression is particularly useful for the evaluation of the borders of nodules and for focal densities that may represent either true lesions or overlapping tissue (Figs. 2.28 and 2.29). Another use of spot compression is in the evaluation of a palpable nodule not clearly seen on mammography. The technologist rotates the palpable lesion into tangent with the beam and spot compresses the area (30). Magnification

(text continues on page 37)

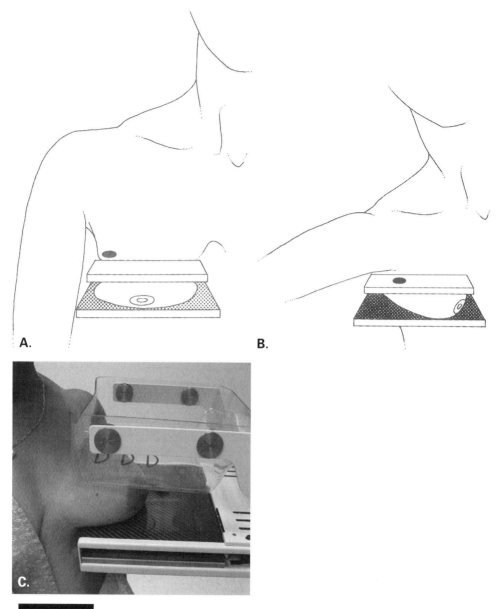

Figure 2.18

On the standard CC view (**A** and **B**), a lesion located posterolaterally may not be included on the image, but by rotating the patient for the XCCL view (**C**), the lesion projects into the radiographic field. For this position, the breast is rotated medially so that the far lateral and posterior aspect of the breast is included in the field of view.

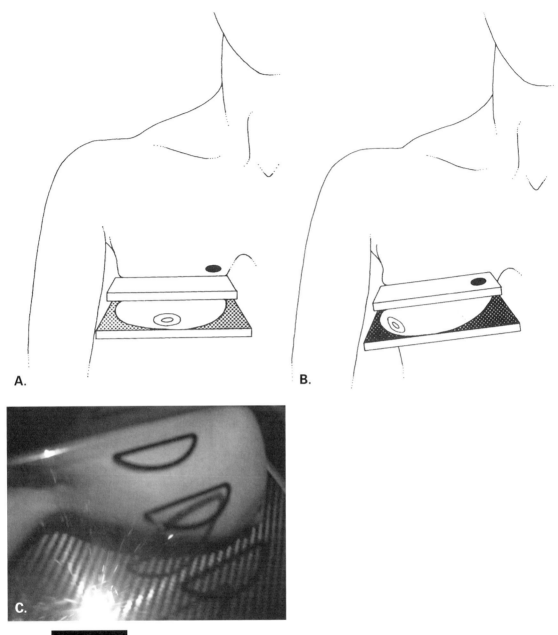

Figure 2.19

On the standard CC view (**A** and **B**), a lesion located posteromedially may not be included on the image, but by rotating the patient forward for the XCCM view (**C**), the lesion projects into the radiographic field. The breast is rotated laterally so that the far medial and posterior aspect is included in the field of view. The opposite breast is draped on the image receptor.

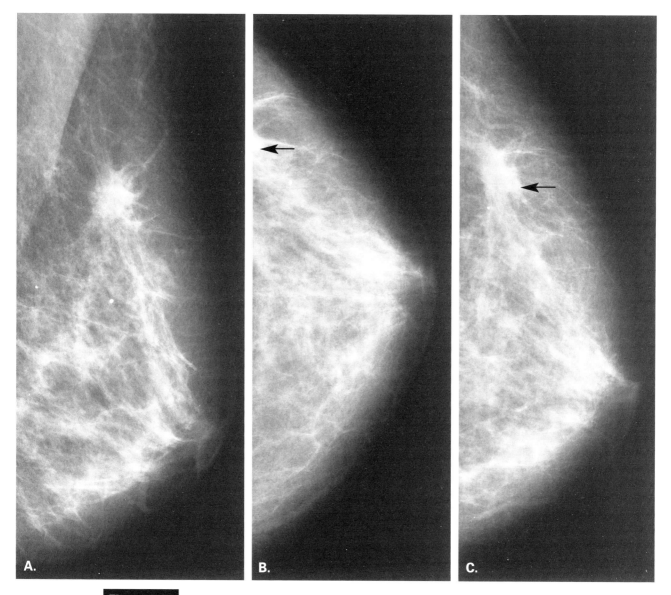

Figure 2.20

HISTORY: A 65-year-old gravida 4, para 3, abortus 1 woman for screening.

MAMMOGRAPHY: Right MLO **(A)**, CC **(B)**, and XCCL **(C)** views. The breast is moderately dense. There is a focal spiculated lesion in the upper aspect of the breast on the MLO view **(A)**, but this lesion is faintly seen **(arrow)** on the CC view **(B)**. The XCCL view **(C)** is performed to demonstrate the location and the appearance of the lesion **(arrow)**. The XCCL view is performed first if a lesion is seen only on the MLO, because more carcinomas occur laterally than medially. If a lesion is not found on the XCCL position, then the XCCM view is performed.

IMPRESSION: Spiculated lesion located posteriorly in the upper outer quadrant, highly suspicious for malignancy.

HISTOPATHOLOGY: Infiltrating lobular carcinoma.

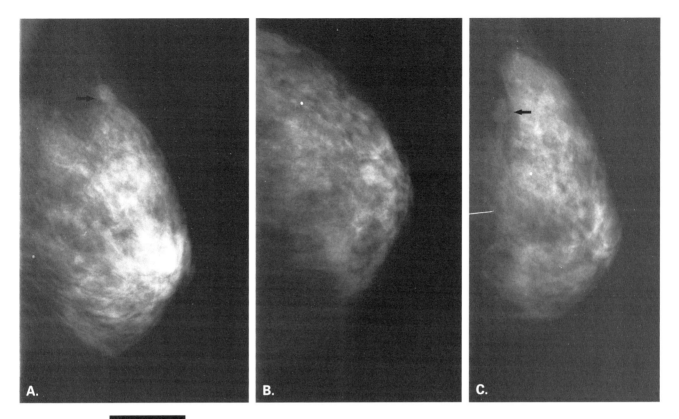

A. B. C.

Figure 2.21

HISTORY: Screening mammogram on a 70-year-old woman.

MAMMOGRAPHY: Right MLO **(A)** and CC **(B)** views show heterogeneously dense tissue. There is a small mass at the superior margin of the parenchyma **(arrow)** seen on the MLO view only. Because the lesion was not seen on the CC view, an XCCL view **(C)** was obtained. This projection shows that the lesion is located far laterally and posteriorly **(arrow)**.

IMPRESSION: Suspicious mass in the right upper-outer quadrant, demonstrated on the XCCL view.

HISTOPATHOLOGY: Invasive ductal carcinoma.

may be combined with spot compression, particularly in the evaluation of a small nodule or calcifications.

When a possible lesion is seen on the CC view but not the MLO view, rolled CC views are useful to determine if the lesion is real and to locate it in the sagittal plane. The rolled CC views are performed by positioning the patient for the CC view and before compressing the breast, slightly displacing the tissue. For the rolled CC medial view, the upper pole of the breast is displaced medially before compression. For the rolled CC lateral view, the upper pole of the breast is displaced laterally (Fig. 2.30).

The interpretation of the rolled views requires an understanding of the displacement for each view. If the "lesion" is still apparent on the rolled CC views, it is a real finding. Its position in the breast is determined by the direction of displacement. If the lesion appears more medial on the rolled medial and more lateral on the rolled lateral, it is in the upper half of the breast (Fig. 2.31). If it moves in the opposite direction from the roll, it is in the inferior pole.

Axillary View

Although the axillary tail of the breast and the inferior aspect of the axilla are seen on the MLO view, it may be necessary to obtain an additional view to evaluate the upper axilla. The tube and cassette are angled 45 to 60 degrees from the superomedial to the inferolateral direction. The patient is turned 15 degrees away from the mammographic unit, and the ipsilateral arm is placed at a 90-degree angle to the breast. The cassette is placed

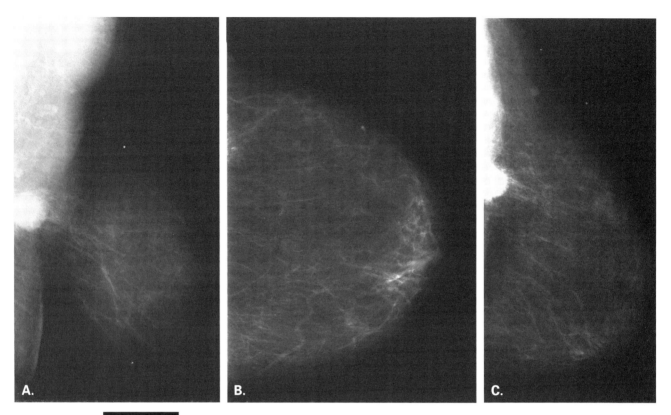

Figure 2.22

HISTORY: A 62-year-old woman with a palpable mass in the right breast.

MAMMOGRAPHY: Right MLO view **(A)** shows a large dense round mass at the chest wall. The lesion was not visible on the CC view **(B)**. The XCCL view is performed to rotate the postero-lateral aspect of the breast forward and to try to image the lesion in a transverse projection. On the XCCL view **(C)**, the spiculated lesion is noted laterally and posteriorly.

IMPRESSION: Highly suspicious for carcinoma.

HISTOPATHOLOGY: Invasive ductal carcinoma.

behind the ribs with the edge just above the patient's humeral head, and the patient leans slightly backward to optimize contact with the cassette (Fig. 2.32). The axilla is the only area to be included on the film. Vigorous compression is not obtained because of the many structures interposed. Imaging of this region is typically performed to evaluate palpable masses or to evaluate a mass or masses seen in the superior aspect of the MLO image (Figs. 2.33 and 2.34).

Tangential Views

The tangential view is an ancillary view that is used primarily to (a) assess a palpable lump, (b) visualize the area of the tumor bed after lumpectomy and radiotherapy, and (c) confirm that calcifications are dermal. For palpable lumps or for lumpectomy scars, the area of interest is placed in tangent to the x-ray beam and is compressed in this orientation (Fig. 2.35).

For possible dermal calcifications, a localization procedure is performed. The localization compression plate is placed over the surface of the breast in which the calcifications are thought to be located, and an image is obtained. The coordinates of the calcifications are identified, and a BB is placed over these coordinates. The localization plate is then removed, and the skin surface beneath the BB is placed in tangent. If the calcifications are dermal, they project at the skin (Fig. 2.36).

IMAGING THE PATIENT WITH IMPLANTS

The presence of breast implants for augmentation poses particular difficulty in obtaining adequate mammographic

(text continues on page 45)

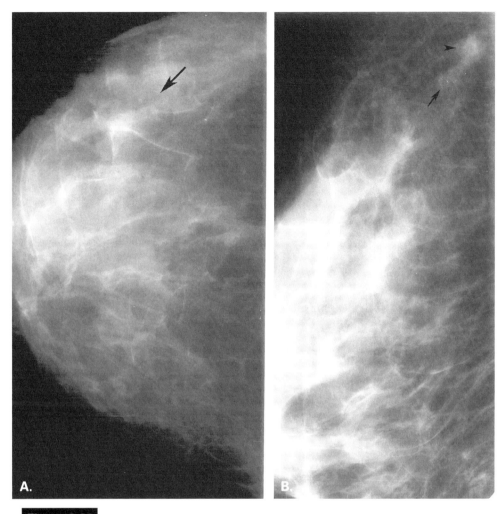

Figure 2.23

HISTORY: A 43-year-old woman for screening mammography.

MAMMOGRAPHY: Left CC view **(A)** shows heterogeneously dense tissue and grouped microcalcifications laterally **(arrow)**. On the left XCCL magnification views **(B)**, groups of pleomorphic microcalcifications **(arrow)** are present. There is also a small spiculated mass located posteriorly **(arrowhead)** that was not visualized on the standard CC view.

IMPRESSION: Highly suspicious for multifocal carcinoma.

HISTOPATHOLOGY: Invasive ductal, nuclear grade 2, and ductal carcinoma in situ.

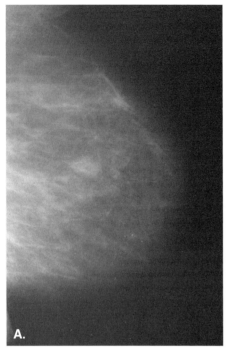

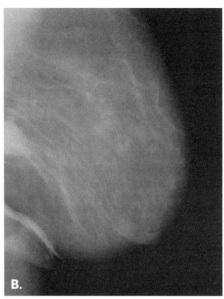

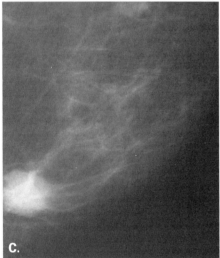

Figure 2.24

HISTORY: A 48-year-old woman with a palpable 4.5-cm mass in the right upper-inner quadrant.

MAMMOGRAPHY: Right MLO (**A**), ML (**B**), and XCCM (**C**) views. The MLO view is not of optimum quality because the posterior aspect of the breast and the pectoralis muscle are not visualized completely. There is a relatively well-defined mass in the midportion of the breast. Posterior to this mass, there is an ill-defined area of increased density extending to the edge of the film. It is important that if one identifies an area of increased density such as this, the breast posterior to it should be evaluated with additional views. On repositioning the breast (**B**), the 3.5-cm high-density mass is identified. XCCM spot (**C**) demonstrates the spiculated lesion in the far posteromedial aspect of the breast.

IMPRESSION: Carcinoma of the breast.

HISTOPATHOLOGY: Infiltrating ductal carcinoma.

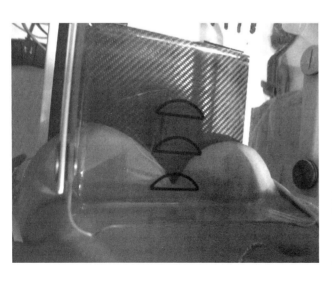

Figure 2.25

Positioning for the cleavage view shows both breasts over the receptor. Phototiming is not used because the automatic exposure control is not positioned over parenchyma.

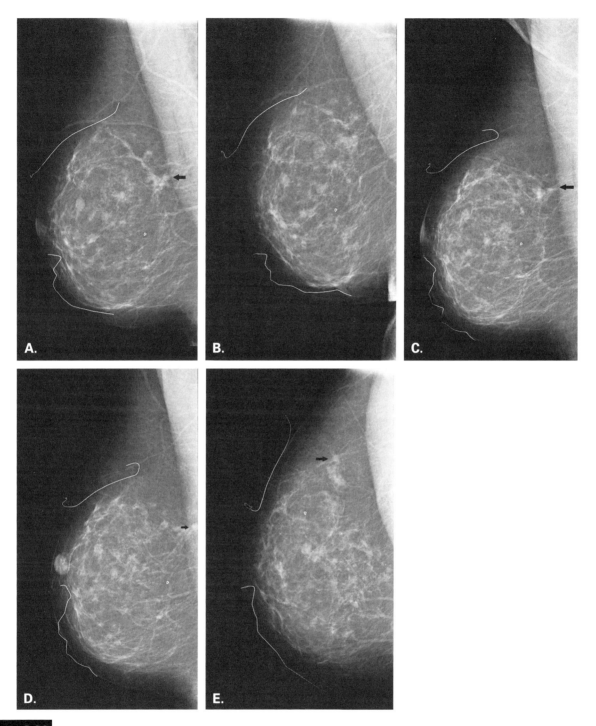

Figure 2.26

HISTORY: Screening mammogram on a 62-year-old patient with a history of multiple cysts and benign biopsies.

MAMMOGRAPHY: Left MLO view **(A)** shows scattered fibroglandular densities and multiple round masses consistent with cysts. In the far posterior aspect of the left axillary tail is a small indistinct density **(arrow)** that was not clearly evident on prior studies. On the ML view **(B)**, the density was not evident. Off-angle obliques obtained at angulation greater than and less than that of the MLO **(C, D)** again show the small density, which persists and has the same shape. It appears to be located more inferiorly on the oblique at 76 degrees **(C)** versus the oblique at 52 degrees, indicating that it is located laterally. This is the same concept as the movement in the position of the lesion on the MLO versus the 90-degree lateral or ML. Lesions located laterally appear lower on the 90-degree lateral than they do on the MLO view. The lesion is confirmed on the XCCL **(E)** view as being located laterally **(arrow)**.

IMPRESSION: Small mass in the axillary tail confirmed with off-angle MLO positioning.

HISTOPATHOLOGY: Invasive ductal carcinoma.

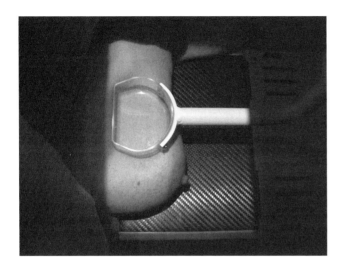

Figure 2.27

Positioning for the spot compression in the MLO projection shows the small compression paddle over the area of interest.

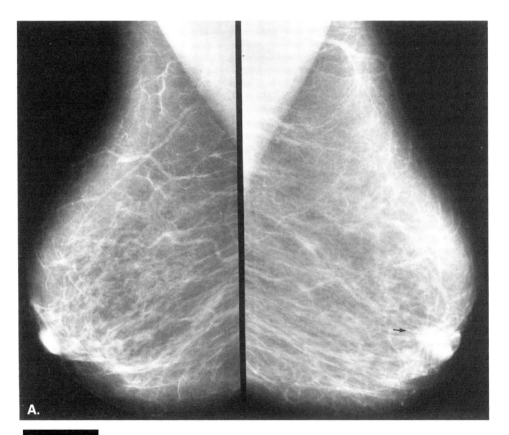

A.

Figure 2.28

HISTORY: A 56-year-old gravida 10, para 10 woman for screening. Bilateral MLO **(A)** view. There is asymmetry between the breasts, with irregular increased density **(arrow)** being noted in the right subareolar area. *(continued)*

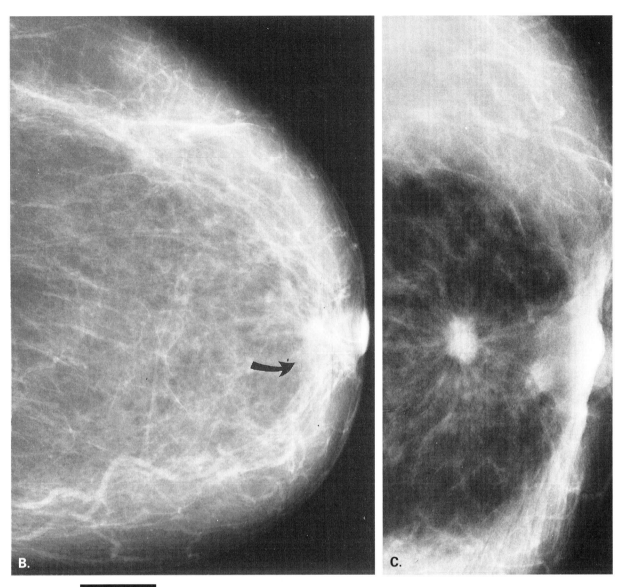

Figure 2.28   (*CONTINUED*)

MAMMOGRAPHY: Right CC (**B**), and spot compression (**C**) views. The area (**arrow**) appears somewhat spiculated on the CC view (**B**). However, a spot compression of the area (**C**) demonstrates
clearly the spiculated mass beneath the nipple. The appearance is highly suspicious for carcinoma.

HISTOPATHOLOGY: Infiltrating ductal carcinoma.

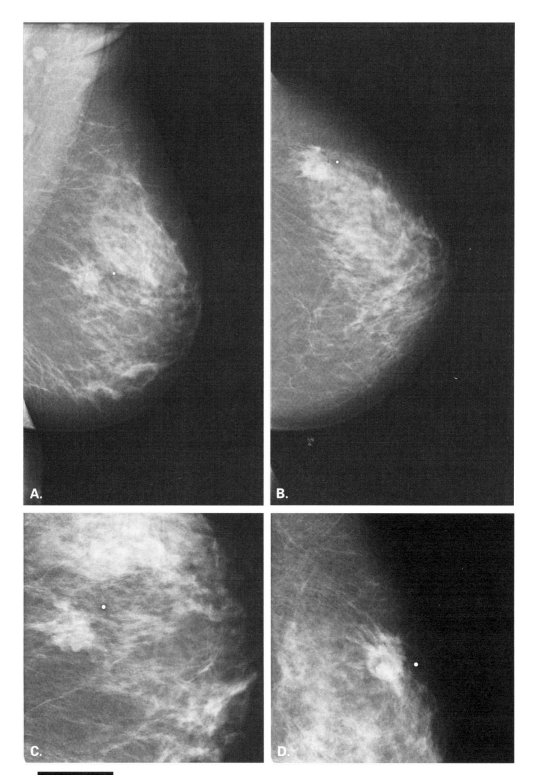

Figure 2.29

HISTORY: A 52-year-old woman for screening mammography.

MAMMOGRAPHY: Right MLO (**A**) and CC (**B**) views show scattered fibroglandular densities. There is an irregular dense mass located in the upper outer quadrant. On spot compression magnification ML (**C**) and XCCL (**D**) views, the mass is better seen to be an irregular lesion with indistinct margins, and it is associated with pleomorphic microcalcifications.

IMPRESSION: Highly suspicious for malignancy.

HISTOPATHOLOGY: Invasive ductal carcinoma with mucinous features.

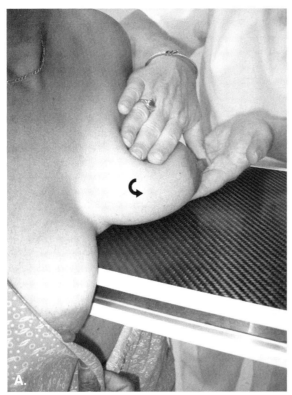
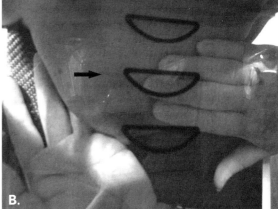

Figure 2.30

Rolled CC views. For a rolled CC medial view **(A)**, the breast is placed in a CC position, and the superior pole is displaced medially as the inferior pole is displaced laterally. For a rolled CC lateral view **(B)**, the breast positioned in a CC orientation, and the superior pole is rolled laterally as the inferior pole is rolled medially. Lesions that are located in the upper aspect of the breast move medially on the rolled medial and laterally on the rolled lateral views. Lesions located inferiorly move in the opposite direction from the roll.

images of the surrounding parenchyma. Standard MLO and CC views using manual techniques are necessary in order to image the posterior aspects of the breast and the implant.

Eklund et al. (37) described a modified positioning technique that allows for better compression and imaging of the anterior parenchymal structures. In positioning the patient for the modified technique, the technologist first palpates the anterior margin of the implant. The breast tissue anterior to the implant is pulled forward and placed over the cassette. For the CC view, the cassette tray is raised more than for standard positioning, and the inferior edge of the implant is displaced behind the cassette tray. As the compression plate is brought down, the technologist gently pulls the parenchyma forward and displaces the implant posteriorly, guiding the superior margin of the implant behind the descending compression device. For the MLO view, the same procedure is used; the

lateral edge is placed behind the cassette holder, and the compression is guided over the medial aspect of the implant (Figs. 2.37 and 2.38).

Well-positioned implant studies show the implant to be included on the standard views, with some visualization of the axillae and axillary tails. On the modified positioning or implant displacement views, the implants are not visible, and the anterior breast tissue is well compressed and visualized (Fig. 2.39).

MAGNIFICATION MAMMOGRAPHY

Direct radiographic magnification results in improved sharpness and detail (38) compared with conventional mammography. There is an improvement in the effective

(text continues on page 49)

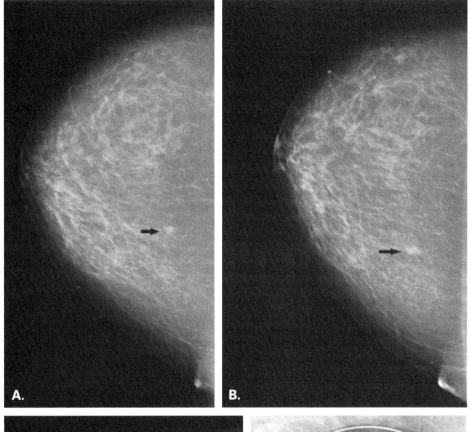

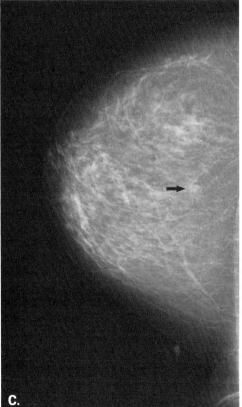

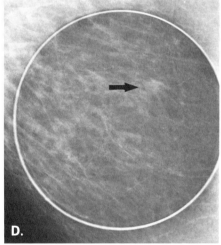

HISTORY: A 56-year-old woman recalled for a left breast density.

MAMMOGRAPHY: Left CC view **(A)** shows a small indistinct mass located medially **(arrow)**. This mass was not seen on the MLO view. Rolled CC views medially **(B)** and laterally **(C)** were obtained and show that the lesion persists **(arrows)** and displaces with the superior pole of the breast. On spot compression **(D)**, the indistinct margins and high density of this small mass are noted.

IMPRESSION: Small mass in the upper inner quadrant, highly suspicious for carcinoma.

HISTOPATHOLOGY: Invasive ductal carcinoma.

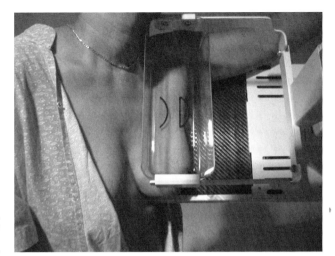

Figure 2.32

Positioning of the patient for the axillary tail view shows the upper aspect of the breast and the axilla included in the field of view.

Figure 2.33

Proper positioning and contrast on the axillary view demonstrate an enlarged axillary node.

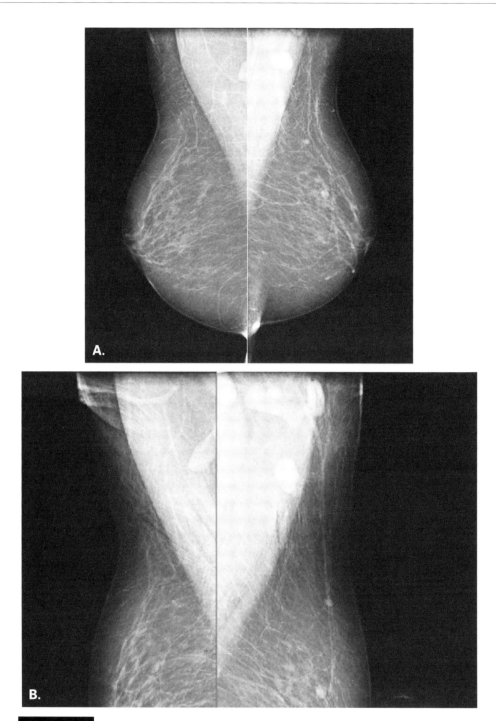

Figure 2.34

HISTORY: An 82-year-old woman for screening mammography.

MAMMOGRAPHY: Bilateral MLO views **(A)** show normal parenchyma and some prominent lymph nodes in the axillae. Axillary views **(B)** include more tissue in the axillae and better demonstrate the adenopathy. The inferior breast is not compressed or positioned in such a way to be evaluated on these views. The axillae are emphasized and are included in the field of view.

IMPRESSION: Axillary views showing mild adenopathy bilaterally.

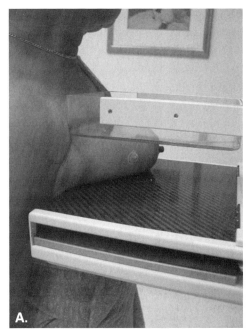
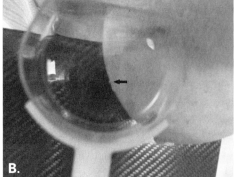

Figure 2.35

Positioning for the tangential view is tailored to the area of interest. A BB is placed over the area of interest, and that area is placed in tangent to the x-ray beam **(A, B)**.

resolution of the recording system, reduction of the effective noise, and reduction of scattered radiation (10). The breast is elevated from the Bucky by placing it on a magnification stand (Fig. 2.40). Small focal spots are used for magnification; because of this, there is a decrease in tube output and increase in exposure time (10). This produces an increase in blur from patient motion and an increase in radiation dose (10). The kVp is increased to compensate for the longer exposure needed for proper optical density. Magnification is of help in defining the borders of mass lesions, morphology, and number of microcalcifications (Figs. 2.41–2.43), and in determining the existence of multicentric tumor (39). There is an increase in radiation dose to the breast of 1.5 to 4 times that of conventional mammography (38).

ASSESSMENT OF IMAGE QUALITY

The role of the radiologist in mammography begins with an assessment of image quality. This must be performed routinely before image interpretation and is critical to the detection of breast cancers. Image quality is assessed, in addition, during the accreditation process for mammography facilities. Clinical image evaluation during the accreditation process includes assessment of positioning, compression, image quality, artifacts, and labeling (22). Imaging of the American College of Radiology Accreditation phantom is used to test the system performance as well by evaluating both contrast and resolution.

(text continues on page 54)

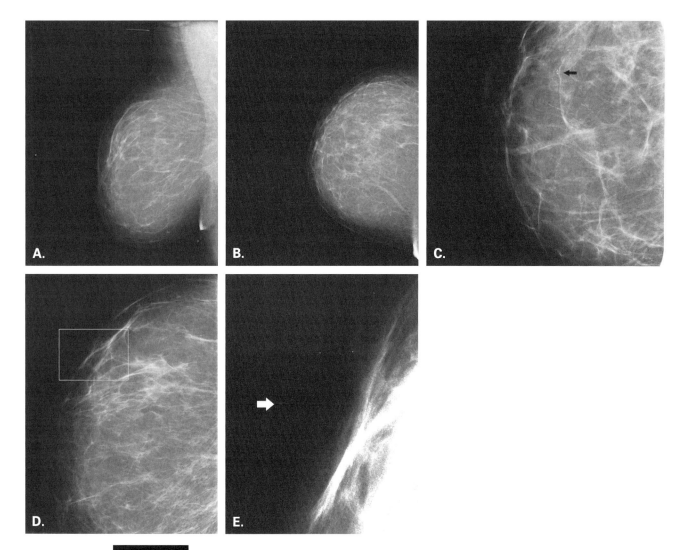

Figure 2.36

HISTORY: A 42-year-old patient referred for evaluation of calcifications seen on screening mammography.

MAMMOGRAPHY: Left MLO **(A)** and CC **(B)** views show a small cluster of calcifications **(arrows)** located at 12 o'clock, somewhat superficially. On the CC magnification view **(C)**, the calcifications are clustered and very well demarcated, suggesting that they are dermal. On the tangential ML view **(D)**, the calcifications are clearly depicted within the skin **(arrow)** seen best on the enlarged image **(E)**.

IMPRESSION: Tangential view demonstrating calcifications to be dermal.

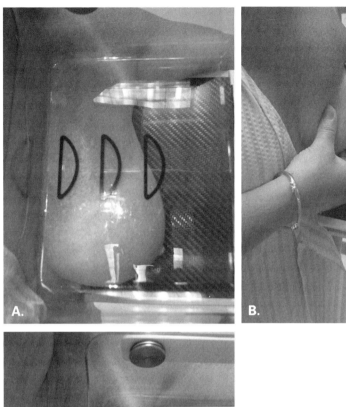

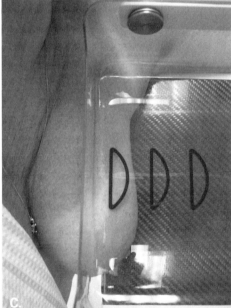

Figure 2.37

Positioning the patient with implants. **(A)** The standard MLO view with the implant in the field of view. **(B)** The technologist is displacing the anterior edge of the implant posteriorly as she is pulling the parenchyma forward. **(C)** The implant-displaced MLO view with only the parenchyma included in the field of view. Much of the parenchyma is included in the image with only the posterior regions not being visible.

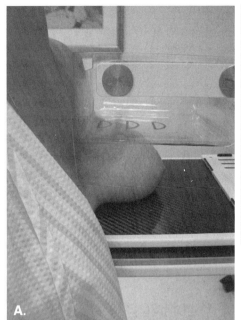

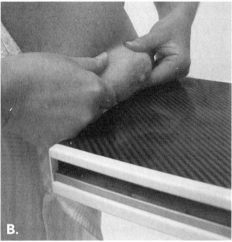

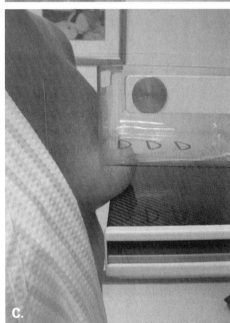

Figure 2.38

Positioning the patient with implants: the CC view. **(A)** The breast including the implant is included in the field of view. **(B)** The technologist is displacing the implant posteriorly as she is pulling the parenchyma anteriorly and placing it over the receptor. **(C)** The implant-displaced CC view includes only the anterior parenchyma in the field of view.

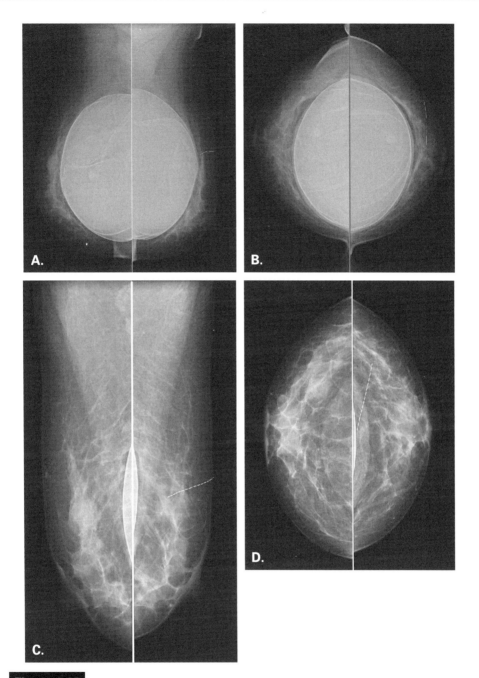

Figure 2.39

Normal implants and mammography. **(A)** Standard MLO views showing the saline implants in the field of view. **(B)** Standard CC views showing the saline implants included. **(C)** Implant-displaced MLO views show the subpectoral implants displaced posteriorly. The parenchyma anterior to the implants is well compressed and visualized. **(D)** Implant-displaced CC views show the pectoralis muscles and the breast parenchyma included and only an edge of the right implant visible. A scar marker indicates a prior benign biopsy site.

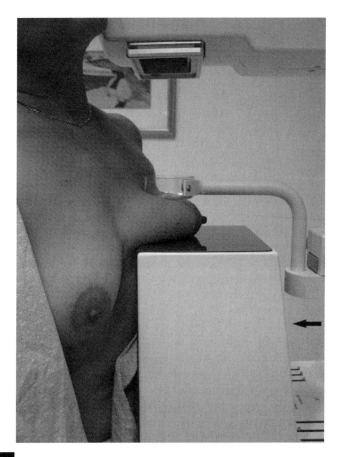

Figure 2.40

Positioning the patient for spot magnification. The breast is elevated away from the receptor on
the magnification stand **(arrow)**, increasing the object-to-receptor distance and creating an air
gap. Spot compression is applied over the area of interest.

Clinical image evaluation should be performed by the technologist and the radiologist on each mammogram. Evaluation of image quality includes an assessment of technical factors, such as exposure, contrast, noise, and sharpness. An underexposed image may have occurred because of incorrect position of the photocell, and such underexposure greatly compromises the detection of masses or calcifications in dense parenchyma. Optimizing contrast in mammography is critical to the visualization of subtle differences in tissue densities. Noise or radiographic mottle is affected by the number of x-rays used to produce the image. Fewer x-rays are associated with increased quantum mottle and decreased ability to visualize fine calcifications (22). Sharpness is related to the geometry of the focal spot, motion unsharpness, and screen unsharpness from poor film screen contrast. Proper compression of the breast is important in reducing motion unsharpness.

The images should be free from artifacts. The types of artifacts visible on mammography may include those related to the patient, such as overlying structures (chin, ear, hair, eyeglasses) (Figs. 2.44 and 2.45), or to substances on the skin (deodorant or powder). Artifacts on film-screen mammography images are different from those on digital mammography. On film-screen mammography, common artifacts that relate to film and cassette handling include dust, fingerprints, and focal fog.

Lastly, the assessment of image quality includes the evaluation of positioning. Factors such as proper positioning and compression on the MLO view to include the posterior tissue and proper positioning on the CC view to include the medial tissue are part of this evaluation. In patients in whom the posterior tissue is very thick relative to the nipple area, uniform compression

(text continues on page 56)

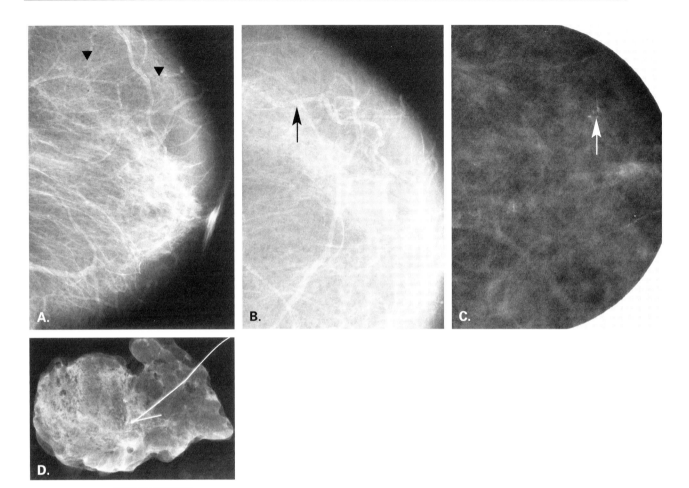

Figure 2.41

HISTORY: A 72-year-old gravida 6, para 4, abortus 2 woman for screening.

MAMMOGRAPHY: Right ML **(A)**, enlarged (1.5X) CC **(B)**, spot magnification (2X) **(C)**, and specimen **(D)** views. There is scattered glandularity present. Extensive vascular calcifications are seen **(arrowheads, A** and **B)**. On the initial CC view **(B)**, there are microcalcifications **(arrow)** that appear to project beyond the lumen of the calcified vessel. These calcifications **(arrow)** are better evaluated with the spot compression magnification view **(C)**, on which they are clearly displaced away from the calcified vessel **(arrowhead)**. Their contour is slightly irregular, and they are, therefore, of moderate suspicion for malignancy. These were biopsied after needle localization **(D)**, and the specimen film demonstrates their clustered nature and slightly irregular morphology.

IMPRESSION: Moderately suspicious calcifications demonstrated on spot compression magnification view.

HISTOPATHOLOGY: Intraductal carcinoma.

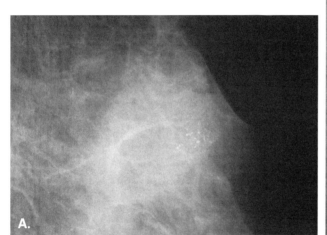
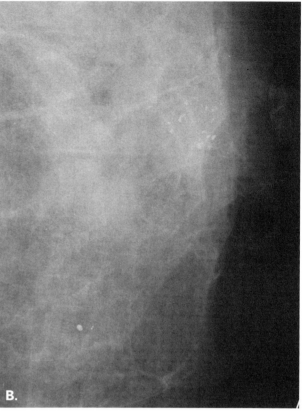

Figure 2.42

HISTORY: A 54-year-old patient recalled for an abnormal screening mammogram.

MAMMOGRAPHY: Right magnification ML **(A)** and CC **(B)** views show highly pleomorphic clustered microcalcifications **(arrow)** at 12 o'clock superimposed on dense parenchyma. The magnification views demonstrate very clearly the shapes and borders of the microcalcifications.

IMPRESSION: Highly suspicious for malignancy.

HISTOPATHOLOGY: High-grade ductal carcinoma in situ.

may not be attainable. Obtaining additional CC and MLO views of the anterior aspects of the breasts in both projections can optimize compression and imaging of both regions of the breast. For lesions that are clinically evident, a tailored examination is necessary to be sure that the palpable area is included in the field of view (Fig. 2.46).

The viewing conditions are also evaluated through MQSA and are critical to the optimization of visualization of breast abnormalities. For film-screen mammography, high-intensity view boxes with shutters to reduce extraneous light are required. The ambient light in the reading room should be kept to a minimum. Likewise, with digital mammography, high-luminance workstations and low ambient light are used for image interpretation. Intensity windowing at the workstation has been shown to improve detection of simulated calcifications in phantoms (40). Kimme-Smith et al. (41) found that the detection of microcalcifications in dense breasts was significantly affected by viewing conditions.

Even with good techniques, 5% to 10% of breast cancers are not detected by mammography. It is of utmost importance that the radiologist maintain high standards of quality, be certain that excellent positioning is performed, and correlate the clinical examination with mammogram in determining that the region of interest is included on the film. By maintaining these standards, the number of cancers not detected by mammography will be kept to a minimum.

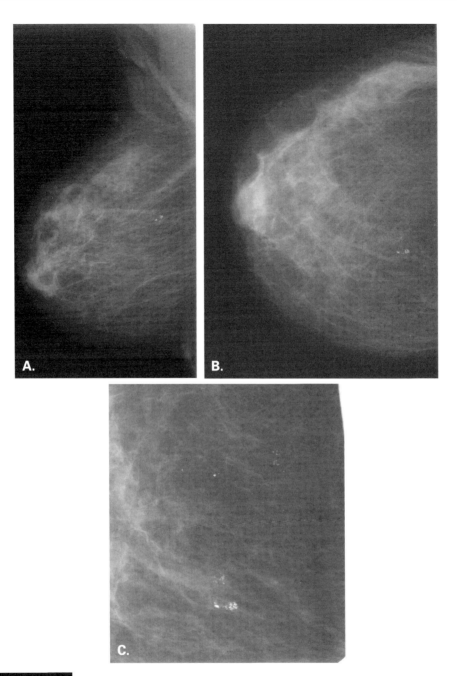

Figure 2.43

HISTORY: Patient recalled from screening for evaluation of microcalcifications.

MAMMOGRAPHY: Left MLO **(A)** and CC **(B)** views show a cluster of microcalcifications at 10 o'clock. A magnification CC **(C)** view demonstrates the morphology and number much more clearly. Magnification mammography is very important in the assessment of microcalcifications and in defining their possible etiologies and management.

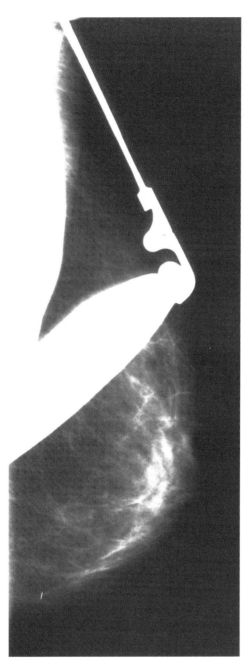

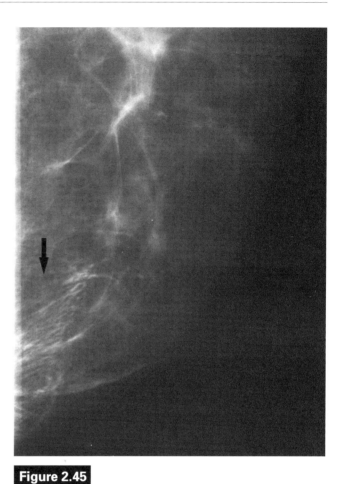

Figure 2.45

Coned-down right CC view showing a striated density **(arrow)** at the chest wall. This is the patient's hair extending forward between the tube and receptor and overlying the field of view.

Figure 2.44

Artifact during positioning the patient for the CC view from her eyeglasses overlying the field of view.

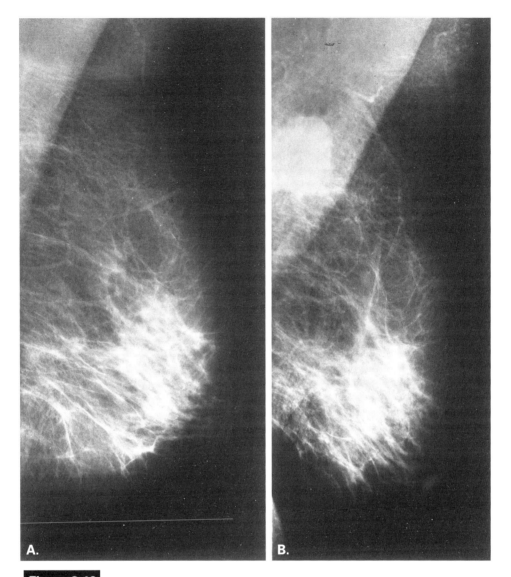

Figure 2.46

HISTORY: A 55-year-old gravida 2, para 2 woman with a large tender mass in the right axillary tail.

MAMMOGRAPHY: Right MLO **(A)** and repositioned right MLO **(B)** views. On the initial view **(A)**, the breast is moderately dense, and no suspicious abnormalities are seen. The patient did have a palpable lump in the axillary tail; for this reason, the technologist repositioned her to bring the mass forward into the field of view **(B)**. More of the axillary area is seen on this view **(B)**, but the breast itself is not compressed as well on the standard MLO **(A)**. A large, partially circumscribed mass with microlobulated borders is present in the right axillary tail and is most consistent with breast carcinoma, although a metastatic node is another consideration.

IMPRESSION: Carcinoma, right axillary tail, demonstrated on a tailored MLO view to demonstrate the palpable mass.

HISTOPATHOLOGY: Poorly differentiated adenocarcinoma.

NOTE: It is critical that the technologist palpate any masses noted by the clinician or patient and be certain that the area of palpable concern is included in the field of view.

REFERENCES

1. Shaw de Paredes E, Frazier AB, Hartwell GD, et al. Development and implementation of a quality assurance program for mammography. *Radiology* 1987;163:83–85.
2. Haus AG. Technologic improvements in screen-film mammography. *Radiology* 1990;174:628–637.
3. PL 102-539: The Mammography Quality Standard Act of 1992.
4. Martin JE, Moskowitz M, Milbrath JR. Breast cancer missed by mammography. *Radiology* 1979;132:737–739.
5. Kalisher L. Factors influencing false negative rates in xeromammography. *Radiology* 1979;133:297–301.
6. Haus AG. Screen-film mammography updates: x-ray units, breast compression, grids, screen-film characteristics, and radiation dose. In: Mulvaney JA, ed. *Medical Imaging and Instrumentation '84 (Proceedings of the SPIE)*. Bellingham, WA: International Society for Optical Engineering, 1984;486.
7. Feig SA. Mammography equipment: principles, features, selection. *Radiol Clin North Am* 1987;25:897–911.
8. National Council on Radiation Protection and Measurements. *Mammography: A User's Guide* (NCRP Report No. 85). Bethesda, MD: National Council on Radiation Protection and Measurements, 1986.
9. Vyborny CJ, Schmidt RA. Mammography as a radiographic examination an overview. *RadioGraphics* 1989;9(4):723–764.
10. Haus AG. Recent advances in screen-film mammography. *Radiol Clin North Am* 1987;25:913–928.
11. Muntz EP, Logan WW. Focal spot size and scatter suppression in magnification mammography. *AJR Am J Roentgenol* 1979;133:453–459.
12. Tabar L, Dean PB. Screen-film mammography: quality control. In: Feig S, McClelland R, eds. *Breast Carcinoma: Current Diagnosis and Treatment*. New York: Masson Publishing USA, 1983:161–168.
13. Fajardo LL, Westerman BR. Mammography equipment: practical considerations for the radiologist. *Appl Radiol* 1990;19:12–15.
14. Egan RL, McSweeney MB, Sprawls P. Grids in mammography. *Radiology* 1983;146:359–362.
15. Sickles EA, Weber WN. High-contrast mammography with a moving grid: assessment of clinical utility. *AJR Am J Roentgenol* 1986;146:1137–1139.
16. Logan WW. Screen-film mammography: technique. In: Feig S, McClelland R, eds. Breast Carcinoma: Current Diagnosis and Treatment. New York: Masson Publishing USA, 1983: 141–160.
17. Kimme-Smith C, Bassett LW, Gold RH, et al. New mammography screen-film combinations: imaging characteristics and radiation dose. *AJR Am J Roentgenol* 1990;154:713–719.
18. Haus AG. Recent trends in screen-film mammography: technical factors and radiation dose. Paper presented at the Third International Copenhagen Symposium on Detection of Breast Cancer; August 1985; Copenhagen, Denmark.
19. Skubic SE, Yagan R, Oravec D, et al. Value of increasing film processing time to reduce radiation dose during mammography. *AJR Am J Roentgenol* 1990;155:1189–1193.
20. Tabar L, Haus AG. Processing of mammographic films: technical and clinical considerations. *Radiology* 1989;173:65–69.
21. Kimme-Smith C, Rothschild PA, Bassett LW, et al. Mammographic film-processor temperature, development time, and chemistry: effect on dose, contrast, and noise. *AJR Am J Roentgenol* 1989;152:35–40.
22. Bassett LW. Clinical image evaluation. *Radiol Clin North Am* 1995;33(6):1027–1039.
23. Yaffe MJ. Physics of mammography: image recording process. *RadioGraphics* 1990;10:341–363.
24. Pisano ED, Gatsonis C, Hendrick E, et al. Diagnostic performance of digital versus film mammography for breast-cancer screening. *N Engl J Med* 2005;353(17):1773–1783.
25. Feig SA, Yaffe MJ. Clinical prospects for full-field digital mammography. *Semin Breast Dis* 1999;2(1):64–72.
26. Williams MB, Fajardo LL. Digital mammography: performance considerations and current detector designs. *Acad Radiol* 1996;3:429–437.
27. Bassett LW, Bunnell DH, Jahanshahi R, et al. Breast cancer detection: one versus two views. *Radiology* 1987;165:95–97.
28. Schmitt EL, Threatt B. Tumor location and detectability in mammographic screening. *AJR Am J Roentgenol* 1982;139: 761–765.
29. Bassett LW, Gold RH. Breast radiography using the oblique projection. *Radiology* 1983;149:585–587.
30. Logan WW, Janus J. Use of special mammographic views to maximize radiographic information. *Radiol Clin North Am* 1987;25:953–959.
31. Sickles EA. Practical solutions to common mammographic problems: tailoring the examination. *AJR Am J Roentgenol* 1988;151:31–39.
32. Feig SA. The importance of supplementary mammographic views to diagnostic accuracy. *AJR Am J Roentgenol* 1988;151: 40–41.
33. Eklund GW, Cardenosa G, Parsons W. Assessing adequacy of mammographic image quality. *Radiology* 1994;190:297–307.
34. Eklund GW, Cardenosa G. The art of mammographic positioning. *Radiol Clin North Am* 1992;30(1):21–53.
35. Gilula LA, Destouet JM, Monsees B. Nipple simulating a breast mass on a mammogram. *Radiology* 1989;170:272.
36. Bassett LW, Hirbawi IA, DeBruhl N, et al. Mammographic positioning: evaluation from the view box. *Radiology* 1993;188:803–806.
37. Eklund GW, Busby RC, Miller SH, et al. Improved imaging of the augmented breast. *AJR Am J Roentgenol* 1988;151:469–473.
38. Sickles EA. Magnification mammography. In: Feig S, McClelland R, eds. *Breast Carcinoma: Current Diagnosis and Treatment*. New York: Masson Publishing USA, 1983:177–182.
39. Sickles EA. Microfocal spot magnification mammography using xeroradiographic and screen-film recording systems. *Radiology* 1979;131:599–607.
40. Pisano ED, Chandramouli J, Hemminger BM, et al. Does intensity windowing improve the detection of simulated calcifications in dense mammograms? *J Digit Imaging* 1997;10(2):79–84.
41. Kimme-Smith C, Haus AG, DeBruhl N, et al. Effects of ambient light and view box luminance on the detection of calcifications in mammography. *AJR Am J Roentgenol* 1997;168:775–778.

Chapter 3

An Approach to Mammographic Analysis

Once the mammographic images are presented to the radiologist for interpretation, an approach to the analysis and interpretation defines how lesions are identified and how they are described and managed. The assessment and description of the mammographic findings are defined in a standardized lexicon known as the Breast Imaging Reporting and Data System (BI-RADS®). BI-RADS® was developed by the American College of Radiology in the mid-1990s (1) and includes a nomenclature for lesion description and overall assessment. BI-RADS® incorporates three basic components: (a) a description of the parenchymal density, (b) specific lesion descriptions for masses, calcifications, and other findings, and (c) an overall assessment or management recommendation for the patient. The use of this lexicon is ideal: The terms are standardized, and the correct use of the terms to describe an abnormality is helpful to the radiologist to correctly manage the case. The use of the standardized terminology and the requirement for an overall assessment are also very helpful for communication of the findings to the referring physician.

As the Mammography Quality Standard Act was redefined with the publication of the final regulations in 1997 (2), so included was the requirement that every mammography report include the final assessment category for the case. Only one final assessment category can be used for the patient's study. The utilization of the final assessment category is important not only for communication of results to the referring physician and the patient, but also for tracking of outcomes and quality-assurance monitoring.

The BI-RADS® reporting includes a description of tissue composition based on the volume of glandular tissue relative to fat. The four categories of composition include (a) almost entirely fat, (b) scattered fibroglandular densities, (c) heterogeneously dense, and (d) extremely dense. The specific descriptions for masses, calcifications, and other findings will be covered later in this chapter and throughout the book.

Based on the findings for the case, a BI-RADS® final assessment category is applied. The final assessment categories are shown in Table 3.1. For screening mammography, the assessment categories may be BI-RADS® 0 (requiring additional evaluation with diagnostic mammography and/or ultrasound) or BI-RADS® 1 (negative) or 2 (benign).

If lesions are identified that could potentially be malignant, additional evaluation should be performed based on the diagnostic mammogram. BI-RADS® categories for diagnostic mammography range from 2 through 6. For BI-RADS® 2 (benign) lesions, routine mammographic follow-up is obtained. For BI-RADS® 3 (probably benign) lesions, the likelihood for malignancy is less than 2% (3), and the lesion is followed at 6-month intervals for 2 years. For BI-RADS® (suspicious) 4 lesions, the possibility for malignancy ranges from 2% to 95%, but the overall positive predictive value is approximately 20% to 25%. Therefore, biopsy is recommended for the BI-RADS® 4 category. Lesions classified as BI-RADS® 5 have a high probability of being malignant (>95%), and biopsy is necessary. Category 6 was added to the BI-RADS® classification and is used for biopsy-proven cancers that are being followed with mammography before surgery. This category may be used for patients who have a biopsy-proven cancer and are being imaged for other possible lesions, or for a patient being treated with neoadjuvant chemotherapy before surgical management.

If there are multiple lesions, the overall assessment for the case is the highest or worst category applicable to any lesion. For example, if one lesion is a BI-RADS® 3 and another lesion on the same mammogram is a BI-RADS® 4, the assessment category for the case is BI-RADS® 4, suspicious.

Lesions that are correctly analyzed and categorized as BI-RADS® 3, probably benign, have a high likelihood of actually being benign. Sickles (3) prospectively evaluated the value of periodic mammographic follow-up over a 3- to 3.5-year period for nonpalpable, mammographically detected, probably benign lesions. The frequency of probably benign interpretations in this study was 11.2%. In this study (3), 17 of 3,184 (0.5%) cases were subsequently found to be malignant, 15 of which were identified by means of a mammographic interval change. The importance of completely evaluating the lesion with diagnostic

▶ TABLE 3.1 BI-RADS® Classification

BI-RADS® Category	Descriptive	Recommendation
0	Incomplete	Needs further evaluation (Additional views, ultrasound, comparison with old films)
1	Negative	Routine annual screening
2	Benign	Routine annual screening
3	Probably benign	Short interval follow-up mammography
4	Suspicious	Biopsy should be considered
5	Highly suspicious	Appropriate action/biopsy
6	Proven malignancy	Appropriate action

mammography before classifying it as probably benign was emphasized in the study.

Vizcaino et al, (4) reported a study of 13,790 women, of whom 795 (5.8%) underwent short-term follow-up for a nonpalpable, probably benign lesion. Only seven lesions (1%) changed and were biopsied. Of these, two cancers were identified (0.3%).

The specific type of lesions considered to be BI-RADS® 3 include clustered round calcifications, a noncalcified circumscribed solid mass, a focal asymmetry, multiple clusters of tiny calcifications, scattered tiny calcifications, and multiple solid circumscribed masses. A suggested algorithm to manage probably benign lesions is shown in Figure 3.1. The importance of performing a diagnostic mammogram and a complete evaluation before classifying a lesion as BI-RADS® 3 cannot be overemphasized. Rosen et al. (5) found that in 52 cancers initially called probably benign, no cases fulfilled the strict criteria for a probably benign lesion. Correct workup and assessment of a lesion to categorize it as BI-RADS® 3 should lead to the follow-up of lesions that are actually benign and—very infrequently—lesions that are malignant.

More recently, Leung and Sickles (6) studied the need for recall or further evaluation in 1,440 consecutive cases of multiple circumscribed masses identified on screening mammography. These cases were prospectively managed as benign and were followed with mammography at 1 year; any that were palpable were aspirated. Two interval cancers (0.14%) were identified, which is less than the incident rate of breast cancer in the United States. Based on this, the authors did not recommend recall for women with multiple, similar nonpalpable, circumscribed masses.

SEARCH PATTERNS

Cancers are missed on mammography for a variety of reasons, including technical, perceptive, and interpretative ones. In a study by Bird et al. (7) of the reasons for missed breast cancers, the authors found that 43% of the errors were caused by the lesions being overlooked by the radiologists. Missed breast cancers were more likely to be manifested as a developing density on mammography. In a study of breast cancers that were missed by radiologists, Goergen et al. (8) found that missed cancers were significantly lower in density than detected cancers, and missed cancers were more often seen on only one of the two views.

Bilateral synchronous breast cancers do occur and are often diagnosed through mammography. However, magnetic resonance imaging (MRI) has made an important impact in this area by detecting mammographically and clinically occult cancers in the contralateral breast. In a study of 77 patients with bilateral breast cancers, 43% were found to be synchronous (9), and the remainder were metachronous. When one lesion of suspicion is identified, it is imperative that the radiologist modify the search pattern to specifically look for other foci of tumor in the same breast and for contralateral disease.

It is important for the radiologist who is interpreting mammography to develop careful and consistent search patterns that will assist one in identifying potential abnormalities. Because the mammographic appearance of the breasts is quite variable from patient to patient, it is important that films be placed as mirror images during interpretation. In this way, one will be able to identify most easily a subtle mass or asymmetry that may be the only sign of carcinoma. With the films placed as mirror images (Fig. 3.2), a systematic comparison of the various areas of each breast should be carried out.

A search pattern that emphasizes the importance of symmetry as a parameter of benignity is as follows. The mediolateral oblique (MLO) views are imaged side by side, and an overall assessment of positioning and image quality is made. Then the images are viewed overall for any obvious abnormalities. Even if an obvious finding is

Screening Mammography

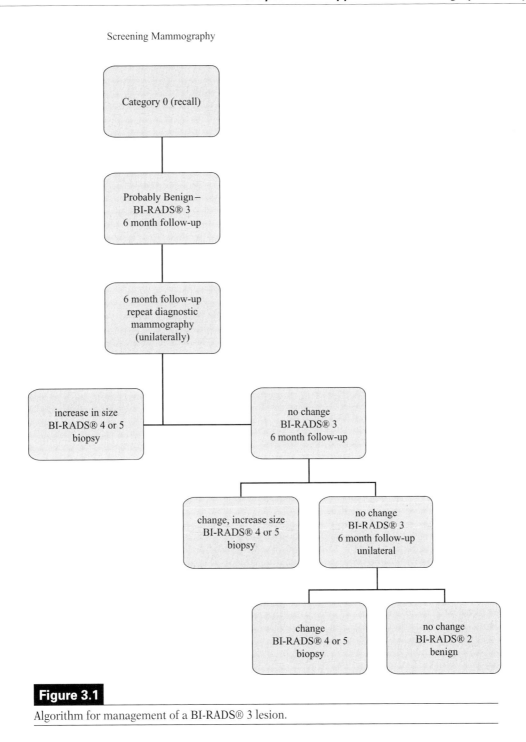

Figure 3.1

Algorithm for management of a BI-RADS® 3 lesion.

identified, a meticulous review of the remainder of the images is performed. By segmenting the image into identical sections, small portions of the breasts are compared with each other. For an experienced reader, this process becomes nearly instantaneous.

Initially, image segmentation can be performed by placing an opaque overlay on the images to emphasize the segment; as one develops the skills, this function is performed subconsciously. In addition to emphasizing the review of the images for symmetry, the amount of information in a segment versus the whole breast is more easily managed by the eye-brain axis (Fig. 3.3). This technique can be performed rapidly and incorporated into the global overview that an experienced breast imager uses

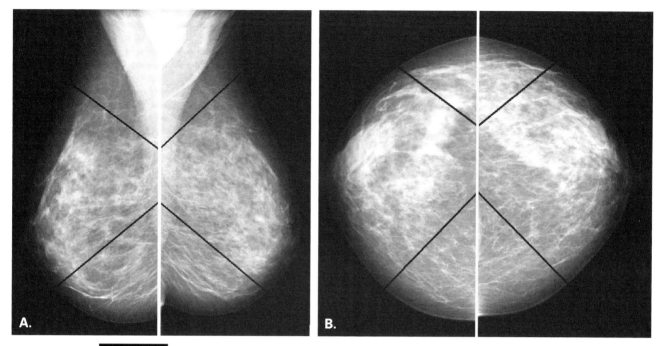

Figure 3.2

Bilateral MLO **(A)** and CC **(B)** views of a screening mammogram. The approach to interpretation begins with viewing the images as mirror images with both MLOs together and both CCs together. Comparison of like areas of each breast is performed using a segmentation approach as shown. By focusing on segments of the breasts together, one may be better able to identify subtle areas of asymmetry or subtle masses.

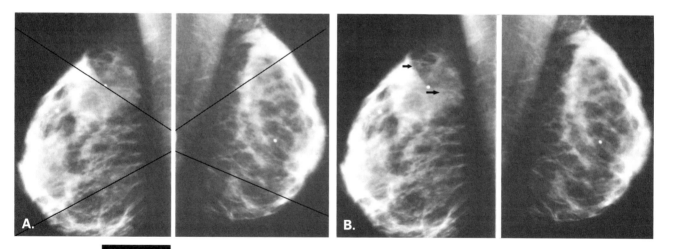

Figure 3.3

Segmentation of MLO images on a patient for screening mammography shows a focal asymmetry located in the axillary tail of the left breast **(arrow)**. Although the area is less dense than some of the surrounding parenchyma, it is clearly asymmetric in comparison with the same region of the opposite breast. Pathology showed invasive lobular carcinoma.

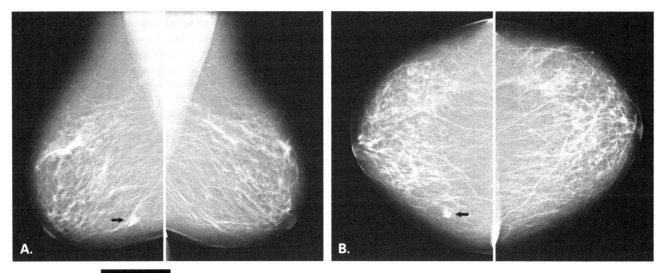

Figure 3.4

The initial step in evaluation of the mammogram, after determining that the quality is adequate, should be to assess the symmetry of the breasts. This can be accomplished best by orienting the images together, as mirror images of each other. The viewer should make a systematic comparison of the breasts from side to side, determining if there are any asymmetries. In **A**, both MLO views are shown, and there is a masslike area of asymmetry in the left lower-inner quadrant **(arrow)**. On the CC views **(B)**, the mass is more clearly seen as being asymmetric **(arrow)** in comparison with the opposite breast. This lesion was an infiltrating carcinoma.

when interpreting a mammogram. The same pattern is used on the craniocaudal (CC) views that are arranged side by side as mirror images of each other (Fig. 3.4).

Literature on search patterns by radiologists has shown that experienced versus nonexperienced readers are different. Mammographic search patterns for different readers vary in terms of duration of gaze, scan pattern, and detection times for abnormalities. Krupinski (10) found that true positives and false positives on mammography were associated with prolonged eye gaze duration, and that false negatives were associated with longer eye gaze durations than true negatives. Therefore, gaze duration was a useful predictor of missed lesions in mammography (10). Barrett et al. (11) showed a rapid identification of microcalcifications by experienced readers as measured by pupil direction and dilatation. Less experienced readers spend more time reviewing images and covering more image area than more experienced radiologists (10).

When a potential abnormality is perceived, an analysis ensues that includes its features, possible etiologies, and a plan for evaluation. Many lesions are benign at this point and do not require further workup. Other lesions are equivocal or suspicious and necessitate further mammographic imaging and possibly imaging with other modalities. If the lesion has various features on additional views, some of which are worrisome and others of which are often associated with benign lesions, biopsy is usually

warranted. When imaging a lesion in the breast, it is best to err on the side of caution by managing the case based on the worst mammographic features (Fig. 3.5).

SELECTION OF APPROPRIATE VIEWS

It is important first to correlate any clinical findings with the mammographic findings. The location of skin lesions, scars, or palpable masses should be indicated by the technologist, and the radiologist must correlate the position of such entities with the imaging findings (Fig. 3.6). A knowledge of the clinical history is also important, particularly when working up clinically suspicious lesions or palpable masses and in the defining the differential diagnosis for certain findings. For example, a history of surgery at the site of an area of spiculation could be compatible with a scar. Without the history of surgery, the same finding is of concern for malignancy (Fig. 3.7).

The mammographic examination should be tailored to the individual patient (12). Particular attention should be paid to the deep aspects of the breasts, and if breast parenchyma extends posteriorly to the edge of the film on both views, exaggerated CC views should be obtained also to evaluate the deep areas completely. In thin patients with small dense breasts, the posterior lower aspect of the breasts may not be adequately visualized on the MLO

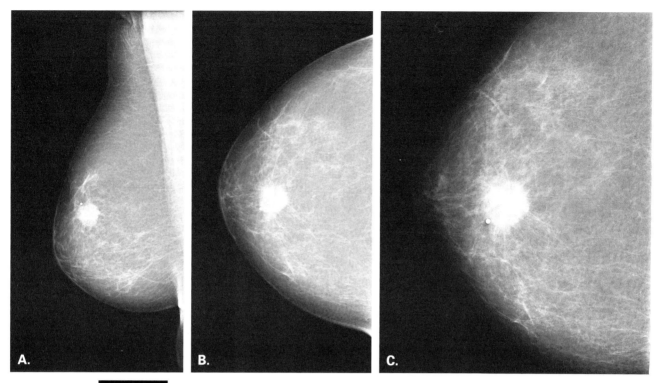

A.   B.   C.

Figure 3.5

HISTORY: A 65-year-old woman with a palpable left breast mass.

MAMMOGRAPHY: Left MLO **(A)** and CC **(B)** views show a round dense mass corresponding to the palpable lesion. The mass is associated with dense coarse calcifications, but its margins are highly spiculated on the magnification CC view **(C)**.

IMPRESSION: Highly suspicious for malignancy.

HISTOPATHOLOGY: Invasive ductal carcinoma.

NOTE: When approaching a lesion, it is important to judge it by its worst features. In this case, the pattern of calcification is benign, but the margins of the mass are very malignant.

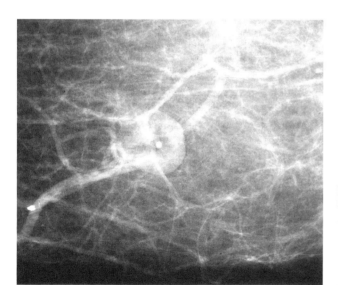

Figure 3.6

A skin lesion is evident on mammography and marked with a BB. It is important for the technologist to document observed skin lesions with a radiopaque marker. Skin lesions are often evident on mammography and may occasionally be confused with parenchymal abnormalities.

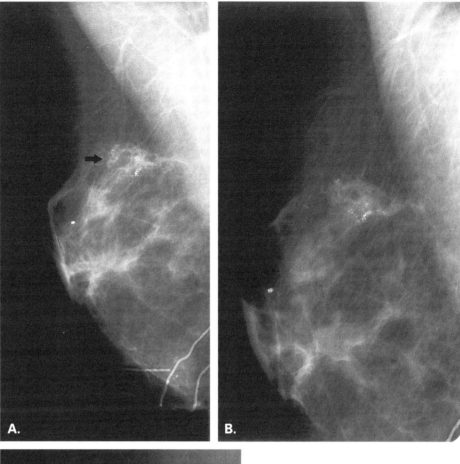

Figure 3.7

HISTORY: A 53-year-old woman who is status post–right mastectomy with reconstruction and left reduction mammoplasty. She presents for routine mammography.

MAMMOGRAPHY: Left MLO **(A)**, ML **(B)**, and MLO spot-magnification **(C)** views. The patient is status post-reduction mammoplasty, and typical postoperative changes are seen. Scars are present inferiorly and in the periareolar area, and there are areas of distortion of the architecture. Clustered microcalcifications are present superiorly and are associated with some distortion **(arrows)** of the parenchyma. On the magnification view **(C)**, these calcifications are coarse and pleomorphic, and they are surrounding a fat-containing round mass. The constellation of findings is consistent with fat necrosis.

IMPRESSION: Fat necrosis, post-reduction mammoplasty.

NOTE: Clinical correlation is key in suggesting the correct diagnosis in this case. The pattern of calcifications could be mistaken for malignant pleomorphic calcifications. The history of surgery and the fat-containing region in the area of calcifications are the factors that are indicative of a benign lesion.

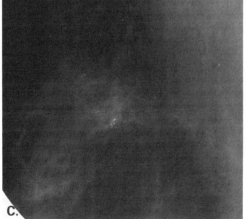

view; an additional mediolateral (ML) view often demonstrates this posterior tissue.

In the evaluation of each breast, attention should be paid to the skin thickness, the symmetry of the subcutaneous fat, and the presence of asymmetric tissue, nodules, or calcifications (13). The architecture of the breasts should be symmetrical, with the fibroglandular tissue oriented to the nipple and with Cooper's ligaments appearing as thin arcs traversing the fat. Correlation with clinical examination and the location of any scars is important in assessing the presence of an area of asymmetry or architectural distortion. Focal distortion—including linear densities oriented in a different direction from the other structures, or focal puckering in or out of the glandular tissue—may indicate an underlying carcinoma. Carcinomas may infiltrate into the fat and parenchyma, producing thickening of Cooper's ligaments. Such involvement can produce skin thickening or retraction that may first be evident on mammography. Central carcinomas also may fix the nipple-areolar complex, which is evident to the technologist on compression of the breast as nipple retraction but which is not evident in the noncompressed state.

Additional positioning, including ML, lateromedial oblique (LMO), or rolled CC views, may be necessary to determine the presence and location of a lesion. An ML view may rotate a lesion in tangent, demonstrating distortion or nodularity obscured by glandular tissue on the MLO view. The ML view is also advantageous to demonstrate (a) the relative medial or lateral location of a lesion based on how it moves in relationship to the MLO position, (b) the posteroinferior aspect of the breast, and (c) the medioposterior aspect of the breast (Fig. 3.8). The LMO view is useful for palpable lesions deep in the inner quadrant not seen on mammography or for lesions identified on mammography deep in the medial aspect of the breast on the CC view not seen on the MLO view.

Spot compression and magnification are used to analyze mass borders, areas of distortion, and microcalcifications. Special views, such as a magnification and spot compression, have been shown to increase the specificity of mammography in one half of patients recalled from screening (14). If a mass or focal area of distortion is found, spot compression views will displace the surrounding tissue and aid in identifying the presence of an underlying lesion. Berkowitz et al. (15) found spot compression was of help in the analysis of 75 lesions in rendering them more or less suspicious than was evident on the routine view. The spot-compression view is useful to determine if (a) a focal density is superimposed tissue or a true lesion, (b) the border of a relatively circumscribed mass identified on the routine view is actually circumscribed, and (c) a focal area of architectural distortion is being produced by a spiculated lesion (Fig. 3.9).

The rolled CC view is performed to determine the relative inferior or superior position of a lesion seen on the CC view but not demonstrated on the MLO view. If the superior aspect of the breast is rolled laterally and the lesion moves laterally from its position on the CC view, it is located in the superior aspect of the breast (Fig. 3.10). If the lesion moves in the opposite direction of the roll, it is located inferiorly.

The radiologist must choose the additional views carefully in order to correctly evaluate a potential lesion. The proper choice of views will answer two questions; (a) Is there a true lesion? and (b) Where is the lesion located? Based on these considerations, further evaluation with ultrasound (Fig. 3.11) or biopsy may be considered.

EVALUATION OF BREAST MASSES

In the evaluation of a mass lesion, an assessment of its margins (16–18), shape, density, location, orientation, presence of a fatty halo, and size is made. Masses may be divided into four groups based on their density relative to the parenchyma: (a) fat containing, (b) low density, (c) isodense, or (d) high density. Fat-containing radiolucent and mixed-density circumscribed lesions are benign (Fig. 3.12), whereas isodense to high-density masses may be of benign or malignant origin. Benign lesions tend to be isodense or of low density, with very-well-defined margins, and surrounded by a fatty halo (Fig. 3.13), but this is certainly not diagnostic of benignancy (19). The halo sign is a fine radiolucent line that surrounds circumscribed masses and is highly predictive that the mass is benign (19). The halo sign is different from the broad band of lucency described by Gordenne and Malchair (20). The broad band is a Mach band effect creating a hyperlucent zone around malignant lesions, but this hyperlucency had an average diameter of 5 to 10 mm.

A spot compression view is important to define the borders of a seemingly circumscribed mass as either completely or partially well defined. Lack of a complete halo should warrant further investigation. The likelihood of a circumscribed mass being benign is great, but various series (21–23) report significant numbers of occult carcinomas presenting as at least partially defined masses. Sickles (22) found that in a series of 300 nonpalpable cancers, only one half of the noncalcified lesions were spiculated, and the remainder were well-defined or poorly defined masses or areas of architectural distortion. Swann et al. (19) found at least a partial halo sign to be associated with 25 of 1,000 breast cancers, and in 60% of these cancers, the halo was complete.

An algorithm that describes the management of a patient with a nonpalpable circumscribed mass is shown in Figure 3.14. Ultrasound plays an integral role in the assessment of a circumscribed isodense mass (24–29). If ultrasound demonstrates a cyst to correspond to a circumscribed mammographic mass (Fig. 3.15), the lesion is benign and is followed annually. If ultrasound does not confirm a cyst, mammographic follow-up is necessary. It is important that in the follow-up of such lesions, the subsequent examinations should be tailored to allow accurate comparisons with the initial study. Noncystic masses that are completely well defined and nonpalpable are considered probably benign and are followed mammographically at 6-month intervals for 2 years (Figs. 3.16 and 3.17) (30).

Although some radiologists routinely biopsy circumscribed solid masses larger than a certain size, others do not. Sickles (31) showed no significant effect of patient age or lesion size on the likelihood of cancer for nonpalpable circumscribed breast masses. Therefore, the decision to

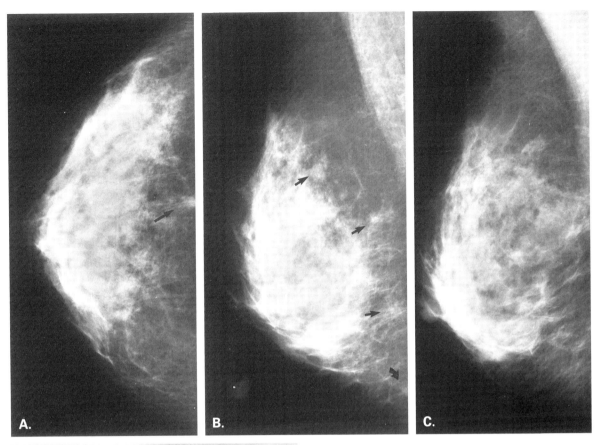

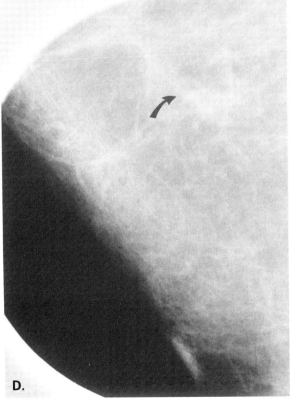

Figure 3.8

HISTORY: A 53-year-old gravida 3, para 0, abortus 3 woman with a positive family history of breast cancer for screening mammography.

MAMMOGRAPHY: Left CC **(A)**, MLO **(B)**, ML **(C)**, and enlarged spot-compression **(D)** views. The breast is dense for the age of the patient. Deep in the central aspect of the breast on the CC view **(A)** is a small, high-density irregular mass **(arrow)**. On the MLO view **(B)**, several nodular densities are seen **(arrows)**, any of which could correspond to the lesion. An ML view **(C)** was obtained but again does not clearly identify the lesion. Spot-compression views were obtained in the ML position, along the plane of the various densities. The spot ML **(D)** view of the lowermost density revealed the lesion.

IMPRESSION: Indistinct mass at the 6 o'clock position of the left breast, highly suspicious for carcinoma.

HISTOPATHOLOGY: Well-differentiated infiltrating ductal carcinoma.

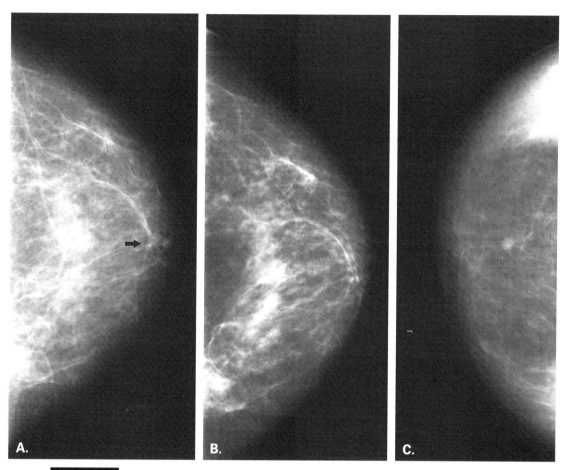

Figure 3.9

HISTORY: A 61-year-old woman for routine screening.

MAMMOGRAPHY: Left CC view **(A)** from 1989 and left CC view **(B)** from 1986. The breast is mildly glandular. In the subareolar area, there is a relatively well-circumscribed 5-mm isodense mass **(A, arrow)**. The nodule was not present on the mammogram **(B)** 3 years earlier. On spot compression, **(C)** the mass is high density and indistinct, which are features suspicious for malignancy. Ultrasound was performed but did not demonstrate the mass. A nodule of this size and in a superficial location would probably be seen on ultrasound if it were cystic; it therefore is presumed to be solid. Because of the interval change from the prior study, the mass should be considered moderately suspicious for malignancy. In this case, the lesion was excised following a needle localization procedure.

IMPRESSION: New indistinct mass, left breast, BI-RADS® 4.

HISTOPATHOLOGY: Infiltrating ductal carcinoma, comedocarcinoma.

biopsy a circumscribed nonpalpable mass should not be made based on its diameter. Palpable masses or dominant masses are usually evaluated by biopsy even if they are circumscribed. The presence of a new palpable mass implies that the mass has developed or changed, so early mammographic follow-up is not the best management plan.

A lesion that is ill-defined or spiculated and in which there is no clear history of trauma to suggest hematoma or fat necrosis suggests a malignant process (Figs. 3.18–3.21). The presence of a central high density with surrounding fine spiculation is a highly suspicious appearance. Spot compression may be of help in elucidating such an appearance within dense parenchyma. Stomper et al. (23), in the evaluation of specimen films and histology of noncalcified nonpalpable carcinomas, found that gross spiculation of >2 mm was microscopically found to represent islands of neoplastic cells surrounded by dense collagenous stroma.

(text continues on page 73)

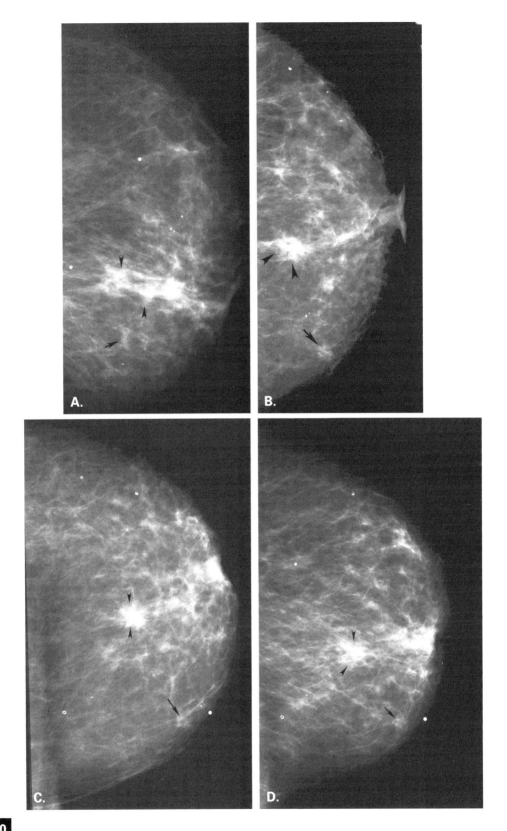

HISTORY: A 70-year-old woman with a palpable mass in the medial aspect of the right breast.

MAMMOGRAPHY: Right ML **(A)** and CC **(B)** views show a small mass medially **(arrow)** that corresponded to the palpable lesion. A second area of increased density is present centrally **(arrowheads)** and is associated with nipple retraction. On rolled CC medial **(C)** and lateral **(D)** views, the palpable mass **(arrow)** and the central indistinct mass **(arrowheads)** are confirmed. Both lesions are displaced eccentrically on the rolled view (moving medially on the lateral roll), indicating that they are located slightly inferiorly.

IMPRESSION: Findings suspicious for multiple carcinomas.

HISTOPATHOLOGY: Multicentric, invasive lobular carcinoma.

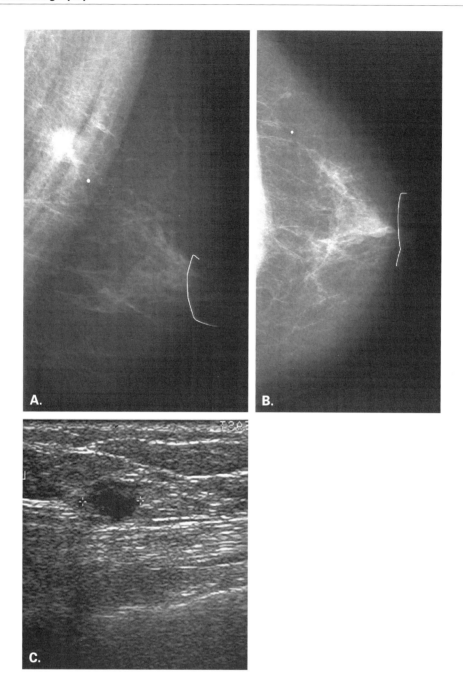

Figure 3.11

HISTORY: A 78-year-old woman who had been followed at 6-month intervals for 5 years for a right breast axillary tail density. She requests second opinion.

MAMMOGRAPHY: Right MLO **(A)** and CC **(B)** views show scattered fibroglandular densities. A BB marks a skin lesion. An indistinct mass is seen on the MLO view only, overlying the pectoralis muscle, but the lesion is not seen on the CC view. This lesion had been considered to be a lymph node at the outside facility and was followed at short intervals. No additional mammographic views had been obtained. Because the lesion is not seen on the CC view, its position on the transverse plane is only speculative. An ML view was obtained showing that the lesion appeared higher than on the MLO, suggesting a medial location. A directed ultrasound **(C)** of the right upper-inner quadrant was performed based on the suspected position of the mass. Ultrasound demonstrates that the lesion is solid and slightly irregular in contour.

IMPRESSION: Indistinct mass in the upper inner quadrant, suspicious for carcinoma.

HISTOPATHOLOGY: Medullary carcinoma.

NOTE: The error made by the initial radiologist was not obtaining additional views to locate the lesion and assuming that it was in the axillary tail. The incomplete workup led to the false assumption that the lesion could be a node. By identifying the position of the lesion with the ML view, the further workup with ultrasound is performed, identifying the mass as likely malignant.

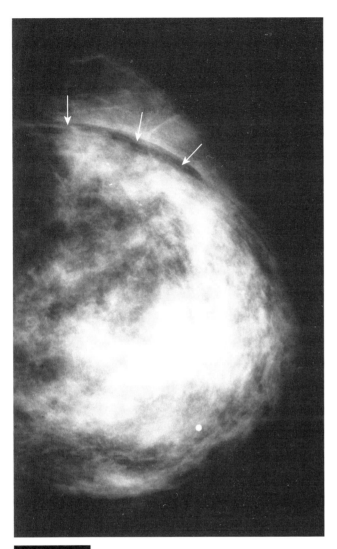

Figure 3.12

A large, heterogeneous fat-containing mass is outlined by a very-well-defined margin with a fatty halo **(arrows)**. The appearance of the lesion is typical of a hamartoma because of its mixed density and its well-circumscribed border.

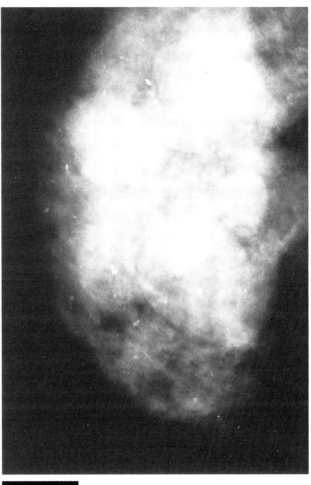

Figure 3.13

Multiple well-circumscribed round masses are outlined by fatty haloes, suggestive of a benign nature, likely cysts. Also noted are scattered benign calcifications.

Ultrasound is used increasingly for masses that are indistinct or even somewhat spiculated. With ultrasound, the level of suspicion is further defined. In addition, sonography is an excellent method for guidance of percutaneous breast biopsy, so ultrasound is performed to determine if this method for biopsy is feasible (Figs. 3.22–3.24).

The additional findings of suspicious microcalcifications also are important in defining the likelihood of malignancy. An indistinct mass that is noncalcified may represent a breast cancer, fibrocystic change, abscess, hematoma, inflamed cyst, lymphoma, or desmoid tumor.

If fine pleomorphic microcalcifications are associated with the lesion, the differential no longer includes most of the lesions, other than cancer and fibrocystic change. Also, secondary signs, such as skin thickening or retraction, nipple retraction, disruption of Cooper's ligaments, or fixation of the pectoralis muscle are all very suspicious features that may be associated with a malignant mass. Biopsy is usually necessary in the evaluation of a poorly defined or spiculated lesion identified on two views.

(text continues on page 76)

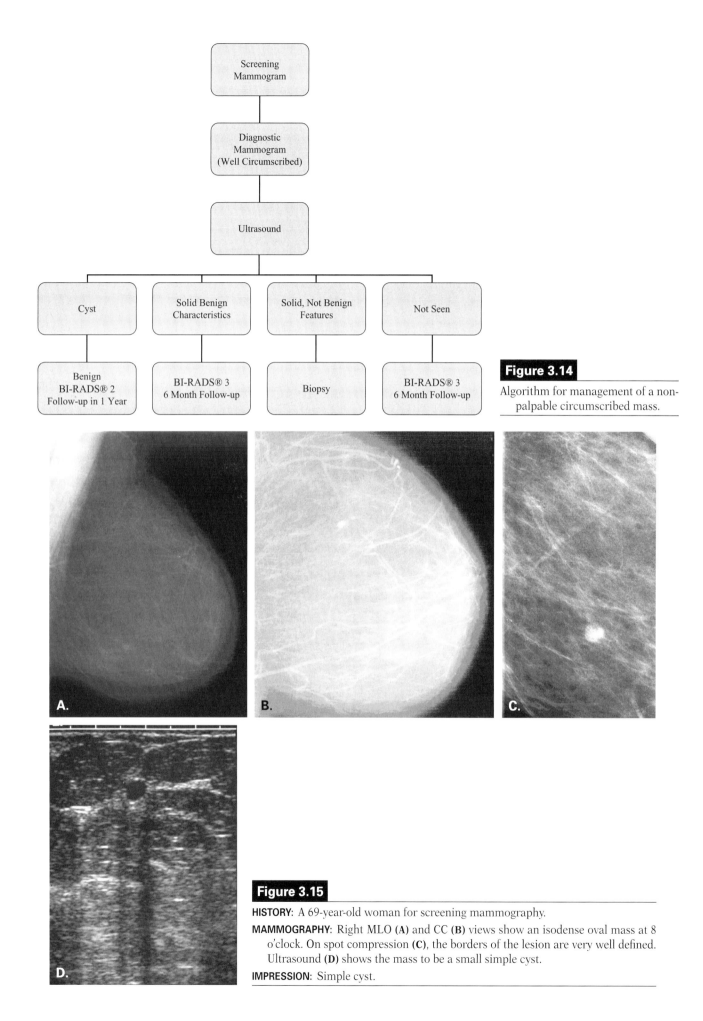

Figure 3.14

Algorithm for management of a non-palpable circumscribed mass.

Figure 3.15

HISTORY: A 69-year-old woman for screening mammography.

MAMMOGRAPHY: Right MLO **(A)** and CC **(B)** views show an isodense oval mass at 8 o'clock. On spot compression **(C)**, the borders of the lesion are very well defined. Ultrasound **(D)** shows the mass to be a small simple cyst.

IMPRESSION: Simple cyst.

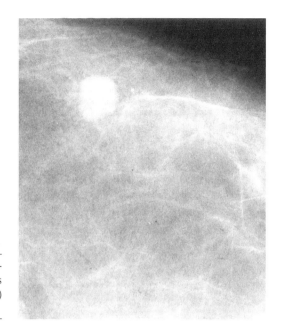

Figure 3.16

Well-defined, isodense round mass. If this mass is seen on a baseline mammogram, ultrasound is performed. If the mass is not a cyst and not suspicious on ultrasound, then it is classified as a probably benign lesion (BI-RADS® 3) and is followed at an early interval.

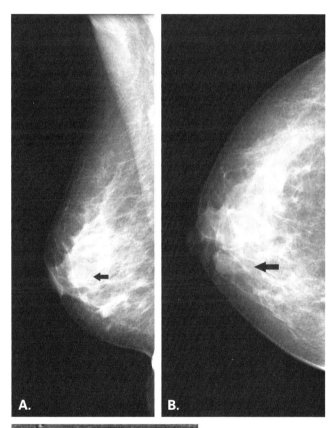

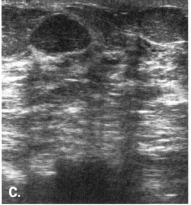

Figure 3.17

HISTORY: A 42-year-old gravida 2, para 2 woman for screening mammography.

MAMMOGRAPHY: Left MLO **(A)** and CC **(B)** views show the breast to be heterogeneously dense. There is a lobular isodense mass with circumscribed margins in the left breast at 9 o'clock. Mammographic features suggest that this is most likely benign. On ultrasound **(C)**, the very-well-defined thin margins of the solid hypoechoic mass are seen. The features are most suggestive of a fibroadenoma. Because the lesion was not palpable, and because of its benign features, 6-month follow-up was performed.

IMPRESSION: Well-defined solid mass, probably benign, BI-RADS® 3; recommend 6-month follow-up.

NOTE: This lesion meets the criteria for a probably benign mass. Its borders are very defined. It is not palpable or enlarging. The sonographic features suggest a benign etiology. Therefore, the likelihood that it is benign is at least 98%, and early mammographic follow-up is performed.

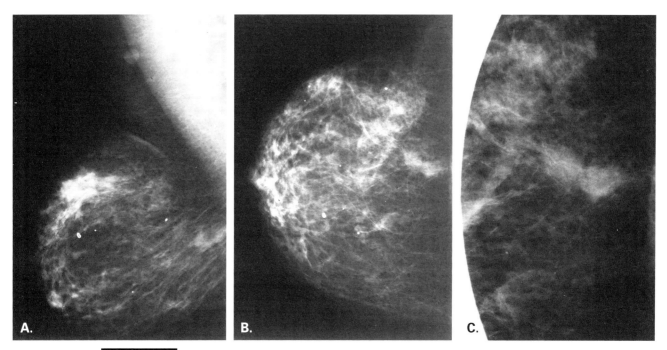

Figure 3.18

HISTORY: A 57-year-old woman for screening.

MAMMOGRAPHY: Left MLO **(A)** and CC **(B)** views show a focal asymmetry located posteriorly. On spot compression **(C)**, this is a true mass that is lobulated with indistinct margins. In this case, spot compression helps with assessment of the patient in predicting the likelihood of malignancy.

IMPRESSION: Indistinct mass, suspicious for carcinoma.

HISTOPATHOLOGY: Invasive ductal carcinoma.

EVALUATION OF ASYMMETRIC DENSITIES

In analyzing all ill-defined area of asymmetric tissue without other associated findings, one should first determine if, in fact, the asymmetry is present on two views or if it merely represents overlapping glandular tissue on one view. Global asymmetry is a large area of parenchymal density in one breast compared with the other, and this finding usually represents asymmetric breast tissue. A focal asymmetry is seen on two views and has a similar configuration, but it lacks the borders and conspicuity of a mass. Architectural distortion is focal spiculation and disruption of the orientation of the normal parenchyma without a central mass.

Focal asymmetries are often benign but occasionally may be a sign of breast cancer. Kopans et al. (32) found that asymmetric glandularity occurred in 3% of patients on mammography; carcinoma was found in only three patients with breast asymmetry without other signs of malignancy but in whom there were concurrent palpable findings. Asymmetries of concern are those that are changing or enlarging or new, those that are palpable, and those that are associated with other findings, such as microcalcifications or architectural distortion. If the patient has a scar or has had trauma to the area, the density may be fat necrosis. If a palpable thickening or mass corresponds to an asymmetric density, the density is regarded with a greater degree of suspicion for malignancy.

If the patient is premenopausal, particularly if she has other fibrocystic changes on mammography, a nonpalpable asymmetry may often be followed in 2 to 3 months, immediately after a menstrual cycle, and may diminish in size or disappear completely. In a postmenopausal patient, if there are no old films for comparison, a focal nonpalpable asymmetric density may be followed or biopsied, depending on the degree of asymmetry and other glandularity in the breast, the risk factors, and the clinical examination. A developing asymmetry in a postmenopausal woman who is not on hormones should be regarded with suspicion and biopsied. However, in the patient who has been placed on

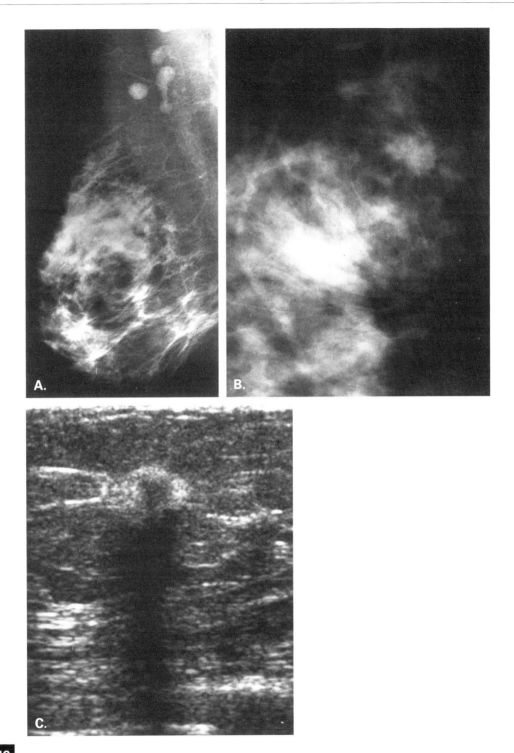

Figure 3.19

HISTORY: A 58-year-old woman for screening mammography.

MAMMOGRAPHY: Left MLO view (**A**) shows heterogeneously dense tissue. There is a small apparent mass located far posteriorly (**arrow**). On spot-compression CC (**B**), the mass is confirmed (**arrow**), and it has a lobular contour with indistinct margins. Sonography of the mass (**C**) confirms that it has suspicious characteristics. On ultrasound, the mass is hypoechoic and irregular with central shadowing, consistent with malignancy.

IMPRESSION: Small mass, suspicious for carcinoma.

HISTOPATHOLOGY: Invasive ductal carcinoma.

NOTE: The workup of this potential mass includes spot compression and ultrasound. These are performed to determine if the density is a true mass and to further characterize it.

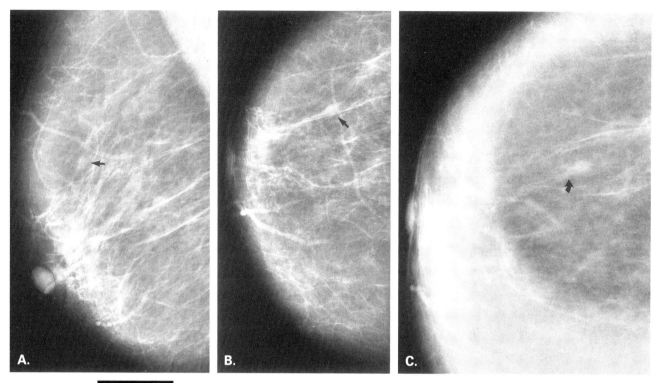

Figure 3.20

HISTORY: A 68-year-old gravida 2, para 2 woman for screening.

MAMMOGRAPHY: Left MLO **(A)**, CC **(B)**, and spot-compression magnification (1.5×) **(C)** views. The breast shows fatty replacement. In the upper outer quadrant, there is a 5-mm, relatively well-circumscribed, isodense mass **(A** and **B, arrow)**. The spot-compression view **(C)** shows the nodule to be smoothly marginated posteriorly, but to have a linear extensions anteriorly **(arrow)**. Because of this finding, the mass is of suspicion for malignancy.

HISTOPATHOLOGY: Infiltrating ductal carcinoma.

NOTE: In the evaluation of a small circumscribed mass, it is important to perform spot compression to evaluate the margins. If the margins are not completely smooth and round, the lesion should be biopsied.

hormone replacement therapy and who develops a focal asymmetry, discontinuation of the hormones and a repeat mammogram after 3 to 4 weeks may demonstrate that the area has diminished in size and is, therefore, parenchymal tissue.

Architectural distortion may be the only manifestation of breast cancer and is a sign that is easily missed. By comparing images using the search patterns described, distortion and asymmetry are more easily identified. Architectural distortion is a finding commonly seen after surgery; however, in the absence of a surgical scar to correspond to the mammographic finding, distortion should be regarded as suspicious for malignancy (Fig. 3.25).

EVALUATION OF CALCIFICATIONS

Calcifications of some type are present on a majority of mammograms, and it necessary to exclude those that are characteristically benign to avoid unnecessary biopsies. Microcalcifications rather than macrocalcifications are the form most often presenting as, or associated with, a carcinoma and represent a greater diagnostic dilemma. An analysis of the calcifications as to their distribution, size, morphology, variability, and the presence of associated findings, such as ductal dilatation or a mass, will assist one in deciding which are benign, which should be

(text continues on page 82)

Figure 3.21

HISTORY: A 67-year-old gravida 0 woman with a left breast lump. No nipple retraction was noted on clinical examination.

MAMMOGRAPHY: Left MLO **(A)** and CC **(B)** views. There is a 2.5-cm spiculated high-density mass in the left subareolar area. Retraction of the left nipple and skin retraction of the areola **(arrow)** are noted with compression of the breast during mammography. It is not unusual for a central carcinoma to produce nipple retraction during compression of the breast, even when it is not evident during clinical examination.

HISTOPATHOLOGY: Infiltrating ductal carcinoma, with macrometastases in 1 of 16 nodes.

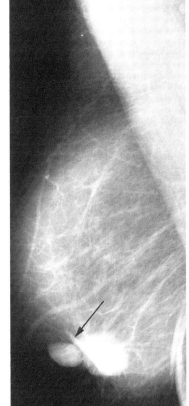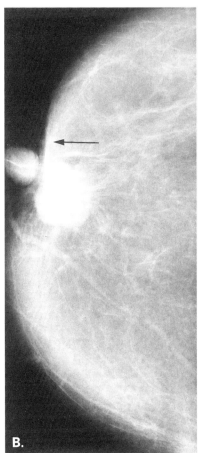

Figure 3.22

HISTORY: A 54-year-old gravida 1, para 1 woman with a palpable left breast mass.

MAMMOGRAPHY: Left MLO view **(A)** shows the palpable mass to be lobular and isodense. On the spot-compression CC **(B)** and MLO **(C)** views, the borders of the mass are indistinct, features that are highly suggestive of malignancy. Ultrasound confirmed that the lesion was solid.

IMPRESSION: Highly suspicious for carcinoma.

HISTOPATHOLOGY: Poorly differentiated carcinoma with extensive necrosis.

NOTE: The margination of a mass is the most important feature to predict its nature. Malignant masses may be round, oval, lobular, or irregular in shape, but the indistinctness of the margins suggests the infiltrative nature of the lesion.

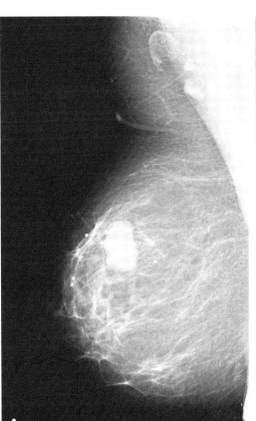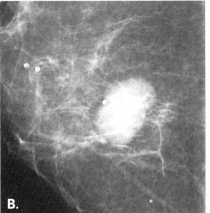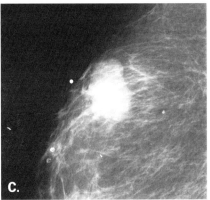

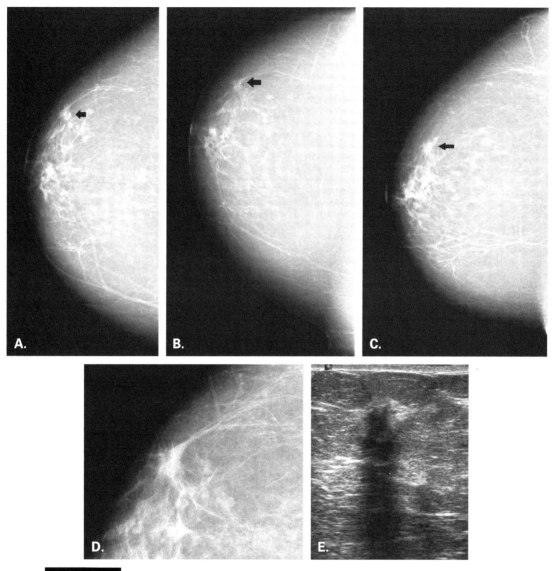

Figure 3.23

HISTORY: A 48-year-old woman for screening mammography.

MAMMOGRAPHY: Left CC view **(A)** shows a focal indistinct density located lateral to the areola **(arrow).** The mass persists on rolled CC medial **(B)** and lateral **(C)** views **(arrows).** On the rolled views, the lesion is displaced in an opposite direction from the direction of displacement, indicating that it is located inferiorly in the breast. On spot compression **(D),** the lesion appears spiculated. Ultrasound **(E)** shows the mass to be solid, irregular, and associated with surrounding edema, all of which are features highly suggestive of malignancy. The lesion was biopsied using a core needle and ultrasound guidance.

IMPRESSION: Highly suspicious mass, left breast.

HISTOPATHOLOGY: Invasive ductal carcinoma.

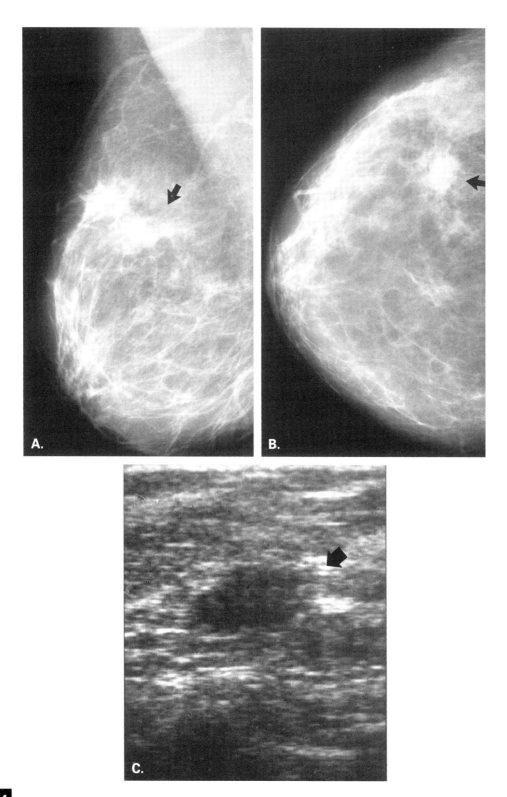

Figure 3.24

HISTORY: A 45-year-old woman after mastectomy for breast cancer on the right and treatment for colon cancer, for routine screening of the left breast.

MAMMOGRAPHY: Left MLO **(A)** and CC **(B)** views and ultrasound **(C)**. There is a high-density mass with indistinct margins in the upper outer quadrant of the left breast **(A** and **B, arrows)**. The mass has a slightly different shape on the two views but nonetheless persists as a high-density lesion. On ultrasound **(C)**, characteristically malignant features are present **(arrow)**: hypoechogenicity, ill-defined borders, and faint shadowing.

IMPRESSION: Carcinoma, left breast.

HISTOPATHOLOGY: Infiltrating ductal carcinoma with 13 negative axillary nodes.

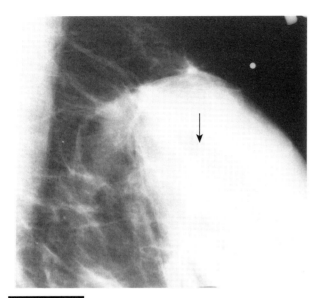

Figure 3.25

Architectural distortion **(arrow)** in a palpable area at the edge of the dense parenchyma causes a fixed, tethered, spiculated appearance of the tissue. This appearance should prompt further assessment with spot compression and ultrasound. In this case, the pathology showed invasive lobular carcinoma.

followed carefully, and which should be biopsied. In conjunction with the analysis of the pattern of calcifications, the radiologist must keep in mind the patient's history and risk factors. A woman with a synchronous contralateral breast cancer or who is otherwise at high risk may be biopsied more readily for clustered microcalcifications of indeterminate nature.

Homogeneous round, smooth microcalcifications, which may be clustered, diffuse, or in tiny florets, usually represent lobular calcifications (33) (Fig. 3.26). Often, such calcifications occur in multiple quadrants and are bilateral. Most often, these represent benign fibrocystic disease—adenosis, sclerosing adenosis, lobular hyperplasia—but they may also occur in lobular neoplasia or lobular carcinoma in situ. For these reasons, such calcifications, when focal or clustered, should be at least followed up carefully with mammography. There are a variety of opinions concerning the recommendation for follow-up about this finding. If a decision is made to follow a patient with mammography rather than to biopsy calcifications, mammograms including magnification views should be obtained at 6-month intervals for at least 2 years and annually thereafter to assess for any increase in number.

Calcifications that are associated with carcinoma tend to lie in the abnormal ducts and assume shapes that are

casts of the irregular malignant epithelial lining of the duct (33). Malignant calcifications can be identified as such when they are pleomorphic, linear, or branching, with irregular, jagged, sharp margins. When this morphology is identified on the mammogram—whether in a tight cluster or distributed in several groups, or even throughout an entire quadrant or an entire breast—biopsy is indicated (Fig. 3.27). Many malignant calcifications, however, may not have these classic features and may be more amorphous in appearance, although they do tend to have variability of size and shape.

Magnification views are particularly useful in the evaluation of the morphology of microcalcifications as well as in the more accurate determination of their distribution. The analysis of calcifications should include careful attention to all areas in each breast. There may be a variety of benign calcifications as well as malignant calcifications occurring synchronously in the same breast, and one must inspect carefully all areas to avoid overlooking an occult calcified malignancy (Fig. 3.28).

Ultrasound has a role in the evaluation of some patients with calcifications. Some calcifications are evident on ultrasound but most are not, so sonography really has no role in diagnosing or analyzing calcifications. The importance of ultrasound is to search for an underlying mass that may be indicative of an invasive cancer when malignant-appearing calcifications are identified in a dense breast (Fig. 3.29). Before biopsy, the identification of a suspicious mass on ultrasound affects the assessment of the case and the plan for the interventional procedure. The presence of a suspicious solid mass implies that an invasive cancer may be present, and the identification of an invasive component rather than pure ductal carcinoma in situ (DCIS) is critical to surgical management. When an invasive cancer is present, pathologic assessment of the axilla is necessary, whereas with pure DCIS, the axillary nodes are usually not sampled.

THE CHANGING MAMMOGRAM

Comparison with a baseline mammogram is of great help in the decision about a focal mammography abnormality. The development of a new mass, an area of asymmetric soft tissue density, an area of architectural distortion, or calcifications should alert the radiologist that there is activity in the area identified and that further evaluation is necessary. Similarly, the change in size, density, or margination of a mass or density or an increase in the number of microcalcifications focally are of concern. Comparison with multiple previous studies, not just the most recent, is important in the determination of any change in a region that is being followed.

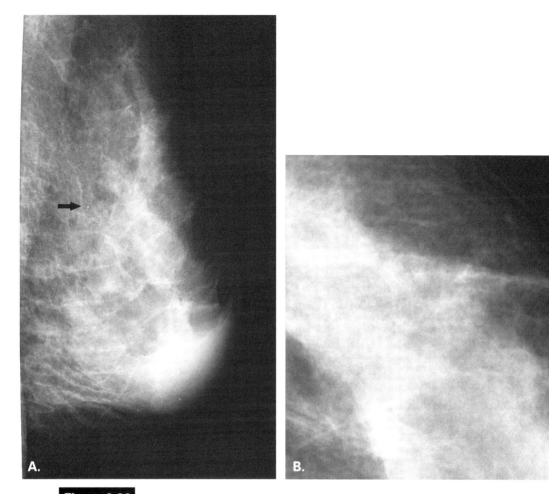

Figure 3.26

HISTORY: A 48-year-old woman recalled from screening mammography for calcifications.

MAMMOGRAPHY: Right ML **(A)** and enlarged CC **(B)** magnification views show dense parenchyma and scattered punctuate calcifications. There are clustered microcalcifications **(arrows)** at 10 o'clock that are a mixture of punctuate and amorphous forms. The morphology of these calcifications is more likely benign, but because of the amorphous type and the clustering, biopsy was performed.

IMPRESSION: Right breast clustered microcalcifications that are indeterminate; recommend biopsy, BI-RADS® 4.

HISTOPATHOLOGY: Fibrocystic changes with calcifications.

The doubling times of breast carcinomas vary greatly, from 44 to 1,869 days (34); therefore, the changes that occur at 6 months or a year may be quite variable. Kusama et al. (35) found the mean doubling time of breast tumors to be 3.5 months but to range from 0.2 to 18 months. The growth rate of breast cancer varies relative to patient age (35), with younger women exhibiting faster growth rates than older women (36). Although not common, it is not unusual to see the development of a 1-cm carcinoma in a 1-year interval, nor is it unusual to identify lack of perceptible change in a cancer over a year (Figs. 3.30 and 3.31). For these reasons, follow-up at 6-month intervals initially, followed by annual mammography after 2 years of stability, is a reasonable approach to management of a circumscribed mass. The lack of interval change of a suspicious lesion after 2 years is not a completely reliable indicator that it is benign, but it is highly suggestive of benignity. Lev-Toaff et al. (37) found that some microcalcifications associated with DCIS did not change for up to 5 years on serial mammograms.

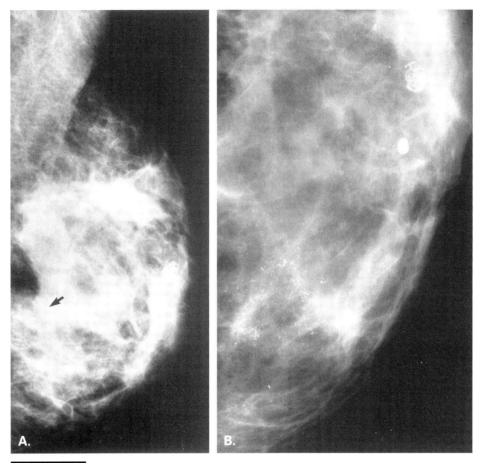

Figure 3.27

HISTORY: A 26-year-old woman with a palpable thickening in the right lower-inner quadrant.

MAMMOGRAPHY: Right MLO **(A)** and magnified (2×) **(B)** views. There are extensive irregular microcalcifications throughout the right lower-inner quadrant **(A, arrow)**. Although the distribution is extensive, the morphology of these is highly malignant. Even if the area were nonpalpable, it should be considered highly suspicious for carcinoma.

IMPRESSION: Extensive calcifications, highly suspicious for carcinoma.

HISTOPATHOLOGY: Comedocarcinoma and infiltrating ductal carcinoma.

The importance of correct use of the information that is gleaned from the prior studies cannot be overemphasized. The documentation of the presence and stability of an equivocal finding on prior studies aids one in avoiding an unnecessary workup for a benign lesion. Any increase in size of a mass requires further evaluation with ultrasound. A noncystic enlarging mass that is circumscribed, indistinct, or spiculated requires biopsy for diagnosis. Microcalcifications that are increasing in number require biopsy unless the morphology is clearly benign. The formation of more benign-appearing calcifications, however, may not necessitate tissue sampling.

When the prior studies show the area in question, routine mammographic follow-up is performed. For many lesions that are cancers, the change in growth is slow, and the management of the lesion is completely affected by this inapparent change in size. For a very suspicious lesion that does not show appreciable change in size on mammography, the lack of change should not dissuade one from performing a biopsy. The radiologist must use the principle of judging a lesion by its worst features when in doubt about its etiology. In this situation, a suspicious morphology overrides a lack of growth or change on mammography.

(text continues on page 87)

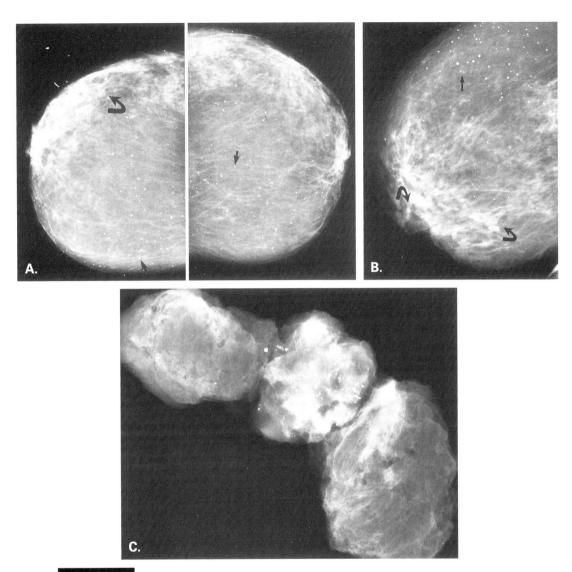

Figure 3.28

HISTORY: A 75-year-old gravida 0, para 0 woman for routine screening mammography.

MAMMOGRAPHY: Bilateral CC views **(A)**, left ML view **(B)**, and specimen film **(C)**. There are extensive benign calcifications of fat necrosis bilaterally **(A and B, arrows)**. In addition, in the left lower-outer quadrant **(A and B, curved arrows)**, there are irregular linear ductal-type microcalcifications extending from the nipple posteriorly. Because of the pleomorphic morphology and linear distribution, these calcifications have an appearance typical of comedocarcinoma. The area was removed following a needle localization procedure, and the specimen film **(C)** demonstrates many of the calcifications.

HISTOPATHOLOGY: Extensive intraductal carcinoma of comedo type, with residual carcinoma in the mastectomy specimen.

NOTE: It is important for the radiologist to evaluate all areas of calcifications independently, because there can be two or more etiologies present.

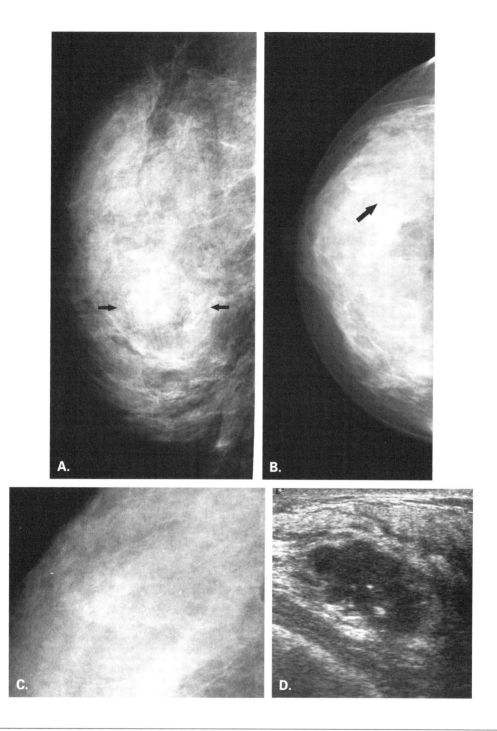

HISTORY: A 49-year-old woman for baseline mammography.

MAMMOGRAPHY: Left MLO **(A)** and CC **(B)** views show heterogeneously dense tissue. There are fine pleomorphic microcalcifications located at 4 o'clock **(arrows)**. On the magnification CC view **(C)**, the microcalcifications are highly pleomorphic and linearly arranged, features that are consistent with ductal carcinoma. Ultrasound **(D)** was performed to assess the region for an underlying mass and demonstrates a hypoechoic irregular mass that is highly suspicious for malignancy.

IMPRESSION: Pleomorphic microcalcifications and solid mass, highly suspicious for invasive ductal carcinoma.

HISTOPATHOLOGY: Invasive ductal carcinoma, DCIS.

NOTE: The use of ultrasound in the assessment of an area of calcifications that are highly suspicious for malignancy is helpful to identify a potentially invasive component. The presence of a solid mass within a region of microcalcifications suggests the possibility of invasive ductal carcinoma. Percutaneous biopsy of this mass is important in treatment planning. The preoperative diagnosis of invasive carcinoma prompts assessment of the axillary nodes pathologically, whereas the diagnosis of pure DCIS on needle biopsy does not usually lead to removal of lymph nodes at the time of lumpectomy. If invasive cancer is found at lumpectomy performed for DCIS, then a second surgical procedure is necessary to assess the axilla. The preoperative diagnosis of invasive carcinoma can reduce the need for a second surgical procedure because lumpectomy with sentinel node biopsy can be performed initially.

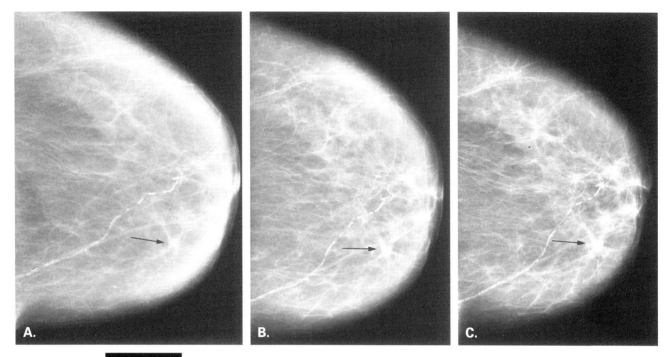

Figure 3.30

HISTORY: An 84-year-old woman after treatment of left breast cancer, for screening of the right breast.

MAMMOGRAPHY: Right CC view **(A)** from February 1987, right CC view **(B)** from December 1988, and right CC view **(C)** from November 1989. The breast shows fatty replacement. There is a small irregular density located medially **(arrow)** that was not identified on the original mammogram **(A)**. Eighteen months later **(B)** it was noted, but because it was unchanged in size and density, biopsy was not recommended. It was followed at 24 months and remained unchanged, but at 30 months **(C)**, it increased in size. The lesion was considered suspicious, and biopsy was recommended.

IMPRESSION: Irregular lesion, suspicious for carcinoma.

HISTOPATHOLOGY: Infiltrating ductal carcinoma, intraductal carcinoma.

NOTE: The lack of change in a nodule over 1 or even 2 years does not confirm a benign nature but suggests it. Carcinomas may grow slowly, and the changes mammographically may be subtle from 6-month interval to 6-month interval. It is important that comparison be made from the most current mammogram and the earliest study to be able to perceive the slight changes that occur in some malignant lesions.

EVALUATION OF A PALPABLE BREAST MASS

Mammography has a significant role to play preoperatively in the presence of a palpable breast mass. The presence of a neoplasm can be confirmed; a clearly benign lesion, such as a lipoma or an oil cyst, which does not require biopsy, can be identified; an ipsilateral multicentric cancer is demonstrated, and an occult contralateral cancer can be detected; and an occult malignancy in a breast in which a palpable mass is to be excised can be demonstrated (38).

The approach to the patient with a palpable mass begins with mammography unless the patient is very young. An algorithm showing the management of the patient with a palpable mass is shown in Figure 3.32. Often, an additional spot-compression tangential view over the lump is performed to evaluate the area of clinical concern (39). Patel et al. (40), in a study of 496 patients with breast cancer, found that mammography was abnormal in

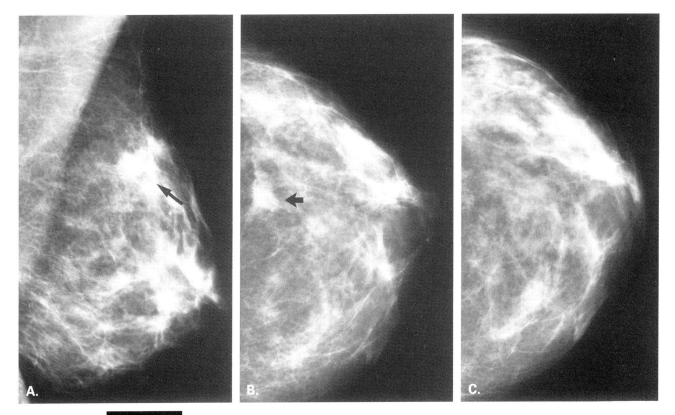

Figure 3.31

HISTORY: A 53-year-old gravida 0 woman presenting with a new 1-cm palpable mass in the right breast at the 12 o'clock position.

MAMMOGRAPHY: Right MLO (**A**) and CC (**B**) views from April 1990 and a right CC (**C**) view from March 1989. On the current study (**A** and **B**), there is a high-density irregular mass (**arrows**) in the upper aspect of the right breast, corresponding in location to the palpable mass. The mass has a highly suspicious mammographic appearance. Comparison with the previous study (**C**) shows development of the lesion over a 1-year interval.

IMPRESSION: New irregular mass, right breast, suspicious for carcinoma.

HISTOPATHOLOGY: Intraductal and infiltrating ductal carcinoma, grade II of III, with peritumoral lymphatic invasion.

NOTE: There is considerable variability in the doubling times of breast carcinomas, some of which may be followed for several years without definite change, whereas others develop over a period of months. For these reasons, it is important not only to perform mammography regularly to detect interval changes but also to compare with studies before the last one in order to detect subtle changes of slowly growing cancers.

92%. In all 14 mammograms with missed cancers, the breast tissue was very dense. The authors (40) emphasized the importance of optimal mammographic techniques and the use of nonmammographic imaging modalities when examining women with dense breasts.

At times, mammography alone may be the only imaging modality used in the patient with a palpable breast mass. However, most often, ultrasound is performed next in this clinical situation. In situations in which the palpable lump is clearly benign—a lipoma, a calcified fibroadenoma, a hamartoma, or a normal lymph node—ultrasound is not necessary and does not change the management of the lesion. If the mass is clearly malignant on mammography, such as a spiculated mass with pleomorphic microcalcifications, ultrasound is not necessary to plan the management. The patient needs a biopsy no matter what the ultrasound shows. However, a reason to perform ultrasound in this situation may be to plan biopsy guidance if ultrasound rather than stereotaxis is preferred for percutaneous breast biopsy.

Patient Over 30 Years

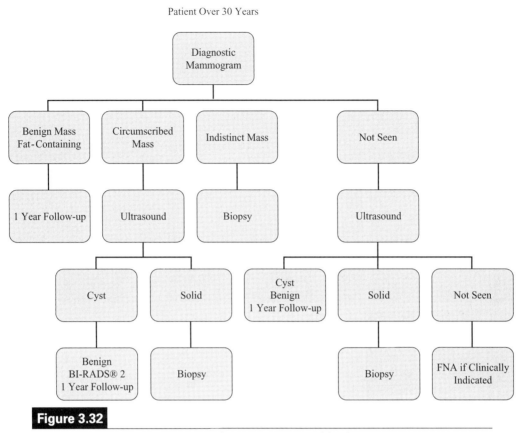

Figure 3.32

Algorithm for management of a palpable mass in a patient older than 30 years.

The importance of mammography is also to evaluate the remainder of the breasts for other clinically occult abnormalities. The mammogram may demonstrate additional clinically occult benign or malignant lesions that certainly affect the management of the palpable lesion itself. Before a needle biopsy of a palpable mass by a clinician, it is best to perform mammography, because the trauma from the biopsy procedure itself may alter the mammographic findings.

If the mammogram demonstrates a round non–fat-containing mass, an indistinct mass, asymmetry, or suspicious microcalcifications in the area of palpable concern, ultrasound is extremely important for further evaluation (Figs. 3.33 and 3.34). It is important that when scanning the patient with a clinical finding that the radiologist palpate the lesion and correlate the clinical finding with the mammographic finding. Sonography is used in the setting of a palpable mass to determine of the lesion is solid, cystic, or not seen. A simple cyst, even a palpable cyst, is benign based on sonography and is followed. A solid mass that is palpable is biopsied.

When mammography is negative and a palpable mass is present, ultrasound is the necessary next step. If ultra-sound demonstrates a solid mass in the patient with a new palpable lesion, needle biopsy is performed (Figs. 3.35 and 3.36). Similarly, if ultrasound is negative and there is a clinically evident palpable lesion that is seen on mammography a needle biopsy is performed. When both mammography and ultrasound are negative, the management of the patient is based on the clinical findings. In a study of 420 patients with 455 palpable breast lesions that were negative on mammography and sonography, Soo et al. (41) found the negative predictive value of the combined mammographic and sonographic modalities was 99.8%. In another study of 600 palpable breast masses and negative mammography and sonography, Dennis et al. (42) found no cancers to occur or develop within 2 years in the women who were not biopsied. Sixty lumps were biopsied because they were clinically suspicious for cancer or occurred in high-anxiety, high-risk patients. Of these 60 palpable lumps, none were found to be malignant on tissue sampling. In a series of 233 women with negative imaging and a palpable lump, Moy et al. (43) found that 2.6% of patients had breast cancer in

(text continues on page 93)

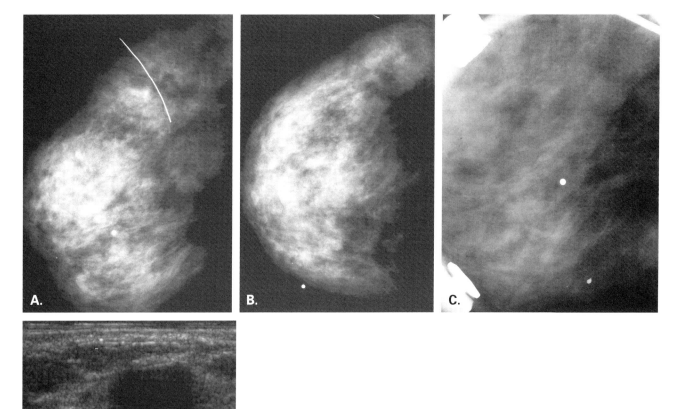

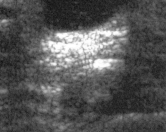

Figure 3.33

HISTORY: A 40-year-old woman with a palpable mass in the left breast at 9 o'clock.

MAMMOGRAPHY: Left MLO (**A**) and CC (**B**) view shows heterogeneously dense tissue. A BB marks the palpable abnormality; however, no abnormality is seen on these routine views nor on the spot compression view (**C**). Ultrasound of the palpable lesion (**D**) shows it to be round and nearly anechoic. However, there are low-level echoes and slightly indistinct margins associated with the mass.

IMPRESSION: Palpable mass, likely complicated cyst; recommend aspiration/biopsy.

HISTOPATHOLOGY: Cyst fluid with proteinaceous debris and histiocytes.

NOTE: The management of the palpable mass includes mammography and ultrasound, particularly when mammography is negative.

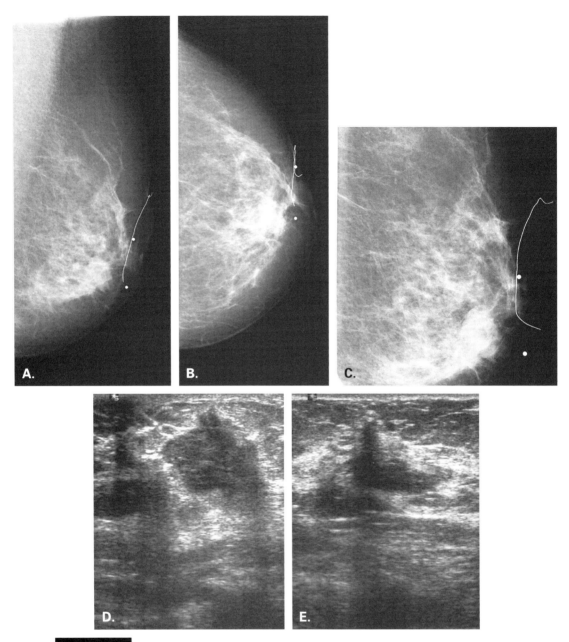

Figure 3.34

HISTORY: A 70-year-old woman with two palpable masses in the right periareolar area. She had a history of prior benign biopsy in the right breast years ago.

MAMMOGRAPHY: Right MLO (**A**) and CC (**B**) views show a wire marking the prior surgical site and two BBs marking the palpable masses. The mass at 5 o'clock is mammographically evident as a lobulated lesion, but the mass located more superiorly is not visible on mammography. A right MLO spot-magnification view (**C**) shows the edges of the palpable mass to be somewhat indistinct and therefore suspicious for malignancy. Ultrasound of the 5 o'clock mass (**D**) shows a hypoechoic, microlobulated mass with angulated margins and some shadowing. Ultrasound of the mammographically occult mass (**E**) located superiorly at 10 o'clock shows a smaller, densely shadowing lesion.

IMPRESSION: Highly suspicious for multicentric carcinoma.

HISTOPATHOLOGY: Five o'clock mass, infiltrating ductal carcinoma; superior mass, fibrosis.

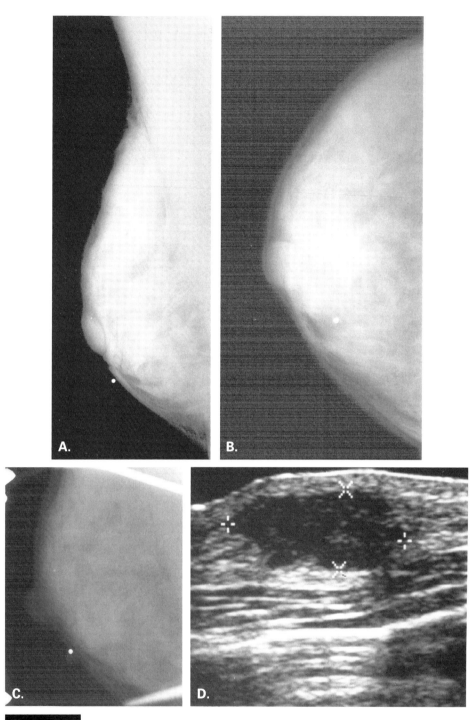

Figure 3.35

HISTORY: A 36-year-old woman with a palpable left breast mass.

MAMMOGRAPHY: Left MLO (**A**) and CC (**B**) views show very dense parenchyma. On spot compression (**C**) over the palpable lump, slight increased density is seen. Sonography of the lump (**D**) shows a hypoechoic mass that is wider than tall and that is associated with slight acoustic enhancement. However, the edges are indistinct, and the echotexture is inhomogeneous, findings that are suspicious for malignancy.

IMPRESSION: Palpable mass, suspicious for carcinoma.

HISTOPATHOLOGY: Mucinous carcinoma.

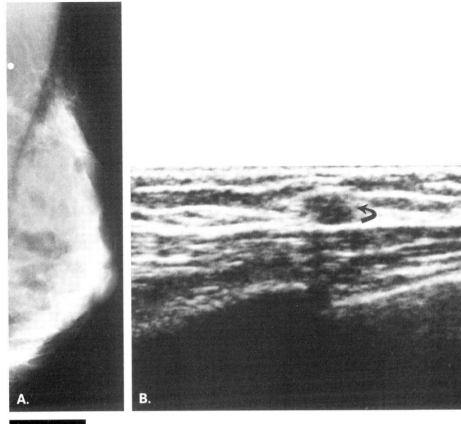

Figure 3.36

HISTORY: A 36-year-old woman with a questionable, small, palpable nodule high in the right upper-inner quadrant.

MAMMOGRAPHY: Right MLO view **(A)** and ultrasound **(B)**. There is a metallic marker overlying the palpable lump **(A)**. No abnormality is seen on the mammogram. The palpable lesion is probably lying posterior to the edge of the film. Lesions high in the upper inner quadrant are difficult to image with the routine MLO and CC views. Ultrasound is of help demonstrating the location and characteristic of a palpable lesion not seen on mammography. On the sonogram **(B)**, the mass, which lies just anterior to the pectoralis major muscle, is hypoechoic, somewhat irregular, and therefore suspicious in nature **(arrow)**. The area was localized under ultrasound guidance before excisional biopsy.

IMPRESSION: Solid mass, suspicious for carcinoma.

HISTOPATHOLOGY: Infiltrating ductal carcinoma.

the palpable area. In all six patients with cancer, the breast tissue was radiographically dense. If the palpable area is clinically of concern, even with negative imaging, fine-needle aspiration biopsy (FNAB) or needle biopsy are performed.

The triple test has been described (44–49) in the management of the patient who presents with a palpable breast lump. The likelihood that a palpable lesion is benign or malignant is predicted by the triple test, and depending on the test outcome, it may be used in lieu of open biopsy for some masses. The triple test consists of mammography, clinical examination, and FNAB. The

addition of ultrasound since the triple test was originally described increases the strength of the combined test reliability. The concept of the triple test is that if all three tests indicate that the palpable mass is benign, the likelihood of malignancy approaches 0%. However, if any of the tests are positive or suspicious for malignancy, further evaluation with open biopsy is necessary.

The accuracy of FNAB is very much related to the technique for biopsy performance, quality of the aspirate, and skill of the pathologist in cytologic diagnosis. The technique includes the vigorous movement of a small-gauge needle throughout the abnormality, shearing cells from the area of concern. Some cancers may be desmoplastic, so the use of a small-gauge needle (25 g) is helpful to mobilize cells.

The sensitivity of FNAB is in the range of 75% to 95% (50–55). The overall accuracy of FNAB for breast masses ranges from 85% to 90% (56–58). Depending on how the atypical smears are categorized (positive or negative) in the data analysis, reported sensitivity and specificity are affected. False negatives can occur, particularly with small lesions, low-grade tumors, fibrous tumors, or invasive lobular carcinomas (46). Therefore, a negative cytology alone is not sufficient to exclude cancer in the face of a palpable suspicious mass. A comprehensive approach to the patient with a palpable mass includes imaging, clinical findings, and cytology or biopsy if necessary.

IMAGING THE SYMPTOMATIC YOUNG PATIENT

The approach to a young (<30 years) patient who is symptomatic, presenting with a palpable mass, is different from that for older patients. Because of the relatively low likelihood of malignancy, mammography is usually not performed first. Ultrasound is performed initially in women younger than 30 years (Fig. 3.37). Typically after age 30, mammography is performed first. If the palpable mass is a cyst, no further imaging evaluation is necessary in the normal-risk patient. If ultrasound demonstrates a solid mass that corresponds to the palpable lump, further management is typically performed. When sonography shows a smoothly marginated, oval, solid lesion, the likelihood is very high that the mass is a fibroadenoma (Fig. 3.38). FNAB or tissue sampling is usually performed to confirm this. Before an intervention, limited mammography can be performed in women older than age 20 to assess the lesion and the remainder of the breast (Fig. 3.39).

If sonography shows the mass to be solid and suspicious because of irregularity of margins and a more rounded, irregular, or microlobulated shape, bilateral diagnostic mammography should be performed before biopsy. The purpose of mammography in this situation is to assess the extent of disease when a palpable cancer is present. Mammography may depict the suspicious lesion identified clinically and on ultrasound, but more impor-

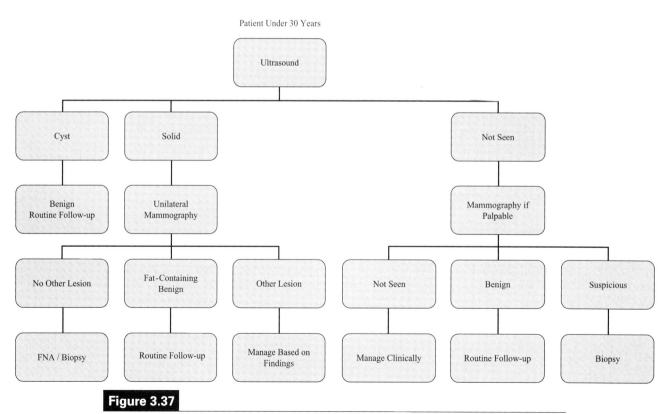

Figure 3.37

Algorithm for management of a palpable mass in a woman younger than 30 years of age.

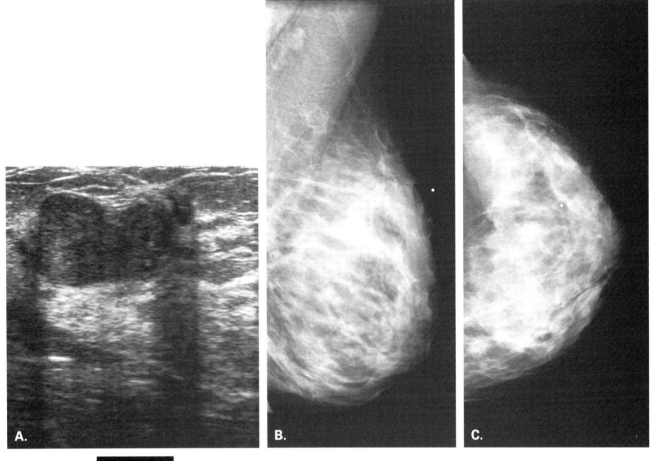

Figure 3.38

HISTORY: A 26-year-old gravida 0, para 0 woman with a new palpable mass in the right breast.

MAMMOGRAPHY: Ultrasound **(A)** was performed first because of the patient's age and demonstrates that the palpable mass is solid, lobular, and hypoechoic with well-defined margins, suggesting that it is most likely a fibroadenoma. Mammography was performed to evaluate this area and to exclude any other lesions before biopsy. Right MLO **(B)** and CC **(C)** views show no focal abnormality.

IMPRESSION: Palpable mass is solid, likely fibroadenoma; recommend biopsy.

HISTOPATHOLOGY: Fibroadenoma.

tantly, mammography may demonstrate other clinically occult foci of malignancy.

Lesions that occur in young patients include fibroadenomas most commonly, with cysts, lymph nodes, and cancer less likely. In patients who are pregnant or lactating, particular lesions related to these states include lactating adenomas (59) and galactoceles. In young and in pregnant patients with breast cancer, the prognosis is similar to that of older patients with similar size and stage of disease (60). However, because of the lower frequency of breast cancer in younger women, the diagnosis may be delayed by not imaging and evaluating the patient (61,62). Because a patient is young and not at high risk because of family history, one should not assume that a palpable mass is not cancer. Although the breast tissue tends to be dense in young women, a majority of breast cancers in this age group are visible on mammography (63).

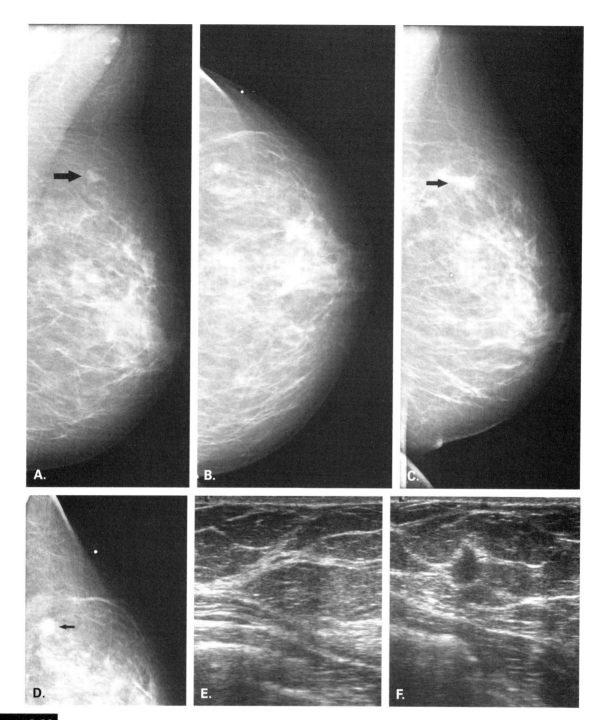

Figure 3.39

HISTORY: A 31-year-old gravida 0, para 0 woman with a palpable thickening in the 9 o'clock position of the right breast.

MAMMOGRAPHY: Right MLO view **(A)** shows a small mass located superiorly in the axillary tail **(arrow)** but no abnormality in the region of palpable concern at 9 o'clock. On the CC view **(B)**, the mass is not clearly seen, but it is evident on the ML view **(C, arrow)**. The lower location of the mass on the ML view compared with the MLO view is consistent with the lesion being in a lateral location. A spot exaggerated CC lateral **(D)** shows the small, high-density indistinct mass **(arrow)**. The BB marking the palpable region, which was located more inferiorly, is also evident. Ultrasound of the palpable region at 9 o'clock **(E)** shows no abnormality. However, ultrasound of the axillary tail **(F)** demonstrates a small solid mass that is a taller-than-wide lesion with angulated margins.

IMPRESSION: Palpable region is not demonstrated on imaging; recommend management based on clinical findings. Solid, clinically occult lesion in the axillary tail is highly suspicious for carcinoma.

HISTOPATHOLOGY: Invasive ductal carcinoma axillary tail, negative sentinel lymph node.

NOTE: The assessment of the patient with a palpable mass requires attention to the area of palpable concern as well as the remainder of the breasts. Our protocol for imaging young women who present with a palpable mass is as follows: ultrasound only for those younger than age 20; ultrasound first, then mammography if needed between ages 20 and 30; mammography first, then ultrasound after age 30.

IMAGING EXTENT OF DISEASE

When an obvious mammographic finding is identified, a satisfaction of search phenomenon can occur and can cause a cancer to be missed. The radiologist's attention is drawn by the obvious finding, and a careful review of the remainder of the images does not occur. It is imperative that when a suspicious abnormality is identified, a complete review of the images be performed to search for other cancers (Fig. 3.40). Ipsilateral multiple cancers and contralateral synchronous cancers are identified frequently, and their diagnosis greatly affects patient management (64–68).

Multiple breast cancers may occur in the same quadrant, which is termed *multifocal disease* (Fig. 3.41), or they may occur in different quadrants, which is *multicentric disease* (Fig. 3.42). The clinical significance of multicentric disease is that this entity is a contraindication to breast conservation therapy, and typically a mastectomy is necessary (Fig. 3.43). Multifocality has been described to occur in 45% of cases of DCIS, and multicentricity has been found in 8% to 23% of cases (69,70). Multiple invasive cancers occur as well in the same and contralateral breasts (Figs. 3.44 and 3.45); in particular, patients with invasive lobular carcinoma are at highest risk of having synchronous contralateral disease (67,68). The incidence of synchronous

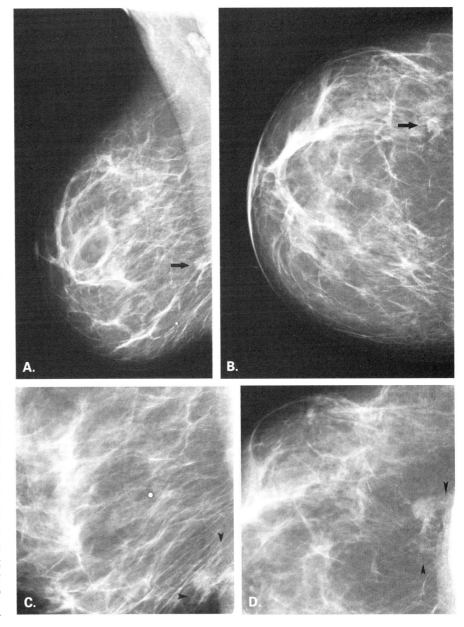

Figure 3.40

HISTORY: A 38-year-old gravida 3, para 3 patient for baseline screening.

MAMMOGRAPHY: Left MLO **(A)** and CC **(B)** views show a small indistinct mass located posteriorly at 5 o'clock **(arrows)**. On the spot-compression magnification ML **(C)** and CC **(D)** views, the mass is dense and indistinct in margination. Within it and extending around it are fine pleomorphic microcalcifications **(arrowheads)** that are highly suspicious for DCIS.

IMPRESSION: Highly suspicious for malignancy, possible extensive intraductal component.

HISTOPATHOLOGY: Infiltrating ductal carcinoma, grade II; DCIS, solid and cribriform types.

NOTE: The identification of a suspicious mass as well as calcifications requires communication regarding the extent of disease for surgical planning. Pleomorphic calcifications extending beyond the mass suggest the possibility of an extensive intraductal component. Depending on the size of the area, percutaneous biopsy of the various components may be necessary. If lumpectomy is performed or attempted, bracketing the perimeters of the abnormality with several wires is helpful to achieve complete excision.

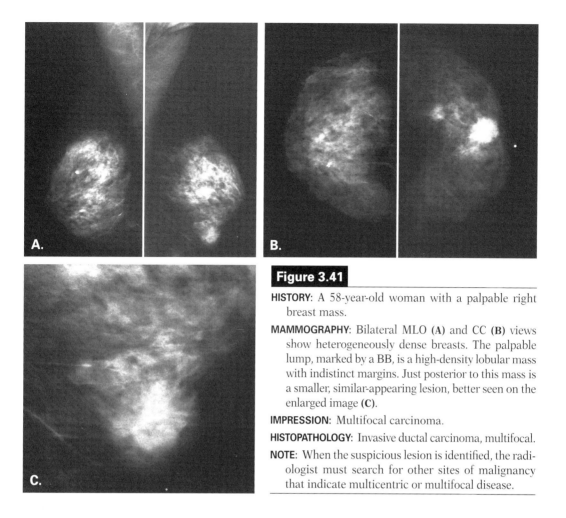

Figure 3.41

HISTORY: A 58-year-old woman with a palpable right breast mass.

MAMMOGRAPHY: Bilateral MLO (**A**) and CC (**B**) views show heterogeneously dense breasts. The palpable lump, marked by a BB, is a high-density lobular mass with indistinct margins. Just posterior to this mass is a smaller, similar-appearing lesion, better seen on the enlarged image (**C**).

IMPRESSION: Multifocal carcinoma.

HISTOPATHOLOGY: Invasive ductal carcinoma, multifocal.

NOTE: When the suspicious lesion is identified, the radiologist must search for other sites of malignancy that indicate multicentric or multifocal disease.

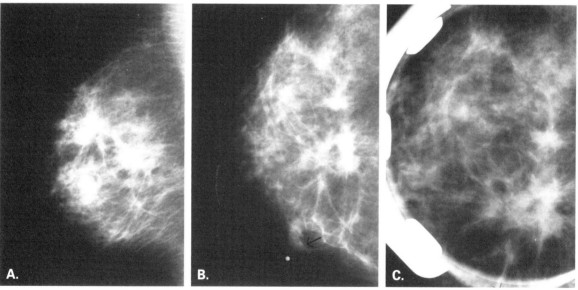

Figure 3.42

HISTORY: A 62-year-old woman who presents with a small palpable lump at the site of a bruise. This is her first mammogram.

MAMMOGRAPHY: Left MLO (**A**) and CC (**B**) views show a lobular isodense mass located superficially at 9 o'clock (**arrow**) and marked by the BB at the site of the palpable lump. In addition, there are multiple, high-density irregular masses with spiculated margins throughout the breast. Spot-compression CC (**C**) shows the highly spiculated appearance of several of these lesions.

IMPRESSION: Highly suspicious for multicentric carcinoma.

HISTOPATHOLOGY: Invasive ductal carcinoma, multiple foci, including the site of the palpable mass.

bilateral breast cancer has been reported in as many as 2% to 9% of patients (66). Modalities other than mammography, particularly MRI, have proven to be helpful in assessing the extent of disease in a patient with what appears to be a unifocal breast cancer (71–76). Regardless, a careful mammographic search pattern when one lesion is identified must be implemented to identify other cancers.

Careful attention to subtle areas of asymmetry, nodules, and the presence of architectural distortion or microcalcifications is necessary in order to detect breast cancers at an early stage. Correlation with the history and physical findings is of help in determining recommendations about equivocal mammographic findings. The use of ultrasound and interventional techniques—such as aspiration, percutaneous breast biopsy, and galactography—as an adjunct to mammography allows the radiologist to make a more accurate diagnosis and plan for patient management.

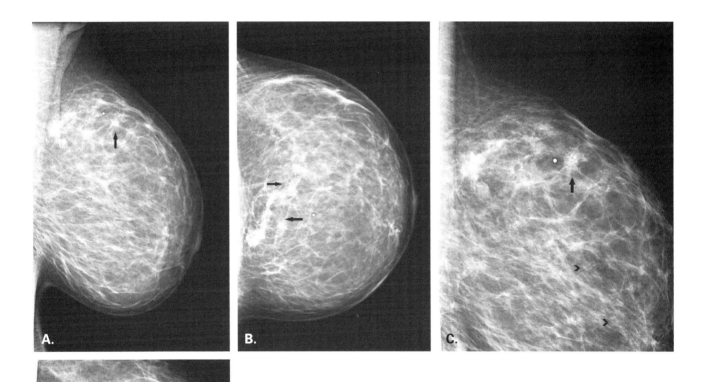

Figure 3.43

HISTORY: A 36-year-old woman for a baseline mammogram. She presents with palpable thickening in the right breast at 12 o'clock.

MAMMOGRAPHY: Right MLO **(A)** and CC **(B)** views show a dense indistinct mass posteriorly that corresponds to the palpable lesion. Anterior to this are multiple groups of pleomorphic fine linear microcalcifications **(arrows)**. On the magnification ML **(C)** and CC **(D)** views, these highly malignant microcalcifications are visible **(arrow)**. In addition, there are two other foci of linear and pleomorphic microcalcifications **(arrowheads)** located anteriorly, remote from the index lesion. These separate foci are very important in treatment planning. Because of their distance from the index lesion, mastectomy is likely necessary.

IMPRESSION: Multicentric ductal carcinoma.

HISTOPATHOLOGY: Ductal carcinoma, high grade, multiple foci with invasive ductal carcinoma.

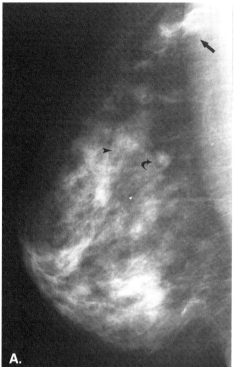

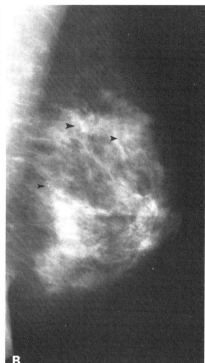

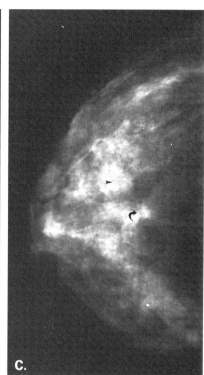

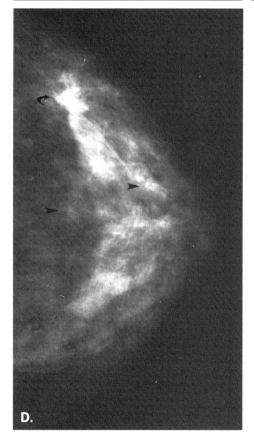

Figure 3.44

HISTORY: A 67-year-old woman who presents with an abnormal screening mammogram.

MAMMOGRAPHY: Left MLO **(A)** and right MLO **(B)** views show heterogeneously dense tissue. Multiple abnormalities are present. Focal asymmetry is present in the left axillary tail **(arrow)**, and a small, dense spiculated mass is noted in the superior posterior region **(curved arrow)** of the left breast. Clustered microcalcifications are present in both breasts **(arrowhead)**. On the left CC view **(C)**, the spiculated mass is noted to contain pleomorphic microcalcifications **(curved arrow)**. On the right CC view **(D)**, the clustered microcalcifications **(arrowheads)** are suspicious. In addition, there is a spiculated area of distortion laterally **(curved arrow)** in the right breast **(D)**.

IMPRESSION: Highly suspicious for multicentric bilateral carcinoma.

HISTOPATHOLOGY: Invasive lobular carcinoma, both breasts, and multiple foci of DCIS (calcifications).

NOTE: When one abnormality that is suspicious for carcinoma is identified, the radiologist must search for other foci that could represent multicentric carcinoma in the same breast as well as the contralateral breast. The correct preoperative assessment of the extent of the disease is critical to achieving the best surgical management for the patient.

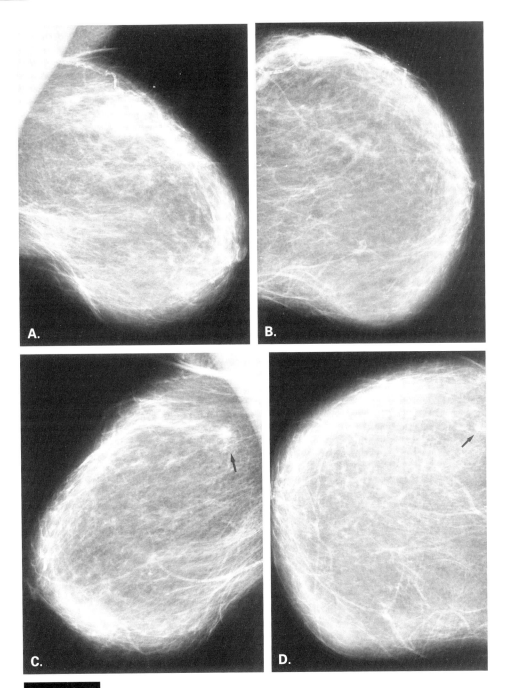

Figure 3.45

HISTORY: A 58-year-old gravida 5, para 5 woman with a firm tender mass in the right breast.

MAMMOGRAPHY: Right MLO **(A)** and CC **(B)** views and left MLO **(C)** and CC **(D)** views. There is a high-density spiculated mass with associated microcalcification in the right upper-outer quadrant **(A** and **B)**. This lesion has an appearance highly suggestive of carcinoma. In the left upper-outer quadrant, there is an 8-mm indistinct mass **(arrows)** that is isodense **(C** and **D)**. Although the mass appears less indistinct and dense on the CC view **(D)**, it nonetheless persists and is therefore of moderate suspicion for a contralateral carcinoma.

IMPRESSION: Carcinoma of the right breast, moderately suspicious mass left breast.

HISTOPATHOLOGY: Right breast: infiltrating lobular carcinoma. Left breast: widespread intraductal carcinoma, lobular carcinoma in situ.

REFERENCES

1. *ACR Breast Imaging and Reporting Data Systems, Breast Imaging Atlas.* 2003. Reston, VA: American College of Radiology.

2. 21 CFR Part 16 and 900: Mammography quality standards: final rule. Federal Register. 1997 Oct 28:62(208): 55851–55994.

3. Sickles EA. Periodic mammographic follow-up of probably benign lesions: results in 3,184 consecutive cases. *Radiology* 1991;179:463–468.

4. Vizcaíno I, Gadea L, Andreo L, et al. Short-term follow-up results in 795 nonpalpable probably benign lesions detected at screening mammography. *Radiology* 2001;219: 475–483.

5. Rosen EL, Baker JA, Soo MS. Malignant lesions initially subjected to short-term mammographic follow-up. *Radiology* 2002;223:221–228.

6. Leung JWT, Sickles EA. Multiple bilateral masses detected on screening mammography: assessment of need for recall imaging. *AJR Am J Roentgenol* 2000;175:23–29.

7. Bird RWE, Wallace TW, Yankaskas BC. Analysis of cancers missed at screening mammography. *Radiology* 1992;184: 613–617.

8. Goergen SK, Evans JE, Cohen GPB, et al. Characteristics of breast carcinomas missed by screening radiologists. *Radiology* 1997;204:131–135.

9. Roubidoux MA, Helvie MA, Lai NE, et al. Bilateral breast cancer: early detection with mammography. *Radiology* 1995; 196:427–431.

10. Krupinski EA. Visual scanning patterns of radiologists searching mammograms. *Acad Radiol* 1996;3:137–144.

11. Barrett JR, de Paredes ES, Dwyer SJ, et al. Unobtrusively tracking mammographers' eye gaze direction and pupil direction. *Acad Radiol* 1994;1:40–45.

12. Sickles EA. Practical solutions to common mammographic problems: tailoring the examination. *AJR Am J Roentgenol* 1988;151:31–39.

13. Egan RL. Fundamentals of mammographic diagnoses of benign and malignant diseases. *Oncology* 1969:23:126–148.

14. Hayes R, Michell M, Nunnerley HB. Evaluation of magnification and paddle compression techniques in the assessment of mammographic screening detected abnormalities. *Clin Radiol* 1991;44:158–160.

15. Berkowitz JE, Gatewood OMB, Gayler BW. Equivocal mammographic findings: evaluation with spot compression. *Radiology* 1989;171:369–371.

16. Gold RH, Montgomery CK, Rambo ON. Significance of margination of benign and malignant infiltrative mammary lesions: roentgenographic pathological correlation. *AJR Am J Roentgenol* 1973;118:881–895.

17. Sickles EA. Evaluation of breast masses. Radiology 1989; 173:297–303.

18. Feig SA. Breast masses: mammographic and sonographic evaluation. *Radiol Clin North Am* 1992;30(1):67–92.

19. Swann CA, Kopans DB, Koerner FC, et al. The halo sign of malignant breast lesions. *AJR Am J Roentgenol* 1987;149: 1145–1147.

20. Gordenne WH, Malchair FL. Mach bands in mammography. *Radiology* 1988;169:55–58.

21. Marsteller LP, Shaw de Paredes E. Well defined masses in the breast. *RadioGraphics* 1989;9(1):13–17.

22. Sickles EA. Mammographic features of 300 consecutive nonpalpable breast cancers. *AJR Am J Roentgenol* 1986;146: 661–663.

23. Stomper PC, Davis SP, Weidner N, et al. Clinically occult, noncalcified breast cancer: serial radiologic-pathologic correlation in 27 cases. *Radiology* 1988;160:621–626.

24. Rubin E, Miller VE, Berland LL, et al. Hand-held real-time breast sonography. *AJR Am J Roentgenol* 1985;144: 623–627.

25. Jackson VP. The role of US in breast imaging. *Radiology* 1990;177:305–311.

26. Hilton SvW, Leopold GR, Olson LK, et al. Real-time breast sonography: application in 300 consecutive patients. *AJR Am J Roentgenol* 1986;145:479–486.

27. Sickles EA, Filly RA, Callen PW. Benign breast lesions: ultrasound detection and diagnosis. *Radiology* 1984;151:467–470.

28. Harper AP, Kelly-Fry E, Noe JA, et al. Ultrasound in the evaluation of solid breast masses. *Radiology* 1983;146:731–736.

29. Fornage BD, Lorigan JG, Andry E. Fibroadenoma of the breast: sonographic appearance. *Radiology* 1989;172:671–675.

30. Adler DD, Helvie MA, Ikeda DM. Nonpalpable, probably benign breast lesions: follow-up strategies after initial detection on mammography. *AJR Am J Roentgenol* 1990;155:1195–1201.

31. Sickles EA. Nonpalpable, circumscribed, noncalcified solid breast masses: likelihood of malignancy based on lesion size and age of patient. *Radiology* 1994;192(2):439–442.

32. Kopans DB, Swann CA, White G, et al. Asymmetric breast tissue. *Radiology* 1989;171:639–643.

33. Tabar L, Dean PB. *Teaching atlas of mammography.* Stuttgart: Georg Thieme Verlag, 1983.

34. Fournier DV, Weber E, Hoeffken W, et al. Growth rate of 147 mammary carcinomas. *Cancer* 1980;45:2198–2207.

35. Kusama S, Spratt JS, Donegan WL, et al. The gross rates of growth of human mammary carcinoma. *Cancer* 1972;30(2): 594–599.

36. Moskowitz M. Breast cancer: age-specific growth rates and screening strategies. *Radiology* 1986;161:37–41.

37. Lev-Toaff AS, Feig SA, Saitas VL, et al. Stability of malignant breast microcalcifications. *Radiology* 1994;192:153–156.

38. Kopans DB, Meyer JE, Cohen AM, et al. Palpable breast masses: the importance of preoperative mammography. *JAMA* 1981;246:2819–2822.

39. Faulk RM, Sickles EA. Efficacy of spot compression-magnification and tangential views in mammographic evaluation of palpable breast masses. *Radiology* 1992;185:87–90.

40. Patel MR, Whitman GJ. Negative mammograms in symptomatic patients with breast cancer. *Acad Radiol* 1998;5(1): 26–33.

41. Soo MS, Rosen EL, Baker JA, et al. Negative predictive value of sonography with mammography in patients with palpable breast lesions. *AJR Am J Roentgenol* 2001;177:1167–1170.

42. Dennis MA, Parker SH, Klaus AJ, et al. Breast biopsy avoidance: the value of normal mammograms and normal sonograms in the setting of a palpable lump. *Radiology* 2001;219: 186–191.

43. Moy L, Slanetz PJ, Moore R, et al. Specificity of mammography and US in the evaluation of a palpable abnormality: retrospective review. *Radiology* 2002;225:176–181.

44. Hermansen C, Poulsen HS, Jensen J, et al. Diagnostic reliability of combined physical examination, mammography, and fine-needle puncture ("Triple-Test") in breast tumors. *Cancer* 1987;60:1866–1871.

45. Butler A, Vargas HI, Worthen N, et al. Accuracy of combined clinical-mammographic-cytologic diagnosis dominant breast masses. *Arch Surg* 1990;125:893–896.

46. Adye B, Jolly PC, Bauermeister DE. The role of fine-needle aspiration in the management of solid breast masses. *Arch Surg* 1988;123:37–39.

47. Abele B, Miller TR, Goodson WH, et al. Breast fine-needle aspiration of palpable breast masses. *Arch Surg* 1983;118:859–863.

48. Frable WJ. Cancer trends: aspiration biopsy of the breast. *Virginia Medical Med* 1982;109:452–455.

49. Kaufman Z, Shpitz B, Shapiro M, et al. Triple approach in the diagnosis of dominant breast masses: combined physical examination, mammography, and fine-needle aspiration. *J Surg Oncol* 1994;56:254–257.

50. Stavric GD, Tevcev DT, Kaftandjiev DR, et al. Aspiration biopsy cytologic method in diagnosis of breast lesions: a critical review of 250 cases. *Acta Cytol* 1973;17:188–190.

51. Franzen S, Zajicek J. Aspiration biopsy in diagnosis of palpable lesions of the breast: critical review of 3,479 consecutive biopsies. *Acta Radiol* 1968;17:241–262.

52. Bjurstam N, Hedberg K, Hultborn KA, et al. Diagnosis of breast carcinoma: evaluation of clinical examination, mam-

mography, thermography, and aspiration biopsy in breast disease. *Prog Surg* 1974;13:1–65.

53. Smith C, Butler J, Cobb C, et al. Fine-needle aspiration cytology in the diagnosis of primary breast cancer. *Surgery* 1988;103:178–183.

54. Boerner S, Sneige N. Specimen adequacy and false-negative diagnosis rate in fine-needle aspirates of palpable breast masses. *Cancer* 1998;84(6):344–348.

55. Wanebo HJ, Feldman S, Wilhelm MC, et al. Fine needle aspiration cytology in lieu of open biopsy in management of primary breast cancer. *Ann Surg* 1984;199:569–578.

56. Norton LW, Davis JR, Wiens JL, et al. Accuracy of aspiration cytology in detecting breast cancer. *Surgery* 1984;96:806–814.

57. Sheikh FA, Tinkoff GH, Kline TS, et al. Final diagnosis by fine-needle aspiration biopsy for definitive operation in breast cancer. *Am Surg* 1987;154:470–474.

58. Kline TS, Neal HS. Needle aspiration biopsy: a critical appraisal. *JAMA* 1978;239:36–39.

59. James K, Bridger J, Anthony PP. Breast tumour of pregnancy ("lactating" adenoma). *J Pathol* 1988;156:37–44.

60. Petrek JA, Dukoff R, Rogatko A. Prognosis of pregnancy-associated breast cancer. *Cancer* 1991;67:869–872.

61. Hoover HC. Breast cancer during pregnancy and lactation. *Surg Clin North Am* 1990;70(5):1151–1163.

62. Donegan WL. Breast cancer and pregnancy. *Obstet Gynecol* 1977;50(2):244–252.

63. Shaw de Paredes E, Marsteller LP, Eden BV. Breast cancers in women 35 years of age and younger: mammographic findings. *Radiology* 1990;177:117–119.

64. Kinne DW. Management of the contralateral breast. In: Harris JR, Hellman S, Henderson IC, et al, eds. *Breast diseases.* Philadelphia: JB Lippincott, 1987:620–621.

65. Kesseler HJ, Grier WRN, Seidman I, et al. Bilateral primary breast cancer. *JAMA* 1976;236(3):278–280.

66. Hungness ES, Safa M, Shaughnessy EA, et al. Bilateral synchronous breast cancer: mode of detection and comparison of histologic features between the two breasts. *Surgery* 2000;128:702–707.

67. Broet P, de la Rochefordiere A, Scholl SM, et al. Contralateral breast cancer: annual incidence and risk parameters. *J Clin Oncol* 1995;13:1578–1583.

68. Healey EA, Cook EF, Orav EJ, et al. Contralateral breast cancer: clinical characteristics and impact on prognosis. *J Clin Oncol* 1993;11:1545–1552.

69. Coombs JH, Hubbard E, Hudson K, et al. Ductal carcinoma in situ of the breast: correlation of pathologic and mammographic features with extent of disease. *Am Surg* 1997; 63:1079–1083.

70. Lagios MD, Westdahl PR, Margolin FR, et al. Ductal carcinoma in situ: relationship of extent of noninvasive disease to the frequency of occult invasion, multicentricity, lymph node metastases, and short-term treatment failure. *Cancer* 1982;50:1309–1314.

71. Berg WA. Imaging the local extent of disease. *Semin Breast Dis* 2001;4:153–173.

72. Berg WA, Gutierrez L, NessAirer MS et al. Diagnostic accuracy of mammography, clinical examination, ultrasound, and MR imaging in preoperative assessment of breast cancer. *Radiology* 2004;233:830–849.

73. Liberman L, Morris EA, Dershaw DD, et al. MR imaging of the ipsilateral breast in women with percutaneously proven breast cancer. *AJR Am J Roentgenol* 2003;180:901–910.

74. Orel SG, Schnall MD, Powell CM, et al. Staging of suspected breast cancer: effect of MR imaging and MR-guided biopsy. *Radiology* 1995;196:115–122.

75. Boetes C, Mus RD, Holland R, et al. Breast tumors: comparative accuracy of MRI imaging relative to mammography and US for demonstrating extent. *Radiology* 1995;197(3): 743–747.

76. Smith M, Allison K, Shaw de Paredes E. Nonmammographic evaluation of the extent of breast carcinoma. *Semin Ultrasound CT MR* 2006;27:308–319.

Chapter 4

Circumscribed Masses

Masses with circumscribed margins are a common finding on mammography. Well-defined lesions are more commonly benign, but it imperative that the radiologist evaluating a mass differentiate those that are characteristically benign from the indeterminate or suspicious lesions. Careful mammographic assessment includes comparison with prior mammography and the use of spot compression to assess the details of the margin of a seemingly circumscribed mass. Sonography (1) plays a key role in the differentiation of solid from cystic masses and greatly facilitates the recommendations for follow-up or further evaluation of the patient.

ASSESSMENT OF CIRCUMSCRIBED MASSES

An approach to the evaluation of a well-defined mass on mammography includes an assessment of the shape, density, margins, size, orientation, presence of a fatty halo, and presence of other findings (i.e., calcifications). Benign lesions tend to be isodense or less dense than the parenchyma and to have very circumscribed margins, whereas malignant masses are more often of greater density and have fine irregularity or micronodularity on their borders.

The shapes of masses that are circumscribed may be round, oval, or lobular. The margination that is described as "circumscribed" allows one to visualize a fine, clear edge around the entire mass. Often masses that are circumscribed may be overlapped by parenchyma in some areas. These are described as obscured or partially circumscribed. A microlobulated margin appears as fine nodularity or undulation of the edge of the lesion and implies a more malignant nature.

A basic division of well-circumscribed masses based on their density is of help in determining possible etiologies of and approach to such lesions. In Table 4.1 the differential diagnosis of circumscribed masses based on their density is shown. Masses that are fatty—lipomas, oil cysts, and galactoceles—and circumscribed masses that are mixed density are characteristically benign. Isodense circumscribed masses include benign and malignant lesions, and an evaluation of the borders is critical to help differentiate these etiologies. Masses that are of high density, particularly for their size, are of concern for malignancies. However, in a study of radiologists' interpretations of mass density, Jackson et al. (2) found that the assessment of mammographic density of masses was quite variable among different readers; in addition, the density assessment was of limited value in the prediction of benign versus malignant for noncalcified breast masses.

The mammographic feature of greatest importance in assessing a relatively circumscribed isodense mass is its margination. Any notching, waviness, or indistinctness of the margins of a mass should be regarded with suspicion (3). The presence of a halo sign, i.e., a fine radiolucent ring surrounding a well-defined mass, has long been considered to be a mammographic sign of benignancy (4). The halo may be due to compression of fat by the mass (5) or to Mach effect (6). Swann et al. (7) have, however, described 25 malignant lesions from approximately 1,000 breast cancers in which a halo sign was present. The presence of a halo suggests but does not guarantee a benign process (7). Certainly, the presence of a partially circumscribed margin and a partially indistinct margin is suspicious, and biopsy is indicated in this situation.

Stability in size from prior mammography is an important factor that suggests that a circumscribed noncystic mass is benign. The growth rates of breast cancers are quite variable. In two series, the mean doubling times for mammary carcinoma have been found to be 212 (8) and 325 (9) days, respectively. The lack of interval change suggests that a well-defined lesion is more likely benign, but this is not confirmatory. Meyer and Kopans (10) reported five cases of occult cancers that did not change in size on follow-up mammography over a minimum of 2 years and a maximum of 4.5 years from the original study. Therefore, if a nodule is followed and there is no interval change in the size at 6 months or 1 year, continued follow-up is necessary. In addition, the other features of density and margination are used to decide whether to follow or biopsy a circumscribed mass.

▌**TABLE 4.1 Differential Diagnosis of Circumscribed Masses**

Density	Type of Lesion	Characteristics
Fat-containing masses	Hamartoma	Encapsulated, large, mixed density
	Lipoma	Encapsulated, radiolucent
	Intramammary node	Mixed density, small, lateral location, subcutaneous
	Fat necrosis (oil cyst)	Radiolucent with eggshell calcification
	Galactocele	Fat density or mixed density, lactating patient
Isodense	Cyst	Round, any size, oriented toward the nipple
	Fibroadenoma	Lobulated, any size, coarse calcification
	Tubular adenoma	Lobular, noncalcified
	Fibrocystic change	Partially circumscribed
	Adenosis tumor	May have microcalcification
	Focal fibrosis	Partially circumscribed
	Papilloma	Small, may calcify, periareolar
	Hematoma	Slightly indistinct, skin thickening
	Hemangioma	Subcutaneous, small
	Metastases	Round, subcutaneous
	Inclusion cyst	Round, subcutaneous, may calcify
	Pseudoangiomatous stromal hyperplasia	Relatively circumscribed, noncalcified
	Lactating adenoma	Pregnant, lactating, lobulated mass
	Skin lesion (neurofibroma, nevus, keratosis)	Crenulated surface, extremely well defined (air halo)
	Nipple out of profile	Different appearance on orthogonal view
High density	Carcinoma	Microlobulated or slightly indistinct, microcalcifications
	Cystosarcoma phylloides	Very large lobulated, may have coarse calcification
	Abscess	Medium to high density, skin thickening
	Hematoma	Slightly indistinct, skin thickening

CIRCUMSCRIBED MASSES OF FAT DENSITY

Lipoma

Lipomas are benign, well-circumscribed radiolucent masses (Figs. 4.1–4.5). Clinically, lipomas are either nonpalpable or, if palpable, soft and freely mobile. Lipomas are visualized more easily in an otherwise dense, glandular breast because of the difference in density. In a fatty breast, this radiolucent mass is perceived because it is surrounded by a thin capsule and, if large, displaces the normal breast around it (11). Often lipomas may be located posteriorly at the chest wall and project forward into the breast. Only the anterior aspect of the capsule may be visible on mammography in these cases. Lipomas may develop coarse calcification, probably secondary to infarction (Fig. 4.6). On ultrasound, lipomas are usually intensely hyperechoic, oval, and well defined.

Fat Necrosis

Posttraumatic oil cysts, a form of fat necrosis, may occur as early as 6 months after breast trauma or surgery. Oil cysts may be evident in a pattern corresponding to the path of the seat belt shoulder restraint in patients who have been in automobile accidents (12). Clinically, an area of fat necrosis may be asymptomatic, or it may be an indurated mass with thickening or retraction of the overlying skin. Histologically, the fat necrosis is characterized by anuclear fat cells, histiocytic giant cells, and foamy phagocytic histiocytes. The necrotic focus may cavitate, forming an oil cyst (13), and the wall of the oil cyst may calcify in an eggshell pattern. This ringlike calcification (Figs. 4.7–4.10) in the wall of an oil cyst, as originally described by Leborgne (14), is characteristic of this form of fat necrosis. Extensive oil cysts in the subcutaneous area of the breast and the soft tissues elsewhere are seen in the condition known as steatocystoma multiplex (15) (Fig. 4.11).

Galactoceles

Galactoceles may be radiolucent masses or they may be of mixed density or isodense, depending on their contents. Galactoceles are benign breast masses that contain inspissated milk; they are commonly found during or after lactation (11). Mammographically, they are small, round often multiple, radiolucent or mixed-density lesions, and they often occur in the retroareolar

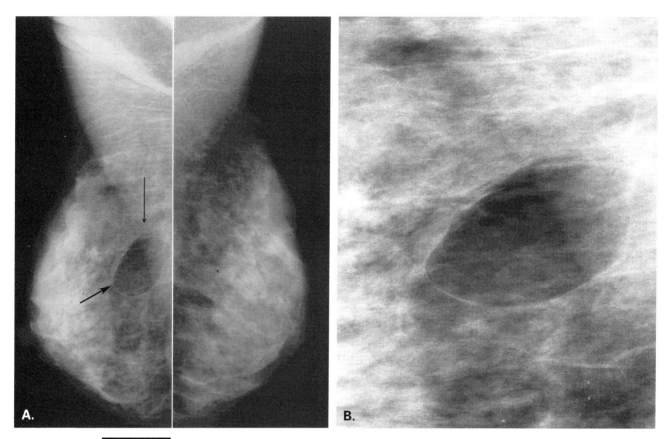

Figure 4.1

HISTORY: A 52-year-old woman with a positive family history of breast cancer for screening mammography.

MAMMOGRAPHY: Bilateral MLO (**A**) and coned left MLO (**B**) views show an oval circumscribed radiolucent mass (**arrows**) in the left breast posteriorly. A thin capsule surrounds the mass, which is characteristic of a lipoma.

IMPRESSION: Lipoma.

area (11). The retention of lactiferous material accounts for the low density of these lesions (16) (Fig. 4.12). A fat-water level within a well-defined mass on a mediolateral view is pathognomonic of a galactocele (17) (Fig. 4.13).

MIXED-DENSITY CIRCUMSCRIBED MASSES

Fibroadenolipoma

A hamartoma or fibroadenolipoma is a benign tumor composed of normal mammary tissue (adipose, fibrous, and glandular), including ducts and lobules of varying amounts. The lesion is relatively uncommon, with a frequency of 16 in 10,000 mammograms in a series by

Hessler et al. (18). In this series, the patients ranged in age from 27 to 88 years and presented with a breast mass of a consistency similar to that of the adjacent tissue (18).

On mammography (Figs. 4.14–4.22), the appearance of a fibroadenolipoma is usually pathognomonic (18–21). Depending on the amount of fat versus parenchymal tissue, the lesion may vary from a relatively radiolucent mass to a relatively radiodense mass. The borders are very well defined, and a thin pseudocapsule may be evident. There is a loss of normal architecture of the mammary tissue with lack of orientation of glandular elements toward the nipple. The hamartoma displaces away the normal parenchyma of the breast, which appears to be draped over the lesion. Helvie et al. (22), however, found the mammographic findings of hamartomas to range from the mixed-density circumscribed mass to the isodense,

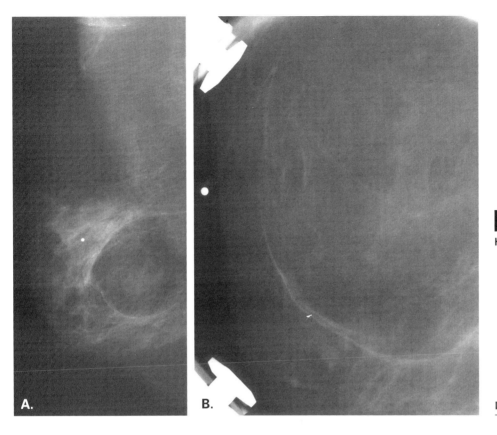

A.

B.

Figure 4.2

HISTORY: A 53-year-old woman with a palpable mobile left breast mass. Mammography: Left MLO (**A**) view shows a large radiolucent round mass extending from the chest wall forward and draping the normal parenchyma over its margin. On spot magnification (**B**), the thin capsule of the mass is evident.

IMPRESSION: Lipoma, BI-RADS® 2.

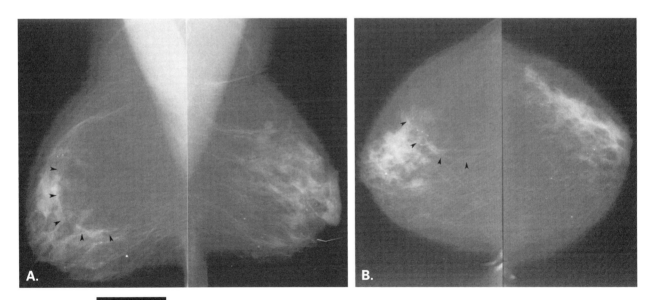

A.

B.

Figure 4.3

HISTORY: A 61-year-old woman for screening mammography.

MAMMOGRAPHY: Bilateral MLO (**A**) and CC (**B**) views show an asymmetric appearance of the breasts. The left breast appears larger and more fatty than the right breast. On close inspection, there is draping of the glandular tissue on the left around a large radiolucent mass (**arrows**).

IMPRESSION: Lipoma.

NOTE: Large benign lesions such as lipomas are often evident because of the displacement and draping of the normal parenchyma around their margin.

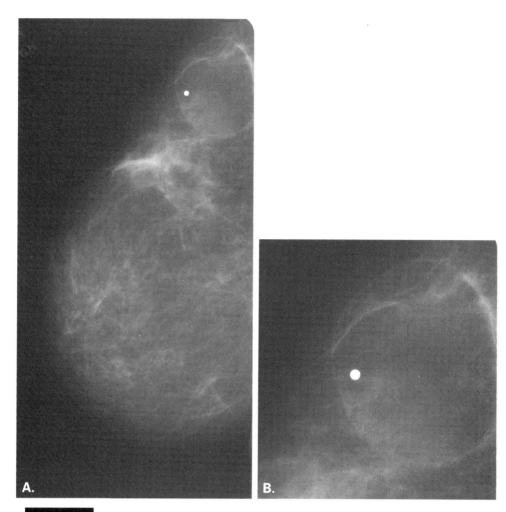

Figure 4.4

HISTORY: A 37-year-old woman with a palpable mass in the upper aspect of the right breast. She had no history of trauma.

MAMMOGRAPHY: Right MLO **(A)** and enlarged MLO **(B)** views. There is a round, circumscribed radiolucent mass in upper aspect of the right breast, marked with a BB. Because of the completely radiolucent characteristics, this mass is a lipoma or a large oil cyst. Without a history of trauma, lipoma is the most likely diagnosis.

IMPRESSION: Lipoma.

more irregular lesions that were biopsied because of the concern of possible malignancy.

On sonography, the lesion is well defined and composed of lobulated sonolucent areas mixed with irregular echogenic planes (23). If large and cosmetically a problem, or if not clearly of mixed density mammographically, the lesion is treated with complete excision and enucleation. No association with malignancy has been described.

Intramammary Nodes

Intramammary lymph nodes have an appearance similar to that of axillary nodes; namely, they are well defined, mixed density or medium to low density, round, ovoid, or reniform nodules with a fatty notch or center (Figs. 4.23–4.27). Intramammary nodes can be found throughout the breast (24) but most commonly are located in the middle- to upper-outer aspect of the breasts and are

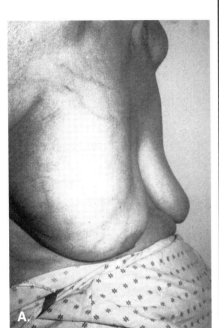
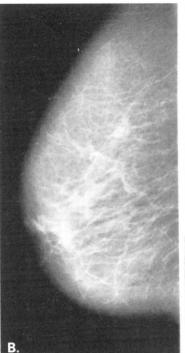
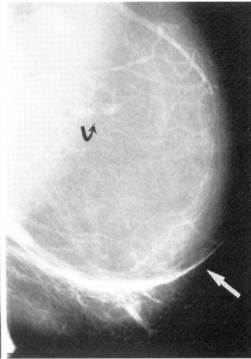

Figure 4.5

HISTORY: A 79-year-old gravida 3, para 3 woman with a history of the right breast being larger than the left for years **(A)**.

MAMMOGRAPHY: Bilateral mediolateral views **(B)**. There is marked asymmetry in the size of the breasts. There is a large radiolucent mass surrounded by a thin capsule **(straight arrow)** in the right upper-outer quadrant. The mass compresses and drapes the normal parenchyma around it. These findings are characteristic of a lipoma. The ovoid nodules present in the superior aspect of the breast **(curved arrow)** are lymph nodes superimposed over the large lipoma.

IMPRESSION: Lipoma.

often multiple and bilateral. Intramammary nodes are located in the superficial soft tissue in the vast majority of cases.

Most intramammary nodes are less than 1 cm in diameter. Nodes may increase in diameter and be benign, although if the mass does not have a fatty hilum, biopsy may be necessary to confirm its etiology. In a study of 158 whole-breast specimens with primary operable carcinoma, Egan and McSweeney (25) found intramammary lymph nodes in 28% and metastatic deposits in intramammary nodes in 10%. Although nodes involved with metastatic disease may enlarge and become more rounded and dense (24), this is not necessarily the case, and nodes of less than 1 cm in diameter can be malignant (25).

On ultrasound, lymph nodes also have a characteristic appearance. They are very well defined and oval or lobular with mixed echogenicity. The cortex is hypoechoic, and the fatty hilum is hyperechoic. Abnormal nodes may lose this appearance and be more rounded and poorly marginated.

Other benign conditions also may be associated with the presence of intramammary nodes as well as axillary adenopathy. These include rheumatoid arthritis (26), sarcoidosis (27), psoriatic arthritis, and systemic lupus erythematosus (24). Enlarged dense nodes may be present in these conditions as well as in lymphoma. Often, in the case of adenopathy, the fatty hilum is lost and the node is isodense or even of high density.

Skin Lesions

It is critical that the technologist indicate any skin lesions on the patient's breasts. Moles, keratoses (Figs. 4.28–4.30), retracted nipples (Figs. 4.31 and 4.32), scars

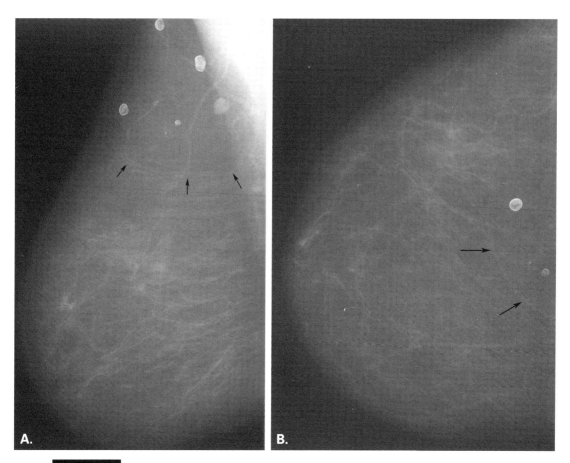

Figure 4.6

HISTORY: A 51-year-old woman with fullness in the left breast superiorly.

MAMMOGRAPHY: Left MLO **(A)** and CC **(B)** views show a fatty replaced breast. There is a large radiolucent mass with circumscribed margins **(arrows)** projecting forward from the chest wall. The mass is associated with eggshell and lucent centered calcifications of fat necrosis.

IMPRESSION: Lipoma with fat necrosis.

NOTE: Lipomas may be associated with small areas of fat necrosis and dystrophic or eggshell calcifications. The observation of a lipoma in a fatty breast is difficult, and the primary finding is the thin capsule.

(Fig. 4.33), and neurofibromas (Fig. 4.34) may appear as very-well-defined masses of mixed or medium density on at least one of the projections. As the lesion is compressed against the breast, air is trapped around it, creating an especially lucent halo. If the surface is irregular, a crenulated appearance is noted, creating a mixed density on mammography. By turning the breast with the lesion in tangent, the well-defined mass disappears or projects at the skin surface. Artifacts on the patient's skin, including electrocardiogram pads and various patches for transdermal medications, may trap air underneath, producing a "mixed-density mass" appearance on mammography (Fig. 4.35).

Isodense to High-Density Masses

There is considerable overlap between the lesions that are of medium density or isodense with the background parenchyma and the lesions that are of high density (2). Cysts and fibroadenomas tend to be of isodense, and the background stromal markings may be visualized through the masses. Carcinomas tend to be of higher density, but these divisions are not absolute, and several benign lesions—including fibroadenomas, hematomas, and abscesses—may be of high density, depending on their

(text continues on page 117)

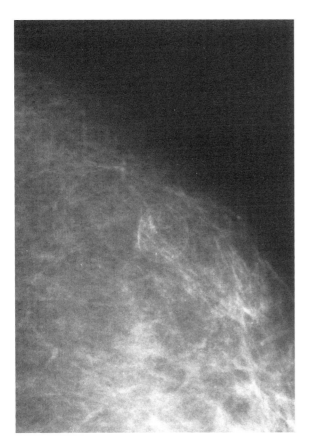

Figure 4.7

HISTORY: Patient recalled for magnification view of the right breast.

MAMMOGRAPHY: Right CC magnification view demonstrates a round, thin-walled lucent mass in the superficial area. Within this mass are a few faint punctuate microcalcifications. The findings are typical of fat necrosis, with formation of an oil cyst and early calcification in its wall.

IMPRESSION: Oil cyst.

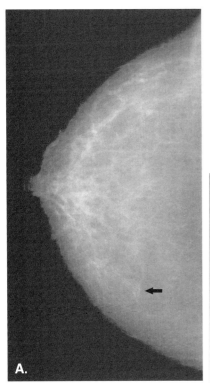

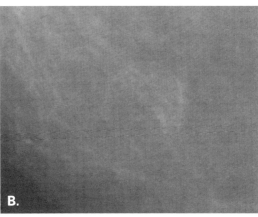

Figure 4.8

HISTORY: A 74-year-old woman for screening mammography.

MAMMOGRAPHY: Left CC (A) view shows a round, circumscribed, fat-containing mass located medially (arrow). On the enlarged image (B), the very-well-demarcated margin of the radiolucent mass is seen. The findings are typical of an oil cyst.

IMPRESSION: Oil cyst.

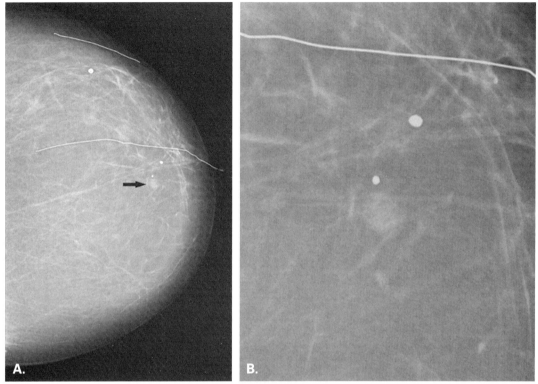

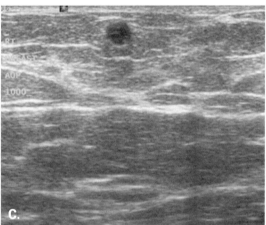

Figure 4.9

HISTORY: A 63-year-old woman who has a small palpable mass in the right breast at 12 o'clock. She had a car accident with bruising of the right breast 1 year ago.

MAMMOGRAPHY: Right CC **(A)** view shows a small round mass **(arrow)** in the subareolar region, corresponding to the palpable lesion. On the enlarged image **(B)**, the circumscribed mass of very low density is seen. The nearly radiolucent lesion implies a fat containing mass. Ultrasound **(C)** shows a complex cystic mass. A fluid level is seen in the cyst, and it is located in the subcutaneous area, all of which are features of fat necrosis.

IMPRESSION: Fat necrosis, oil cyst.

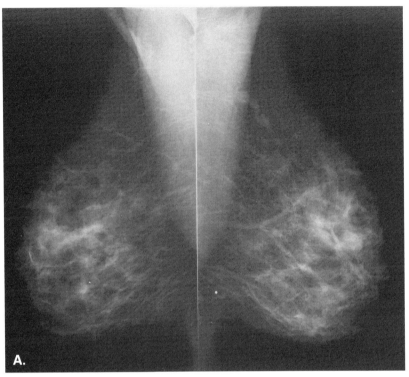

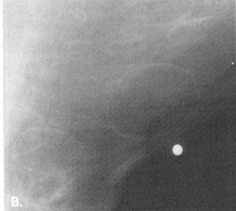

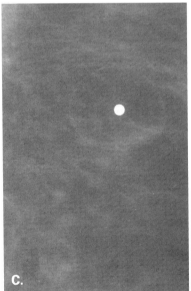

Figure 4.10

HISTORY: A 50-year-old woman with a palpable mass in the inferior aspect of the right breast.

MAMMOGRAPHY: Bilateral MLO **(A)** views show heterogeneously dense breasts. There is a small round mass marked by a BB in the right breast at 6 o'clock in the area of palpable concern. On spot-magnification ML **(B)** and CC **(C)** views, the area contains multiple round circumscribed fat containing masses with thin rims.

IMPRESSION: Oil cysts, BI-RADS® 2.

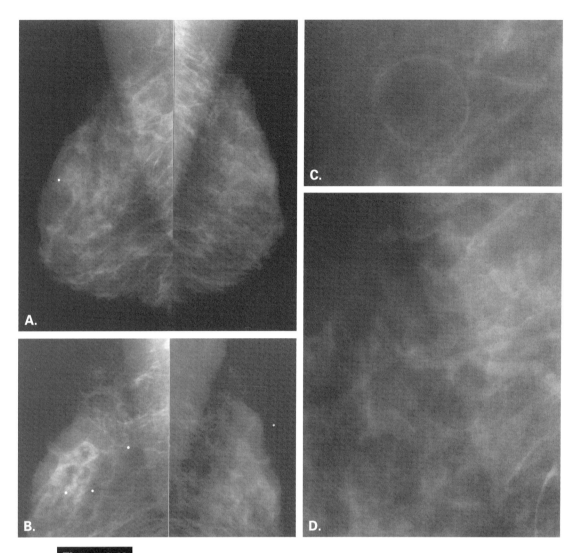

Figure 4.11

HISTORY: A 41-year-old woman with multiple small palpable masses bilaterally. There is no history of trauma.

MAMMOGRAPHY: Bilateral MLO (**A**) views show multiple round masses marked by BBs in the breasts and axillae. On enlarged images (**B, C, D**), the masses are very well circumscribed and radiolucent, consistent with oil cysts. Because of the extensive nature of these, the findings are consistent with steatocystoma multiplex.

IMPRESSION: Steatocystoma multiplex.

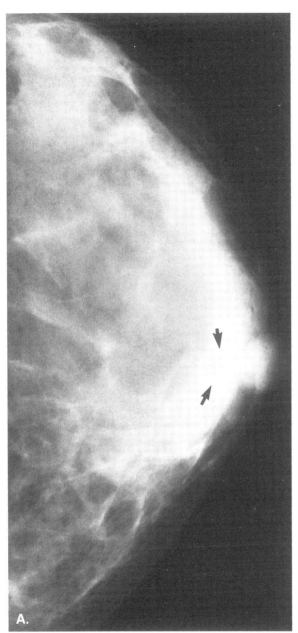
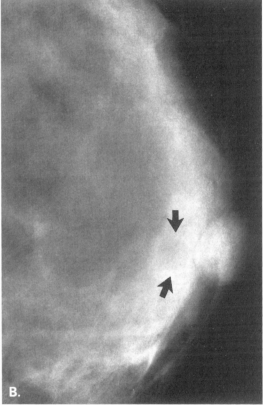

Figure 4.12

HISTORY: A 32-year-old gravida 1, para 1 patient who stopped nursing 4 months earlier, presenting with a small right subareolar nodule.

MAMMOGRAPHY: Right CC (**A**) and enlarged (2×) CC (**B**) views. The breast is quite dense, consistent with the patient's age and her recent lactating state. In the subareolar area, corresponding to the palpable nodule, there is a small circumscribed radiolucent nodule **(arrows)**. The differential for this nodule includes a lipoma, an oil cyst, or a galactocele, and given the clinical history, a galactocele is most likely. The lesion appears radiolucent because of the fat content of the milk it contains.

IMPRESSION: Galactocele.

NOTE: The patient was followed clinically, and the nodule resolved.

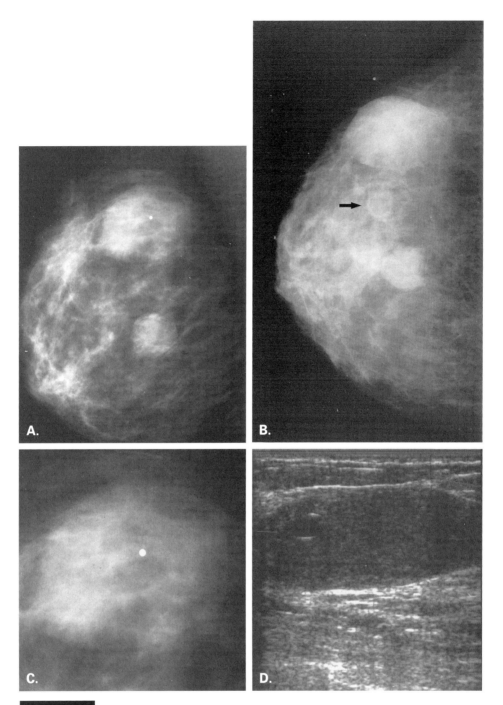

Figure 4.13

HISTORY: A 38-year-old woman who is lactating and presents with a palpable mass in the left breast.

MAMMOGRAPHY: Left MLO **(A)**, CC **(B)**, and enlarged ML **(C)** views and ultrasound **(D)**. There is a round circumscribed mixed-density mass in the left upper-outer quadrant **(A, B)** marked with a BB. In addition, there is a second smaller isodense mass located medially. In the center of the breast is a small radiolucent mass **(arrow)** that has a circumscribed margin. Ultrasound of the palpable mass shows it to be echogenic and to contain a small cystic area. Based on the history of the patient and the findings, the masses are most consistent with galactoceles. The patient underwent drainage of the two larger lesions, revealing milk contents.

IMPRESSION: Galactoceles.

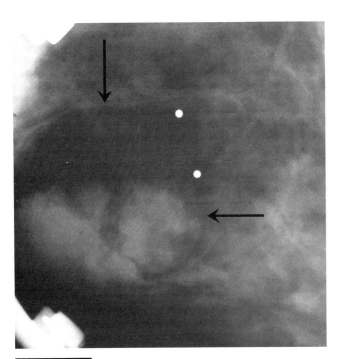

Figure 4.14

HISTORY: A 45-year-old woman with a palpable left breast mass.

MAMMOGRAPHY: Left spot compression MLO view shows a very-well-circumscribed mass of mixed density. This mass is composed of fat as well as fibrous and glandular tissues and is surrounded by a thin capsule **(arrows).**

IMPRESSION: Fibroadenolipoma (hamartoma).

size. Margination of the mass is important in suggesting a malignant etiology. Also, a multimodality approach to these masses, including physical examination, mammography, and ultrasound, is important in determining the approach for further evaluation (28).

The sonographic features of a benign solid mass are a thin pseudocapsule (29), an ellipsoid shape, fewer than four gentle lobulations, and extensive hyperechogenicity (30). Based on these criteria, Stavros et al. (30) found the negative predictive value to be 99%. Although sonography cannot definitely differentiate benign from malignant solid masses, the correlation of a circumscribed mass that has not enlarged on mammography and benign sonographic characteristics can be used to follow rather than biopsy a nonpalpable lesion.

Malignant sonographic criteria (30) include spiculation, a taller-than-wide shape, angular margins, shadowing, branching pattern, hypoechoicity, duct extension, and microlobulation. The presence of these features, even in the face of a relatively circumscribed mass on mammography, should prompt biopsy.

Cysts

One of the manifestations of fibrocystic disease is simple cysts that may vary from 3 mm to several centimeters in diameter. Cysts are more commonly seen in women 30 to 50 years old. Pain and tenderness may accompany the development of a cyst, and the symptoms may occur just before and with the menstrual cycle. There appears to be a relationship between caffeine consumption and fibrocystic disease. Boyle et al. (31) found that women who consumed 31 to 250 mg of caffeine per day had a 1.5-fold increase and those who consumed more than 500 mg/day had a 2.3-fold increase in the odds of fibrocystic disease. Allen and Froberg (32), however, found in a study of patients with suspected benign proliferative breast disease that a decrease in caffeine consumption did not result in a significant reduction of palpable breast nodules or in lessening of breast pain.

Cysts are derived from the lobules and may be lined by ordinary mammary epithelium or by an apocrine-type epithelium (33). A tension cyst is an apocrine cyst that contains fluid under pressure, secondary to obstruction of the outflow tract (33). Clinically, cysts are tender, circumscribed masses that are mobile, ranging from soft to firm, depending on the degree of distension.

On mammography, cysts (Figs. 4.36–4.43) are very well-defined, round or ovoid masses that may vary from several millimeters to 5 cm or more in diameter (34). The density is usually equal to or slightly greater than that of parenchyma. A halo sign is often present, and the orientation of the cyst is along the path of the ducts. Cysts may be multilocular or multiple and may be associated with other findings of fibrocystic disease. It is important when multiple masses are present that each lesion be evaluated individually so that a well-defined carcinoma not be missed.

On sonography, cysts are well defined and anechoic, with well-defined walls and good through-transmission of sound. If echoes are present within a lesion thought to be a cyst, aspiration should be performed for complete evaluation. Pneumocystography also may be performed at the time of aspiration to outline the internal aspect of the cyst wall. When sonography demonstrates a complicated cyst (imperceptible wall, acoustic enhancement, and low-level echoes) or a cluster of microcysts, the likelihood of malignancy is very low.

Cystic masses with thick walls, thick septae, or an intracystic solid component or predominately solid masses with cystic foci are categorized as complex cysts. Complex cysts may be malignant, and biopsy is warranted. In a study of cystic lesions, Berg et al. (35) found that none of the 38 complicated cysts or the 16 clustered microcysts were malignant; however, 18 of the 79 complex masses were malignant. Papillomas and intracystic papillary carcinomas may develop within a cyst and usually cannot be

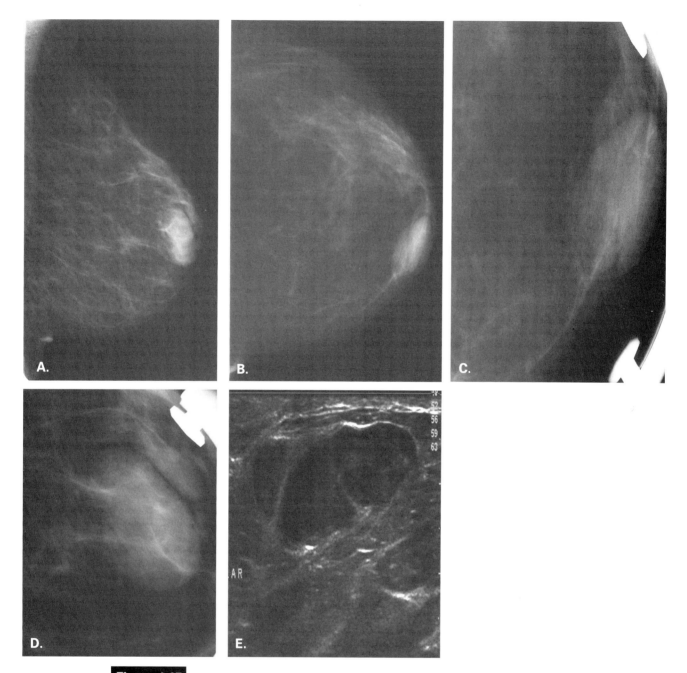

Figure 4.15

HISTORY: A 30-year-old woman with a palpable mass in the right subareolar area.

MAMMOGRAPHY: Right MLO **(A)** and CC **(B)** views show a lobular circumscribed mass in the sub-areolar area. On spot compression **(C, D)**, the mass is of mixed density and is surrounded by a thin capsule. On ultrasound **(E)**, the mass is very well defined and elliptical in shape. The echo pattern is mixed, with echogenic bands traversing a primarily hypoechoic mass. The mammographic and sonographic findings are typical of a hamartoma.

IMPRESSION: Hamartoma (fibroadenolipoma), BI-RADS® 2.

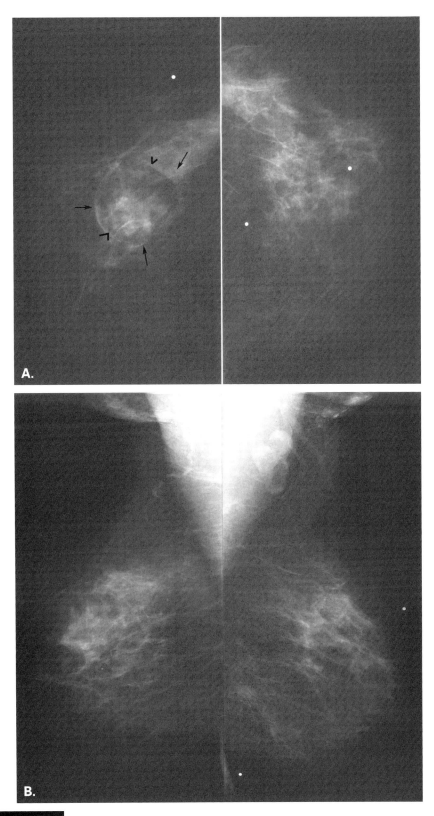

Figure 4.16

HISTORY: A 62-year-old woman with a palpable mass in the right breast at 6 o'clock.

MAMMOGRAPHY: Bilateral CC **(A)** and MLO **(B)** views show a circumscribed, round mixed-density mass in the left breast at 12 o'clock **(arrows)**. On the right, there is a BB marking the palpable mass posteriorly. The palpable mass is radiolucent and has a thin pseudocapsule **(arrowhead)**. (*continued*)

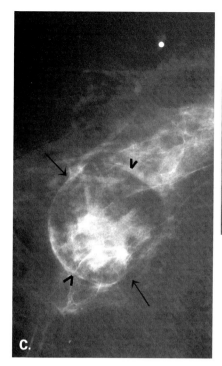

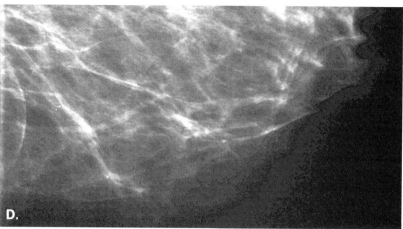

Figure 4.16   *(CONTINUED)*

Enlarged image **(C)** of the left breast mass shows its thin capsule **(arrow)** and heterogeneous composition, consistent with a hamartoma. Enlarged ML image **(D)** of the right breast mass shows it to be completely radiolucent, which is consistent with a lipoma.

IMPRESSION: Left breast hamartoma, right breast lipoma.

differentiated radiographically (36). Invasive papillary carcinomas tend to present as multiple, relatively well-defined masses. If a cyst contains an intracystic lesion, lobulation or slight irregularity of the wall may be seen on mammography. On pneumocystography, papillary lesions are seen as a polypoid filling defect within the cyst cavity.

Fibroadenoma

A fibroadenoma is a benign tumor of the breast, usually presenting with a well-defined mass. The term *fibroadenoma* was first used by Bilroth in 1880 (37). Being estrogen-sensitive tumors, fibroadenomas usually appear in adolescents and young women before the age of 30 years. Their growth may be enhanced by pregnancy or lactation (38). After menopause, these tumors undergo mucoid degeneration, hyalinize, and eventually develop characteristic coarse calcifications.

Dupont et al. (39), in a study of 1,835 patients with fibroadenomas, found that there was a slight increase in the risk of breast cancer in women diagnosed with fibroadenoma. However, the histologic features of the fibroadenoma influenced the risk of breast cancer. Fibroadenomas with associated proliferative disease in the epithelium or in those patients with positive family history of breast cancer were considered to be at increased long-term risk.

In a study of the follow-up of fibroadenomas, Carty et al. (40) found that at 5 years after diagnosis, 52% of the fibroadenomas had reduced in size, 16% were unchanged, and 32% had grown. When fibroadenomas have been diagnosed based on a triple test of mammography, clinical examination, and cytology, or have been diagnosed on percutaneous tissue sampling with a core needle, usual management is follow-up rather than excision. If an incidental nonpalpable fibroadenoma is identified at mammography and confirmed as having benign sonographic features (30), early imaging follow-up rather than biopsy is typically performed.

On histology, fibroadenomas are composed of dense, connective-tissue stroma surrounding canaliculi or tubules lined with ductal epithelium (41). On clinical examination, these tumors are smooth and of firm or rubber consistency and freely movable. In young patients, fibroadenomas may reach a very large size. This variant, sometimes termed the *juvenile fibroadenoma*, is characterized by rapid growth rate in young women and an increase in stromal cellularity (42).

The mammographic findings (Figs. 4.44–4.51) of a fibroadenoma are an isodense, very-well-defined, round, ovoid, or smoothly lobulated mass (43). A fatty halo surrounds the lesion and may be the key to identifying a

(text continues on page 124)

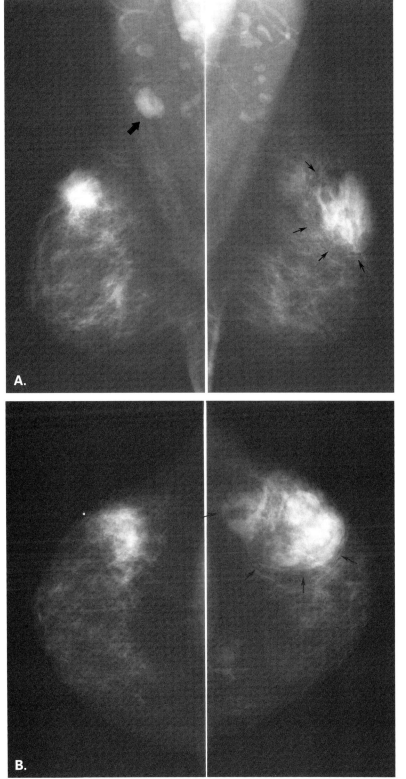

Figure 4.17

HISTORY: A 49-year-old woman with a palpable left breast mass.

MAMMOGRAPHY: Bilateral MLO **(A)** and CC **(B)** views show masses in both upper-outer quadrants. On the right, a large circumscribed mixed-density mass **(arrow)** is present, consistent with a hamartoma. On the left, the palpable mass is high density and irregular with indistinct margins. An enlarged lymph node is also seen in the left axilla.

IMPRESSION: Hamartoma, right breast, carcinoma left breast, metastatic to the axillary nodes.

HISTOPATHOLOGY: Left breast: Invasive ductal carcinoma with metastatic nodes in the left axilla.

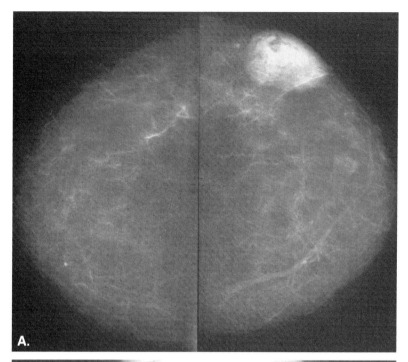

A.

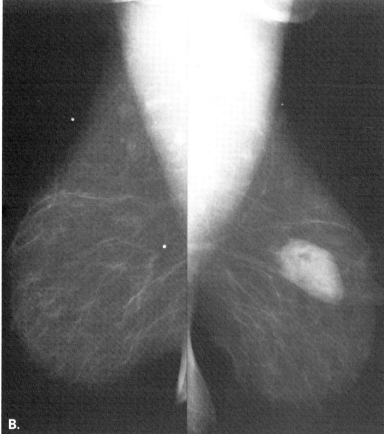

B.

Figure 4.18

HISTORY: A 57-year-old woman for screening mammography.

MAMMOGRAPHY: Bilateral MLO **(A)** and CC **(B)** views show an oval circumscribed mass in the right upper-outer quadrant. Fat is interspersed with the dense components of the mass, indicating a benign nature.

IMPRESSION: Hamartoma (fibroadenolipoma).

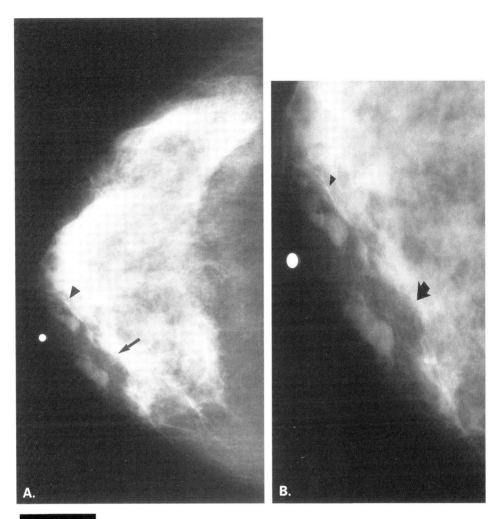

Figure 4.19

HISTORY: A 53-year-old gravida 8, para 4, abortus 4 woman with a 4-cm palpable soft mass in the left middle-inner quadrant.

MAMMOGRAPHY: Left CC **(A)** and enlarged (2.5×) CC **(B)** views. The breast is dense for the age and parity of the patient. A BB was placed over the palpable lesion. Beneath the BB, there is striking area of asymmetry **(arrow)** that is fatty in contrast to the background of dense parenchyma; within this fatty mass are two lobulated isodense nodules. Portions of a capsule are seen **(arrowhead)** surrounding this heterogeneous mass. The appearance is characteristic of a fibroadenolipoma of the breast.

IMPRESSION: Fibroadenolipoma (hamartoma).

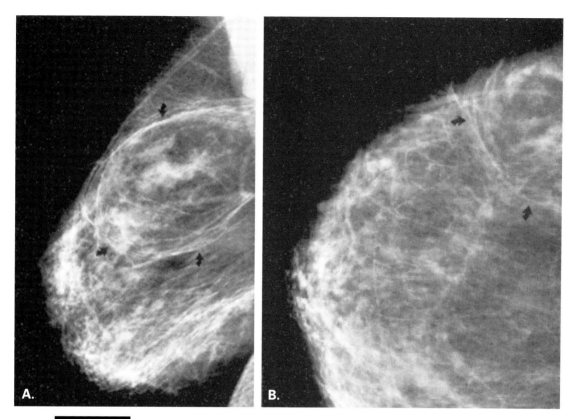

Figure 4.20

HISTORY: A 52-year-old gravida 0 woman for screening.

MAMMOGRAPHY: Left MLO **(A)** and CC **(B)** views. Scattered fibroglandular tissue is present. In the upper-outer quadrant, there is a large, mixed-density circumscribed mass. A thin pseudo-capsule **(arrows)** surrounds the lesion that is primarily fatty but contains some glandular elements. The lesion is very smoothly marginated and drapes the background parenchyma over it. The appearance of this lesion is characteristic of a benign hamartoma or fibroadenolipoma.

IMPRESSION: Hamartoma.

fibroadenoma in a young dense breast. Calcifications may vary from punctuate peripheral deposits to the typical coarse popcornlike morphologies that are characteristic of fibroadenomas. On ultrasound, fibroadenomas are usually smooth, hypoechoic masses of homogeneous echo-texture with well-defined margins and no attenuation or enhancement of sound posteriorly (44) (Figs. 4.52 and 4.53).

Rarely, a fibroadenoma may contain or be associated with malignancy (45,46), usually an in situ carcinoma. Fibroadenomas containing malignancy may be indistinguishable from benign fibroadenomas, but features that Baker et al. (47) found of concern were the large size of the mass, indistinct margins, and clustered microcalcifications. Even so, a palpable solid mass having an appearance consistent with a fibroadenoma or a nonpalpable enlarging mass are often biopsied because a well-circumscribed malignancy can have a similar appearance.

Large fibroadenomas has been described (48–50) to develop in transplant patients who are on cyclosporin A therapy. Weinstein et al. (48), in a study of five patients with cyclosporin-induced fibroadenomas, found that the masses ranged from 4 cm to 16 cm in diameter. In another study of renal transplant patients aged 27 to 50 years, Baildam et al. (49) found that 13 of 29 patients on cyclosporin developed fibroadenomas, in comparison with 0 of 10 patients not on cyclosporin.

Phylloides Tumor

Phylloides tumor is a fibroepithelial breast tumor that has malignant potential. Previously called cystosarcoma

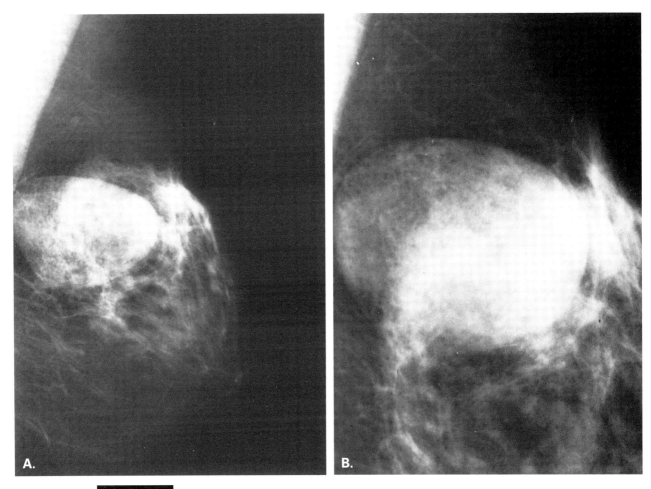

Figure 4.21

HISTORY: Baseline screening mammogram on a 40-year-old woman. There were no abnormalities noted on physical examination of the breasts.

MAMMOGRAPHY: Right MLO **(A)** and enlarged MLO **(B)** views show a large oval circumscribed mass in the upper aspect of the breast. Key to the diagnosis in this case is the density of the mass and the physical examination. The mass is of mixed density with small pockets of fat interspersed within the dense tissue. The lack of a palpable finding to correspond to such a large mammographic mass suggests a benign etiology.

IMPRESSION: Fat-containing mass consistent with a hamartoma (fibroadenolipoma).

NOTE: The mass was stable on subsequent routine mammography.

phylloides, the name refers to the leaflike pattern of growth of the epithelial elements, not to prognosis. Most phylloides tumors are benign or have limited invasion into the surrounding parenchyma. If the tumors are not completely excised, they may recur (51). When the lesions are malignant, metastases most often occur to lung, pleura, and bone (52).

Phylloides tumors are rare, presenting at a mean age of 40.5 years (53). On palpation, a firm, mobile, smooth mass is found; the lesion may be rapidly enlarging. Mammographically, the tumor is well circumscribed, large, and dense, having an appearance similar to that of a large fibroadenoma (54,55) (Figs. 4.54–4.56). Coarse calcification within a large circumscribed tumor should suggest, more likely, a fibroadenoma. When calcification occurs in a phylloides tumor, it has been described as plaquelike (11). Histologically, a phylloides tumor has a more cellular, pleomorphic connective tissue component than a fibroadenoma. Epithelially lined clefts are present within the lesion. The microscopic features of the connective-tissue component determine if the lesion is considered benign or malignant (56).

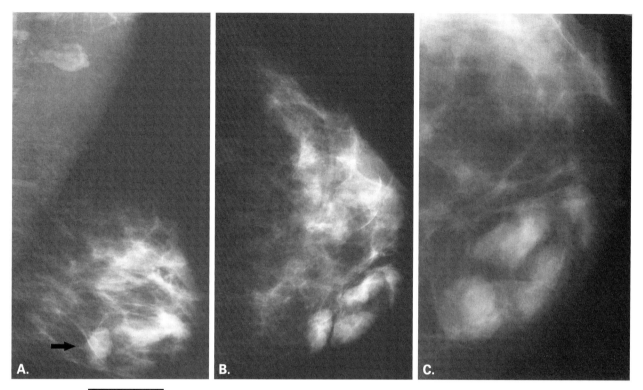

Figure 4.22

HISTORY: Screening mammogram on a premenopausal patient.

MAMMOGRAPHY: Right MLO **(A)**, CC **(B)**, and enlarged CC **(C)** views show a mixed-density mass in the lower-inner quadrant **(arrow)**. The lesion contains fat as well as multiple isodense lobulated masses, and it is surrounded by a fatty halo. The findings are characteristic of a fibroadenolipoma or hamartoma.

IMPRESSION: Hamartoma.

Other Benign Masses

Other benign lesions that may present mammographically as well-defined isodense masses include focal fibrocystic lesions, papillomas, hematomas, abscesses, pseudoangiomatous stromal hyperplasia, vascular tumors, sclerosing lobular hyperplasia, tubular adenomas, lactating adenomas, and epidermal inclusion or sebaceous cysts.

Occasionally, focal fibrosis, sclerosing adenosis, or areas of ductal hyperplasia can present as well-circumscribed masses (Figs 4.57–4.61). The mammographic appearance is nonspecific, and many of these lesions are associated with microcalcifications. Focal fibrosis is characterized by abundant connective tissue with intervening ducts and lobules that are atrophic (57). Focal fibrosis is common in young women with a palpable lump and is frequently diagnosed on core needle biopsy of solid circumscribed lesions. The most common presentations of focal fibrosis are a mass that is relatively circumscribed and

solid or a developing density (58). Biopsy is usually necessary to exclude a malignant process. Nodular adenosis or "adenosis tumor" is a confluent area of sclerosing adenosis that forms a mass. The mammographic appearance is usually a circumscribed ellipsoid or hypodense mass (59,60).

Intraductal papillomas are benign intraductal lesions characterized by a frondlike epithelium on a fibrovascular core. Most authors (61,62) do not consider papillomas to be precursors to papillary carcinoma or to elevate the risk of developing breast cancer, although some do suggest that papillomas increase the risk of cancer somewhat (63).

Solitary intraductal papillomas are often not evident on the mammogram and instead are detected on galactography. When small, these lesions present typically with a nipple discharge, usually sanguineous or serosanguineous (64). If papillomas are identified on mammography (Fig. 4.62), they generally are small, well-defined

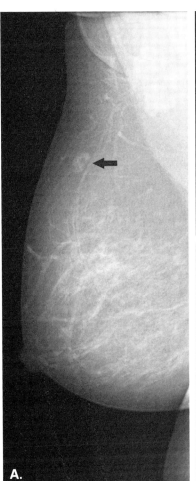

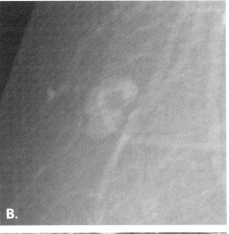

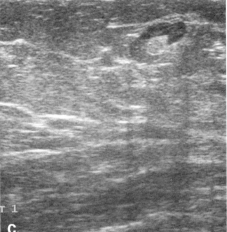

A.

B.

C.

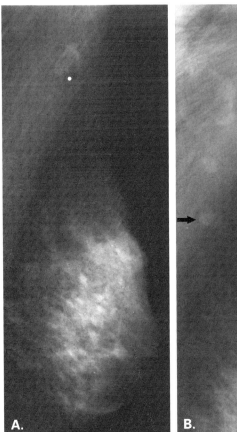

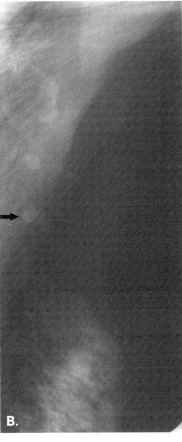

A.

B.

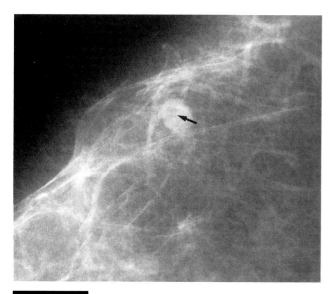

Figure 4.25

HISTORY: A 54-year-old woman for screening.

MAMMOGRAPHY: Left CC magnification (1.5×) view. There is a circumscribed nodule located superficially in the outer aspect of the breast. The fatty hilum **(arrow)** is characteristic of an intramammary lymph node.

IMPRESSION: Intramammary lymph node.

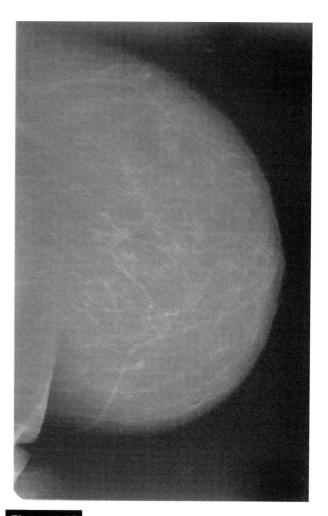

Figure 4.26

HISTORY: A 54-year-old woman for screening.

MAMMOGRAPHY: An enlarged CC image of the lateral aspect of the right breast shows a circumscribed round mass located superficially. The lesion has a radiolucent center, consistent with the hilum of a normal intramammary lymph node.

IMPRESSION: Intramammary node.

lesions oriented along the path of the ducts and often located in the subareolar area. A tubular shape should suggest the possibility of a papilloma. Because papillomas have a delicate blood supply via their stalk, they have a tendency to infarct (64). Calcification that is nonspecific may occur in infarcted papillomas.

A hematoma may be lobulated and appear as a circumscribed mass or be interstitial and dissect through the tissues, creating a diffuse increased density (Figs. 4.63–4.65). The density of a hematoma is the same or slightly greater than that of the parenchyma. The margins of the lesion are often slightly indistinct, but particularly in the case of a postoperative hematoma or seroma, the initial finding is that of a well-circumscribed mass. As a hematoma contracts, it may appear more indistinct in margination. Overlying skin edema is usually present in the acute stage with the bruising noted on the clinical examination. Follow-up examinations will show gradual resolution of the fluid collection.

Pseudoangiomatous stromal hyperplasia (PASH) is a benign stromal proliferation with a probable hormonal etiology. The lesion is composed of a complex pattern of anastomosing channels lined by spindle-shaped stromal cells that simulate endothelium. The lesion can be mis-

taken for a vascular lesion on histology because of this pattern. Polger et al. (65) described the imaging findings associated with PASH. The authors described seven patients with this entity and found that 5 of 7 cases were either circumscribed or partially circumscribed noncalcified masses on mammography.

Lactating adenoma is a benign mass that occurs in response to the physiologic changes that affect the breast during pregnancy and lactation (66). The lactating adenoma usually has a mammographic and sonographic appearance similar to a fibroadenoma, namely a well-circumscribed, hypoechoic mass (67). However, in some

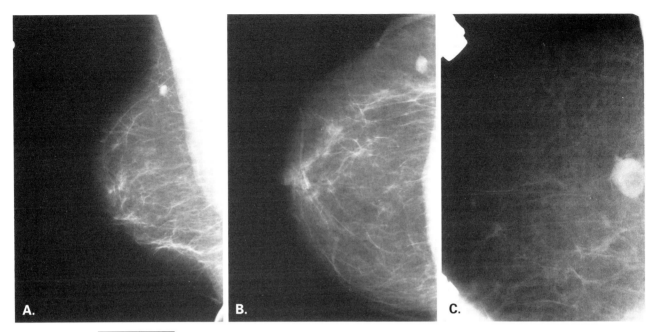

Figure 4.27

HISTORY: Baseline screening mammogram.

MAMMOGRAPHY: Left MLO **(A)**, and CC **(B)** views show essentially fatty replaced tissue. There is an oval circumscribed mass in the superficial aspect of the axillary tail. On spot compression **(C)**, the fatty hilum is seen, confirming that this is a node.

IMPRESSION: Normal intramammary node.

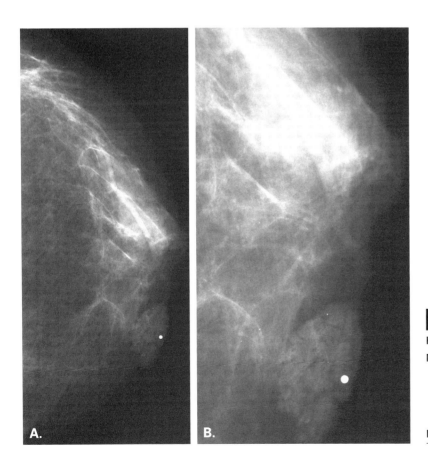

Figure 4.28

HISTORY: Screening mammogram.

MAMMOGRAPHY: Right CC **(A)** view and enlarged CC view **(B)** show a BB marking a pedunculated skin lesion. The crenulated surface is easily visible because of air trapped within the crevices of the keratosis.

IMPRESSION: Keratosis.

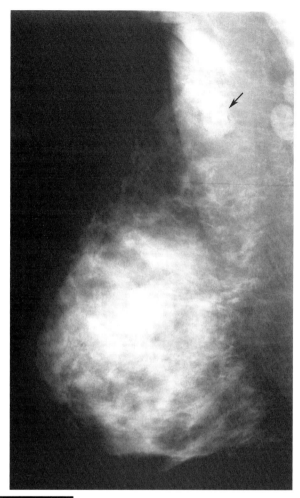

Figure 4.29

HISTORY: A 38-year-old woman for screening.

MAMMOGRAPHY: Left MLO view shows heterogeneously dense tissue. A BB marks a very-well-demarcated mass **(arrow)** in the axillary tail. This represented a large pedunculated skin lesion on clinical examination.

IMPRESSION: Skin lesion.

cases, the margins of the adenoma are more indistinct. Because of the similarity to the appearance of a circumscribed cancer, biopsy is usually necessary (67).

Sclerosing lobular hyperplasia is a benign lesion that most commonly occurs in young black women (68). The lesion typically presents as a palpable mobile mass. Sclerosing lobular hyperplasia is similar to a fibroadenoma both in its presentation and in its mammographic appearance.

Tubular adenomas are rare benign tumors that occur in women younger than 35 years. Histologically, these masses are related to fibroadenomas. However, instead of containing large ducts, as are found in fibroadenomas, the tubular adenomas are composed of acinar or lobular units

as the epithelial component. In young women, tubular adenomas look like noncalcified fibroadenomas, but in older women, they may resemble malignant masses with microcalcifications (69).

Epidermal inclusion cysts or sebaceous cysts are of skin origin; therefore, they are superficially located. Sebaceous cysts are palpated as smooth, firm cutaneous nodules. These very-well-defined lesions are often located in the areolar area or in the lower aspect of the breast and are contiguous with the skin on mammography (4) (Figs. 4.66–4.68). Epidermal inclusion cysts usually appear as a circumscribed mass that is noncalcified, although occasionally heterogeneous microcalcifications may be noted on mammography within the mass (70). On ultrasound, the inclusion cyst is hypoechoic depending on the amount of debris, with good through-transmission of sound. Extension of the mass into the dermis is often seen as well (70).

Moles and skin lesions, if smoothly marginated, appear as isodense superficial masses on mammography. A normal structure that may stimulate a well-defined mass is the nipple out of profile. With care taken to keep the nipple in profile on both views or at least on one view, there should not be any doubt as to whether a well-defined lesion represents the nipple. If there is a question, a radiopaque marker may be placed on the nipple and the film repeated with the nipple in profile.

An acute breast abscess is usually suspected in clinical examination because of the associated findings of inflammation: a painful tender breast, redness of the skin, and fever. Abscesses most often occur in the postpartum patient, but they also may occur in older patients as well. Because of the inflammation associated with an acute abscess, skin thickening and a surrounding edema pattern are present and may obscure the abscess itself. Mammography with good compression is difficult to perform because of the severe breast tenderness present. When the abscess is visualized, it is usually a relatively well-defined mass (11) (Figs. 4.69 and 4.70). After an abscess has resolved completely, repeat mammography should be performed to exclude an underlying malignancy, particularly in a nonlactating patient.

Vascular tumors of the breast are rare. Most often vascular masses that are located in the subcutaneous area, superficial to the anterior pectoralis fascia, are benign (71). Hemangiomas are superficial, circumscribed masses that are round or lobular (72,73). On ultrasound, hemangiomas may be hypoechoic or intensely hyperechoic (71). Hemangiopericytoma may also rarely occur in the breast (74) and present as a circumscribed soft tissue mass.

(text continues on page 135)

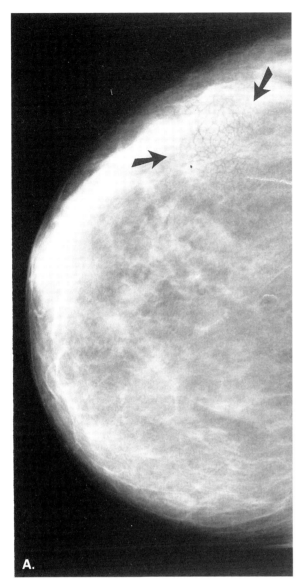

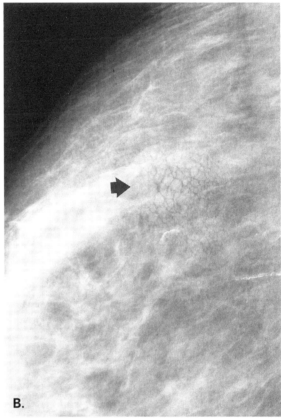

Figure 4.30

HISTORY: A 77-year-old gravida 3, para 3 woman for screening mammography.

MAMMOGRAPHY: Left CC **(A)** and enlarged (2×) **(B)** views. The breast is heterogeneously dense. There is a mixed-density lesion **(arrows)** in the outer aspect of the breast. The crackled appearance is typical of air in the surface of a skin lesion.

IMPRESSION: Skin lesion (seborrhea keratosis) simulating a breast mass.

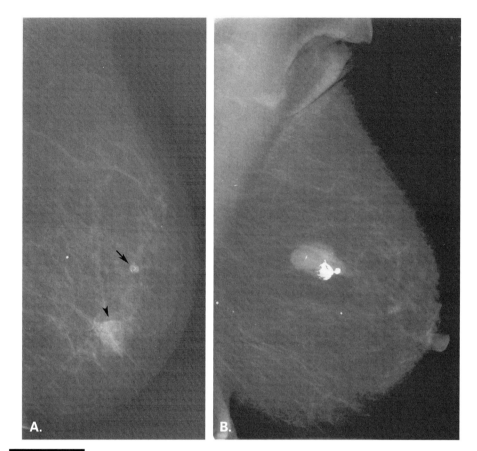

Figure 4.31

HISTORY: A 69-year-old woman for screening.

MAMMOGRAPHY: Right anterior MLO **(A)** view shows a small calcified mass superiorly **(arrow)**. There is also a more indistinct lobular mass inferiorly **(arrowhead)**. Repeat MLO **(B)** view, which is better positioned, shows that the inferior "mass" represents the nipple out of profile. The subareolar calcified mass and a larger calcified fibroadenoma posteriorly are seen.

IMPRESSION: Nipple out of profile, calcified fibroadenomas.

Figure 4.32

HISTORY: A 56-year-old woman for follow-up of a nonpalpable right breast nodule that had been stable for 5 years.

MAMMOGRAPHY: Right MLO **(A)** and CC **(B)** views. In the central aspect of the breast, there is a well-circumscribed ovoid nodule **(straight arrow)** that was stable from prior examinations and presumed to be a fibroadenoma **(A and B)**. A second nodule **(curved arrow)**, seen superiorly on the MLO view **(A)**, disappears on the CC view **(B)**. This represents the nipple out of profile, simulating a breast lesion.

IMPRESSION: Nipple out of profile, stimulating a breast lesion.

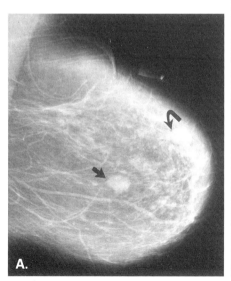

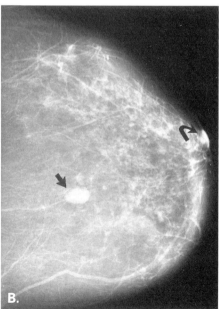

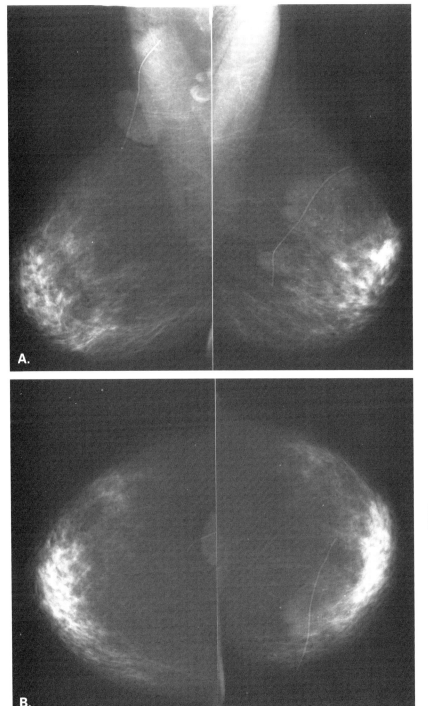

Figure 4.33

HISTORY: A 70-year-old woman with a history of benign breast biopsies, for screening mammography.

MAMMOGRAPHY: Bilateral MLO **(A)** and CC **(B)** views show very-well-defined densities bilaterally, marked with wires indicating the biopsy sites. These densities have very defined edges, suggesting that the lesions are on the skin and are demarcated by air haloes. Clinical examination confirmed keloids.

IMPRESSION: Keloids at biopsy sites.

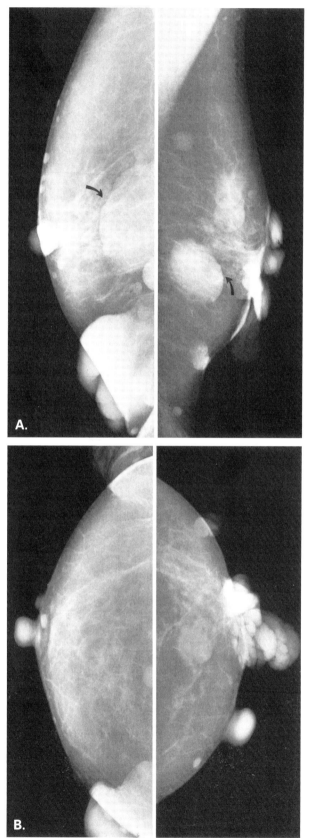

A.

B.

Figure 4.34

HISTORY: A 57-year-old woman with neurofibromatosis, for screening mammography.

MAMMOGRAPHY: Bilateral MLO **(A)** and CC **(B)** views. The breasts are fatty replaced. There are multiple, very-well-defined masses of varying size projected over the skin surfaces of both breasts, compatible with the obvious cutaneous lesions on physical examination. Note on the MLO views **(A)** that the lesions that superimpose over the breast have strikingly lucent haloes **(curved arrows)**, more lucent than is seen with a fatty halo. This appearance is created by air surrounding the nodule compressed against the surface of the breast.

IMPRESSION: Multiple cutaneous lesions of neurofibromatosis.

Well-Circumscribed Carcinoma

Primary breast carcinoma characteristically presents mammographically as a spiculated mass. However, some carcinomas are relatively well defined or even very sharply marginated, and these lesions may be confused with benign masses, such as fibroadenomas, radiographically. Radiologists must be aware of the subtle features of breast cancer, which include relatively circumscribed masses, to avoid the pitfall of missing carcinomas presenting in this way (75) (Figs. 4.71–4.86).

It has been said (11) that approximately 2% of carcinomas are very-well-defined masses. Moskowitz (76) found 2% of carcinomas to be very well defined and 5% to 10% to be partially well defined. Marsteller and Shaw de Paredes (77) found that 4.1% of relatively circumscribed lesions were carcinomas, and an additional 4% were atypical hyperplastic lesions. If one considers nonpalpable breast cancers only, however, a greater percentage (4%) appear very sharply marginated (78). Most relatively circumscribed carcinomas are ductal carcinomas, which are the most frequently occurring primary carcinomas of the breast. Intraductal or infiltrating ductal carcinomas can be well defined on mammography, although there is usually some indistinctness of the margins of the infiltrating lesions. In a series of 350 cases of intraductal carcinomas, Mitnick et al. (79) found that 13 lesions were sharply circumscribed lesions simulating benign masses. Calcifications within these masses tend to be pleomorphic, amorphous and asymmetric in location within the nodules.

The types of carcinomas that more characteristically appear as well-defined masses are medullary mucinous and papillary cancers, which are subtypes of invasive ductal carcinoma. However, because invasive ductal carcinoma not otherwise specified (NOS) accounts for the vast majority of breast cancers, a frequent histologic type of cancer that presents as a well-circumscribed mass is invasive ductal NOS. It is very uncommon that invasive lobular carcinoma appears as a circumscribed mass (80).

Medullary carcinoma accounts for 3% of all breast cancers (81). Clinically, the lesions are soft and movable, and unlike the irregular scirrhous carcinomas, medullary carcinomas do not necessarily palpate as larger than they appear mammographically. The lesions tend to be located either deep in the breast or in the subareolar or subcutaneous areas (82). Histologically, medullary carcinoma is a variety of ductal carcinoma characterized by a growth pattern of syncytial, solid sheetlike areas of malignant cells. Necrosis is frequent; calcification does not usually occur (83). The mammographic appearance is of a well-circumscribed, medium- to high-density noncalcified mass. Faint indistinctness of the borders may be detected, indicating a suspicious nature. On ultrasound,

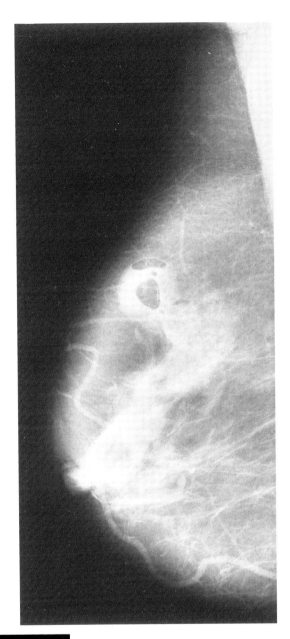

Figure 4.35

HISTORY: A 65-year-old woman with angina, for screening mammography. She had had no recent breast interventional procedures.

MAMMOGRAPHY: Left MLO view. There is a very-well-circumscribed mixed-density mass superimposed over the upper aspect of the left breast. The lucencies within the mass are more radiolucent than fat, suggesting air beneath a device on the skin. An unusual appearance of a pneumocystogram or air within a mass or hematoma from recent biopsy would also be a consideration with an appropriate clinical history.

IMPRESSION: Air trapped beneath a Nitro-Bid patch on the skin, simulating a breast lesion.

NOTE: The patient had placed the new patch on her breast just before the mammogram and refused to have the technologist remove it for the study.

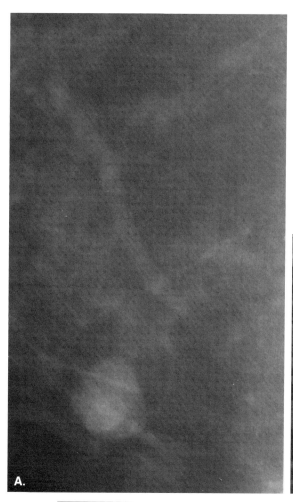

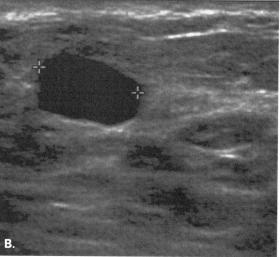

Figure 4.36

HISTORY: A 64-year-old woman with an abnormal screening mammogram.

MAMMOGRAPHY: Left CC spot compression **(A)** view shows a circumscribed lobulated mass medially. Ultrasound **(B)** demonstrates that the lesion is anechoic, smoothly marginated, with a thin wall and acoustic enhancement.

IMPRESSION: Simple cyst.

medullary carcinomas are well-defined, inhomogeneous hypoechoic masses that show enhanced through-transmission (84).

Mucinous or colloid carcinomas also may present as well-circumscribed masses (82) (Fig. 4.87). However, in a study of 10 patients with pure mucinous carcinoma, Cardenosa et al. (85) found that the majority of masses were poorly defined and lobulated. The density of these lesions tends to be medium to low because of the presence of mucin (82). Mucinous carcinomas, like medullary cancers, tend to be peripherally located.

Pure mucinous carcinoma is a well-differentiated subtype of invasive ductal carcinoma that has a better survival rate than other less differentiated carcinomas (86,87).

Wilson et al. (88) found that the mammographic findings in pure mucinous carcinomas were masses with circumscribed, lobular contours that were the result of the expansile growth pattern. Patients with mixed mucinous tumors had masses with more irregular margins than those with pure mucinous carcinoma.

Metastases

Metastases from extramammary primary carcinomas are unusual, accounting for about 1% to 2% (89) of all breast malignancies. The mammographic presentation of a metas-

(text continues on page 142)

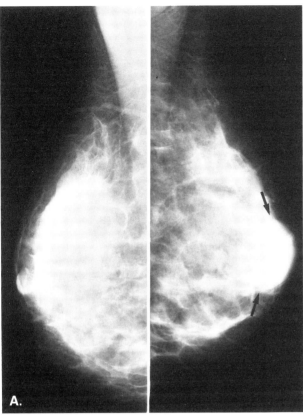

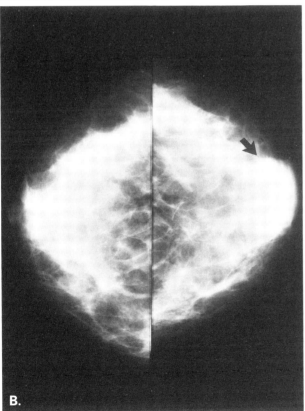

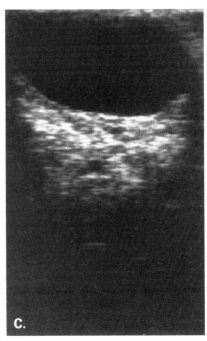

Figure 4.37

HISTORY: A 41-year-old gravida 3, para 4 woman with a right subareolar mass.

MAMMOGRAPHY: Bilateral MLO (**A**) and CC (**B**) views and ultrasound (**C**). The breasts are dense and glandular for the age and parity of the patient. In the right subareolar area, there is an isodense, relatively circumscribed mass (**arrows**) (**A** and **B**). A halo is present around the anterior aspect of the lesion, but its posterior margin is indistinct. Ultrasound (**C**) demonstrates the anechoic nature of the lesion.

IMPRESSION: Simple cyst.

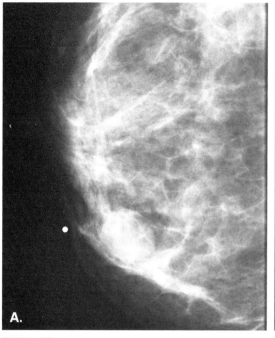

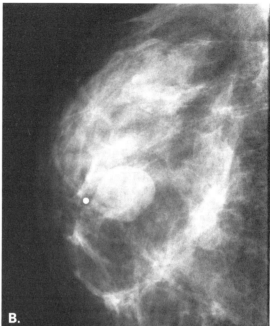

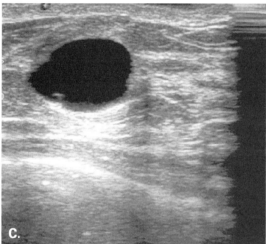

Figure 4.38

HISTORY: A 38-year-old woman with a solitary palpable left breast mass.

MAMMOGRAPHY: Left MLO **(A)** and CC **(B)** spot views show the BB marking a palpable mass. The edges are very well defined and the mass is isodense. On ultrasound **(C)**, the mass is well defined and anechoic, consistent with a simple cyst.

IMPRESSION: Simple cyst.

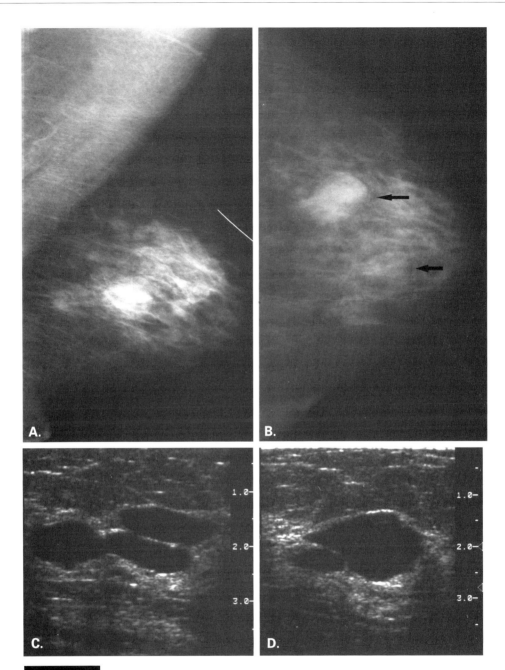

Figure 4.39

HISTORY: A 73-year-old woman with a history of fibrocystic disease, for routine mammography.

MAMMOGRAPHY: Right MLO **(A)** and CC **(B)** views show the breast to be heterogeneously dense. There are several partially obscured, round, isodense masses **(arrows)**. The multiplicity of the findings and the appearance suggests that these are most likely cysts. Sonography **(C, D)** confirms that the masses are simple cysts. They are oval, well defined, and anechoic.

IMPRESSION: Simple cysts bilaterally, BI-RADS® 2.

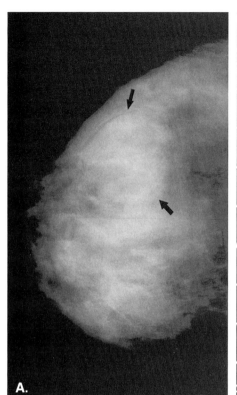

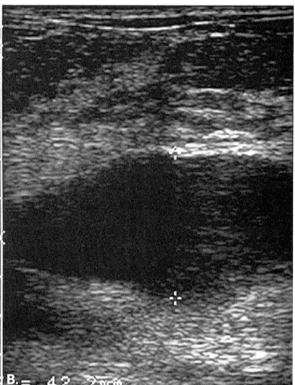

Figure 4.40

HISTORY: A 62-year-old woman with a palpable mass in the right breast.

MAMMOGRAPHY: Right CC **(A)** view shows very dense tissue. In the lateral aspect of the breast is a large, round isodense mass that has a fatty halo surrounding its border **(arrows)**. On ultrasound **(B)**, an anechoic oval lesion is seen.

IMPRESSION: Simple cyst.

Figure 4.41

HISTORY: A 42-year-old woman who presents with a new palpable mass in the right breast.

MAMMOGRAPHY: Right MLO **(A)** view shows a BB overlying the palpable mass in a heterogeneously dense breast. The mass is large, somewhat high density, round, and circumscribed. Just posterior to it is another lower-density round mass **(arrow)**. Ultrasound **(B)** demonstrates the palpable lesion to be a simple cyst: anechoic and well defined with increased through-transmission of sound. The more posterior mass was also identified as a smaller cyst on ultrasound.

IMPRESSION: Simple cyst.

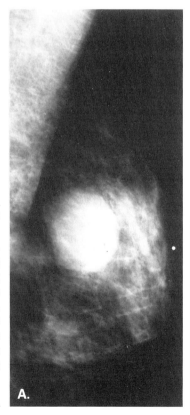

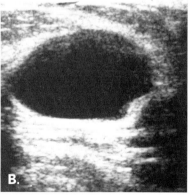

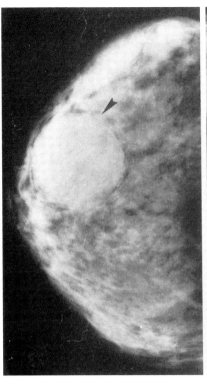
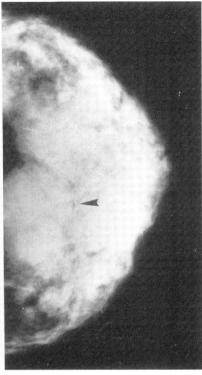

Figure 4.42

HISTORY: A 51-year-old gravida 1, para 2 woman with a history of fibrocystic disease and lumpy breasts on physical examination.

MAMMOGRAPHY: Bilateral CC views. The breasts are dense and glandular for the age and parity of the patient. There are bilateral, well-defined round masses surrounded by fatty haloes **(arrow)** and oriented in the direction of the ducts. The multiplicity of findings and the similarity in appearance of the lesions suggest fibrocystic changes. Ultrasound confirmed the cystic nature of the masses.

IMPRESSION: Bilateral cysts, diffuse fibrocystic changes.

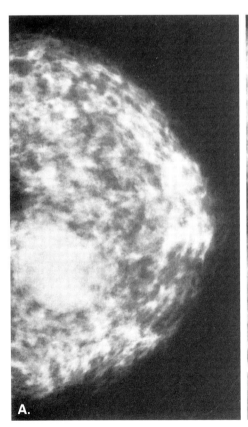
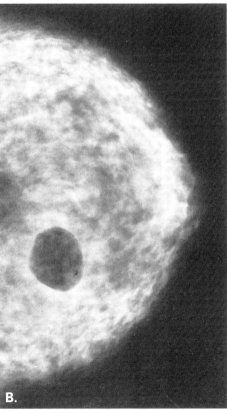

A. B.

Figure 4.43

HISTORY: A 42-year-old gravida 3, para 3 woman with a lump in the right breast.

MAMMOGRAPHY: Right CC view **(A)** and pneumocystogram **(B)**. The breast is dense and diffusely nodular. There is a moderately high-density, very-well-defined round mass surrounded by a fatty halo. Sonography revealed a cyst. The pneumocystogram **(B)** shows a normal, thin-walled cavity.

IMPRESSION: Cyst.

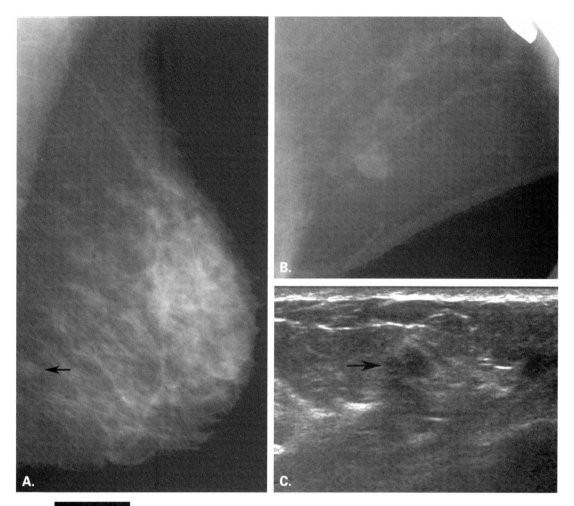

Figure 4.44

HISTORY: A 64-year-old woman for screening mammography.

MAMMOGRAPHY: Right MLO (**A**) view shows a small oval mass located posteriorly (**arrow**). On spot compression (**B**), the mass is circumscribed and slightly lobulated. On ultrasound (**C**), the mass is lobulated, hypoechoic, and slightly taller than wide. Sonographic findings are suspicious and necessitate biopsy.

IMPRESSION: Solid mass, BI-RADS® 4. Biopsy recommended,

HISTOPATHOLOGY: Fibroadenoma.

tasis may be as a very well-defined mass having an appearance similar to that of fibroadenoma. Although it is more common for a patient presenting with a metastatic lesion in the breast to have a known carcinoma, it is not necessarily the case (89). The most common sites of origin of metastases to the breast are lymphoma, melanoma, sarcoma, lung, stomach, prostate, and ovary (90) (Figs. 4.88–4.92). In most series (90–92), a solitary well-defined mass is the most common presentation, with multiple masses and diffuse involvement of the breast being less likely; others have described diffuse involvement more frequently (92). The lesions tend to be superficially located (90) and may have an appearance similar to that of sebaceous cyst (Figs. 4.77 and 4.78).

Lymphoma may occur as a primary or secondary lesion in the breast. Lymphomas may produce axillary or intramammary adenopathy or may present with circumscribed or poorly marginated breast nodules (Figs. 4.79 and 4.80). In a study of 29 women with non-Hodgkin lymphoma affecting the breast, Liberman et al. (93) found that solitary masses were the most frequent presentation. Although mammography showed indistinct or partially circumscribed masses in the majority of cases, well-circumscribed masses were the presentation in 28% of the patients. The development of numerous new round masses bilaterally in a patient who is not on hormone replacement therapy should suggest the possibility of lymphoma.

(References begin on page 184.)

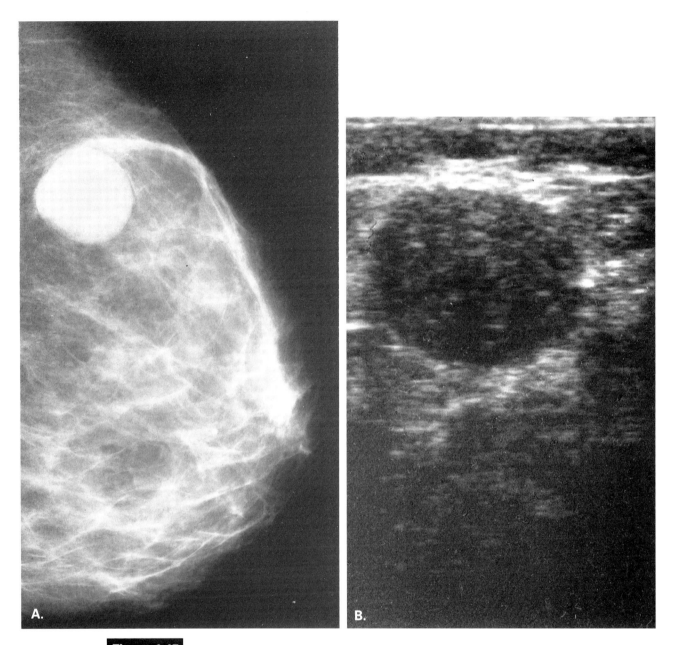

Figure 4.45

HISTORY: A 30-year-old gravida 2, para 2 patient with a right breast mass.

MAMMOGRAPHY: Right CC view **(A)** and ultrasound **(B)**. There is an isodense, very-well-circumscribed mass in the right upper-outer quadrant. A halo surrounds the lesion. On sonography **(B)**, the mass is circumscribed, solid, and of relatively homogeneous hypoechogenicity, suggesting a fibroadenoma.

IMPRESSION: Solid mass, favoring fibroadenoma.

HISTOPATHOLOGY: Fibroadenoma.

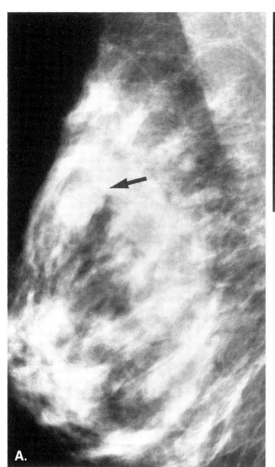

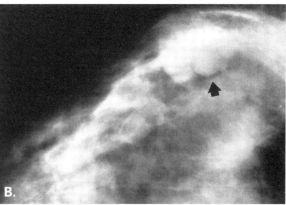

Figure 4.46

HISTORY: A 33-year-old gravida 3, para 0, abortus 3 woman with a palpable mass in the left breast.

MAMMOGRAPHY: Left MLO **(A)** and enlarged CC **(B)** views. The breast is dense, compatible with the age of the patient. There is a very-well-circumscribed, lobulated, isodense mass **(arrow)** in the upper-outer quadrant of the left breast. The lobulated contour suggests that this is most likely a fibroadenoma. Ultrasound confirmed the solid nature of the lesion.

IMPRESSION: Solid mass, probable fibroadenoma.

HISTOPATHOLOGY: Fibroadenoma.

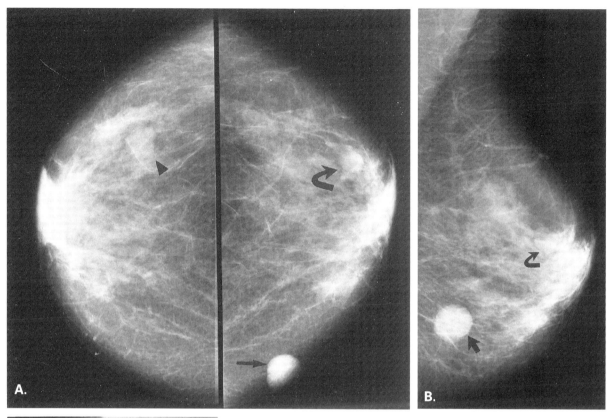

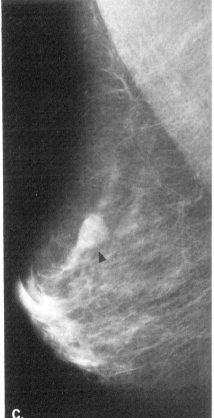

HISTORY: A 57-year-old gravida 7, para 7 woman with a palpable nodule in the right lower-inner quadrant.

MAMMOGRAPHY: Bilateral CC views **(A)**, right MLO view **(B)**, and left MLO view **(C)**. There are three relatively well-circumscribed masses present. In the right inner quadrant **(A** and **B)**, there is a very-well-marginated high-density mass **(straight arrow)** located in the subcutaneous area and corresponding to the palpable nodule. *(continued)*

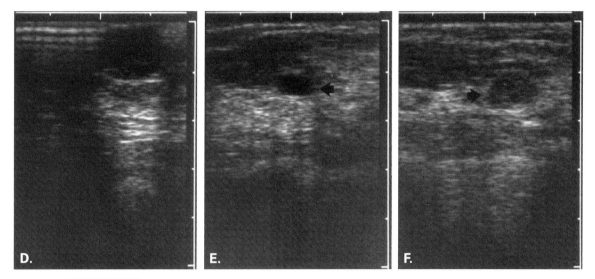

Figure 4.47   *(CONTINUED)*

Ultrasound of the right (**D** and **E**) and left (**F**) breasts. On ultrasound (**D**), this mass is complex; there is a fluid component with debris layering in the base. This mass, particularly because of its location, is most consistent with an inclusion or sebaceous cyst. In the right upper-outer quadrant (**A** and **B**), there is an isodense circumscribed mass **(curved arrow)**, which on ultrasound (**E**) is a simple cyst. In the left upper-outer quadrant, a third mass is noted (**A** and **C**) **(arrowhead)**. This mass is of isodense and has well-circumscribed lobulated margins, suggesting that the lesion may be a fibroadenoma. Sonography (**F**) reveals the lesion to be hypoechoic and well marginated, consistent with a fibroadenoma.

IMPRESSION: Three circumscribed masses: simple cyst and sebaceous cyst on the right and fibroadenoma on the left.

HISTOPATHOLOGY: Right epidermal cyst, left fibroadenoma.

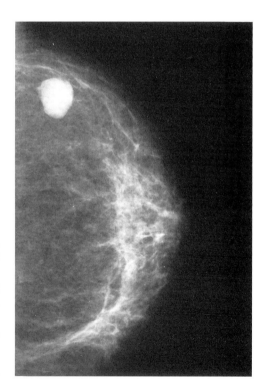

Figure 4.48

HISTORY: Baseline mammogram in a patient who presents with a new palpable lump in the right breast.

MAMMOGRAPHY: Right CC view shows a lobulated, circumscribed, somewhat dense mass in the outer quadrant. Sonography showed the mass to be solid. The lesion has very-well-defined margins, suggesting a benign etiology.

IMPRESSION: Circumscribed mass, favor fibroadenoma. Recommend biopsy to confirm.

HISTOPATHOLOGY: Fibroadenoma.

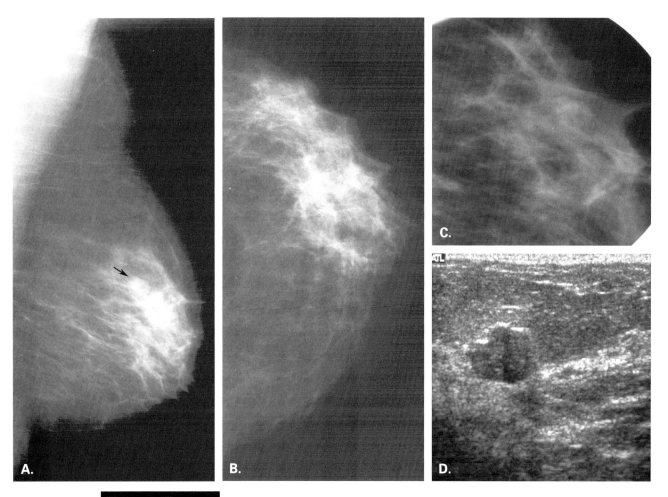

Figure 4.49

HISTORY: A 35-year-old woman with palpable nodularity in the upper-outer quadrant.

MAMMOGRAPHY: Right MLO **(A)** and CC **(B)** views show dense parenchyma. In the 10 o'clock position, there is a circumscribed mass **(arrow)** present. Spot compression **(C)** shows the mass to be lobular, isodense, and partially circumscribed; however, some of the borders are obscured. Ultrasound **(D)** demonstrates a solid lobular lesion that is somewhat vertical in orientation with a multilobulated border.

IMPRESSION: Solid mass, possible fibroadenoma. Recommend biopsy because of borders on mammography and ultrasound.

HISTOPATHOLOGY: Fibroadenoma.

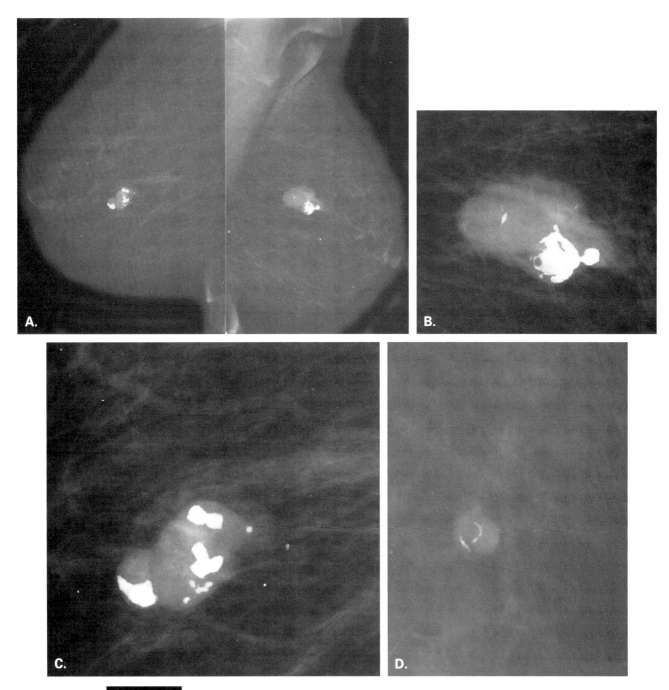

Figure 4.50

HISTORY: A 69-year-old woman for screening mammography.

MAMMOGRAPHY: Bilateral MLO view **(A)** shows lobulated masses containing coarse calcifications bilaterally. On spot magnification views **(B, C, D)**, the masses are circumscribed and lobulated. Coarse and dystrophic calcifications are present in all three masses, and the calcifications are located in the periphery of the lesions.

IMPRESSION: Calcified fibroadenomas.

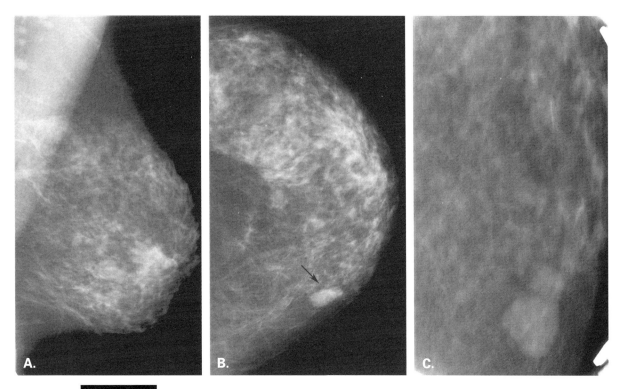

Figure 4.51

HISTORY: A 49-year-old woman for screening mammography.

MAMMOGRAPHY: Right MLO **(A)** and CC **(B)** views show a lobular isodense mass at the 3 o'clock position **(arrows)**. Spot compression **(C)** shows that the mass is lobular, isodense, and well circumscribed. Sonography was performed and demonstrated a solid lesion. The mass had developed from a prior study, so biopsy was performed.

IMPRESSION: Circumscribed mass, possible fibroadenoma.

HISTOPATHOLOGY: Fibroadenoma.

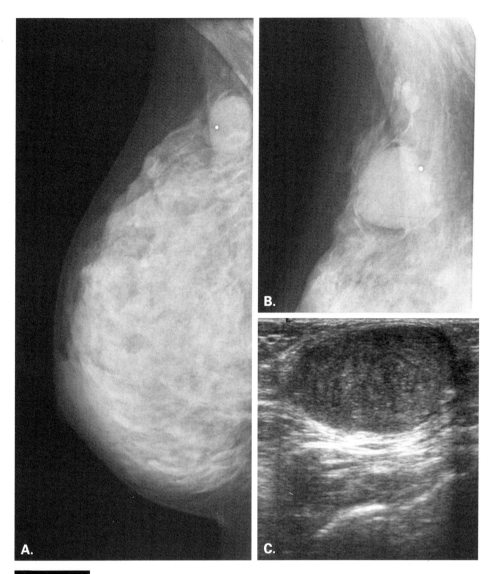

Figure 4.52

HISTORY: A 37-year-old gravida 0, para 0 patient with a palpable mass in the left axillary tail.

MAMMOGRAPHY: Left MLO **(A)** view shows extremely dense breast tissue. A BB marks the palpable mass, which is a circumscribed, isodense lobular lesion. On the spot magnification view **(B)**, the very-well-defined margins are seen. On ultrasound **(C)**, the mass is hypoechoic, well defined, and somewhat oval.

IMPRESSION: Solid palpable mass, likely fibroadenoma. Recommend biopsy.

HISTOPATHOLOGY: Fibroadenoma.

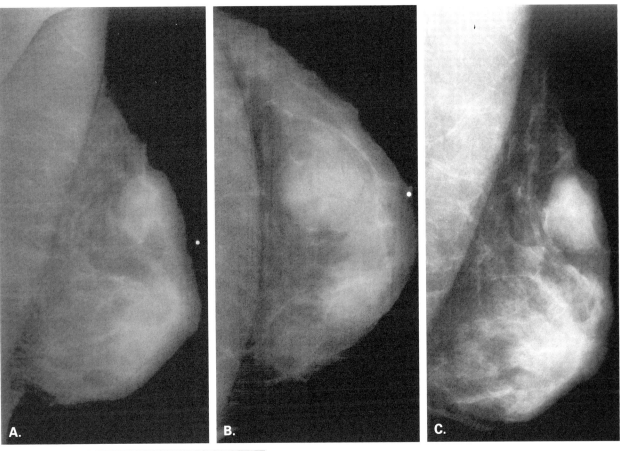

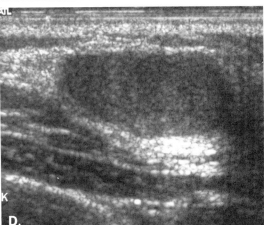

Figure 4.53

HISTORY: A 29-year-old woman with a new palpable right breast mass.

MAMMOGRAPHY: Right MLO **(A)**, CC **(B)**, and ML **(C)** views show heterogeneously dense tissue. There is partially obscured, partially circumscribed, isodense lobular mass in the 12 o'clock position corresponding to the palpable lesion. Ultrasound **(D)** shows the mass to be solid, hypoechoic, elliptical in shape, and well defined. Because it was palpable, biopsy was performed.

IMPRESSION: Solid palpable mass, likely fibroadenoma.

PATHOLOGY: Fibroadenoma with epithelial hyperplasia.

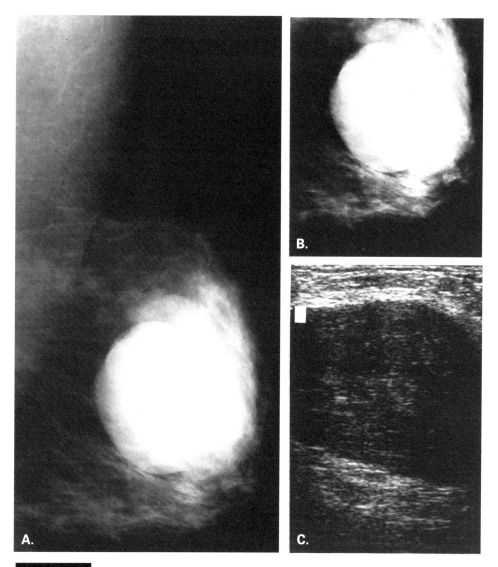

Figure 4.54

HISTORY: A 47-year-old woman with a positive family history of breast cancer presents with a palpable right breast mass.

MAMMOGRAPHY: Right MLO (**A**) view shows a high-density round mass in the superior aspect of the breast. Enlarged image (**B**) shows the circumscribed margins around a portion of the mass, which is otherwise obscured. On ultrasound (**C**), the lesion is hypoechoic and somewhat inhomogeneous. Because of the large size and its appearance, a phylloides tumor is a likely possibility. Also included in the differential diagnosis are a giant fibroadenoma and a primary breast carcinoma.

IMPRESSION: Phylloides tumor.

HISTOPATHOLOGY: Phylloides tumor.

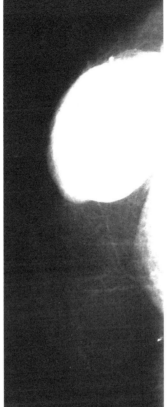 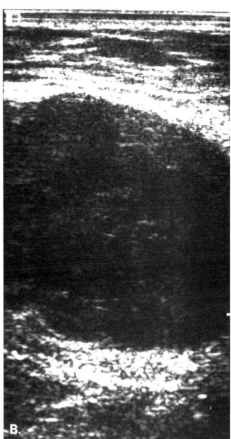

Figure 4.55

HISTORY: A 26-year-old woman with a large, growing palpable mass in the left axillary tail.

MAMMOGRAPHY: Left MLO (**A**) view shows the breast to be fatty replaced. In the upper-outer quadrant is a high-density, very-large-circumscribed mass. On ultrasound (**B**), the mass is noted to be solid and well defined. Based on the size of the lesion, a giant fibroadenoma or a phylloides tumor is most likely.

IMPRESSION: Probable phylloides tumor.

HISTOPATHOLOGY: Malignant cystosarcoma phylloides.

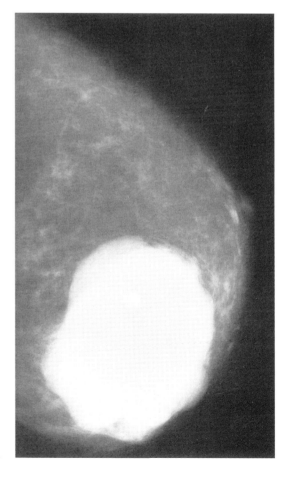

Figure 4.56

HISTORY: An 84-year-old woman with a large palpable mass in the right breast.

MAMMOGRAPHY: Right CC view. There is a large mass in the inner quadrant of the right breast with lobulated but well-defined margins. Some dense coarse calcification is present within the lesion. The well-defined contours and the coarse calcification suggest the possibility of a cystosarcoma phylloides, particularly in an elderly patient. Less likely in the differential diagnosis are a fibroadenoma (which probably would have degenerated to a greater degree and calcificd) and a well-circumscribed carcinoma.

IMPRESSION: Cystosarcoma phylloides versus fibroadenoma.

HISTOPATHOLOGY: Malignant cystosarcoma phylloides.

NOTE: The calcifications in a cystosarcoma are described as plaquelike and coarse.

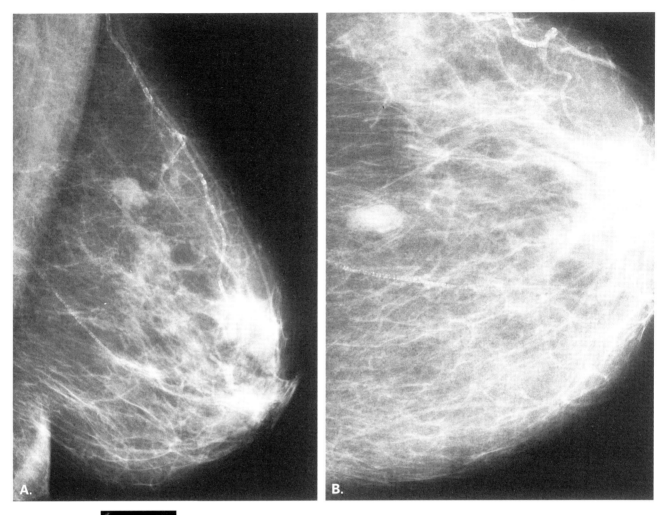

Figure 4.57

HISTORY: A 66-year-old woman for screening mammography.

MAMMOGRAPHY: Right MLO **(A)** and CC **(B)** views. There is a relatively circumscribed, 1.2-cm, oval isodense mass in the 12 o'clock position of the right breast. Sonography did not reveal a solid or cystic lesion. Because of the size of the lesion and the slight indistinctness of some of its margins, it was regarded with a moderate degree of suspicion.

HISTOPATHOLOGY: Sclerosing adenosis (adenosis tumor).

NOTE: It is unusual for sclerosing adenosis to present mammographically as a circumscribed mass. Generally, the appearance is that of an ill-defined lesion with lobular-type microcalcifications.

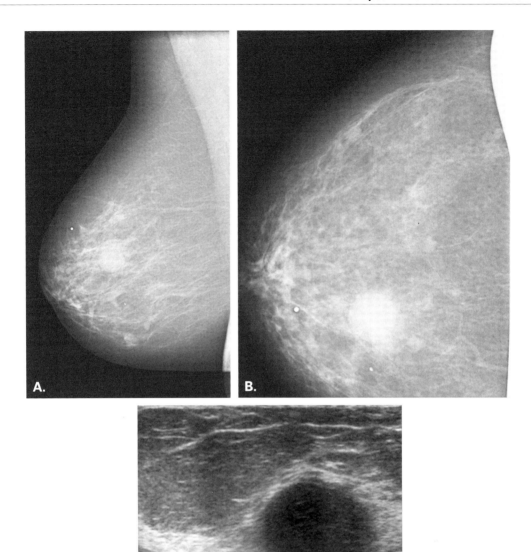

Figure 4.58

HISTORY: A 56-year-old woman with a history of uterine cancer who presents with a palpable left breast mass.

MAMMOGRAPHY: Left MLO **(A)** and spot magnification CC **(B)** views show the palpable mass to be round, very circumscribed, and isodense. Ultrasound **(C)** demonstrates the lesion to be hypoechoic, round, partially well defined, and to enhance the sound slightly. Because the sonographic features are not those of a simple cyst, but likely a complicated cyst, aspiration was performed. Thick turbid fluid was removed, and the lesion collapsed.

CYTOLOGY: Benign cyst fluid with histiocytes.

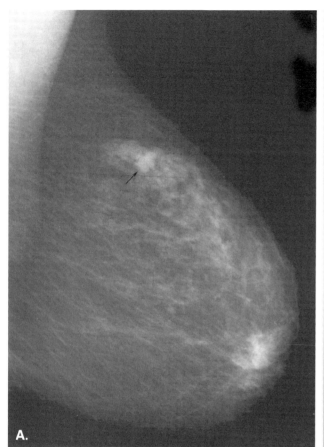

A.

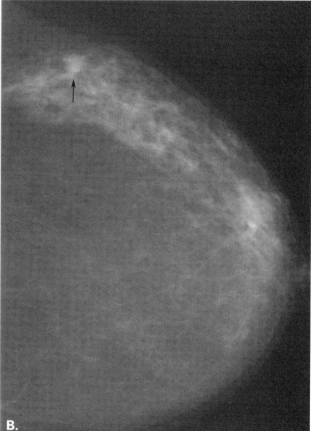

B.

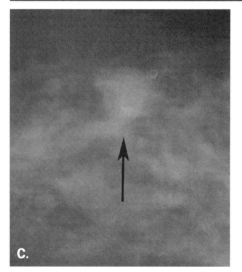

C.

Figure 4.59

HISTORY: A 51-year-old woman for screening mammography.

MAMMOGRAPHY: Right MLO **(A)** and CC **(B)** views show a small, dense, round, relatively circumscribed mass at the 11 o'clock position **(arrows)**. On the spot-compression CC view **(C)**, the borders appear microlobulated, which is suspicious. This mass is associated with focal density containing some punctuate microcalcifications.

IMPRESSION: Microlobulated mass, suspicious for malignancy.

HISTOPATHOLOGY: Focal intraductal hyperplasia, adenosis, apocrine metaplasia, and microcalcifications.

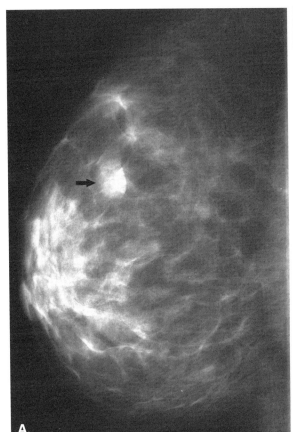

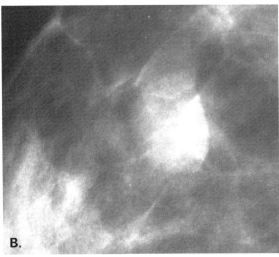

Figure 4.60

HISTORY: A 49-year-old woman for screening mammography.

MAMMOGRAPHY: Left MLO (**A**) and enlarged MLO (**B**) views show the breast to be heterogeneously dense. There is a lobulated isodense mass at 12 o'clock (**arrow**) with relatively circumscribed margins. Ultrasound showed the mass to be solid. Based on these findings, core needle biopsy was performed.

HISTOPATHOLOGY: Sclerosing adenosis, fibrocystic change.

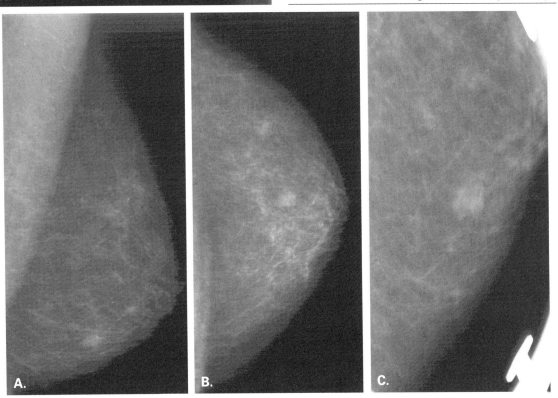

Figure 4.61

HISTORY: A 52-year-old woman for screening mammography.

MAMMOGRAPHY: Right MLO (**A**) and CC (**B**) views show scattered fibroglandular densities. There are two masses in the right breast. In the lateral area is a small lobulated mass that was stable from prior studies. At 6 o'clock is a lobular, isodense mass that appears circumscribed on spot compression (**C**). Ultrasound did not clearly demonstrate the lesion.

IMPRESSION: New solid circumscribed mass, right breast at 6 o'clock. Recommend biopsy.

HISTOPATHOLOGY: Fibrocystic changes with papillary apocrine metaplasia.

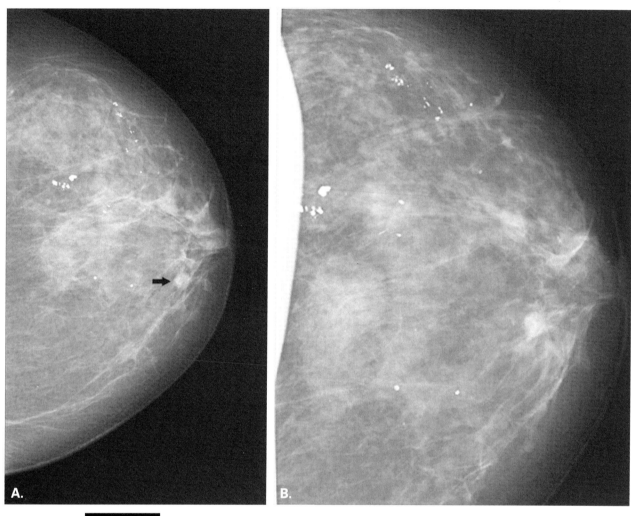

Figure 4.62

HISTORY: A 77-year-old woman with clear nipple discharge from the right breast.

MAMMOGRAPHY: Right CC **(A)** view demonstrates numerous dystrophic, coarse, and rodlike calcifications that are benign. In the right subareolar area medially is a small circumscribed mass **(arrow)**. On the magnification CC view **(B)**, the relatively circumscribed margin is seen, as well as vague, faint amorphous microcalcifications within the lesion.

IMPRESSION: Small subareolar mass, likely papilloma versus ductal carcinoma in situ. Recommend biopsy.

HISTOPATHOLOGY: Intraductal papilloma with atypical ductal hyperplasia.

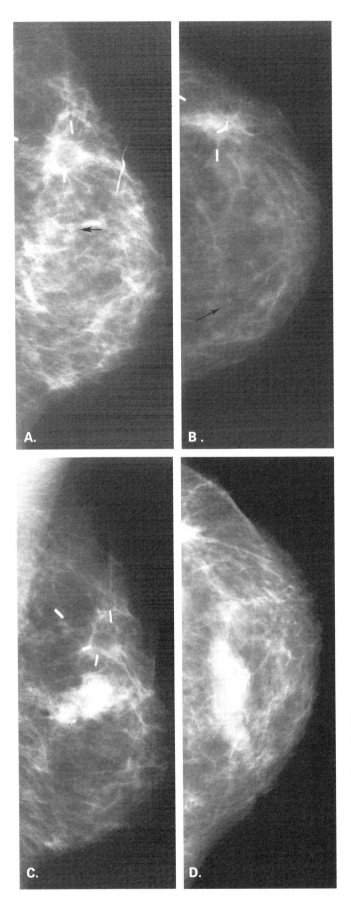

Figure 4.63

HISTORY: A 44-year-old patient postlumpectomy and in radiation therapy for breast cancer.

MAMMOGRAPHY: Right ML (**A**) and CC (**B**) views show the post-surgical scar as well as clustered microcalcifications located at 3 o'clock (**arrows**). Core needle biopsy of the calcifications was performed. On the immediate postprocedure ML and CC images (**C, D**), a marker is noted at the biopsy site. Surrounding the clip is a lobulated isodense mass that has developed since the prebiopsy images.

IMPRESSION: Hematoma secondary to needle biopsy.

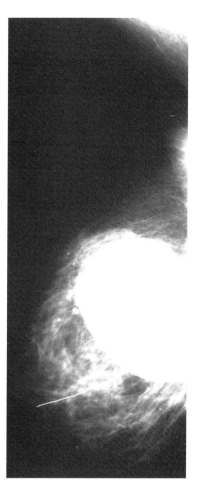

Figure 4.64

HISTORY: A 57-year-old woman who is recently postlumpectomy for breast cancer. The pretreatment mammogram has been performed to assess for residual carcinoma.

MAMMOGRAPHY: Left MLO view shows a large oval mass beneath the surgical scar. This mass has circumscribed margins and is isodense. Scattered benign calcifications are noted throughout the breast.

IMPRESSION: Normal postoperative change with hematoma/seroma at the lumpectomy site.

Figure 4.65

HISTORY: A 76-year-old woman 8 months after a lumpectomy for lobular carcinoma in situ in the left breast, with no palpable masses on physical examination.

MAMMOGRAPHY: Left MLO **(A)** and CC **(B)** views. There is a well-defined, moderately dense, round mass demonstrated on both views. This mass is situated directly beneath the surgical scar **(arrow)** from lumpectomy. Considering the history of recent biopsy in this region, a well-circumscribed hematoma was considered most likely.

IMPRESSION: Hematoma.

HISTOPATHOLOGY: Fibrous-walled cyst containing old blood.

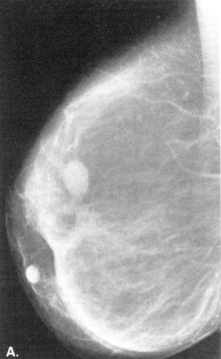
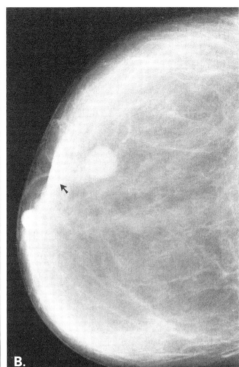

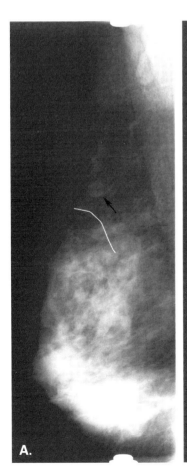
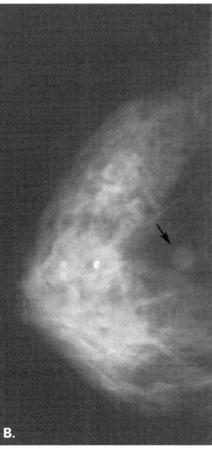
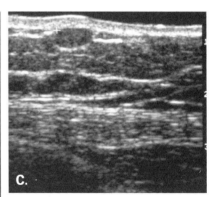

Figure 4.66

HISTORY: A 67-year-old with a small palpable mass in left breast at 12 o'clock.

MAMMOGRAPHY: Left MLO **(A)** and CC **(B)** views show a round circumscribed mass in the superior aspect of the breast **(arrow)**. Ultrasound **(C)** shows the mass to be hypoechoic, smoothly marginated, and located within the dermis. There is no separation between the skin line and the anterior surface of the lesion, suggesting a dermal origin.

IMPRESSION: Sebaceous cyst.

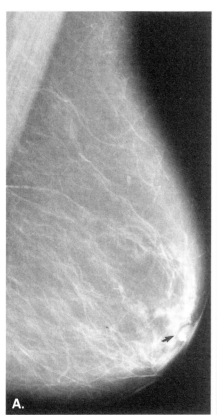

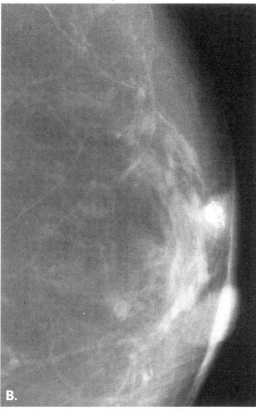

Figure 4.67

HISTORY: A 65-year-old gravida 1, para 1 woman for routine screening.

MAMMOGRAPHY: Right MLO **(A)** and enlarged (2×) CC **(B)** views. There is scattered fibroglandular tissue present. In the right supra-areolar area, there is a well-circumscribed mass attached to the skin **(arrow) (A)**. Coarse calcifications are present within the mass **(A and B)**. The subcutaneous location of the mass is key to the diagnosis of a sebaceous cyst. Clinical examination also showed a firm nodule within the skin. The calcifications are dystrophic, related to chronically retained secretions.

IMPRESSION: Sebaceous cyst of right breast.

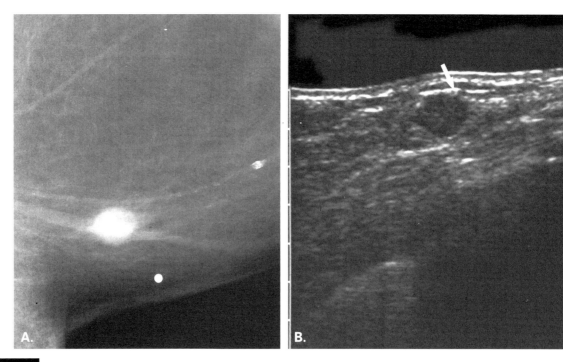

Figure 4.68

HISTORY: A 74-year-old woman with a small palpable mass in the parasternal area of the right breast.

MAMMOGRAPHY: Right CC spot view **(A)** shows a BB demonstrating the palpable lump, which is a small, dense, round circumscribed mass located superficially. On ultrasound **(B)**, the mass is hypoechoic and smoothly marginated, and it is located in the subcutaneous area. There is an extension **(arrow)** from the mass to the skin, typical of the findings in a sebaceous cyst. Clinical exam confirmed the presence of an occluded pore in the skin over the lesion.

IMPRESSION: Sebaceous cyst.

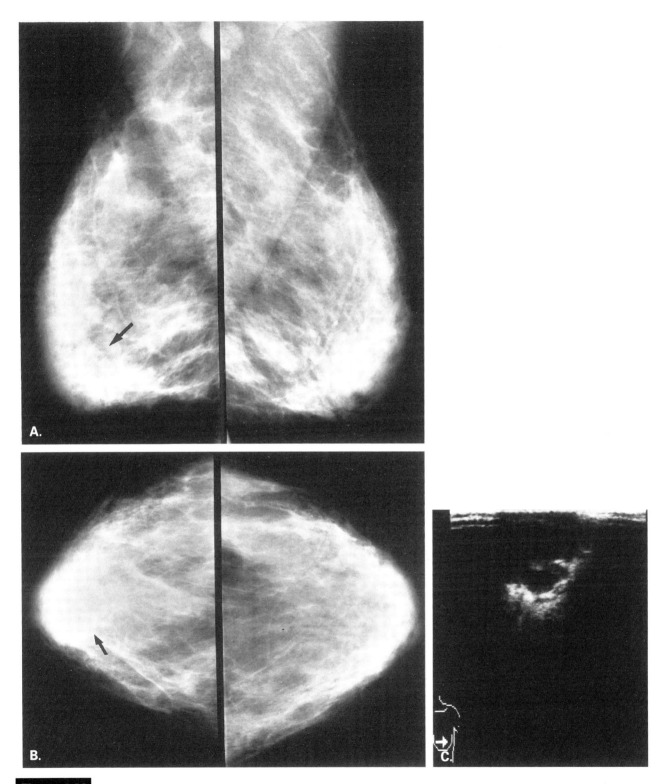

Figure 4.69

HISTORY: A 46-year-old woman with an acute, very tender, indurated mass in the left subareolar area.

MAMMOGRAPHY: Bilateral MLO (**A**) and CC (**B**) views and left breast ultrasound (**C**). Asymmetry in the appearance of the breasts is present (**A** and **B**), with the left breast being more dense, particularly in the subareolar area, than the right. Beneath the left nipple is a well-circumscribed isodense mass (**arrow**). On ultrasound (**C**), the mass is complex, having an irregular wall and some internal echoes. The combination of findings on imaging and clinical examination is most consistent with a breast abscess.

IMPRESSION: Abscess.

NOTE: The lesion was aspirated of purulent material and resolved after treatment with antibiotics.

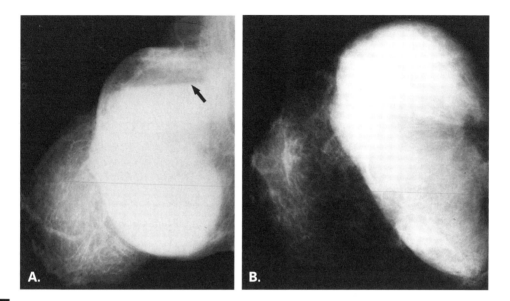

Figure 4.70

HISTORY: A 71-year-old woman who had been in a car accident several weeks earlier and sustained a puncture wound to the left breast. She presents now with a large painful mass.

MAMMOGRAPHY: Left MLO **(A)** and CC **(B)** views show a very large, isodense lobular mass that has well-defined margins. An air-fluid level **(arrow)** is seen in the superior aspect of the mass. The clinical history and symptoms and the mammographic findings were most consistent with either an abscess or a large hematoma with air related to the puncture. The cavity was drained of purulent material.

IMPRESSION: Breast abscess secondary to trauma.

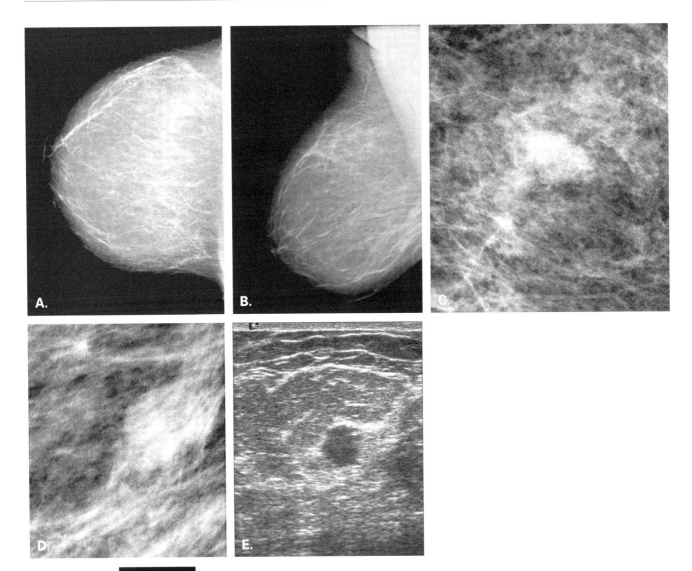

Figure 4.71

HISTORY: A 49-year-old woman with a positive family history of breast cancer, for screening.

MAMMOGRAPHY: Left CC (**A**) and MLO (**B**) views show a small oval mass in the lower-outer quadrant. On the enlarged images (**C, D**), the relatively circumscribed margins of the mass are seen. Ultrasound (**E**) shows the mass to be round and hypoechoic with irregular margins and surrounding hyperechogenicity. The sonographic features are much more suspicious than the mammographic findings.

IMPRESSION: Solid mass, highly suspicious for carcinoma.

HISTOPATHOLOGY: High-grade invasive ductal carcinoma.

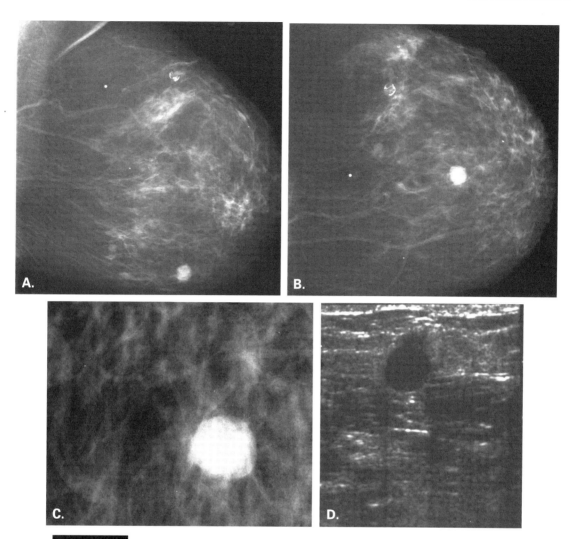

Figure 4.72

HISTORY: A 63-year-old woman with a small palpable mass in the right breast.

MAMMOGRAPHY: Right MLO **(A)** and CC **(B)** views show a round, relatively circumscribed, high-density mass at 5 o'clock. On spot compression **(C)**, the circumscribed border is seen, with slight indistinctness at the posterior edge. On ultrasound **(D)**, the mass is very hypoechoic, taller than wide, and slightly irregular in contour. The high density of the mass on mammography and the sonographic features are very suspicious for malignancy.

IMPRESSION: Highly suspicious for carcinoma, BI-RADS® 5.

HISTOPATHOLOGY: High-grade invasive ductal carcinoma.

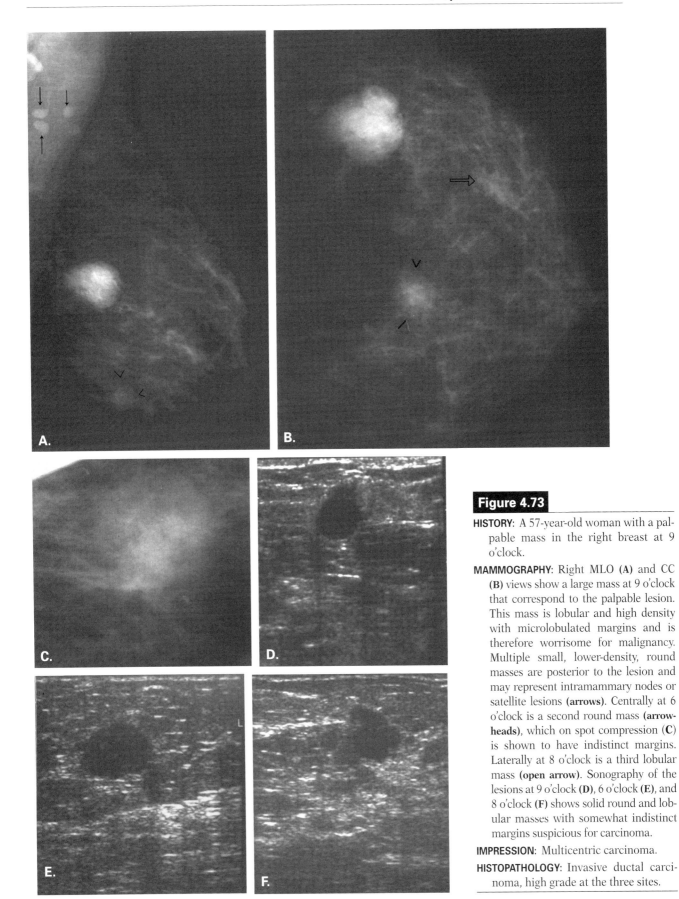

Figure 4.73

HISTORY: A 57-year-old woman with a palpable mass in the right breast at 9 o'clock.

MAMMOGRAPHY: Right MLO (**A**) and CC (**B**) views show a large mass at 9 o'clock that correspond to the palpable lesion. This mass is lobular and high density with microlobulated margins and is therefore worrisome for malignancy. Multiple small, lower-density, round masses are posterior to the lesion and may represent intramammary nodes or satellite lesions (**arrows**). Centrally at 6 o'clock is a second round mass (**arrowheads**), which on spot compression (**C**) is shown to have indistinct margins. Laterally at 8 o'clock is a third lobular mass (**open arrow**). Sonography of the lesions at 9 o'clock (**D**), 6 o'clock (**E**), and 8 o'clock (**F**) shows solid round and lobular masses with somewhat indistinct margins suspicious for carcinoma.

IMPRESSION: Multicentric carcinoma.

HISTOPATHOLOGY: Invasive ductal carcinoma, high grade at the three sites.

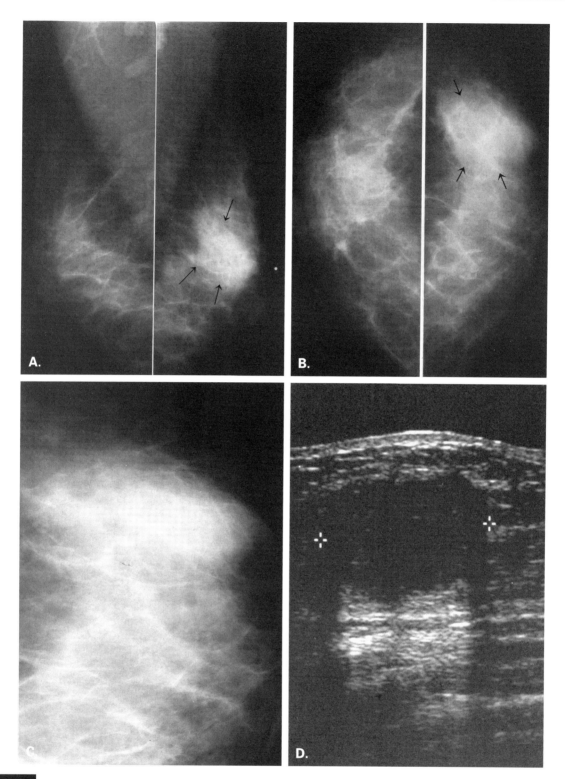

Figure 4.74

HISTORY: A 41-year-old woman with a palpable right breast mass.

MAMMOGRAPHY: Bilateral MLO (A) and CC (B) views show an obscured round mass (arrow) at the site of palpable abnormality. On spot compression (C), the borders remain obscured. Ultrasound (D) shows a markedly hypoechoic round mass with slightly irregular margins and acoustic enhancement. The low-level echoes, round shape, and slightly indistinct edges are suspicious for malignancy.

IMPRESSION: Mass, suspicious for carcinoma.

HISTOPATHOLOGY: Invasive ductal carcinoma.

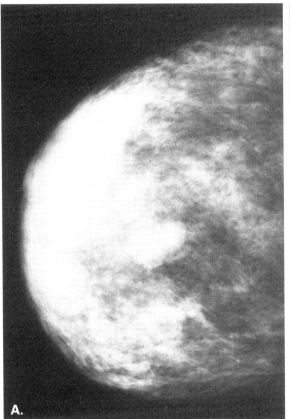

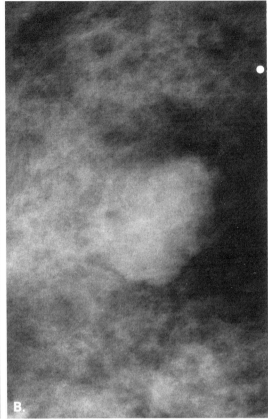

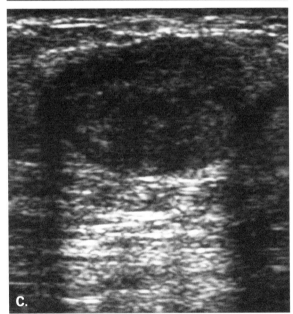

Figure 4.75

HISTORY: A 76-year-old woman with a left palpable mass.

MAMMOGRAPHY: Left CC (**A**) view shows a lobular isodense mass marked with a BB. On spot compression (**B**), the mass is noted to have microlobulated margins, which is a suspicious finding. Ultrasound (**C**) shows the mass to be relatively circumscribed, round, and associated with increased transmission of sound. The finding could represent a fibroadenoma, circumscribed malignancy, or complicated cystic lesion. Because of the microlobulation and the somewhat rounded appearance on ultrasound, malignancy is most likely.

IMPRESSION: Microlobulated mass suspicious for carcinoma.

HISTOPATHOLOGY: Invasive ductal carcinoma with extensive mucinous features.

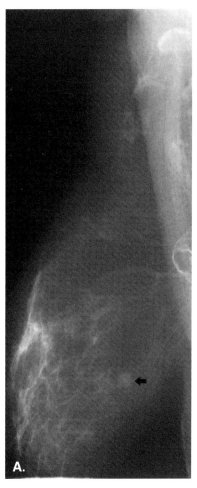

A.

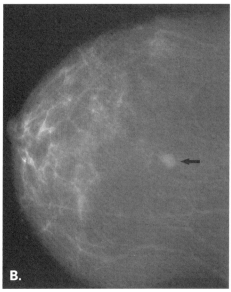

B.

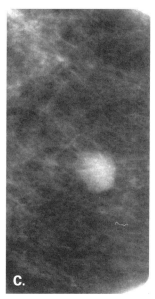

C.

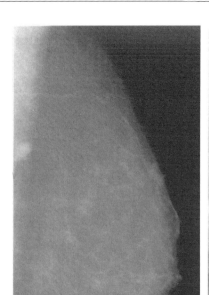

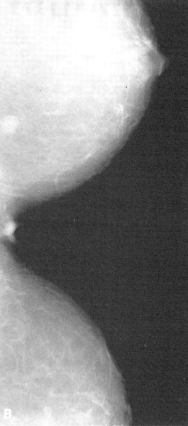

A.

B.

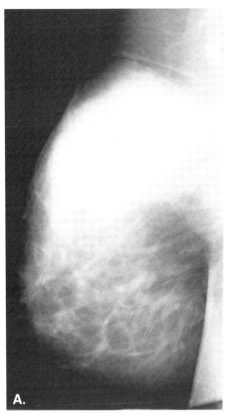

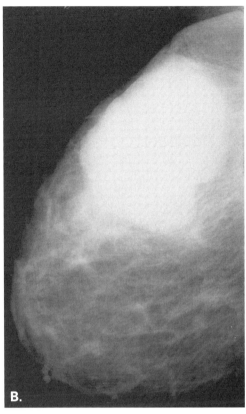

Figure 4.78

HISTORY: A 46-year-old woman with a palpable mass in the upper-outer aspect of the left breast.

MAMMOGRAPHY: Left MLO (**A**) and CC (**B**) views show a large, high-density, lobular mass with relatively circumscribed margins. In some areas, the borders are somewhat indistinct. The differential diagnosis included phylloides tumor versus carcinoma.

IMPRESSION: Highly suspicious for malignancy, BI-RADS® 5.

HISTOPATHOLOGY: Medullary carcinoma.

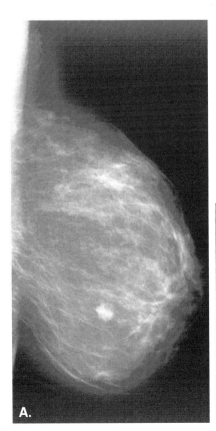

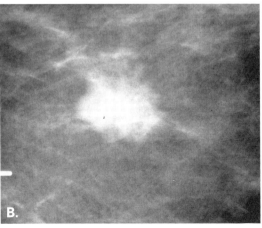

Figure 4.79

HISTORY: A 49 year-old woman recalled from screening for a right breast mass.

MAMMOGRAPHY: Right ML view (**A**) shows a small round mass with microlobulated margins in the central aspect of the breast. On a spot digital image (**B**), the undulating border associated with microlobulation is evident and is suspicious for carcinoma.

IMPRESSION: Microlobulated mass, suspicious for carcinoma.

HISTOPATHOLOGY: Invasive ductal carcinoma, nuclear grade 2.

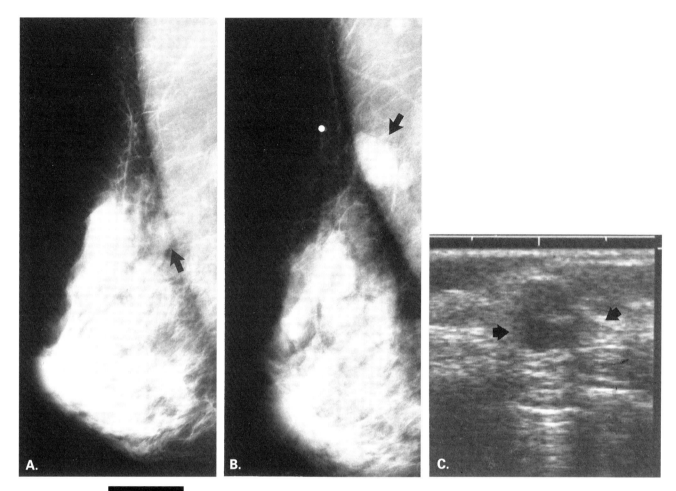

Figure 4.80

HISTORY: A 37-year-old gravida 1, para 1 woman with a positive family history of breast cancer and a palpable 2-cm lump in the left upper-outer quadrant.

MAMMOGRAPHY: Left MLO **(A)** and exaggerated CC lateral **(B)** views and ultrasound **(C)**. There is a relatively well-circumscribed mass in the left upper-outer quadrant **(arrow) (A** and **B)**. The mass is of medium to high density, and although it is relatively circumscribed, its borders are microlobulated, suggesting a malignant etiology. On ultrasound **(C)**, the mass is hypoechoic with mixed echogenicity, and it has irregular borders **(arrow)**. Such findings are more consistent with a malignant lesion than with a benign lesion such as a fibroadenoma.

IMPRESSION: Highly suspicious for primary carcinoma.

HISTOPATHOLOGY: Adenocarcinoma with 24 nodes negative.

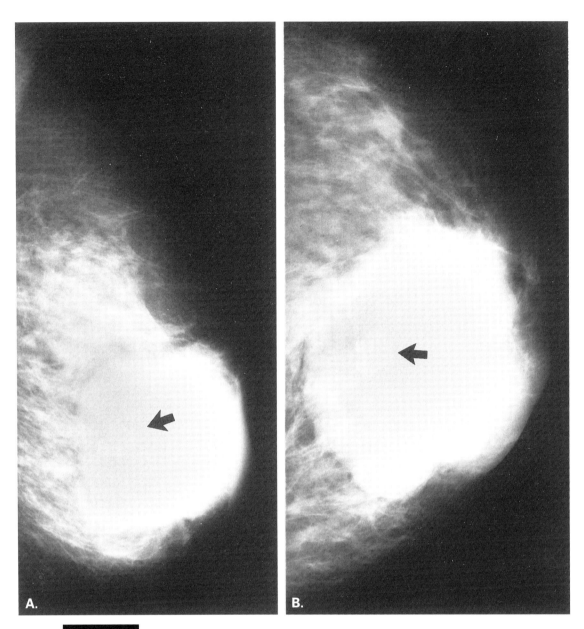

Figure 4.81

HISTORY: A 73-year-old woman with a large palpable right breast mass.

MAMMOGRAPHY: Right MLO **(A)** and CC **(B)** views. There is a large, high-density, relatively circumscribed mass in the central aspect of the right breast. The borders of the mass are microlobulated and poorly defined in areas. A single area of coarse calcification **(arrow)** is present within the lesion. The differential diagnosis for the mass includes cystosarcoma phylloides, primary breast cancer, and a calcifying fibroadenoma; the favored diagnosis is a cystosarcoma phylloides because of the borders, large size, and the coarse calcification.

HISTOPATHOLOGY: Infiltrating ductal carcinoma.

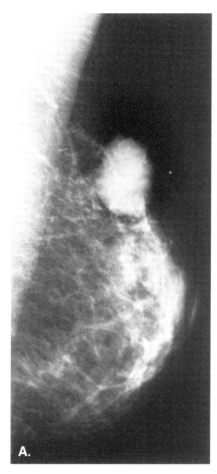

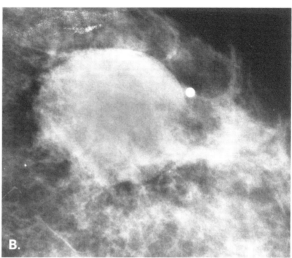

HISTORY: Elderly patient who presents with a new palpable lump in the right breast.

MAMMOGRAPHY: Right MLO **(A)** and spot-magnification CC **(B)** views over the palpable lesion show an oval, relatively circumscribed isodense mass. On the spot view, some of the borders are very well defined, but others are more indistinct or obscured. Because of the partially indistinct margins, carcinoma is of concern. Sonography showed the mass to be solid.

IMPRESSION: Suspicious for carcinoma.

HISTOPATHOLOGY: Invasive ductal carcinoma.

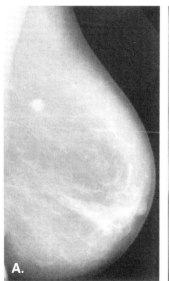

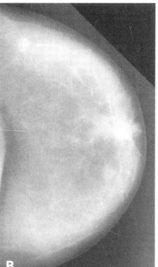

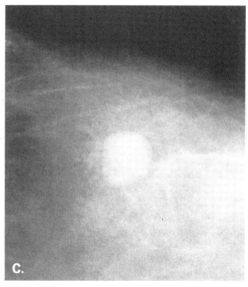

HISTORY: A 74-year-old woman with a tender right breast and no palpable findings.

MAMMOGRAPHY: Right MLO **(A)** and CC **(B)** views and magnified image **(C)**. There is a very-well-defined 1-cm mass in the right upper-outer quadrant. A magnified view shows the very-well-defined margins and fatty halo, suggesting a benign nature. Because of the location of the lesion, a primary consideration was an enlarged intramammary lymph node. Other considerations were fibroadenoma, cyst, and well-circumscribed malignancy.

IMPRESSION: Well-defined mass of low suspicion for malignancy.

HISTOPATHOLOGY: Adenoid cystic carcinoma.

NOTE: The prognosis for a patient with adenoid cystic carcinoma is excellent. Axillary node metastasis is rare, and distant metastases occur in less than 10% of cases.

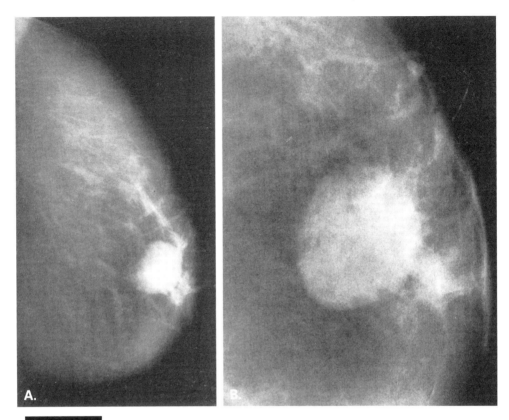

Figure 4.84

HISTORY: A 69-year-old gravida 0 woman with adenocarcinoma in a right axillary node.

MAMMOGRAPHY: Right MLO view **(A)** and magnified image **(B)**. The breasts show fatty replacement compatible with the age of the patient. There is relatively well-defined, moderately dense 2.5-cm mass in the subareolar area. A magnified image demonstrates fine irregularity of the borders of the lesion, rendering it suspicious in nature. Particularly in a patient of this age group, carcinoma is the most likely consideration.

IMPRESSION: Well-circumscribed carcinoma, possibly of medullary or mucinous type.

HISTOPATHOLOGY: Medullary carcinoma.

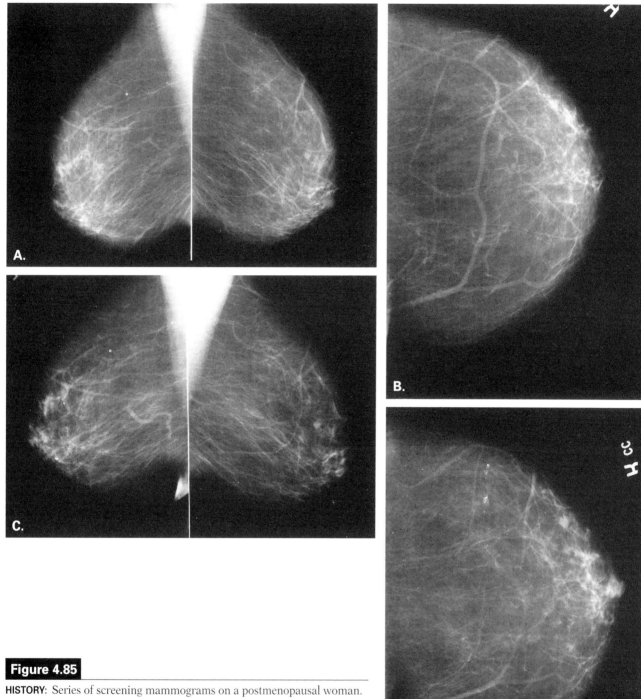

Figure 4.85

HISTORY: Series of screening mammograms on a postmenopausal woman.

MAMMOGRAPHY: Initial bilateral MLO and right CC views **(A, B)**, MLO and right CC views 1 year later **(C, D)**, and bilateral MLO and right CC views **(E, F)** 2 years later. On the initial study, a small, isodense, relatively circumscribed mass is noted at 10 o'clock in the anterior third of the right breast **(arrows)**. No additional evaluation was performed. On subsequent study at 1 **(C, D)** year, the mass has increased in size and density. (*continued*)

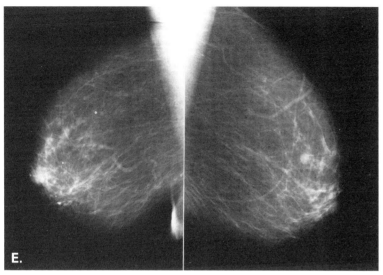

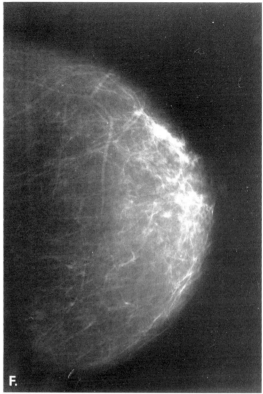

Figure 4.85 *(CONTINUED)*

On subsequent study at 2 years **(E, F)**, the mass has increased in size and density. Because of the change on the final study, biopsy was performed.

IMPRESSION: Suspicious for carcinoma. BI-RADS® 4.

HISTOPATHOLOGY: Intracystic papillary carcinoma.

NOTE: Papillary carcinoma is one of the types of cancer that tends to be well defined. On the initial study, further workup—including spot compression and ultrasound—should have been performed. Any increase is sign of a circumscribed mass and warrants biopsy if the mass is not a cyst.

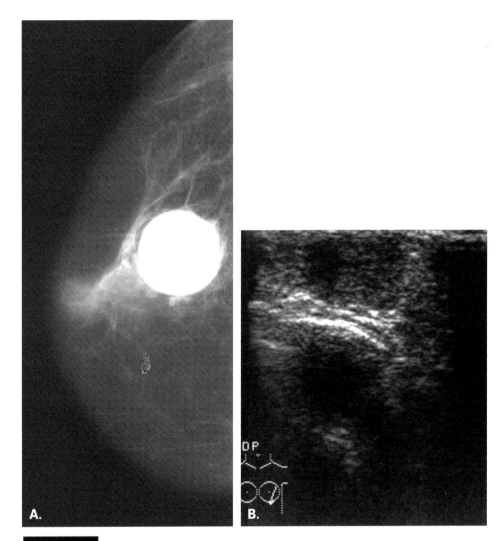

Figure 4.86

HISTORY: A 62-year-old woman with a palpable left breast mass.

MAMMOGRAPHY: Left CC **(A)** view shows a large, very dense round mass in the center of the breast. The borders are slightly indistinct in areas, but the mass is relatively circumscribed. Sonography **(B)** reveals the mass to be isoechoic, rounded, and well defined. Based on the slight indistinctness of the margins on mammography and the rounded appearance on ultrasound, malignancy of concern. Biopsy was performed.

IMPRESSION: Solid circumscribed mass, suspicious: carcinoma versus fibroadenoma versus phylloides tumor.

HISTOPATHOLOGY: Intracystic papillary carcinoma.

NOTE: Sometimes on ultrasound, the cystic and solid components of an intracystic neoplasm are evident. In other cases, as in this patient, the tumor completely fills the cyst cavity and the fluid is no longer evident. (Case courtesy of Dr. Axel Ongre, Oslo, Norway.)

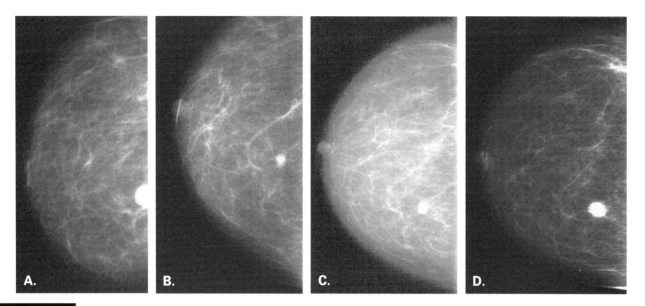

Figure 4.87

HISTORY: An 87-year-old woman with a series of screening mammograms.

MAMMOGRAPHY: Left CC views in 1989 (**A**), 1990 (**B**), 1992 (**C**), and 1995 (**D**). There is a dense, round, circumscribed mass in the left inner quadrant on the initial study (**A**). This was not further evaluated and decreased in size on the study 2 years later (**B**). It remained stable the next year (**C**) and subsequently increased in size and density on the study 3 years later. At this point, it was excised.

HISTOPATHOLOGY: Mucoepidermoid carcinoma.

NOTE: Although it is rare for a breast cancer to decrease in size, those with a mucinous component may do so. On the initial study, further evaluation should have been performed because of the suspicious density of the lesion. (Case courtesy of Dr. Thomas Poulton, Canton, Ohio.)

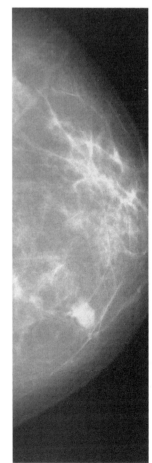

Figure 4.88

HISTORY: A 47-year-old woman with a history of carcinoma of the fallopian tube.

MAMMOGRAPHY: Right coned-down CC view shows heterogeneously dense tissue. There is an oval, dense, relatively circumscribed mass located medially in the anterior third of the breast. The mass was not cystic on ultrasound. Because of the indistinct posterior edge, biopsy was performed.

IMPRESSION: Mass, slightly indistinct. Recommend biopsy.

HISTOPATHOLOGY: Metastatic carcinoma from the fallopian tube.

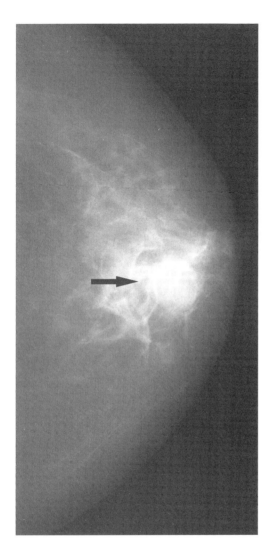

Figure 4.89

HISTORY: A 61-year-old woman with a history of ovarian cancer and a firm lump in the right breast.

MAMMOGRAPHY: Right CC view. There is a 2-cm, well-defined radiodense mass **(arrow)** in the right breast at 12 o'clock. There is a fatty halo around a portion of the lesion. The primary differential diagnoses include cyst, fibroadenoma, well-defined primary breast cancer, and metastasis to the breast. In a patient of this age, a fibroadenoma would very likely have begun to calcify. Therefore, malignancy, either primary or secondary, is more likely.

HISTOPATHOLOGY: Adenocarcinoma metastatic from ovarian primary.

NOTE: Metastatic disease to the breast may present as a solitary well-defined mass, usually located in the subcutaneous fat layer. More common primary sites for metastases to the breast are melanoma, lymphoma, sarcoma, lung, and gynecologic cancers.

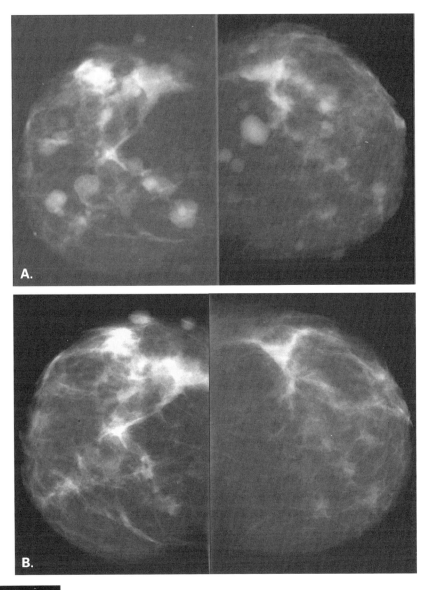

Figure 4.90

HISTORY: A 61-year-old woman for routine screening mammography. She was not on hormonal replacement therapy.

MAMMOGRAPHY: Bilateral CC views **(A)** and CC views 1 year earlier **(B)**. On the current study **(A)**, there are numerous dense, round, circumscribed masses in both breasts. These masses had developed since the prior study. Multiple cysts are included in the differential for round masses; however, the postmenopausal state of the patient and the lack of hormonal replacement therapy make cysts an unlikely etiology. Ultrasound showed solid masses.

IMPRESSION: Numerous new round masses favor metastases or lymphoma.

HISTOPATHOLOGY: Non-Hodgkin's lymphoma.

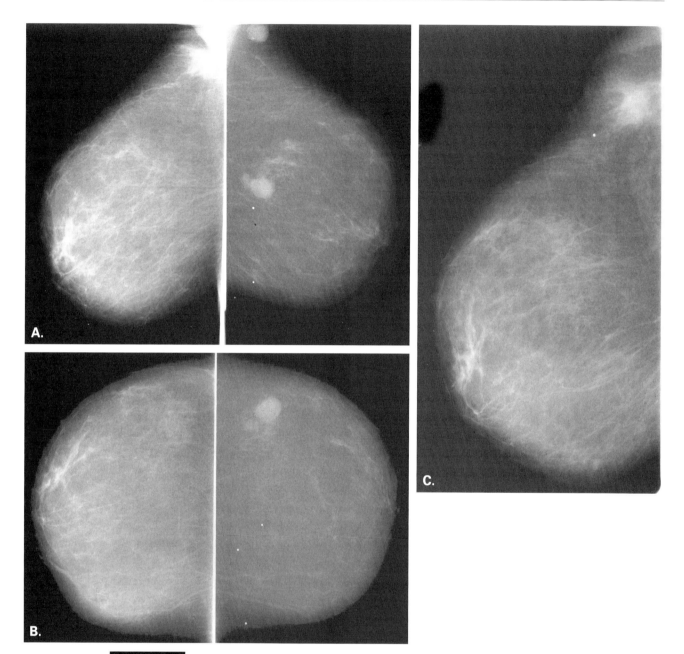

Figure 4.91

HISTORY: A 40-year-old woman with history of melanoma, for screening mammography.

MAMMOGRAPHY: Bilateral MLO (**A**) and CC (**B**) views show multiple abnormalities bilaterally. In the left axillary tail is a spiculated mass, appearing more vague on the exaggerated CC lateral (**C**) view. This was the site of lymph-node dissection following the prior melanoma resection. On the right, there are three round circumscribed masses, one of which is located in the axilla. These were solid on sonography. Although these could be benign—lymph nodes or fibroadenomata—metastatic melanoma is a likely possibility.

IMPRESSION: Left axillary node dissection scar, metastatic melanoma to the right breast.

HISTOPATHOLOGY: Metastatic melanoma, right breast.

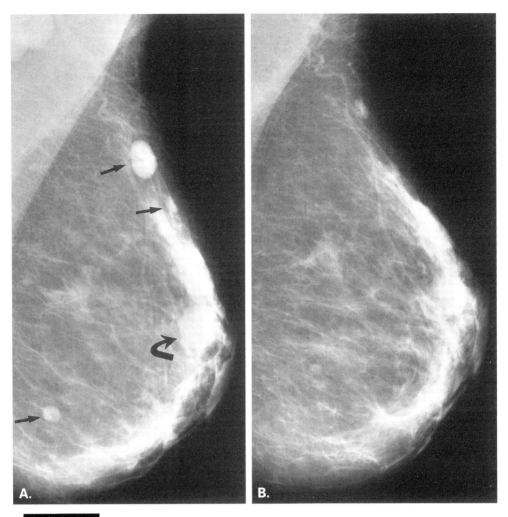

Figure 4.92

HISTORY: A 45-year-old gravida 3, para 3 patient with a history of lymphoma and a palpable nodule in the right retroareolar area.

MAMMOGRAPHY: Right MLO views from April 1989 **(A)** and July 1989 **(B)**, after chemotherapy for lymphoma. On the initial study, there are three bean-shaped, very-well-circumscribed nodules **(straight arrows)** in the right breast, as well as a partially circumscribed, round isodense mass **(curved arrow)** in the subareolar area. The subareolar mass was shown to be a simple cyst on ultrasound. The bean-shaped nodules are most consistent with adenopathy related to the patient's known lymphoma. Following chemotherapy **(B)**, the nodes decreased in size to a normal range. Mammography may be useful for monitoring the response to chemotherapy in patients in whom there is axillary or intramammary adenopathy.

IMPRESSION: Adenopathy secondary to lymphoma.

REFERENCES

1. Teixidor HS, Kazam E. Combined mammographic-sonographic evaluation of breast masses. *AJR Am J Roentgenol* 1977;128:409–417.
2. Jackson VP, Dines KA, Bassett LW, et al. Diagnostic importance of the radiographic density of noncalcified breast masses: analysis of 91 lesions. *AJR Am J Roentgenol* 1991;157:25–28.
3. Gershon-Cohen J, Schorr S. The diagnostic problems of isolated circumscribed breast tumors. *AJR Am J Roentgenol* 1969;106:863–870.
4. Martin JE. *Atlas of Mammography.* Baltimore: Williams & Wilkins, 1982.
5. Wolfe JN. *Xeroradiography of the Breast.* Springfield, IL: Charles C. Thomas, 1972.
6. Lane EJ, Proto AV, Phillips TW. Mach bands and density perception. *Radiology* 1976;121:9–17.
7. Swann CA, Kopans DB, Koerner FC, et al. The halo sign and malignant breast tissues. *AJR Am J Roentgenol* 1978;149:1145–1147.
8. Fournier DV, Weber W, Hoeffken M, et al. Growth rate of 147 mammary carcinomas. *Cancer* 1980;45:2198–2207.
9. Heuser L, Spratt J, Polk H. Growth rates of primary breast cancer. *Cancer* 1979;43:1888–1894.
10. Meyer JE, Kopans DB. Stability of a mammographic mass: a false sense of security. *AJR Am J Roentgenol* 1981;137:595–598.
11. Wolfe J. *Xeroradiography: Uncalcified Breast Masses.* Springfield, IL: Charles C. Thomas, 1977.
12. DiPiro PJ, Meyer JE, Frenna TH, et al. Seat belt injuries of the breast: findings on mammography and sonography. *AJR Am J Roentgenol* 1995;164:317–320.
13. Bassett LW, Gold RH, Cove HC. Mammographic spectrum of traumatic fat necrosis: the fallibility of "pathognomonic" sign of carcinoma. *AJR Am J Roentgenol* 1978;130:119–122.
14. Leborgne R. Esteato necrosis quistica calcificade de la mama. *Torace* 1967;16:172–175.
15. Park KY, Oh KK, Noh TW. Steatocystoma multiplex: mammographic and sonographic manifestations. *AJR Am J Roentgenol* 2003;180(1):271–274.
16. Gomez A, Mata JM, Donoso L, et al. Galactocele: three distinctive radiographic appearances. *Radiology* 1986;158:43–44.
17. Salvador R, Salvador M, Jimenez JA, et al. Galactocele of the breast: radiologic and ultrasonographic findings. *Br J Radiol* 1990;63:140–142.
18. Hessler C, Schnyder P, Ozzello L. Hamartoma of the breast: diagnostic observation of 16 cases. *Radiology* 1978;126:95–98.
19. Anderson I, Hildell J, Linell F, et al. Mammary hamartomas. Acta Radiol (Diagn) 1979;20:712–720.
20. Ljungqvist U, Anderson I, Hildell J, et al. Mammary hamartoma, a benign breast lesion. *Acta Chir Scand* 1979;145:227–230.
21. Abbitt PL, Shaw de Paredes E, Sloop FB. Breast hamartoma: a mammographic diagnosis. *South Med J* 1988;8:167–170.
22. Helvie MA, Adler DD, Rebner M, et al. Breast hamartomas: variable mammographic appearance. *Radiology* 1989;170:417–421.
23. Kopans DB, Meyer JE, Proppe KH. Ultrasonographic, xeromammographic and histologic correlation of a fibroadenolipoma of the breast. *J Clin Ultrasound* 1982;10:409–411.
24. Andersson I. Mammography in clinical practice. *Med Radiogr Photogr* 1986;62:2.
25. Egan RL, McSweeney MB. Intramammary lymph nodes. *Cancer* 1983;51:1838–1842.
26. Andersson I, Marshall L, Nilsson B, et al. Abnormal axillary lymph nodes in rheumatoid arthritis. *Acta Radiol (Diagn)* 1980;21:645–649.
27. Lazarus AA. Sarcoidosis. *Otolaryngol Clin North Am* 1982;15:621–633.
28. van Dam PA, Van Goethem MLA, Kersschot E, et al. Palpable solid breast masses: retrospective single- and multimodality evaluation of 201 lesions. *Radiology* 1988;166:435–439.
29. Skaane P, Engedal K. Analysis of sonographic features in the differentiation of fibroadenoma and invasive ductal carcinoma. *AJR Am J Roentgenol* 1998;170:109–114.
30. Stavros AT, Thickman D, Rapp CL, et al. Solid breast nodules: use of sonography to distinguish between benign and malignant lesions. *Radiology* 1995;196:123–134.
31. Boyle CA, Gertrud BS, LiVoisi VA, et al. Caffeine consumption and fibrocystic breast disease: a case-control epidemiologic study. *J Natl Cancer Inst* 1984;72:1015–1019.
32. Allen SS, Froberg DG. The effect of decreased caffeine consumption on benign proliferative breast disease: a randomized clinical trial. *Surgery* 1987;101(6):720–730.
33. Azzopardi JG. Cystic disease: duct ectasia: fat necrosis: fibrous disease of the breast. In: *Problems in Breast Pathology,* vol. 11: *Major Problems in Pathology.* London: WB Saunders, 1979, 57–89.
34. Gershon-Cohen J, Ingleby H. Roentgenography of cysts of the breast. *Surg Gynecol Obstet* 1953;97:483–489.
35. Berg WA, Campassi CI, Ioffe OB. Cystic lesions of the breast: sonographic-pathologic correlation. *Radiology* 2003;227:183–191.
36. Mitnick JS, Vazquez MF, Harris MN, et al. Invasive papillary carcinoma of the breast: mammographic appearance. *Radiology* 1990;177:803–806.
37. Bilroth CAT. Die Krankheiten der Weiblichen Brustdrush. *Disch Chir* 1880;41:32,72.
38. Hoeffken W, Lanyi M. Fibroadenoma. In: *Mammography.* Philadelphia: WB Saunders, 1977.
39. Dupont WD, Page DL, Parl FF, et al. Long-term risk of breast cancer in women with fibroadenoma. *N Engl J Med* 1994;331:10–15.
40. Carty NJ, Carter C, Rubin C, et al. Management of fibroadenoma of the breast. *Ann R Coll Surg Engl* 1995;77:127–130.
41. McDivitt RW, Stewart FW, Berg JW. Tumors of the breast. Bethesda, MD: Armed Forces Institute of Pathology, 1968.
42. Foster ME, Garrahan N, Williams S. Fibroadenoma of the breast: a clinical and pathological study. *JR Coll Surg Edinb* 1988;33:16–19.
43. Gershon-Cohen J. Ingleby H. Roentgenography of fibroadenoma of the breast. *Radiology* 1952;59:77–87.
44. Fornage BD, Lorigan JG, Andry E. Fibroadenoma of the breast: sonographic appearance. *Radiology* 1989;172:671–675.
45. Buzanowski-Konakry K, Harrison EG, Payne WS. Lobular carcinoma arising in fibroadenoma of the breast. *Cancer* 1975;35:450–456.
46. McDivitt RW, Stewart FW, Farrow JH. Breast carcinoma arising in solitary fibroadenomas. *Surg Gynecol Obstet* 1967;125:572–576.
47. Baker KS, Monsees BS, Diaz NM, et al. Carcinoma within fibroadenomas: mammographic features. *Radiology* 1990;176:371–374.
48. Weinstein SP, Orel SG, Collazzo L, et al. Cyclosporin A—induced fibroadenomas of the breast: report of five cases. *Radiology* 2001;220:465–468.
49. Baildam AD, Higgans RM, Hurley E, et al. Cyclosporin A and multiple fibroadenomas of the breast. *Br J Surg* 1996;83:1755–1757.
50. Rolles K, Caine RY. Two cases of benign lumps after treatment with cyclosporin A [Letter]. *Lancet* 1980;2:795.
51. Hajdu SI, Espinosa MH, Robbins GF. Recurrent cystosarcoma phylloides: a clinicopathologic study of 32 cases. *Cancer* 1976;38:1402–1406.
52. D'Orsi CJ, Feldhaus L, Sonnenfeld M. Unusual lesions of the breast. *Radiol Clin North Am* 1983;21:67–80.
53. Haagensen CD. Cystosarcoma phylloides. In: *Diseases of the Breast.* Philadelphia: WB Saunders, 1986.
54. Gershon-Cohen J, Moore L. Roentgenography of giant fibroadenoma of the breast (cystosarcoma phylloides). *Radiology* 1960;74:619–625.
55. Page JE, Williams JE. The radiological features of phylloides tumour of the breast with clinico-pathological correlation. *Clin Radiol* 1991;44:8–12.
56. Azzopardi JG. Sarcomas of the Breast. In: *Breast Pathology,* vol. 11: *Major Problems in Pathology.* London: WB Saunders, 1979.
57. Tavassoli FA. *Pathology of the Breast.* Norwalk, CT: Appleton & Lange, 1992;50–51.

58. Rosen EL, Soo MS, Bentley RC. Focal fibrosis: a common breast lesion diagnosed at imaging-guided core biopsy. *AJR Am J Roentgenol* 1999;173:1657–1662.

59. DiPiro PJ, Gulizia JA, Lester SC, et al. Mammographic and sonographic appearances of nodular adenosis. *AJR Am J Roentgenol* 2000;175:31–34.

60. Nielsen SM, Nielsen BB. Mammographic features of sclerosing adenosis presenting as a tumour. *Clin Radiol* 1986;37:371–373.

61. Page DL, Salhany KE, Jensen RA, et al. Subsequent breast carcinoma risk after biopsy with atypia in a breast papilloma. *Cancer* 1996;78:258–266.

62. Kraus FT, Neubecker RD. The differential diagnosis of papillary tumours of the breast. *Cancer* 1962;15:444–455.

63. Gutman H, Schachter J, Wasserberg N, et al. Are solitary breast papillomas entirely benign? *Arch Surg* 2003;138(12):1330–1333.

64. Haagenson CD. Solitary intraductal papilloma. In: *Diseases of the Breast*. Philadelphia: WB Saunders, 1986.

65. Polger MR, Denison CM, Lester S, et al. Pseudoangiomatous stromal hyperplasia: mammographic and sonographic appearances. *AJR Am J Roentgenol* 1996;166:349–352.

66. James K, Bridger J, Anthony PP. Breast tumour of pregnancy ('lactating' adenoma). *J Pathol* 1988;156:37–44.

67. Sumkin JH, Perrone AM, Harris KM, et al. Lactating adenoma: US features and literature review. *Radiology* 1998;206:271–274.

68. Kavi J, Chu HB, Leefall L. Sclerosing lobular hyperplasia manifesting as a palpable mass of the breast in young black women. *Hum Pathol* 1984;15:336–340.

69. Soo MS, Dash N, Bentley R, et al. Tubular adenomas of the breast: imaging findings with histologic correlation. *AJR Am J Roentgenol* 2000;174:757–762.

70. Denison CM, Ward VL, Lester SC, et al. Epidermal inclusion cysts of the breast: three lesions with calcifications. *Radiology* 1997;204:493–496.

71. Glazebrook KN, Morton MJ, Reynolds C. Vascular tumors of the breast: mammographic, sonographic, and MRI appearances. *AJR Am J Roentgenol* 2005;184:331–338.

72. Siewert B, Jacobs T, Baum JK. Sonographic evaluation of subcutaneous hemangioma of the breast. *AJR Am J Roentgenol* 2002;178:1025–1027.

73. Jozefczyk MA, Rosen PP. Vascular tumors of the breast: II. Perilobular hemangiomas and hemangiomas. *Am J Surg Pathol* 1985;9:491–503.

74. van Kints MJ, Tham RO, Klinkhamer PJJM, et al. Hemangiopericytoma of the breast: mammographic and sonographic findings. *AJR Am J Roentgenol* 1994;163:61–63.

75. Shaw de Paredes E. Pitfalls in mammography. *Imaging* 1994;6:1–14.

76. Moskowitz M. The predictive value of certain mammographic signs in screening for breast cancer. *Cancer* 1983;51:1007–1911.

77. Marsteller LP, Shaw de Paredes E. Well-defined masses in the breast. *RadioGraphics* 1989;9(1):13–37.

78. Sickles EA. Mammographic features of 300 conservative nonpalpable breast cancers. *AJR Am J Roentgenol* 1986;146:661–663.

79. Mitnick JS, Roses DF, Harris MN, et al. Circumscribed intraductal carcinoma of the breast. *Radiology* 1989;170:423–425.

80. Feig SA. Breast masses: mammographic and sonographic evaluation. *Radiol Clin N Am* 1992;30(1):67–92.

81. D'Orsi CJ, Weissman BNW, Berkowitz DM, et al. Correlation of xeroradiography and histology of breast disease. *CRC Crit Rev Diagn Imaging* 1978;11:75–119.

82. Martin J. Malignant breast masses: In: *Atlas of Mammography*. Baltimore: Williams & Wilkins, 1982.

83. Azzopardi JC. Special problems in breast pathology. In: *Problems in Breast Pathology*, vol. 11: *Major Problems in Pathology*. London: WB Saunders, 1979;250–328.

84. Meyer JE, Amin E, Lindfors KK, et al, Medullary carcinoma of the breast: mammographic and US appearance. *Radiology* 1989;170:79–82.

85. Cardenosa G, Doudna C, Eklund GW. Mucinous (colloid) breast cancer: clinical and mammographic findings in 10 patients. *AJR Am J Roentgenol* 1994;162:1077–1079.

86. Silverberg SG, Kay SC, Chitale AR, et al. Colloid carcinoma of the breast. *Am J Clin Pathol* 1971;55:355–363.

87. Rasmussen BB, Carsten R, Christensen IB. Prognostic factors in primary breast carcinoma. *Am J Clin Pathol* 1987;87:155–160.

88. Wilson TE, Helvie MA, Oberman HA, et al. Pure and mixed mucinous carcinoma of the breast: pathologic basis for differences in mammographic appearance. *AJR Am J Roentgenol* 1995;165:285–289.

89. Hajdu SI, Urban JA. Cancers metastatic to the breast. *Cancer* 1972;29:1691–1696.

90. Toombs BD, Kalisher L. Metastatic disease to the breast: clinical, pathologic, and radiographic features. *AJR Am J Roentgenol* 1977;129:673–676.

91. Bohman LG, Bassett LW, Gold RH, et al. Breast metastases from extramammary malignancies. *Radiology* 1982;144:309–312.

92. McCrea ES, Johnston C, Haney PJ. Metastases to the breast. *AJR Am J Roentgenol* 1983;141:685–690.

93. Liberman L, Giess CS, Dershaw DD, et al. Non-Hodgkin lymphoma of the breast: imaging characteristics and correlation with histopathologic findings. *Radiology* 1994;192:157–160.

Indistinct and Spiculated Masses

A poorly defined mass on mammography is a primary sign of breast carcinoma. The majority of breast carcinomas have an infiltrative, irregular appearance with spiculation (1). A variety of benign lesions, including fibrocystic changes (fibrosis, cysts, hyperplasia), radial scars, fat necrosis, hematomas, abscesses, and scars may also present as poorly defined masses radiographically. In addition to the mammographic findings, clinical history and physical examination may be of help in differentiating these lesions. However, in many cases, biopsy is necessary to confirm the etiology of a poorly defined mammographic lesion.

The BI-RADS® Lexicon (2) defines mass shapes as round, oval, lobular, and irregular and mass margins as circumscribed, obscured, microlobulated, indistinct, and spiculated. Indistinct masses are those in which a lesion or portion of the margin is fuzzy or poorly defined (Fig. 5.1). The shape of an indistinct mass may be any of those listed above. The importance of identifying an indistinctly marginated mass is that biopsy is necessary unless the mass represents a postsurgical finding. A spiculated mass (Fig. 5.2) has a margin that is composed of fine tendrils that surround the lesion. This pattern is highly suggestive of malignancy unless it represents a postsurgical scar. Therefore, history and clinical examination confirming the location of the scar are key to suggesting the correct diagnosis.

It is important to determine that an ill-defined lesion can be identified on two projections and is a true mass. Overlying glandular tissue can be visualized on one projection as an irregular density but on the orthogonal view is seen to disperse. If a density has a similar configuration on two projections, more complete evaluation is necessary. Spot-compression views of the lesion may be of help in evaluating its central density and in displacing the surrounding glandular tissue. The presence of a radiolucent center within a poorly defined density suggests a fibrocystic process as a likely etiology (3) or a radial scar, but it is not confirmatory. Ultrasound is also helpful in the assessment of a poorly defined mass. In particular, if a solid mass is identified on ultrasound, percutaneous biopsy with ultrasound guidance can be performed.

Secondary signs of malignancy, such as architectural distortion or microcalcifications associated with an irregular mass, are highly suspicious for carcinoma. The presence of pleomorphic or linear calcifications within and/or adjacent to an indistinct or spiculated mass increase the probability that the lesion is malignant. Even without secondary signs, if an irregular mass has high-density center and fine surrounding spicules, it is regarded as suspicious for carcinoma.

FIBROCYSTIC CHANGE

Cancer must be considered first when an indistinct or spiculated mass is identified on mammography. However, several benign lesions can be pseudoinfiltrative on pathology and produce an appearance on mammography that is suspicious for malignancy. Most often, false positives that manifest as suspicious mammographic masses are some form of fibrocystic change, including radial scar. These lesions may be associated with microcalcifications as well, which can increase the level of suspicion for malignancy.

Hermann et al. (4) found that lesions that mimic breast cancer on mammography because they present as indistinct or spiculated masses include fibrocystic changes, fibroadenomas, or residual parenchyma in an involuting breast. Keen et al. (5) described nine lesions that presented as masses simulating carcinoma because of their margination. Indurative mastopathy (radial scar) or sclerosing papillary proliferation were the diagnoses in four patients, infarcted papilloma in one, sclerosing adenosis in three, and fat necrosis in one. In these cases, the margins of the lesion on pathologic examination were irregular and pseudoinfiltrative, and this correlates with the mammographic appearance.

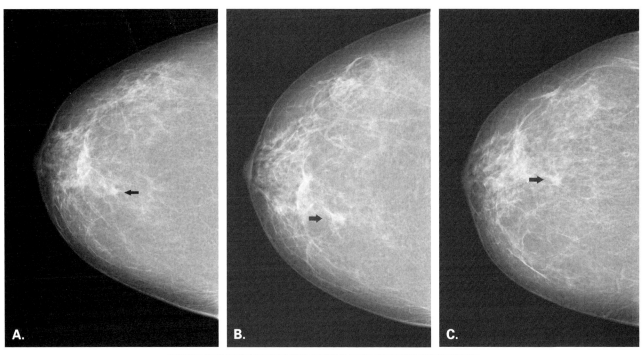

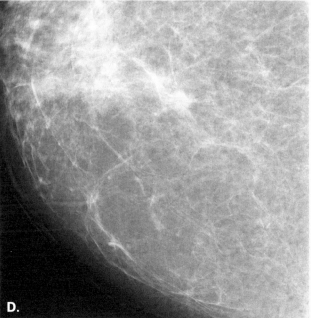

Figure 5.1

HISTORY: A 46-year-old woman for baseline screening.

MAMMOGRAPHY: Left CC **(A)** and rolled CC medial **(B)** and lateral **(C)** views demonstrate a small indistinct mass located medially **(arrows)**. The lesion was not observed on the MLO view, so rolled CC views were obtained to assess its location. The lesion persists on these views and moves with the superior pole of the breast. Spot-compression magnification **(D)** confirms the indistinct, nearly spiculated aspect of this lesion.

IMPRESSION: Highly suspicious for malignancy.

HISTOPATHOLOGY: Invasive ductal carcinoma.

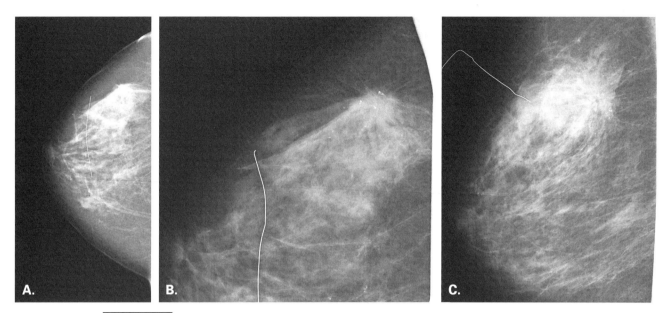

Figure 5.2

HISTORY: A 64-year-old woman with a palpable thickening in the left breast laterally.

MAMMOGRAPHY: Left CC **(A)** and spot-magnification CC **(B)** and ML **(C)** views show a high-density spiculated mass in the outer aspect of the breast. On the magnification views **(B, C)**, the fine spicules surrounding the lesion are evident, and the pleomorphic microcalcification with it and adjacent to it are also seen. The combination of findings is highly predictive of malignancy.

IMPRESSION: Spiculated mass, highly suggestive of carcinoma.

HISTOPATHOLOGY: Invasive ductal carcinoma with DCIS.

Sclerosing adenosis is a form of fibrocystic change characterized by a proliferation of lobules with surrounding fibrous sclerosis (6). When the condition is localized, it may masquerade as cancer on mammography and has been confused with carcinoma on histologic examination. In the early stages, there is a florid proliferation of epithelial cells. In later stages, stromal fibrosis occurs, in which coalescence of adjacent lobules produces areas of fibroepithelial proliferation and loss of normal lobular architecture (1). If the process is diffuse, the mammographic finding is diffuse, and small nodules with microcalcifications may be present. If the condition is localized, a mass with indistinct margins is often seen (1) (Figs. 5.3 and 5.4). In a series of 27 cases of sclerosing adenosis, Nielsen and Nielsen (7) reported an irregular density as the most frequent finding, but circumscribed and stellate masses were also seen. Although the density of the center of an area of sclerosing adenosis may not be as great as that of a malignancy, and the spicules may not radiate completely around the lesion, it is often impossible on mammography to differentiate such an area with certainty from a carcinoma. Therefore, sclerosing adenosis is a diagnosis made by biopsy and not by imaging alone.

A variety of forms of focal fibrocystic changes may appear as ill-defined lesions on mammography (Figs. 5.5–5.10). Focal fibrosis is a benign condition in which there is dense stromal fibrous tissue without cysts or epithelial changes (8). On mammography, fibrosis appears as dense tissue that is often irregularly marginated (9). Irregular microcalcifications that have a coarse pleomorphic appearance may be associated with fibrosis, and these may occasionally simulate carcinoma. Although biopsy is often necessary to confirm the nature of the lesion, the lack of fine linear tendrils around the border of the lesion suggests that malignancy is a somewhat less likely diagnosis. Harvey et al. (10) found that fibrous nodules that were diagnosed on core biopsy were most often masses with circumscribed or indistinct margins, but in about one fourth of cases, the findings were suspicious for malignancy.

An area of common epithelial hyperplasia or atypical ductal hyperplasia may occasionally present in a variety of ways, including as a small indistinct mass. Even a cyst or collection of cysts associated with surrounding fibrous stroma or inflammation may appear as a poorly defined

(text continues on page 193)

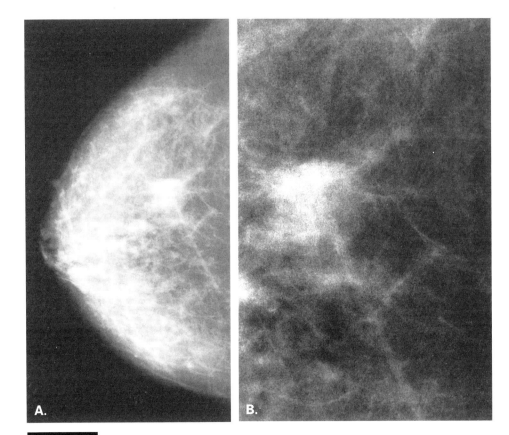

Figure 5.3

HISTORY: A 52-year-old woman with no palpable findings.

MAMMOGRAPHY: Left CC view (A) and magnified image (B). The breast is heterogeneously dense. There is an ill-defined 2-cm mass of moderately high density in the outer aspect of the breast. A coned-down image shows the irregularity of the margins but lack of fine surrounding spiculations that would be more characteristic of malignancy. This finding suggests more likely a fibrocystic etiology.

IMPRESSION: Ill-defined mass, more likely fibrocystic; malignancy cannot be excluded.

HISTOPATHOLOGY: Sclerosing adenosis with epithelial hyperplasia.

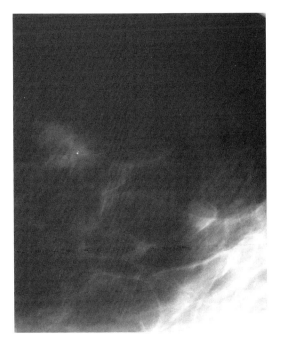

Figure 5.4

HISTORY: A 38-year-old woman recalled from screening mammography for a nonpalpable mass.

MAMMOGRAPHY: Right CC spot view of the mass shows it to be isodense and lobular shaped. The margins are indistinct, and there are a few punctuate microcalcifications associated with the lesion.

IMPRESSION: Suspicious mass; recommend biopsy.

HISTOPATHOLOGY: Sclerosing adenosis.

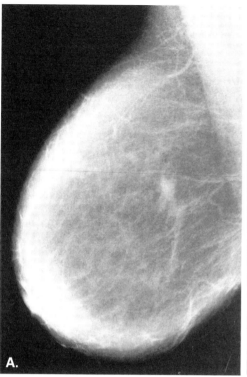

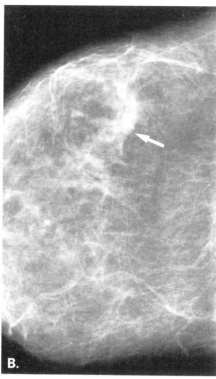

Figure 5.5

HISTORY: A 51-year-old asymptomatic woman for a screening mammogram.

MAMMOGRAPHY: Left MLO (**A**) and CC (**B**) views. The breast is fatty replaced. In the upper outer quadrant, there is an ill-defined mass of moderate to high density with a denser center and coarse spiculation (**arrow**). This has a similar appearance on the MLO (**A**) and CC (**B**) views, suggesting that it is not superimposition of normal glandular structures.

IMPRESSION: Moderately suspicious, indistinct mass; carcinoma versus focal fibrocystic disease.

HISTOPATHOLOGY: Fibrocystic changes, fibrosis.

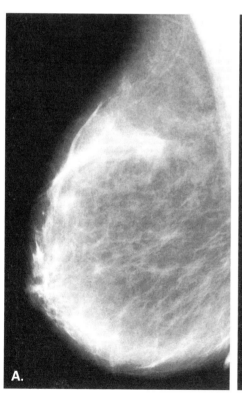

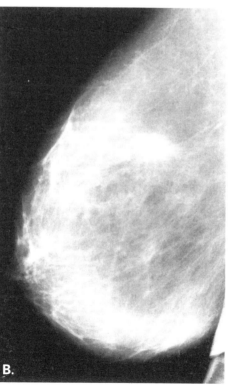

Figure 5.6

HISTORY: A 59-year-old woman with a family history of breast cancer.

MAMMOGRAPHY: Left MLO (**A**) and ML (**B**) views. There is a 2-cm, irregular, high-density lesion in the upper outer quadrant. There are a few lucencies within the mass that might suggest that it is benign; however, because of the overall density and irregular margins, biopsy was performed.

IMPRESSION: Irregular lesion, left breast, of mild to moderate suspicion for malignancy.

HISTOPATHOLOGY: Microglandular adenosis.

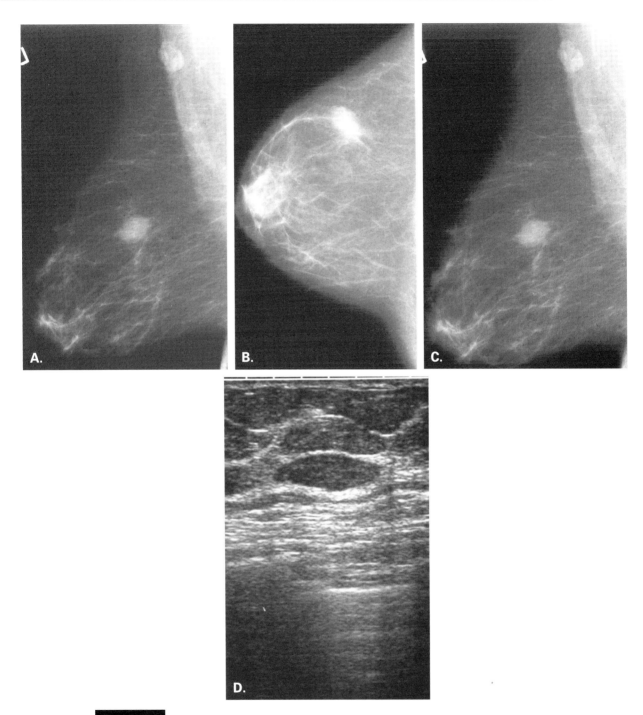

Figure 5.7

HISTORY: A 50-year-old woman for screening mammography.

MAMMOGRAPHY: Left MLO **(A)** and CC **(B)** views show an oval high-density mass in the upper outer quadrant. On the ML **(C)** view, the mass appears dense and somewhat indistinct. Further evaluation with ultrasound **(D)** shows the mass to be oval, circumscribed, and hypoechoic. The sonographic features suggest a benign etiology, but the high density and indistinct margin on mammography warrant biopsy.

IMPRESSION: High-density mass, recommend biopsy.

HISTOPATHOLOGY: Adenosis.

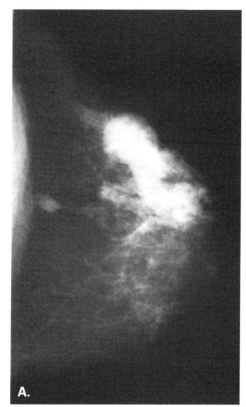

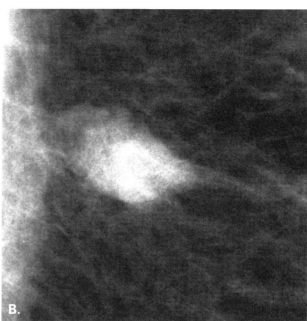

Figure 5.8

HISTORY: A 55-year-old patient with a history of fibrocystic changes.

MAMMOGRAPHY: Right CC (**A**) and spot-magnification CC (**B**) views show a mass that is dense and oval located posteriorly in the right breast. The margins are indistinct on the magnification view, and the posterior location increases the possibility for malignancy.

IMPRESSION: Indistinct dense mass, suspicious for malignancy.

HISTOPATHOLOGY: Sclerosing adenosis.

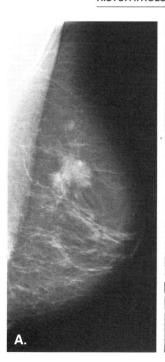

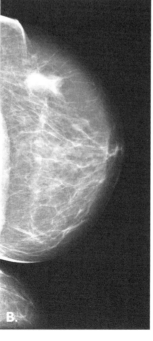

Figure 5.9

HISTORY: A 68-year-old woman for screening mammography.

MAMMOGRAPHY: Right MLO (**A**) and CC (**B**) views show an irregular mass with indistinct margins in the upper outer quadrant. The mass is somewhat high density and has a slightly different shape on the two views. No abnormality was found on ultrasound.

IMPRESSION: Irregular mass suspicious for carcinoma. (Because the ultrasound was negative, the probability for malignancy is less).

HISTOPATHOLOGY: Fibrocystic change.

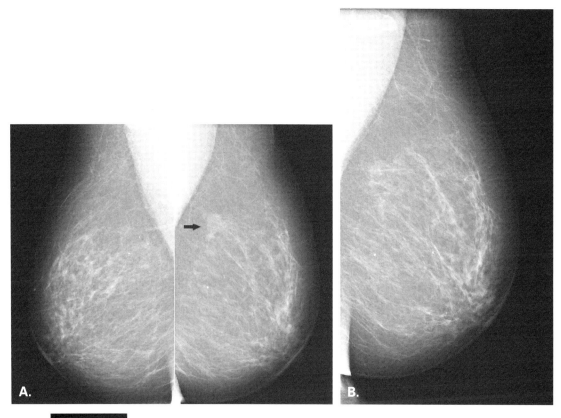

Figure 5.10

HISTORY: A 56-year-old woman with a family history of breast cancer for routine screening mammography.

MAMMOGRAPHY: Bilateral MLO **(A)** and right ML **(B)** views show a focal asymmetry **(arrow)** in the right upper-outer quadrant. The lesion has the appearance of a low-density indistinct mass. The area was new in comparison with a prior study, and therefore it was biopsied.

IMPRESSION: Indistinct mass, suspicious for carcinoma.

HISTOPATHOLOGY: Fibrocystic changes with calcifications.

lesion. Because of the similarities in appearance of many types of fibrocystic change and in breast cancer, many biopsies performed for indistinct lesions are found to represent fibrocystic change on pathology.

PSEUDOANGIOMATOUS STROMAL HYPERPLASIA

Pseudoangiomatous stromal hyperplasia (PASH) is a benign lesion first described by Vuitch et al. in 1986 (11). PASH may mimic breast cancer, because it may present as an irregular or indistinctly marginated mass, although often the lesion is circumscribed (12). PASH is a benign mesenchymal neoplasm composed of myofibroblasts sometimes with glandular hyperplasia.

PASH typically occurs in women younger than age 50 who typically present with a palpable mass. On mammography, PASH may present as a lobular circumscribed mass or as an indistinct distorted mass. The striking histologic feature is the complex pattern of large, empty anastomosing spaces in the dense collagenous stroma. Because of this appearance, PASH is sometimes mistaken for angiosarcoma on histology (13).

RADIAL SCAR

Radial scar is a rosettelike proliferative breast lesion (14) that has also been described as sclerosing papillary proliferation (15), benign sclerosing ductal proliferation (16), nonencapsulated sclerosing lesion (17), infiltrating epithelio-

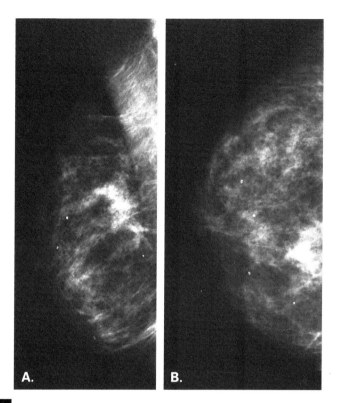

Figure 5.11

HISTORY: A 77-year-old woman who presents for screening mammography.

MAMMOGRAPHY: Left MLO (**A**) and CC (**B**) views show an irregular indistinct masslike density in the upper inner quadrant. The area appears to be distorting the architecture. Considerations for this appearance are carcinoma, especially invasive lobular carcinoma; fibrocystic change with sclerosing adenosis; and radial scar.

IMPRESSION: Indistinct mass with distortion; recommend biopsy.

HISTOPATHOLOGY: Radial scar.

sis, and indurative mastopathy (18). The lesion has been confused with cancer by mammographers (19) and pathologists.

In a study of 32 cases of radial scar, Andersen and Gram (14) found most lesions to be small (mean diameter of 7 mm) and in a stellate configuration. On histology, a fibroelastic center is surrounded by lobules and ducts radiating outward. In 93% of cases, either papillomatosis or a benign epithelial proliferation was present. Small round microcalcifications were seen in 63% of cases (14). Because of the presence of elastosis with sclerosis and ductal distortion, a pseudoinfiltrative pattern occurs, and the lesion may be confused with carcinoma histologically (18).

On mammography, a radial scar is a spiculated defined lesion that produces retraction and distortion of surrounding structure (20) (Fig. 5.11). Microcalcifications may be associated with radial scar. Mitnick et al. (21) found mammography to be unreliable in differentiating radial scar from infiltrating carcinomas. The presence of

small radiolucencies with the lesion are more in favor of a radial scar than of malignancy (3), but histologic examination is necessary to confirm the diagnosis (20,21).

POSTTRAUMATIC CHANGES

Intraparenchymal scars after biopsy appear as poorly defined masses, often with spiculated margins (22) (Figs. 5.12–5.14). Scars and posttraumatic changes are more visible in the first 6 months after biopsy and are less prominent after several years (23). A feature of scars that may help to differentiate them from cancers on mammography is that a scar tends to have a different configuration and density on the orthogonal views of the breast. In patients who have undergone lumpectomy and radiation therapy for treatment of primary breast carcinoma, a prominent area of scarring at the surgical site may resemble recurrent carcinoma (24,25). In these patients, it is particularly

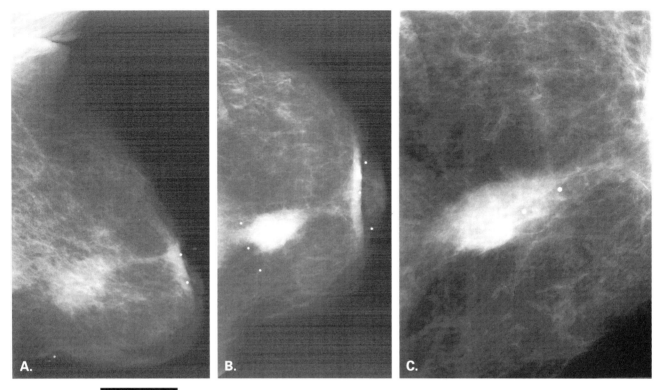

Figure 5.12

HISTORY: Patient with a history of lumpectomy and radiotherapy on the right for routine follow-up.

MAMMOGRAPHY: Right MLO **(A)** and CC **(B)** views show an indistinct oval mass in the center of the right breast located behind the postsurgical skin site. The area appears dense and indistinct on the spot magnification CC view **(C)**, but on the MLO view **(A)**, the shape is more elongated and more dispersed. These features are most suggestive of a postsurgical site. Comparison with the prior films is essential to verify stability of the finding.

IMPRESSION: Postsurgical seroma and fat necrosis.

NOTE: The area had decreased in size in comparison with the prior postoperative study.

useful to have an initial mammogram after surgery, before radiation therapy is started (26), to serve as a basis for future comparisons of the irregular postoperative density that may be present at the lumpectomy site.

An acute response to trauma, such as a hematoma, may also appear as an indistinct mass (Fig. 5.15) or as a diffuse increase in density. Another radiographic feature of a hematoma that may simulate a cancer is the overlying skin thickening from the edema and bruising. Hematomas tend to resolve over a period of 3 to 4 weeks (27) but may occasionally persist for a longer time, particularly if they are of a large size. Clinical correlation is important in suggesting the correct diagnosis. Ultrasound also is helpful in demonstrating a fluid collection.

Fat necrosis is a nonsuppurative inflammatory response to trauma. Particularly if the area is associated

with a desmoplastic reaction, fat necrosis may be confused with carcinoma on clinical examination. One manifestation of fat necrosis mammographically is an irregular mass that simulates carcinoma (1) (Figs. 5.16–5.23). Thickening and retraction of overlying skin may occur. On histologic examination of an area of fat necrosis, fibrous connective tissue proliferates at the periphery of the necrotic debris. The extent of fibrous response correlates with mammographic image. A marked response may appear on mammography as a spiculated mass resembling carcinoma, whereas a mild response occurs when a thin-walled radiolucent oil cyst is seen (26). Correlation with clinical history is the key in suggesting the presence of fat necrosis. The history of

(text continues on page 201)

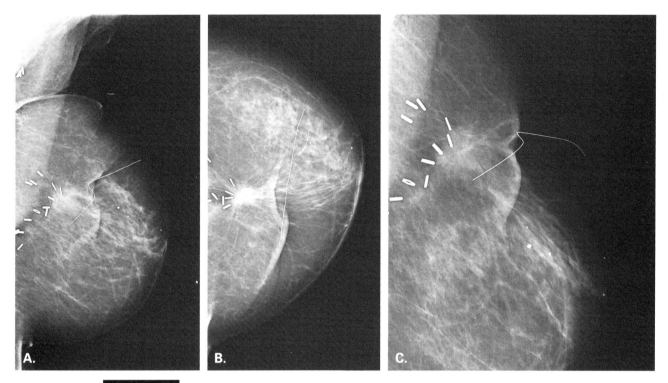

Figure 5.13

HISTORY: A 64-year-old woman with a status post–lumpectomy and radiotherapy on the right.

MAMMOGRAPHY: Right MLO (**A**) and CC (**B**) views show an irregular masslike density at the lumpectomy site, demarcated by the surgical clips. The area appears more dense and spiculated on the CC than the MLO, suggesting that it is more likely a scar. On the spot MLO magnification view of the tumor bed (**C**), the area appears less dense.

IMPRESSION: Postsurgical scar.

NOTE: The area had diminished in size from prior studies, confirming that it is a scar.

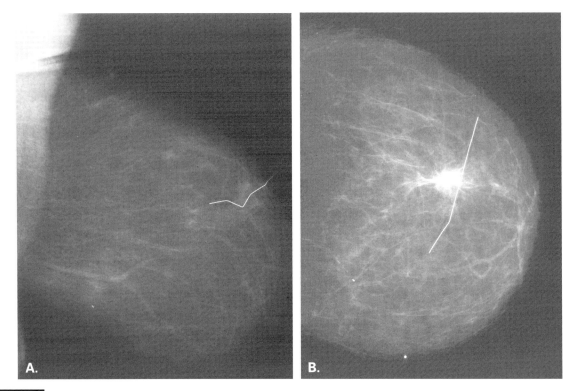

Figure 5.14

HISTORY: A 51-year-old woman status post–benign right breast biopsy.

MAMMOGRAPHY: Right MLO **(A)** and CC **(B)** views show an essentially fatty-replaced breast. The postsurgical site is indicated by a wire marker. This appears dense and spiculated on the CC view **(B)**, but is more amorphous and vertically oriented on the MLO **(A)** view. The differing appearance on the two projections is typical of a scar.

IMPRESSION: Postsurgical scar.

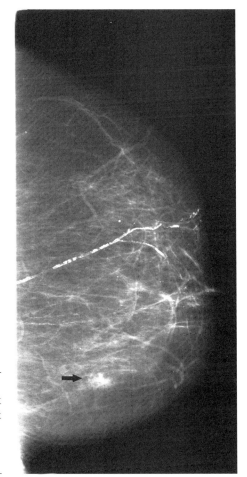

Figure 5.15

HISTORY: A 75-year-old woman with a history of blunt trauma to the right breast.

MAMMOGRAPHY: Right ML view shows fatty replacement. There is a small indistinct mass located inferiorly **(arrow)**. This lesion is oval with indistinct margins, and it is heterogeneous in density. This was located in the area of bruising on the skin.

IMPRESSION: Small indistinct mass, consistent with hematoma.

NOTE: Short-term follow-up mammogram showed resolution of the lesion.

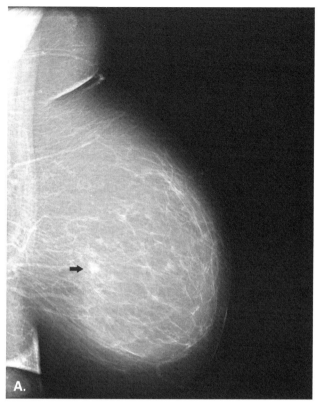

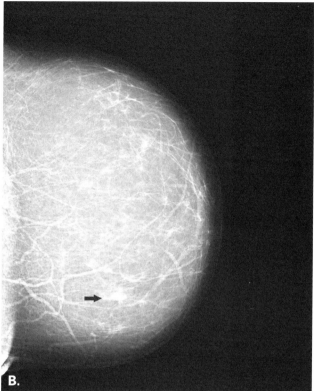

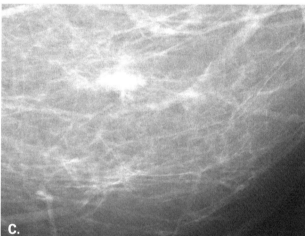

Figure 5.16

HISTORY: A 57-year-old woman for screening mammography.

MAMMOGRAPHY: Right MLO **(A)** and CC **(B)** views show a fatty-replaced breast. There is a small, dense, indistinct mass located medially. The spot view **(C)** demonstrates the indistinct aspect of the lesion, which had developed from the mammogram a year earlier.

IMPRESSION: Suspicious mass; recommend biopsy, BI-RADS® 4.

HISTOPATHOLOGY: Fat necrosis.

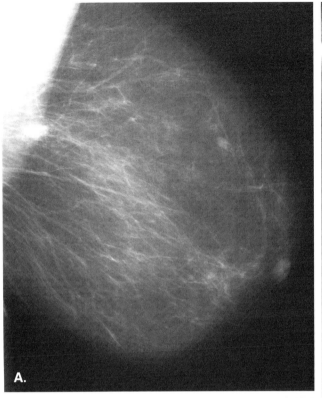

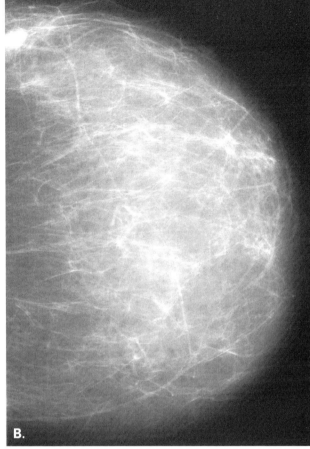

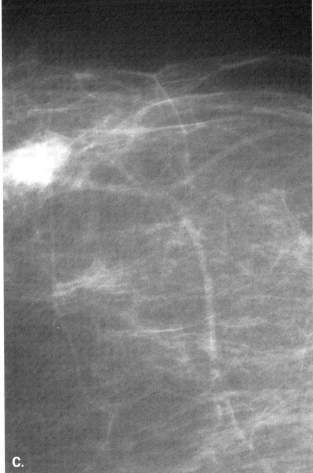

HISTORY: A 58-year-old patient who presents for screening mammography.

MAMMOGRAPHY: Right MLO (**A**) and CC (**B**) views show a small dense mass located posterolaterally in the left breast. On spot magnification (**C**), the indistinct margin of this somewhat high-density mass is noted. Excisional biopsy was performed.

HISTOPATHOLOGY: Fat necrosis.

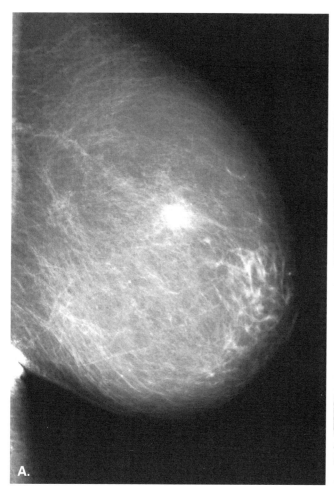

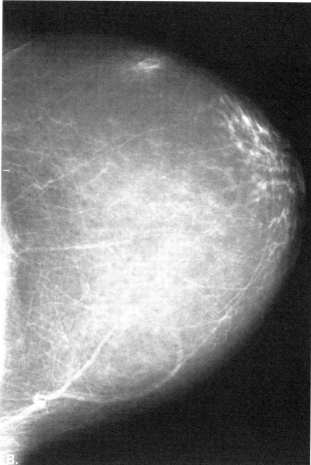

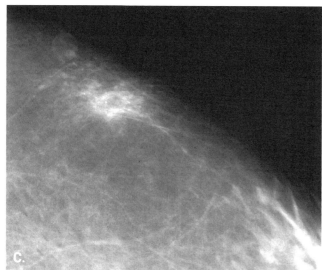

Figure 5.18

HISTORY: A 35-year-old woman for screening mammography.

MAMMOGRAPHY: Right ML (**A**) and CC (**B**) views show an indistinct mass in the 9 o'clock position. On the ML view, this appears dense, but on the CC view, it is less dense and more heterogeneous in appearance. On the magnified CC view (**C**), the area is noted to contain a fatty center, suggestive of fat necrosis. Because the patient reported no history of trauma, needle localization and excision were performed.

IMPRESSION: Indistinct mass, possible fat necrosis; recommend biopsy.

HISTOPATHOLOGY: Fat necrosis with microcalcifications.

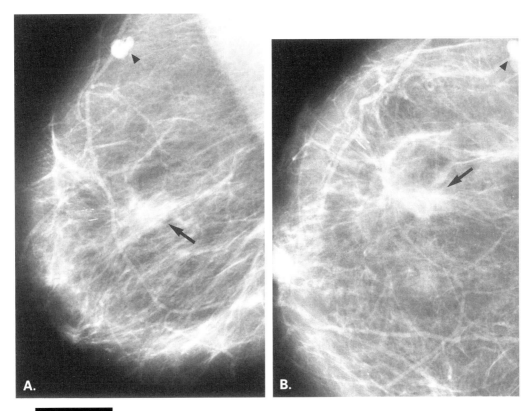

Figure 5.19

HISTORY: A 52-year-old gravida 7, para 7 woman after right breast cancer and left breast biopsy for a benign lesion.

MAMMOGRAPHY: Left MLO **(A)** and enlarged CC **(B)** views. There is an indistinct 2-cm area of increased density **(arrow)** in the upper outer quadrant of the left breast. This density had increased in size since a prior examination and, because of the interval change, was regarded with a moderate degree of suspicion for malignancy. Benign secretory calcifications are adjacent to the lesion. An enlarged intramammary node **(arrowhead)** is present in the upper outer quadrant.

IMPRESSION: New focal area of increased density, of moderate suspicion for malignancy.

HISTOPATHOLOGY: Fat necrosis, chronic inflammation.

NOTE: Areas of fat necrosis are usually most prominent immediately after biopsy and gradually decrease in size and density over time. Occasionally, such an area may increase in size, and biopsy is usually warranted to exclude a neoplastic process.

a recent biopsy or severe blunt trauma in the area of abnormality should alert one to the possibility of fat necrosis. If there is any doubt about the location of a spiculated mass relative to a surgical scar, metallic markers or a wire should be placed over the scar and the film repeated to verify its position.

ABSCESS

A breast abscess is often suspected on clinical examination because of the very tender, red, hot indurated area.

Abscesses tend to occur in lactating breasts, but occasionally may occur in nonlactating women. If a lesion having the clinical appearance of an abscess is found in a nonlactating patient, it should be regarded with suspicion. Most abscesses occur in the subareolar area (20), and skin and areolar thickening may be present (Figs. 5.24–5.26). Because of the extreme tenderness and the level of clinical suspicion in patients with breast abscesses, mammography may not be performed in the acute stages. The clinical appearance of a breast abscess

(text continues on page 206)

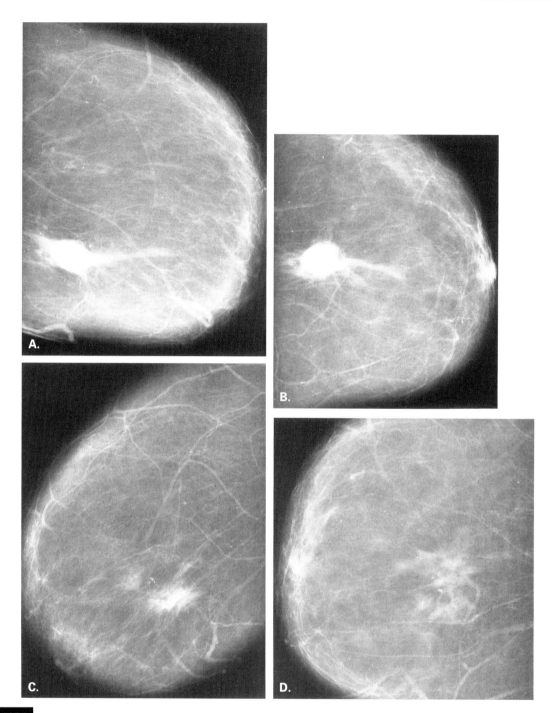

Figure 5.20

HISTORY: A 70-year-old gravida 6, para 6 woman for routine screening.

MAMMOGRAPHY: Right ML (**A**) and CC (**B**) views and left MLO (**C**) and CC (**D**) views. The breasts show fatty replacement. In the 6 o'clock position of the right breast (**A** and **B**), there is a high-density mass appearing circumscribed on some margins and indistinct in other areas. Coarse microcalcifications are present in the periphery of this lesion. On the left (**C** and **D**) in the 6 o'clock position, there is a poorly defined mass, having a differing shape and density on the two views. Similar coarse calcifications are associated with this lesion. On both sides, but particularly on the left, some of the calcifications are round or ringlike, suggesting fat necrosis as the etiology of these densities. Because there was no definite history of trauma, biopsy was performed.

IMPRESSION: Bilateral masses, favoring fat necrosis.

HISTOPATHOLOGY: Bilateral fat necrosis.

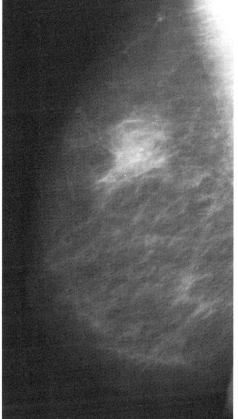

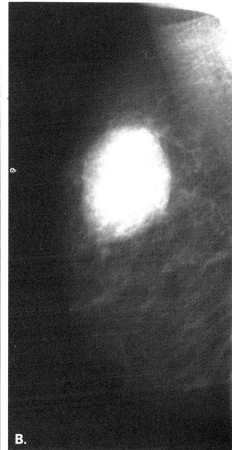

A.   B.

Figure 5.21

HISTORY: A 46-year-old woman who is status post–left lumpectomy and radiotherapy. Prior films are available for comparison.

MAMMOGRAPHY: Left MLO **(A)** and left MLO from 1 year earlier **(B)** show an indistinct mass in the superior region. On the prior study, the mass was larger and more circumscribed, consistent with postsurgical seroma that is evolving into a scar.

IMPRESSION: Postsurgical scar.

Figure 5.22

HISTORY: Postmenopausal patient with a history of right breast benign biopsy.

MAMMOGRAPHY: Right MLO **(A)** and CC **(B)** views show the breast to contain scattered fibroglandular densities. There is a mass present in the upper inner quadrant that has a differing appearance on the two views. On the CC view, the lesion is high density and spiculated, but on the MLO view, an oval fatty center is noted, typical of fat necrosis.

IMPRESSION: Postsurgical scar with fat necrosis.

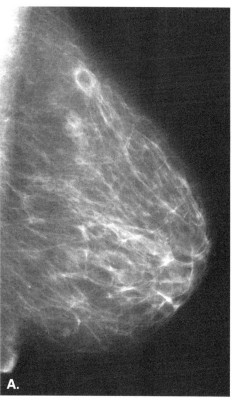

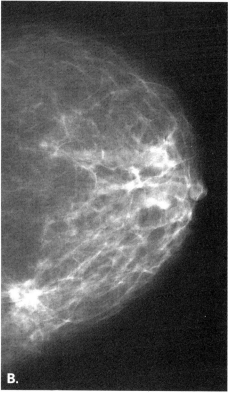

A.   B.

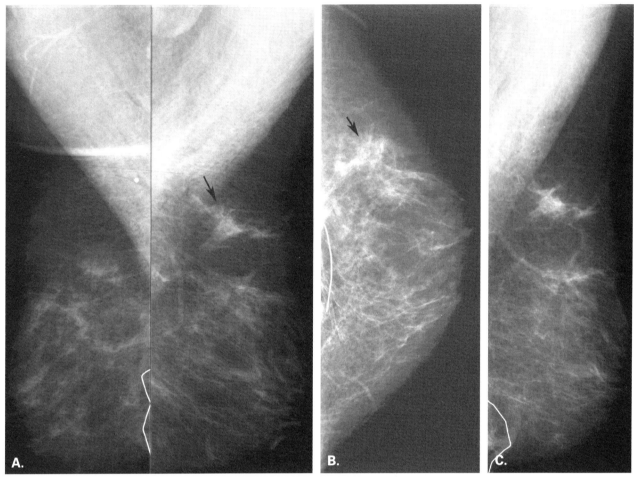

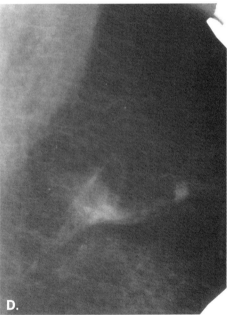

Figure 5.23

HISTORY: A 59-year-old woman who is status post–bilateral implant removal 1 year earlier.

MAMMOGRAPHY: Bilateral MLO views **(A)** show a focal asymmetry **(arrow)** in the right breast superiorly. This area is less dense on the CC view **(B, arrow)**. On the ML view **(C)**, it persists, and on spot compression **(D)**, it appears dense and indistinctly marginated.

IMPRESSION: Indistinct mass; recommend biopsy.

HISTOPATHOLOGY: Fat necrosis and foreign-body giant-cell reaction.

NOTE: This is most likely related to the prior implants; however, its location is a somewhat unusual for the implant site.

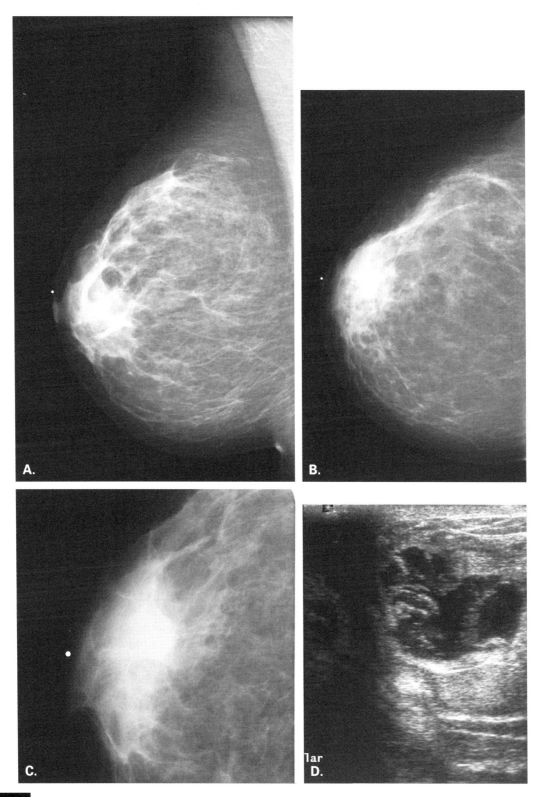

Figure 5.24

HISTORY: A 26-year-old woman with a palpable mass in the left subareolar area.

MAMMOGRAPHY: Left MLO (**A**) and CC (**B**) views show an indistinct density in the left subareolar area. On the spot magnification CC view (**C**), the high-density lesion has indistinct margins posteriorly. Ultrasound (**D**) demonstrates that the mass is complex, and the differential diagnosis includes abscess versus tumor.

IMPRESSION: Palpable mass, possible abscess; recommend biopsy/drainage.

HISTOPATHOLOGY: Abscess.

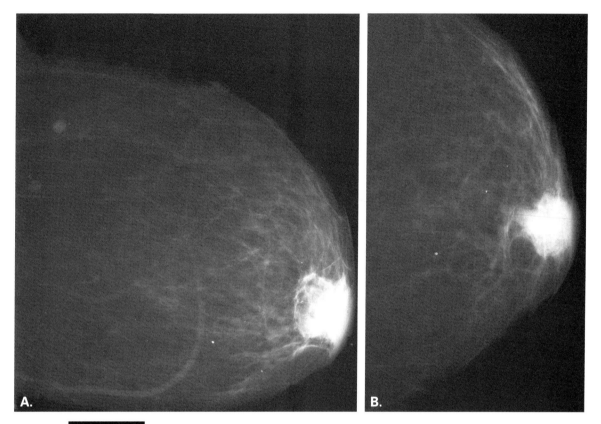

Figure 5.25

HISTORY: A 44-year-old woman with a painful mass in the right breast.

MAMMOGRAPHY: Coned-down right MLO **(A)** and CC **(B)** views show a high-density irregular mass in the subareolar area. There are linear extensions from the mass posteriorly, suggesting distended ducts. The skin of the areolar area is thickened. The findings of the mass and associated skin thickening are most consistent with an abscess or tumor. The patient was treated with antibiotics and drainage, and the area resolved.

IMPRESSION: Subareolar abscess.

may be difficult to differentiate from an inflammatory carcinoma, and needle biopsy is usually performed in the acute stages. Mammography is necessary after therapy to evaluate the remainder of the breast. In an older patient, in particular, abscesses are not common and may be associated with a nearby malignancy or a papilloma obstructing a duct (Fig. 5.27).

A chronic abscess, although associated at times with some thickening and induration of the skin, does not present with the redness and tenderness found in the acute stages. A chronic abscess is usually imaged as a poorly marginated lesion in the subareolar region that may be associated with skin thickening. Sonography reveals an irregular, complex fluid-filled mass with debris. Abscesses may occur elsewhere in the breast and may be related to direct extension of infection from the skin or from surgery or trauma. In addition, infection in a lymph node may lead to suppuration and abscess formation (Fig. 5.28).

GRANULAR CELL TUMOR

Granular cell tumor was first described by Abrikossoff in 1926 (28). Granular cell tumor, also called myoblastoma, is a rare benign tumor that occurs in the tongue most frequently, but also is found in the bronchus, bile duct, or subcutaneous tissues (29). Only about 5% to 6% of granular cell tumors occur in the breast (30). The patient often presents with a firm palpable lump that may be suspicious for malignancy on clinical examination. Granular cell tumors are thought to develop from Schwann cells (13), and they are located in the subcutaneous area of the breast. These lesions are benign but locally infiltrative, and they are treated with excision.

Adeniran et al. (31), in a review of 17 cases of granular cell tumor, found that in three patients, the lesions were multifocal, occurring in the breast and elsewhere. In this

(text continues on page 209)

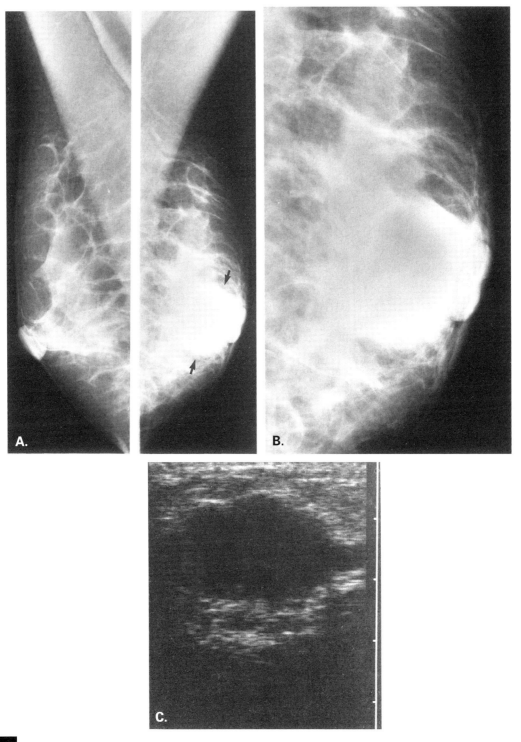

Figure 5.26

HISTORY: A 35-year-old gravida 4, para 3, abortus 1 woman with a family history of breast cancer who presented with an indurated tender mass in the right subareolar area.

MAMMOGRAPHY: Bilateral MLO views **(A)**, right CC view **(B)**, and ultrasound **(C)**. The breasts are heterogeneously dense, consistent with the age and parity of the patient. Marked asymmetry is present, with an indistinct mass **(arrows)** in the right subareolar area **(A and B)**. Nipple retraction and areolar thickening are associated with the mass. Sonography **(C)** shows the mass to be slightly irregular and to contain some internal echoes, suggesting thick fluid. Particularly because of the ultrasound, the favored diagnosis is an abscess; aspiration revealed purulent material.

IMPRESSION: Mass in the right breast, favoring abscess.

HISTOPATHOLOGY: Acute mastitis, breast abscess.

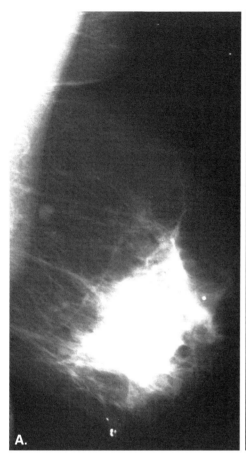

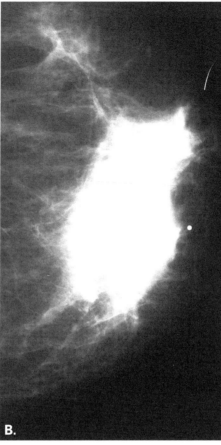

A.

B.

Figure 5.27

HISTORY: Baseline mammogram on a postmenopausal patient who presents with a tender palpable right breast mass.

MAMMOGRAPHY: Right MLO (**A**) and CC (**B**) views show an irregular, very-high-density mass with indistinct margins. The lesion occupies the central, medial aspect of the breast, and the margins are very indistinct. Excision was performed.

IMPRESSION: Highly suspicious for carcinoma.

HISTOPATHOLOGY: Abscess, small focus of DCIS.

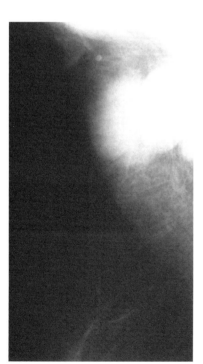

Figure 5.28

HISTORY: A 36-year-old woman with a tender mass in the left axilla.

MAMMOGRAPHY: Left axillary view shows a high-density lesion with spiculated margins in the axilla. There are also several enlarged, dense nodes behind the mass. Differential diagnosis for the lesion includes tumor versus abscess versus hematoma.

IMPRESSION: Spiculated mass in the left axilla, suspicious for carcinoma.

HISTOPATHOLOGY: Lymph node with acute inflammation and abscess formation.

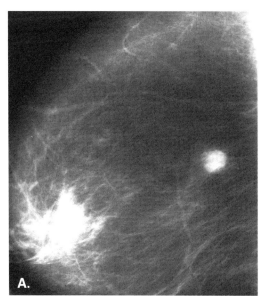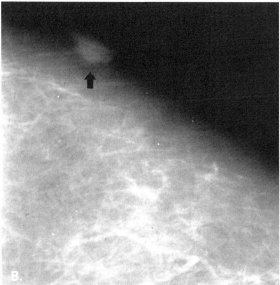

Figure 5.29

HISTORY: A 39-year-old woman with a palpable mass laterally in the left breast.

MAMMOGRAPHY: Left MLO **(A)** and coned-down CC **(B)** views. There is a slightly irregular, high-density mass in the left-mid outer quadrant located in the subcutaneous area **(B, arrow)**. Lesions that most frequently occupy the subcutaneous region are sebaceous cysts and metastatic deposits. Another unusual lesion that may occur here is the granular cell tumor, a benign tumor of the tongue and subcutaneous tissues.

HISTOPATHOLOGY: Granular cell tumor. (Case courtesy of Dr. Stephen Edge, Charlottesville, VA.)

series, the mammographic findings include round circumscribed masses, indistinct densities, or spiculated masses (31). Other authors (29,30) have described a spiculated or indistinct lesion having a malignant appearance on mammography (Figs. 5.29 and 5.30).

FIBROMATOSIS

A rare cause of an ill-defined lesion of the breast is fibromatosis (32). Fibromatosis or desmoid tumor most often occurs in the abdominal wall or in the superficial aponeurosis of the limbs (33). Fibromatosis can also occur in the breast, where it is thought to represent an extension from the pectoralis fascia (33,34). This is a fibroblastic lesion that behaves in a locally invasive but nonmetastasizing manner and may be associated with trauma (34,35). Microscopically, fibromatosis is composed of interlocking proliferating fibroblasts with varying amounts of collagenization and areas of myxoid degeneration and extension into the surrounding fat (36).

Fibromatosis has an appearance on mammography similar to that of carcinoma (Fig. 5.27), namely, a poorly defined or irregular mass (Figs. 5.31–5.34).

Because of the involvement of the pectoralis fascia, fibromatosis is located posteriorly and is fixed. This lesion may cause both retraction of the pectoralis major muscle and the nipple because of the desmoplasia. Three cases of mammary fibromatosis were described by Yiangou et al. (33), who found that the mammographic findings were suspicious for malignancy. Cederlund et al. (37) described a case in a 28-year-old woman who had a small mass with strands extending toward the pectoralis muscle.

Fibromatosis is treated with wide local excision. The lesion may recur locally in about 25% of cases (38). In a study of 28 examples of fibromatosis, Wargotz et al. (38) found that in all cases of recurrence, the lesion was inadequately excised initially, and all the surgical margins were not clear initially.

CARCINOMA

Primary invasive breast cancers are divided into three categories: invasive, or infiltrating ductal carcinoma (IDC), invasive lobular carcinoma (ILC), and the rare carcinosarcomas. The most common type by far is invasive ductal carcinoma, not otherwise specified type. A classic appear-

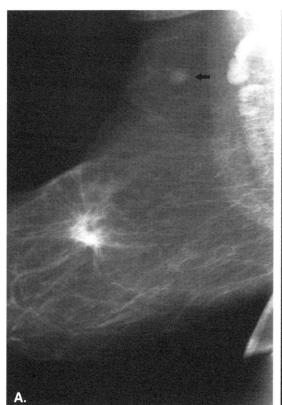
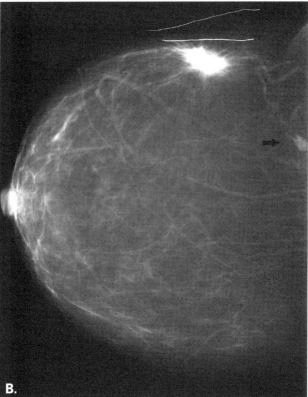
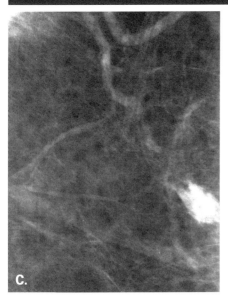

Figure 5.30

HISTORY: A 61-year-old patient with a history of benign surgical biopsy on the left.

MAMMOGRAPHY: Left MLO **(A)** and CC **(B)** views show a spiculated mass at the surgical site marked by the wires on the skin, consistent with postsurgical scar. There is also a small dense mass **(arrow)** in the 1 o'clock position posteriorly. The mass has indistinct margins, seen best on the magnification view **(C)**.

IMPRESSION: Postsurgical scar or posterior lesion suspicious for carcinoma.

HISTOPATHOLOGY: (Posterior lesion): Granular cell tumor.

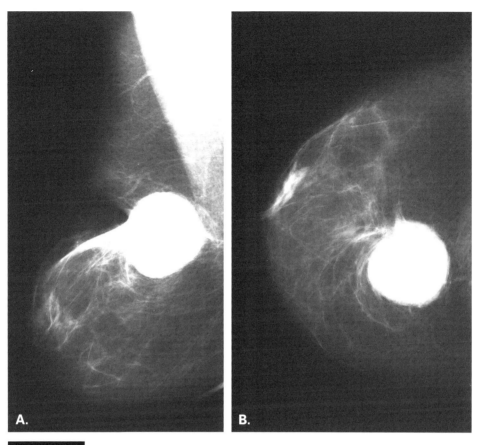

Figure 5.31

HISTORY: A 64-year-old gravida 2, para 2 woman with a history of carcinoid tumor and a left breast biopsy 1 year ago. The biopsy was performed for a nonpalpable mass that was confirmed on specimen radiography and found to represent sclerosing adenosis.

MAMMOGRAPHY: Left MLO **(A)** and CC **(B)** views. There is a large, very-high-density, round, slightly indistinct mass in the upper inner quadrant, producing marked skin retraction. (This mass was in the region of previous biopsy.) Ultrasound showed the lesion to be solid. Because of the history of biopsy for a benign lesion, the favored diagnosis is hematoma with fat necrosis; however, neoplasia is a definite consideration because of the skin changes and high density of the mass.

IMPRESSION: Large mass, favoring postoperative changes, fat necrosis.

HISTOPATHOLOGY: Fibromatosis.

NOTE: Fibromatosis is a benign lesion that occurs in the area of fascia and may be related to trauma. Although rare, when it does occur in the breast, it is more often an indistinct lesion. In this case, the mass was found to be completely attached to the deep fascia at the time of resection.

ance of primary breast carcinoma on mammography is spiculated mass. The density of the lesion is as dense as or more dense than the parenchyma. Fine linear tendrils extend around the border of the lesion (39,40). These findings are related to the growth patterns of infiltrating carcinomas. Gross examination of these tumors reveals a firm, white gritty mass with tendrils radiating into the adjacent breast tissue. Histologic examination shows

nests and cords of malignant cells associated with fibrous stroma infiltrating into the normal breast tissue (1).

On physical examination, carcinomas usually are palpated as larger than they appear on mammography. The fine extensions of tumor cells into the surrounding tissue and the fibrotic, desmoplastic reaction account for

(text continues on page 214)

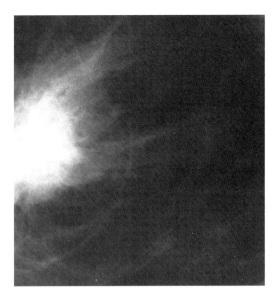

Figure 5.32

HISTORY: A 26-year-old woman with a firm, palpable, right breast mass and nipple retraction.

MAMMOGRAPHY: Right spot CC view of the mass located far posteriorly and laterally shows the lesion to be very high density and spiculated. The lesion is tethering the pectoralis major muscle and is extending anteriorly as well.

IMPRESSION: Highly suspicious for malignancy.

HISTOPATHOLOGY: Fibromatosis.

NOTE: Fibromatosis or extra-abdominal desmoid tumor is associated with the pectoralis fascia and is therefore often located far posteriorly. Because of its highly infiltrative nature, it may retract the nipple or skin, even though it is not located in the retroglandular area.

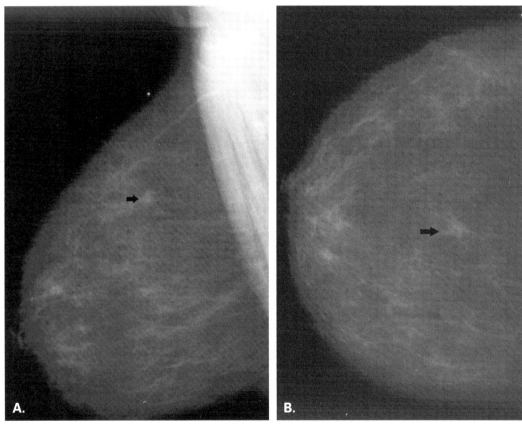

A.

B.

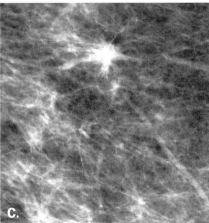

C.

Figure 5.33

HISTORY: A 47-year-old woman for screening.

MAMMOGRAPHY: Left MLO **(A)** and CC **(B)** views show a small indistinct mass **(arrows)** in the 12 o'clock position. On close inspection **(C)**, long, thin tendrils surround the lesion and extend far anteriorly and posteriorly.

IMPRESSION: Suspicious for carcinoma.

HISTOPATHOLOGY: Fibromatosis (desmoid tumor).

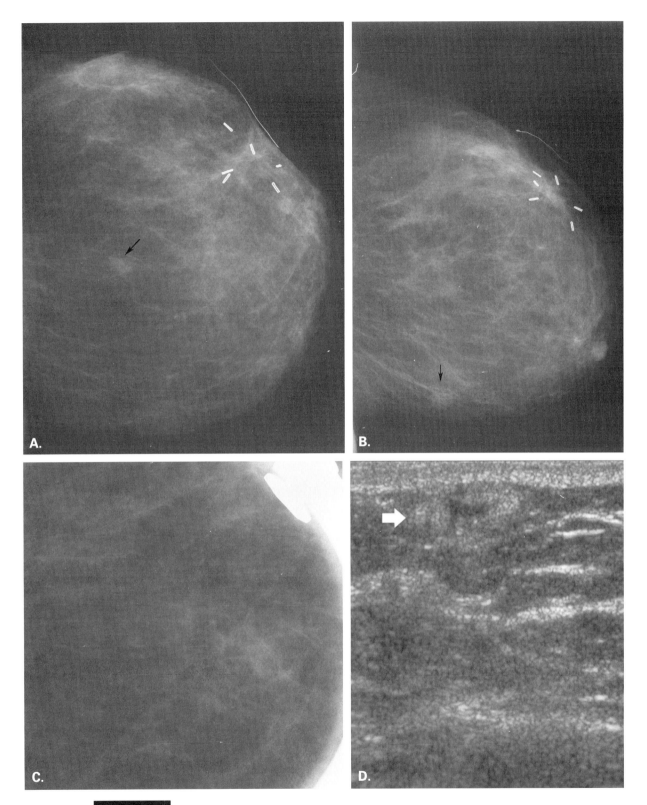

HISTORY: A 52-year-old woman who is status postlumpectomy. Radiotherapy (RT) on the right.

MAMMOGRAPHY: Right CC **(A)** and MLO **(B)** views show an oval mass with indistinct margins in the 6 o'clock position. Spot-magnification view **(C)** shows the very indistinct margination of the lesion. Ultrasound **(D)** shows the mass **(arrow)** to be hyperechoic with a hypoechoic band traversing the center.

IMPRESSION: Suspicious mass right breast.

HISTOPATHOLOGY: Desmoid tumor (fibromatosis).

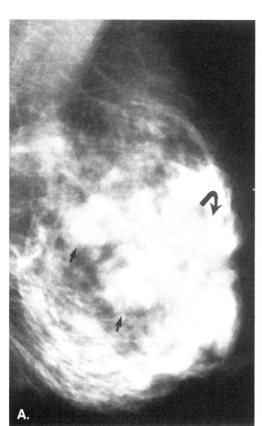
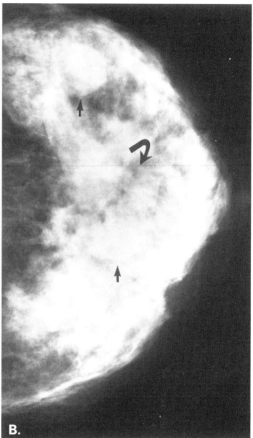

Figure 5.35

HISTORY: A 55-year-old gravida 2, para 2 woman with a history of multiple cysts, for routine screening.

MAMMOGRAPHY: Right MLO **(A)** and CC **(B)** views. The breast is very dense for the patient's age. There are multiple circumscribed masses **(arrows)** that were shown to be cystic by ultrasound. Scattered microcalcifications are present. There is a focal area of architectural distortion **(curved arrow)** in the 12 o'clock position. This area is spiculated, although there is no high-density center to suggest a tumor. The area had developed since a prior mammogram 18 months earlier and was, therefore, regarded with a moderate degree of suspicion for malignancy. The differential includes a radial scar versus a carcinoma.

HISTOPATHOLOGY: Intraductal carcinoma, extensive papillary and cribriform patterns.

the larger palpable mass than is evident at mammography (41).

The specified forms of invasive ductal carcinoma include tubular, medullary, mucinous, metaplastic, and adenoid cystic subtypes. In invasive ductal carcinoma, the malignant cells have extended through the duct wall and basement membrane and are invading the periductal tissues. Invasive ductal carcinoma is a solid dense tumor that may be firm or hard from the scirrhous stroma (13). The tumor cell nuclei are graded into three categories: well differentiated, intermediate, and poorly differenti-

ated. Histologic grading describes the microscopic growth pattern and the cytologic features of differentiation (13), and includes an assessment of the extent of tubule formation by the invading malignant cells, the nuclear features, and the mitotic rate (42). The formation of tubular structures by the invading malignant cells is a good prognostic factor.

Although an intraductal carcinoma—ductal carcinoma in situ (DCIS)—occasionally presents mammographically as a small indistinct mass (43) (Fig. 5.35), this finding is more typical of infiltrating breast cancers. Infiltrating

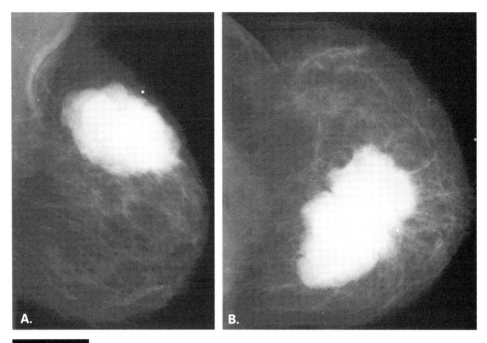

Figure 5.36

HISTORY: A 72-year-old woman with a palpable mass in the right breast.

MAMMOGRAPHY: Right MLO **(A)** and CC **(B)** views show a high-density lobular mass with microlobulated and indistinct margins. A few large round calcifications are associated with the mass and are unusual for a malignant lesion. These may be benign calcifications that were in an area occupied by the tumor, or they may be dystrophic calcifications within the malignancy.

IMPRESSION: Mass suspicious for invasive carcinoma.

HISTOPATHOLOGY: Invasive ductal carcinoma.

---

ductal carcinoma (IDC) accounts for the largest group of malignant mammary tumors and makes up 70% to 80% of breast malignancies (44). IDCs can generally be divided into two categories based on their gross appearance: spiculated and indistinct or relatively circumscribed and microlobulated. Tumors that are spiculated in configuration have been found to be more likely associated with axillary metastases than are circumscribed tumors (44,45).

IDCs more typically have the sunburst appearance and the fibrotic response that lends the name *scirrhous* to these lesions. Scirrhous carcinomas have a marked number of fibrous stroma and elastosis, accounting for some of the spiculation seen on mammography (Figs. 5.36–5.46). Newstead et al. (46) found that a spiculated mass with or without microcalcifications was the presentation of 37.8% of IDCs, and an ill-defined mass with or without microcalcifications accounted for an additional 33.6% of cases. In 85% of the cases of IDC, the density of the lesion was higher than that of the parenchyma (46).

Many cancers—especially small, mammographically detected, and clinically occult cancers—present with fewer classical features of malignancy. Instead of appearing spiculated, these lesions are partially or completely indistinctly marginated. Often the density of the cancer is greater than expected for its size and volume and greater than that of benign lesions. Because many invasive cancers are associated with DCIS, malignant microcalcifications may occur in or adjacent to the mass. The presence of pleomorphic, amorphous or linear microcalcifications associated with a poorly marginated mass increases the probability that the lesion is malignant.

Tubular (well-differentiated) carcinoma is characterized microscopically by neoplastic elements that resemble normal breast ductules (44) because the cells are forming

(text continues on page 222)

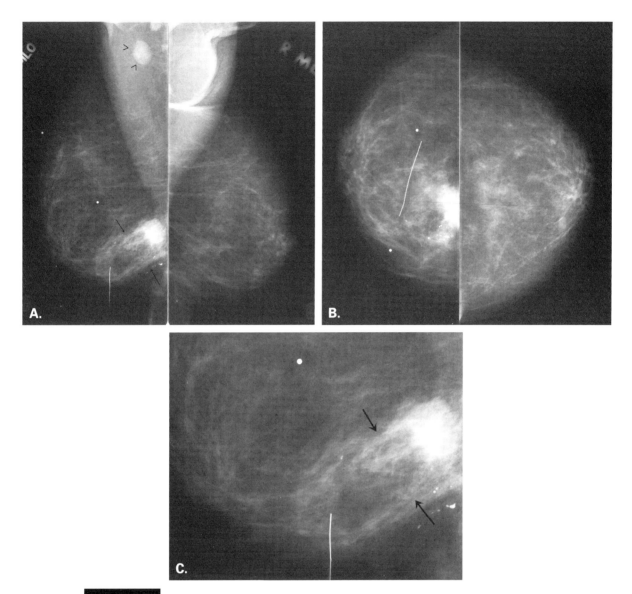

Figure 5.37

HISTORY: A 55-year-old woman with a palpable mass in the left breast.

MAMMOGRAPHY: Bilateral MLO **(A)** and CC **(B)** views show a high-density, indistinct lobular mass in the left breast at 6 o'clock. On the coned-down MLO view **(C)**, the lesion is associated with adjacent dystrophic calcifications and linear extensions anteriorly **(arrow)**, suggesting intraductal extension of tumor. A prominent lymph node **(arrowhead)** is present in the left axilla.

IMPRESSION: Invasive carcinoma with DCIS.

HISTOPATHOLOGY: Invasive ductal carcinoma and micropapillary DCIS with no metastatic carcinoma in the axillary nodes.

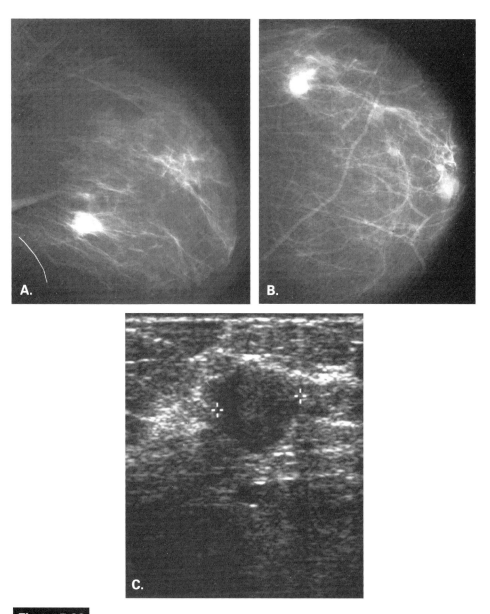

Figure 5.38

HISTORY: A 60-year-old woman for screening.

MAMMOGRAPHY: Right ML (A) and CC (B) views demonstrated a high-density round mass with indistinct margins. The high density and the margination are suspicious for carcinoma. Sonography (C) shows the mass to be solid, slightly irregular, and associated with posterior shadowing, all of which are suspicious features.

IMPRESSION: Mammographic and sonographic findings suspicious for carcinoma.

HISTOPATHOLOGY: Infiltrating ductal carcinoma and DCIS, solid type.

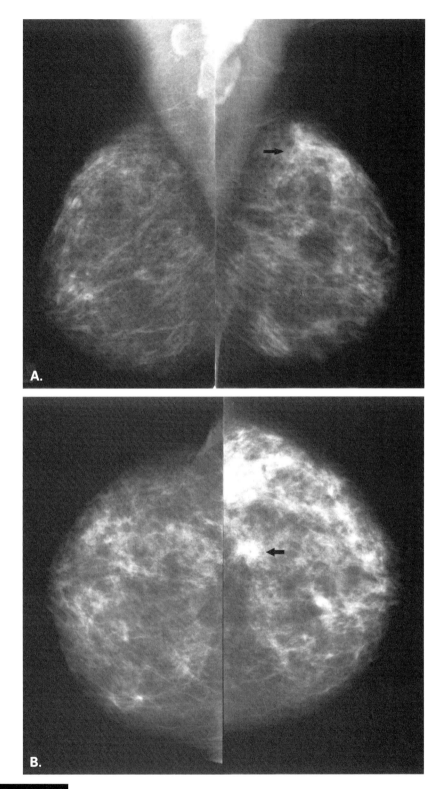

Figure 5.39

HISTORY: A 56-year-old woman for screening mammography.

MAMMOGRAPHY: Bilateral MLO **(A)** and CC **(B)** views show a focal asymmetry **(arrow)** in the right breast at 11 o'clock posteriorly. (*continued*)

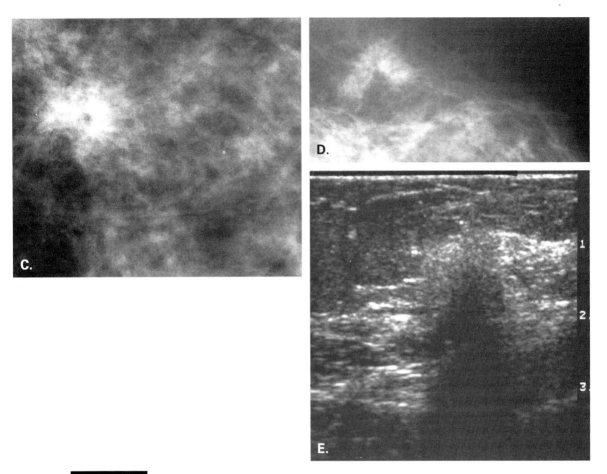

Figure 5.39 *(CONTINUED)*

On the enlarged image **(C)**, the lesion is associated with spiculation and architectural distortion. An ML magnification view **(D)** shows the lesion to be more masslike and spiculated and to be located superiorly in the breast. Sonography **(E)** shows the lesion to be solid, irregular, and densely shadowing, all features of malignancy.

IMPRESSION: Highly suspicious for carcinoma.

HISTOPATHOLOGY: Invasive ductal carcinoma.

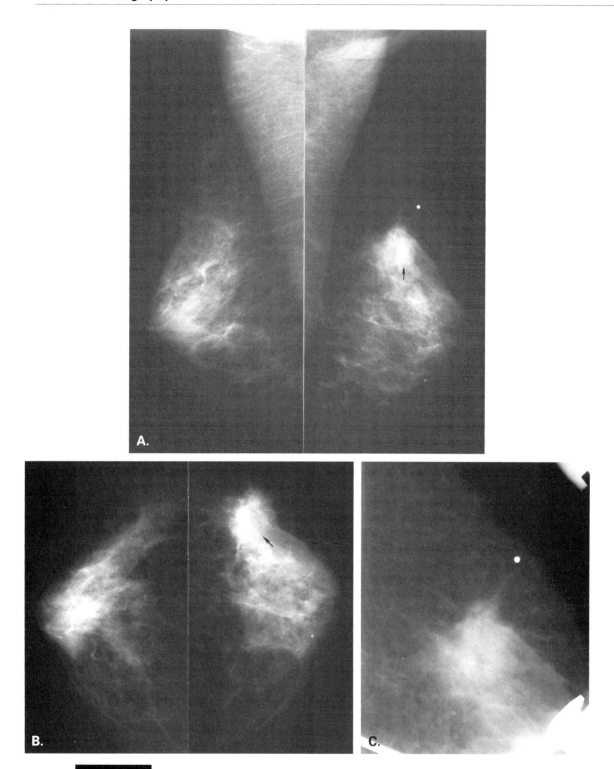

Figure 5.40

HISTORY: 59-year-old woman with a palpable mass in the right breast.

MAMMOGRAPHY: Bilateral MLO **(A)** and CC **(B)** views show heterogeneously dense breasts. There is a focal asymmetry **(arrow)** corresponding to the palpable mass in the right upper outer quadrant, marked by a BB. On spot compression **(C)**, the irregular mass with spiculated margins is seen.

IMPRESSION: Highly suspicious for carcinoma.

HISTOPATHOLOGY: Invasive ductal carcinoma.

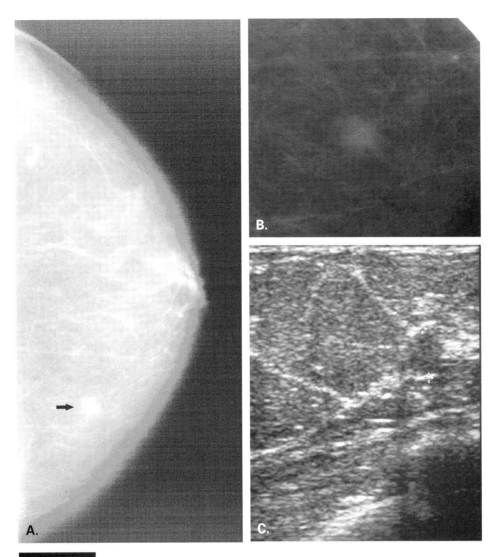

Figure 5.41

HISTORY: A 62-year-old for screening mammography.

MAMMOGRAPHY: Right CC view **(A)** demonstrates an oval mass **(arrow)** in the 3 o'clock position and some normal-appearing lymph nodes laterally. On a spot-CC magnified view **(B)**, the mass is low density, but it has indistinct margins. On ultrasound **(C)**, the mass is hypoechoic, taller than wide, and is associated with slight acoustic shadowing, all of which are suspicious for malignancy.

IMPRESSION: Mass, suspicious for carcinoma.

HISTOPATHOLOGY: Mucinous carcinoma.

NOTE: Mucinous carcinoma is a specialized type of invasive ductal carcinoma that is often somewhat circumscribed. Because of the mucin contents, these tumors may be of low density.

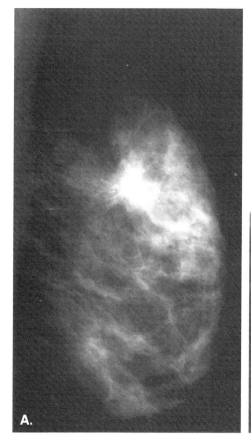
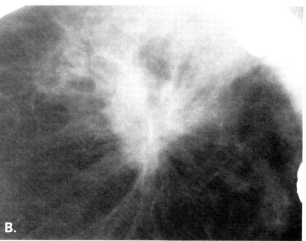

Figure 5.42

HISTORY: A 48-year-old woman with a palpable mass with right breast at 1 o'clock.

MAMMOGRAPHY: Right ML **(A)** views show a high-density, irregular mass superiorly. On spot compression **(B)**, the mass is noted to have markedly spiculated margins and to be associated with some faint amorphous microcalcifications.

IMPRESSION: Highly suspicious for malignancy.

HISTOPATHOLOGY: Infiltrating ductal carcinoma, intermediate nuclear grade.

tubules. The prognosis of pure or nearly pure tubular carcinomas is excellent, and the likelihood of axillary metastases is low. Assessment of the axilla in patients with tubular carcinoma may not be necessary according to some authors (47), but others have described axillary metastases even in pure tubular cancers (48). Tubular carcinoma has a typical appearance of a spiculated mass or architectural distortion (49). Tubular carcinomas tend to be detected when small (<1 cm) (49) and are most often detected on screening mammography as clinically occult lesions (50). These lesions are characterized histologically by orderly elongated tubules arranged in an irregular radiating manner and infiltrating into the surrounding parenchyma (49). There is a marked desmoplastic reaction (49,51). The lesion must be distinguished microscop-

ically from sclerosing adenosis, which it resembles (44). There has been controversy as to whether (52) or not (53) tubular carcinomas may arise from radial scars.

Medullary carcinoma accounts for about 5% of all breast cancers (44) and tends to be a relatively circumscribed rather than a spiculated lesion. Mucinous or colloid carcinomas represent about 1% to 2% of breast carcinomas and, like medullary carcinomas, are circumscribed (44).

Multicentric and multifocal breast cancer occur more frequently than suspected earlier, in part because of detection with magnetic resonance imaging (MRI). Multicentric carcinoma is the occurrence of two or more cancers in different quadrants, whereas multifocal carcinoma is two or more lesions in the same quadrant

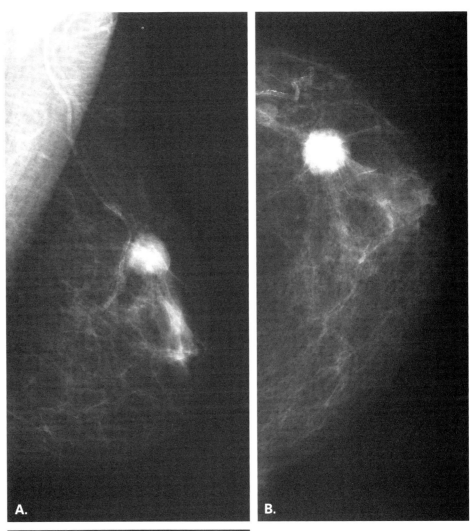

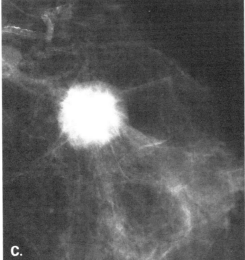

Figure 5.43

HISTORY: A 60-year-old woman with a palpable mass in the right breast.

MAMMOGRAPHY: Right MLO **(A)** and CC **(B)** view show a high-density round mass in the upper outer quadrant. Of particular concern are the margins, which are indistinct and spiculated in areas and better seen on the enlarged CC image **(C)**.

IMPRESSION: Highly suspicious for malignancy.

HISTOPATHOLOGY: Invasive carcinoma with ductal and lobular features.

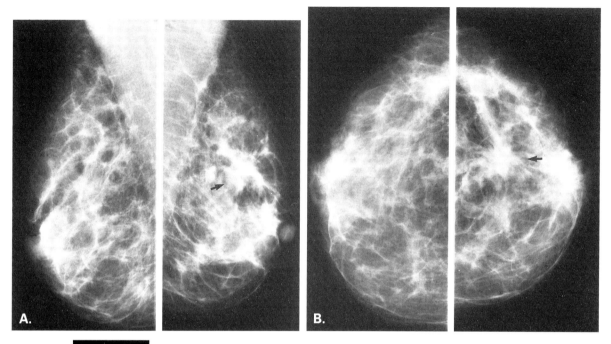

Figure 5.44

HISTORY: A 70-year-old woman with a palpable mass in the right upper-outer quadrant.

MAMMOGRAPHY: Right MLO **(A)** and CC **(B)** views. The breasts are moderately dense. In the upper outer quadrant of the right breast, there is a high-density spiculated mass **(arrows)**. This lesion has a similar shape and density on the two views and, even if it were nonpalpable, would be highly suspicious for malignancy.

IMPRESSION: Spiculated mass in the right breast, highly suspicious for carcinoma.

HISTOPATHOLOGY: Poorly differentiated infiltrating ductal carcinoma, with metastases in five of five axillary nodes.

(Figs. 5.47–5.49). The clinical significance of these entities is immense, especially to the woman with newly diagnosed breast cancer who is contemplating breast conservation. A wide excision or quadrantectomy is feasible in many cases of multifocal cancer. However, multicentric carcinoma is considered a contraindication to breast conservation therapy because of the extent of surgical resection required to remove the tumors. When the radiologist observes one lesion that is suspicious for malignancy, a search for other lesions in the ipsilateral or contralateral breast is necessary. In many cases, mammography detects others, but MRI and ultrasound are also very helpful to define the extent of disease (54). In a study of mastectomy specimens of patients preoperatively diagnosed with unifocal breast cancer, Holland et al. (55) found that only 37% actually had unifocal disease. Additional malignant foci were found in 20% of cases within 2 cm of the index lesion, and in 43%, the addi-

tional tumor deposit was more than 2 cm from the index cancer (55). Both invasive ductal and ILCs can be unifocal, multifocal, or multicentric, and there can be a mixture of types as well as in situ carcinoma.

Infiltrating lobular carcinomas, representing 8% to 10% of all breast malignancies, are characterized by a linear arrangement of tumor cells, a tendency to grow circumferentially around ducts and lobules, and an accompanying desmoplastic reaction (44). ILC is composed of a population of small monomorphic cells that diffusely invade the tissue. Instead of forming a dense mass like invasive ductal carcinoma, ILC diffusely invades the normal parenchyma. Mammographically, ILC is often an asymmetry or architectural distortion, but sometimes it produces the appearance of a spiculated or indistinct mass (56). In comparison with ductal carcinoma, ILC has an increased likelihood for multifocal or multicentric disease, as well as contralateral

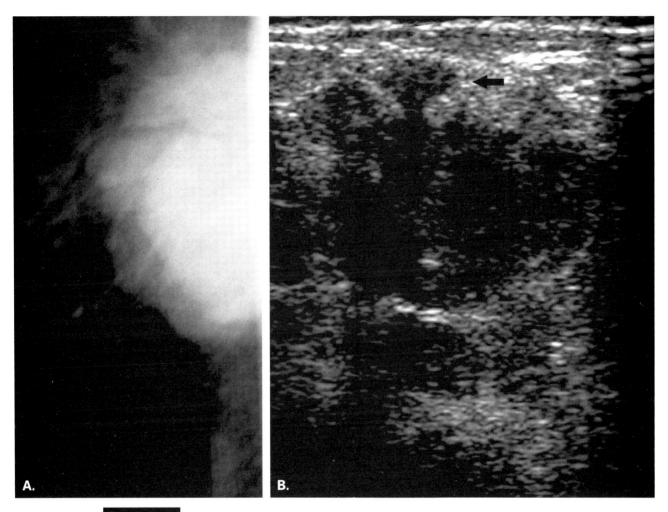

Figure 5.45

HISTORY: A 40-year-old woman with a palpable mass in the left breast.

MAMMOGRAPHY: Left ML spot view **(A)** shows a very-high-density mass with microlobulated margins, highly suspicious for malignancy. On ultrasound **(B)**, the mass is of mixed echogenicity and has irregular margins with nodular extensions **(arrow)**.

IMPRESSION: Highly suspicious for carcinoma.

HISTOPATHOLOGY: Infiltrating ductal carcinoma and DCIS, with one positive node.

malignancy (57–60). Because of the diffuse nature of ILC, it also has a higher chance of having positive margins on excision or lumpectomy (61).

Occasionally, ILCs may produce a scirrhous response (41). A spiculated lesion may extend through the subcutaneous fat to the skin, tethering it and producing the dimpling or puckering noted as secondary signs of malignancy. More often, however, the mammographic appearance is that of a subtle derangement of parenchymal architecture (62) (Figs. 5.50–5.53). Mendelson et al. (62) found that microcalcifications occurred in 25% of patients with lobular carcinoma, but the pattern of calcification was nonspecific.

OTHER MALIGNANCIES

An unusual form of IDC is metaplastic carcinoma. These tumors may have squamous or pseudosarcomatous changes (44). Those tumors with pseudosarcomatous metaplasia may contain areas of cartilage or bone formation and are demonstrated mammographically as unusual patterns of calcification.

Primary lymphoma of the breast is an unusual lesion with the breast being an uncommon site of extranodal involvement. The most common histology of primary lymphoma in the breast was found to be diffuse histocytic lymphoma (63). Lymphoma of the breast presents as a diffuse

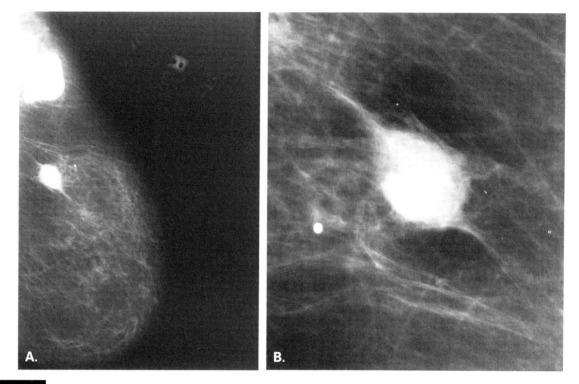

Figure 5.46

HISTORY: Palpable masses in the right axilla and in the right breast.

MAMMOGRAPHY: Right exaggerated CC lateral view **(A)** shows multiple enlarged lymph nodes in the axilla. These are very dense and somewhat indistinct, all features of malignancy. In the breast at the site of the palpable mass is a high-density oval lesion. On spot compression **(B)**, the borders are indistinct, and the overall appearance is malignant.

IMPRESSION: Carcinoma of the right breast with metastatic nodes.

HISTOPATHOLOGY: Invasive ductal carcinoma with multiple lymph nodes involved with tumor.

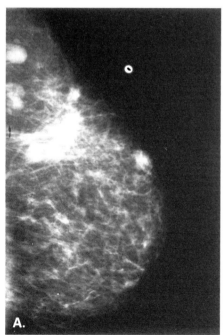

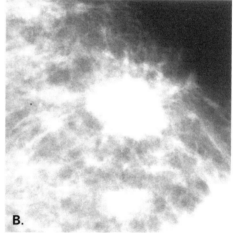

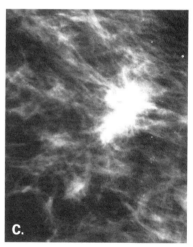

Figure 5.47

HISTORY: A 53-year-old woman with a palpable mass in the right breast laterally.

MAMMOGRAPHY: Right exaggerated CC lateral view **(A)** shows multiple high-density masses. There is a lobular mass located anteriorly, which on spot compression **(B)** appears high density and indistinct. In the central aspect of the breast is a high-density irregular mass with several small adjacent satellite lesions. On spot compression **(C)**, the irregular lesion is high density and spiculated, and there are pleomorphic microcalcifications in the vicinity.

IMPRESSION: Multicentric carcinoma.

HISTOPATHOLOGY: Invasive duct carcinoma with multiple foci of DCIS and invasive carcinoma.

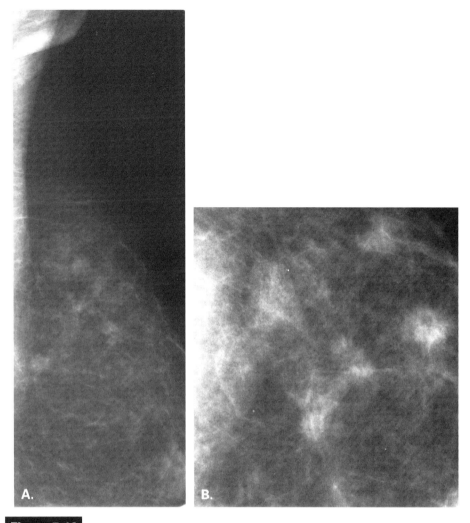

Figure 5.48

HISTORY: A 42-year-old woman recalled from an abnormal baseline mammogram.

MAMMOGRAPHY: Right axillary tail view **(A)** shows several small indistinct densities in the upper outer quadrant of the breast. Right exaggerated CC lateral magnification view **(B)** shows that there are five separate, small, indistinctly marginated masses in the breast, suspicious for malignancy.

IMPRESSION: Multiple indistinct masses, suspicious for multifocal carcinoma.

HISTOPATHOLOGY: Multifocal invasive ductal carcinoma.

increase in density of the breast or as nodules that are either well circumscribed or poorly defined but are not spiculated (64) (Figs. 5.54 and 5.55). In another series, Paulus (65) found that 21 of 23 patients with primary lymphoma had non-Hodgkin's disease, and 16 of these had diffuse large-cell lymphoma. In most cases, the mammographic findings were round, fairly circumscribed masses, but some patients had indistinct masses, focal asymmetries, and areas of increased density. No calcifications were associated with

these tumors. Ten of 24 patients also had ipsilateral axillary adenopathy, and one patient had unilateral adenopathy.

DiPiro et al. (66) also found in a study of 18 women with 21 non-Hodgkin's lymphomas of the breast that 62% presented as palpable masses. Mammographic findings ranged from well-defined to poorly defined masses, and all were hypoechoic on ultrasound. Another feature of lymphoma

(text continues on page 231)

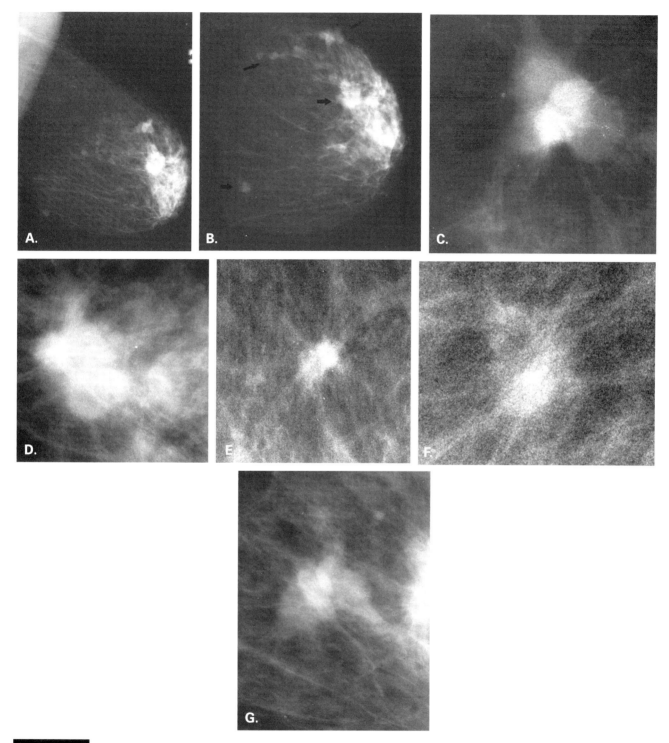

Figure 5.49

HISTORY: Palpable mass in the right breast.

MAMMOGRAPHY: Right MLO **(A)** and CC **(B)** views show dense tissue anteriorly and fatty replacement elsewhere. Multiple masses are identified, all of which are somewhat dense and irregular **(arrows)**. Spot-compression magnification views **(C, D, E, F, G)** of the various masses show the indistinct and spiculated margins associated with these as well as the associated pleomorphic and amorphous microcalcifications.

IMPRESSION: Multicentric carcinoma.

HISTOPATHOLOGY: Multicentric invasive ductal carcinoma.

NOTE: When one suspicious lesion is identified, the radiologist must carefully search for other abnormalities that could represent multicentric or multifocal carcinoma.

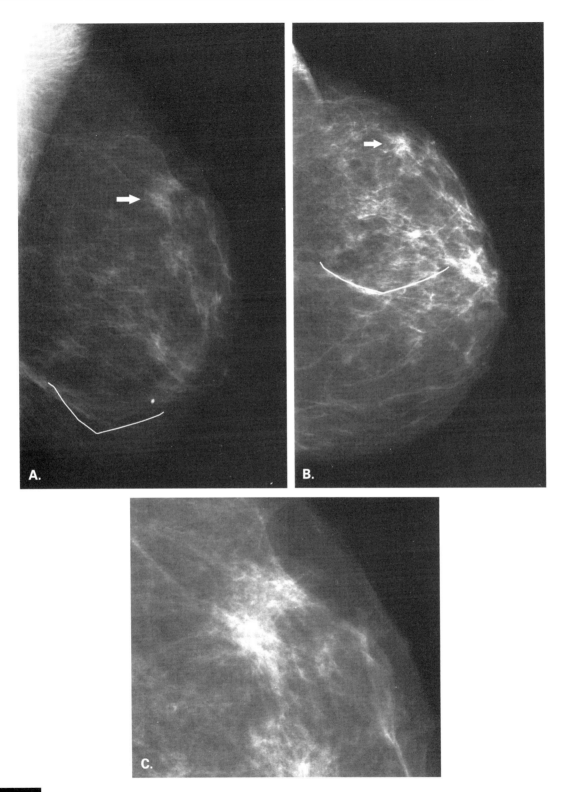

Figure 5.50

HISTORY: A 74-year-old woman for screening mammography.

MAMMOGRAPHY: Right MLO **(A)** and CC **(B)** views show a relatively fatty-replaced breast. There is a focal asymmetry **(arrow)** in the right upper-outer quadrant, which on spot compression **(C)** appears more visible. The margins are indistinct. and the lesion is iso-dense.

IMPRESSION: Indistinct mass; recommend biopsy.

HISTOPATHOLOGY: Invasive lobular carcinoma.

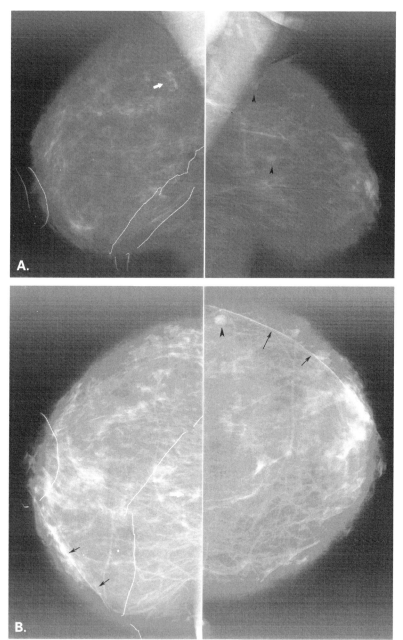

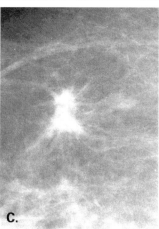

Figure 5.51

HISTORY: A 41-year-old woman who is status post reduction mammoplasty, for screening mammography.

MAMMOGRAPHY: Bilateral MLO **(A)** and CC **(B)** views show scattered fibroglandular densities and scars bilaterally **(arrows)**. There are several intramammary lymph nodes on the right **(arrowheads)**. On the left at 12 o'clock is a small area of architectural distortion **(white arrow)**. The spot-compression MLO view **(C)** of this area shows a persistent, small irregular mass with spiculated margins.

IMPRESSION: Postreduction mammoplasty changes, spiculated mass left breast, highly suspicious for malignancy.

HISTOPATHOLOGY: Invasive lobular carcinoma.

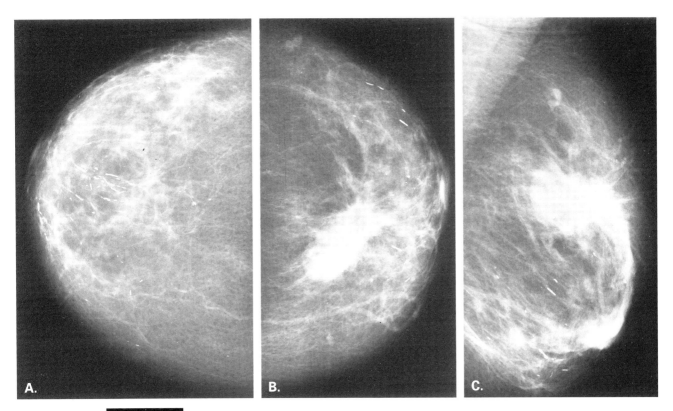

Figure 5.52

HISTORY: An 80-year-old gravida 0 woman with a 4-cm, palpable right breast mass.

MAMMOGRAPHY: Left **(A)** and right **(B)** CC and right MLO **(C)** views. There are bilateral smooth linear calcifications present, consistent with secretory disease. In the right upper-inner quadrant, there is a large, high-density spiculated mass highly suspicious for carcinoma. Incidental note is made of a normal-sized intramammary node in the upper outer quadrant.

HISTOPATHOLOGY: Infiltrating lobular carcinoma, with a large component of mucinous carcinoma. No evidence of carcinoma in 14 nodes.

that may be observed on mammography is enlarged axillary nodes. These nodes are usually dense, bulky, and relatively circumscribed, unlike metastatic nodes from breast cancer, in which the margins are more indistinct.

OTHER UNUSUAL LESIONS

Other unusual lesions that can occur in the breast rarely and can be manifested as a poorly defined mass include lesions such as cholesterol granuloma, tuberculosis, actinomycosis, amyloidosis, and Wegener's granulomatosis. These reactive, inflammatory, or infective lesions all can appear both clinically and mammographically as suspicious for carcinoma.

Tuberculosis involving the breast is very rare in western countries, occurring in fewer than 0.1% of breast biopsies; however, in developing countries, the incidence is 3% to 4.4% of all breast diseases treated (67). Tuberculosis has a predilection for the patient who is lactating. Bodur et al. (68) described a 40-year-old woman with polyarticular and breast involvement with tuberculosis. Mammography showed a suspicious mass that was complex on ultrasound.

Inflammatory conditions that affect the arteries, which are the vasculitides associated with collagen vascular disease, can affect the breast rarely. Wegener's granulomatosis or necrotizing vasculitis may rarely involve the breast (Fig. 5.56). Both clinically (69) and mammographically (70), this lesion is suspicious for malignancy. The tumor is usually tender and has an irregular or spiculated contour.

Amyloid deposits in the breast can occur in patients with the predisposing systemic diseases, such as rheumatoid arthritis, multiple myeloma, and Waldenstrom's macroglobulinemia (13). Clinically, the amyloidosis of the breast is a firm, palpable mass that may contain calcifications on mammography (71).

Plasma cell mastitis and duct ectasia are common, yet the presentation as a spiculated mass is infrequent. Rarely, these patients may present with a palpable subareolar mass that contains cholesterol crystals; this is termed a *cholesterol granuloma* (72).

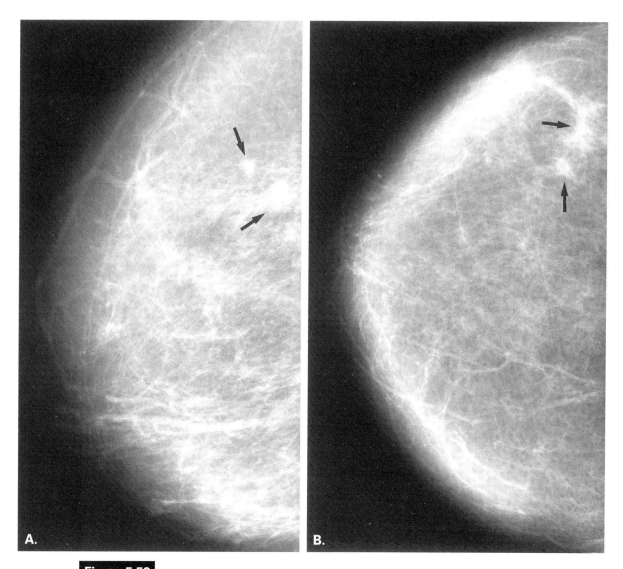

Figure 5.53

HISTORY: A 66-year-old gravida 8, para 6, abortus 2 patient for screening mammography.

MAMMOGRAPHY: Left ML **(A)** and CC **(B)** views. There are two indistinct masses **(arrows)** in close proximity in the upper outer quadrant of the left breast. The masses are of relatively high density for their small size and in comparison with the background parenchymal density. There is a slight difference in the shape of each mass on the two views; nonetheless, these remain very focal and irregular.

IMPRESSION: Two indistinct masses, highly suspicious for multifocal carcinoma.

HISTOPATHOLOGY: Infiltrating lobular carcinoma, intraductal carcinoma, lobular carcinoma in situ, no evidence of carcinoma in 21 axillary nodes.

A variety of vascular lesions can occasionally occur in the breast. The malignant vascular tumor is angiosarcoma, which typically presents as a large, indistinctly marginated mass that may contain microcalcifications (73). A bluish discoloration of the skin has been described in 17% of patients (73), which is thought to be related to the vascular nature of the lesion. Angiosarcoma can develop after breast irradiation for treatment of breast cancer; the prognosis is poor.

Benign vascular tumors include hemangiomas, subcutaneous hemangiomas, and angiomatosis. Many hemangiomas are detected on mammography (Fig. 5.57) and are not clinically evident, but large lesions may be palpable. Often these are circumscribed masses with calcifications (74), but some lesions may be indistinct or even appear as tortuous vessels (13).

(text continues on page 235)

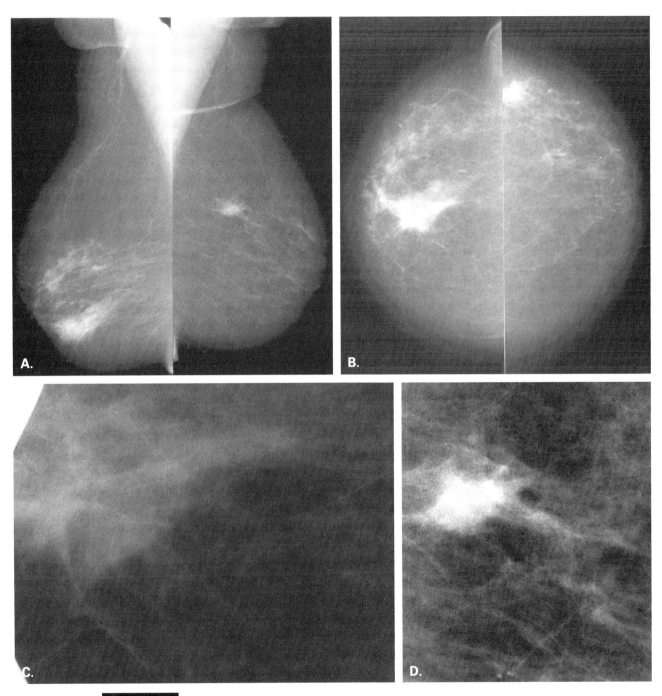

Figure 5.54

HISTORY: A 68-year-old woman with a history of lymphoma of the right eye who presents for screening.

MAMMOGRAPHY: Bilateral MLO **(A)** and CC **(B)** views show irregular indistinct masses in both breasts. On spot-compression left CC **(C)** and spot-compression right MLO **(D)**, the indistinct margins of the masses are seen.

IMPRESSION: Bilateral indistinct masses, lymphoma versus carcinoma.

HISTOPATHOLOGY: Non-Hodgkin's lymphoma.

NOTE: Lymphoma in the breast most often presents as circumscribed or indistinct masses. Adenopathy also may be associated or may be the sole presentation.

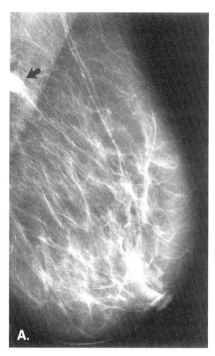

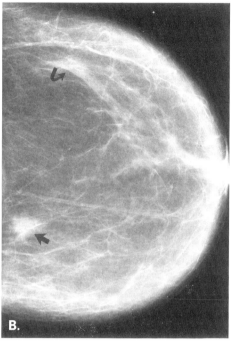

Figure 5.55

HISTORY: A 75-year-old woman with history of lymphoma, for routine screening mammography.

MAMMOGRAPHY: Right MLO (**A**) and CC (**B**) views. There is an isodense indistinct mass located in the posterior upper aspect of the right breast (**arrow**) on the MLO view (**A**). On the CC view (**B**), the lesion is located medially (**arrow**). A second, smaller irregular lesion is also presented laterally (**curved arrow**). Although these lesions could represent lymphoma, the favored diagnosis is a primary breast carcinoma.

IMPRESSION: Two irregular lesions, probably neoplastic: primary carcinoma versus lymphoma.

HISTOPATHOLOGY (BOTH SITES): Malignant lymphoma, mixed small- and large-cell type.

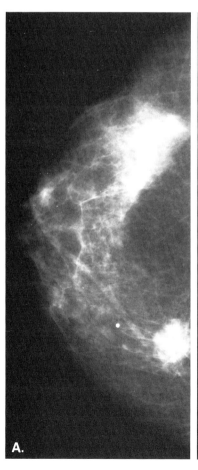

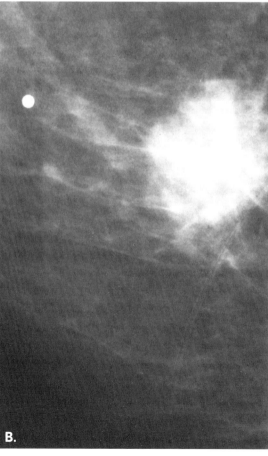

Figure 5.56

HISTORY: A 50-year-old woman with history of Wegener's granulomatosis, who presents with a palpable left breast mass.

MAMMOGRAPHY: Left CC view (**A**) and enlarged CC view (**B**) show the palpable mass to be round and high density but to have very indistinct margins. The primary consideration is breast carcinoma, although occasionally other lesions can have this appearance.

HISTOPATHOLOGY: Vasculitis, consistent with Wegener's granulomatosis.

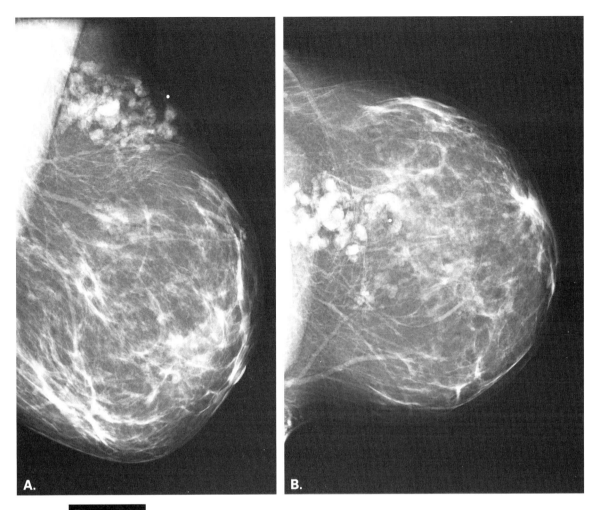

Figure 5.57

HISTORY: A 23-year-old woman with a palpable mass in the superior aspect of the right breast.

MAMMOGRAPHY: Right MLO **(A)** and CC **(B)** views show an irregular, high-density large mass in the 12 o'clock position of the breast. The mass has a tubulonodular appearance and indistinct margination, suggesting that it is either ductal or vascular in origin.

IMPRESSION: Right breast mass, suspicious for an intraductal lesion or vascular lesion.

HISTOPATHOLOGY: Hemangioma.

REFERENCES

1. Gold RH, Montgomery CK, Rambo ON. Significance of margination of benign and malignant infiltrative mammary lesions: roentgenographic-pathological correlation. *AJR Am J Roentgenol* 1973;118:881–893.
2. American College of Radiology. *Breast Imaging Reporting and Data System (BIRADS)*. Reston, VA: ACR, 2003.
3. Tabar L, Dean PB. *Teaching Atlas of Mammography*. Stuttgart: Georg Thieme Verlag, 1983.
4. Hermann G, Janus C, Schwartz IS, et al. Nonpalpable breast lesions: accuracy of prebiopsy mammographic diagnosis. *Radiology* 1987;165:323–326.
5. Keen ME, Murad TM, Cohen MI, et al. Benign breast lesions with malignant clinical and mammographic presentations. *Hum Pathol* 1985;16:1147–1152.
6. Urban JA, Adair FE. Sclerosing adenosis. *Cancer* 1949;2: 625–634.
7. Nielsen NSM, Nielsen BB. Mammographic features of sclerosing adenosis presenting as a tumour. *Clin Radiol* 1986; 37:371–373.
8. Cotron RS, Kumar V, Robbins SL. *Robbins Pathologic Basis of Disease*. Philadelphia: WB Saunders, 1989:1188.
9. Heimann G, Schwartz IS. Focal fibrous disease of the breast: mammographic detection of an unappreciated condition. *AJR Am J Roentgenol* 1983;140:1245–1246.
10. Harvey SC, Denison CM, Lester SC. Fibrous nodules found at large-core needle biopsy of the breast: imaging features. *Radiology* 1999;211:535–540.
11. Vuitch MF, Rosen PP, Edmondson RA. Pseudoangiomatous hyperplasia of mammary stroma. *Hum Pathol* 1986;17: 185–191.
12. Ortiz-Rey JA, Alvarez A, Valbuena L, et al. Pseudoangiomatous hyperplasia of mammary stroma. *Breast Dis* 1995;8:295–299.
13. Rosen PP. *Rosen's Breast Pathology*, 2nd ed. Philadelphia: Lippincott Williams & Wilkins, 2001.

14. Anderson JA, Gram JB. Radial scar in the female breast: a long-term follow-up study of 32 cases. *Cancer* 1984;53: 2557–2560.

15. Fenoglic C, Lattes R. Sclerosing papillary proliferations in the female breast. *Cancer* 1974;33:691–700.

16. Tremblay G, Buell RH, Seemayer TA. Elastosis in benign sclerosing ductal proliferation of the female breast. *Am J Surg Pathol* 1977;1:155–159.

17. Fisher ER, Palekar AS, Kotwal N, et al. A nonencapsulated sclerosing lesion of the breast. *Am J Clin Pathol* 1979;71: 240–246.

18. Rickert RR, Kalisher L, Hutter RVP. Indurative mastopathy: a benign sclerosing lesion of breast with elastosis which may simulate carcinoma. *Cancer* 1981;47:561–571.

19. Cohen MI, Matthies HJ, Mintzer RA, et al. Indurative mastopathy: a cause of false positive mammograms. *Radiology* 1985;155:69–71.

20. Anderson I. Mammography in clinical practice. *Med Radiogr Photogr* 1986:62.

21. Mitnick JS, Vazquez MF, Harris MN, et al. Differentiation of radial scar from scirrhous carcinoma of the breast: mammographic-pathologic correlation. *Radiology* 1989;173:697–700.

22. Stigers KB, King JG, Davey DD, et al. Abnormalities of the breast caused by biopsy: spectrum of mammographic findings. *AJR Am J Roentgenol* 1991;156:287–291.

23. Sickles EA, Herzog KA. Mammography of the postsurgical breast. *AJR Am J Roentgenol* 1981;136:585–588.

24. Clarke D, Curtis JL, Martinez A, et al. Fat necrosis of the breast simulating recurrent carcinoma after primary radiotherapy in the management of early stage breast carcinoma. *Cancer* 1983;52:442–445.

25. Dershaw DD, McCormick R, Cox L, et al. Differentiation of benign and malignant local tumor recurrence after lumpectomy. *AJR Am J Roentgenol* 1990;155:35–38.

26. Bassett LW, Gold RH, Cove HC. Mammographic spectrum of traumatic fat necrosis: the fallibility of "pathognomonic" signs of carcinoma. *AJR Am J Roentgenol* 1978;130:119–122.

27. Mendelson EB. Imaging the post surgical breast. *Semin Ultrasound CT MR* 1989;10(2):154–170.

28. Abrikossoff A. Über myome, ausgehand von der quergestreiften, willkarlichen muskulatur. *Virchows Arch Pathol Anat* 1926: 260:215–233.

29. D'Orsi CJ, Feldhaus L, Sonnenfeld M. Unusual lesions of the breast. *Radiol Clin North Am* 1983;21:67–69.

30. Bassett LW, Cove HC. Myoblastoma of the breast. *AJR Am J Roentgenol* 1979;132:122–123.

31. Adeniran A, Al-Ahmadie H, Mahoney MC, et al. Granular cell tumor of the breast: a series of 17 cases and review of the literature. *Breast J* 2004;10(6):528–531.

32. Ali M, Fayemi AO, Braun EV, et al. Fibromatosis of the breast. *Am J Surg Pathol* 1979;3:501–505.

33. Yiangou C, Fadl H, Sinnett HD, et al. Fibromatosis of the breast or carcinoma. *J R Soc Med* 1996;89:638–640.

34. Kalisher L, Long JA, Peyster RG. Extra-abdominal desmoid of the axillary tail mimicking breast carcinoma. *AJR Am J Roentgenol* 1976;126:903–906.

35. Bogomoletz WV, Boulenger E, Simatos A. Infiltrating fibromatosis of the breast. *J Clin Pathol* 1981;34:30–34.

36. Rosen PP, Ernsberger D. Mammary fibromatosis: a benign spindle-cell tumor with significant risk for local recurrence. *Cancer* 1989;63:1363–1369.

37. Cederlund CG, Gustavasson S, Linell F, et al. Fibromatosis of the breast mimicking carcinoma at mammography. *Br J Radiol* 1984;57:98–101.

38. Wargotz ES, Norris HJ, Austin RM, et al. Fibromatosis of the breast. *Am J Surg Pathol* 1987;11(1):38–45.

39. Leborgne R. Diagnosis of tumors of the breast by simple roentgenography: calcifications in carcinoma. *AJR Am J Roentgenol* 1951;65:1–11.

40. Lundgren B. Malignant features of breast tumours at radiography. *Acta Radiol (Diagn)* 1978;19:623–633.

41. Sadowsky N, Kopans DB. Breast cancer. *Radiol Clin North Am* 1983;21:51–65.

42. Bloom HJG, Richardson WW. Histologic grading and prognosis in breast cancer: a study of 1049 cases of which 359 have been followed 15 years. *Br J Cancer* 1957;11:359–377.

43. Reiff DB, Cooke J, Griffin M, et al. Ductal carcinoma in situ presenting as a stellate lesion on mammography. *Clin Radiol* 1994;49:393–399.

44. Rosen PP. The pathology of breast carcinoma. In: Harris JR, Hellman S, Henderson IC, et al., eds. *Breast Diseases*. Philadelphia: JB Lippincott, 1987:147–209.

45. Gold RH, Main G, Zippin C, et al. Infiltration of mammary carcinoma as an indicator of axillary metastases: a preliminary report. *Cancer* 1972;29:35–40.

46. Newstead GM, Baute PB, Toth HK. Invasive lobular and ductal carcinoma: mammographic findings and stage at diagnosis. *Radiology* 1992;184:623–627.

47. Peters GN, Wolff M, Haagensen CD. Tubular carcinoma of the breast: Clinical pathologic correlations based on 100 cases. *Ann Surg* 1981;193(2):138–149.

48. Winchester DJ, Sahin AA, Tucker SL, et al. Tubular carcinoma of the breast: predicting axillary nodal metastases and recurrence. *Ann Surg* 1996;223(3):342–347.

49. Feig SA, Shaber GS, Patchefsky AS, et al. Tubular carcinoma of the breast: mammographic appearance and pathological correlation. *Radiology* 1978;129:311–314.

50. Elson BC, Helvie MA, Frank TS, et al. Tubular carcinoma of the breast: mode of presentation, mammographic appearance, and frequency of nodal metastases. *AJR Am J Roentgenol* 1993;161:1173–1176.

51. Jao W, Recant W, Swerdlow MA. Comparative ultrastructure of tubular carcinoma and sclerosing adenosis of the breast. *Cancer* 1976;38:180–186.

52. Linell F, Ljungberg O. Breast carcinoma: progression of tubular carcinoma and a new classification. *Acta Pathol Microbiol Scand (A)* 1980;88:59–60.

53. Wellings SR, Alpers CE. Subgross pathologic features and incidence of radial scars in the breast. *Hum Pathol* 1984;15: 475–479.

54. Berg WA. Imaging the local extent of disease. *Semin Breast Dis* 2001;153–173.

55. Holland R, Veling SH, Mravunac M, et al. Histologic multifocality of Tis, T1-2 breast carcinomas: implications for clinical trials of breast-conserving surgery. *Cancer* 1985;56(5):979–990.

56. Sickles EA. The subtle and atypical mammographic features of invasive lobular carcinoma. *Radiology* 1991;178:25–26.

57. Cornford EJ, Wilson AR, Athanassiou E, et al. Mammographic features of invasive lobular and invasive ductal carcinoma of the breast: a comparative analysis. *Br J Radiol* 1995;68:450–453.

58. Dixon JM, Anderson TJ, Page DL, et al. Infiltrating lobular carcinoma of the breast: an evaluation of the incidence and consequence of bilateral disease. *Br J Surg* 1983;70:513–516.

59. Lesser ML, Rosen PP, Kinne DW. Multicentricity and bilaterality in invasive breast carcinoma. *Surgery* 1982;91:234–240.

60. Lesser ML, Rosen PP, Kinne DW. Multicentricity and bilaterality in invasive breast carcinoma. *Surgery* 1982;91:234–240.

61. Moore MM, Borossa G, Imbrie JZ, et al. Association of infiltrating lobular carcinoma with positive surgical margins after breast-conservation therapy. *Ann Surg* 2000;231(6):877–882.

62. Mendelson EB, Harris KM, Doshi N, et al. Infiltrating lobular carcinoma: mammographic patterns with pathologic correlation. *AJR Am J Roentgenol* 1989;153:265–271.

63. Schouten JT, Weese JL, Carbone PP. Lymphoma of the breast. *Ann Surg* 1981;194(6):749–753.

64. Meyer JE, Kopans DB. Xeromammographic appearance of lymphoma of the breast. *Radiology* 1980;135:623–626.

65. Paulus DD. Lymphoma of the breast. *Radiol Clin North Am* 1990;28(4):833–840.

66. DiPiro PJ, Lester S, Meyer JE, et al. Non-Hodgkin lymphoma of the breast: clinical and radiologic presentations. *Breast J* 1996;2(6):380–384.

67. Al-Marri MR, Almosleh A, Almosimeni Y. Primary tuberculosis of the breast in Qatar: ten year experience and the literature. *Eur J Surg* 2000;166(9):687–690.

68. Bodur H, Erbay A, Bodur H, et al. Multifocal tuberculosis presenting with osteoarticular and breast involvement. *Annals of Clinical Microbiology and Antimicrobials* 2003;2(6):1–4.

69. Göbel U, Kettritz R, Kettritz U, et al. Wegener's granulomatosis masquerading as breast cancer. *Arch Intern Med* 1995;155:205–207.

70 Deininger HZ. Wegener's granulomatosis of the breast. *Radiology* 1985;154:59–60.

71. Hecht AH, Tan A, Slen JF. Case report: primary systemic amyloidosis presenting as breast masses, mammographically simulating carcinoma. *Clin Radiol* 1991;44:123–124.

72. Reynolds HE, Cramer HM. Cholesterol granulomas of the breast: a mimic of carcinoma. *Radiology* 1994;191:249–250.

73. Liberman L, Dershaw DD, Kaufman RJ, et al. Angiosarcoma of the breast. *Radiology* 1992;183:649–654.

74. Webb LA, Young JR. Case report: hemangioma of the breast: appearances on mammography and ultrasound. *Clin Radiol* 1996;51:523–524.

Analysis of Calcifications

Some form of calcification is identified on the majority of mammograms. Many calcifications are clearly benign and require no further workup, whereas others are highly suggestive of malignancy. Between these two groups are various patterns of microcalcifications that are indeterminate in etiology and that often require biopsy for diagnosis.

Calcifications in breast tumors were described in early work by Leborgne (1) in 1951. In 1962, Gershon-Cohen et al. (2) described the forms of microcalcifications that were associated with breast malignancies as irregular in size and shape and ranging from minute to 3 mm in diameter. Approximately 50% of breast cancers are associated with calcifications (3), and as many as 98% of intraductal carcinomas contain microcalcifications (4). In cancers manifesting solely as microcalcifications, as many as 69% are noninvasive (5).

Since the early descriptions of breast calcifications, mammography has advanced, and higher image quality is attainable, thereby enhancing the visibility and detectability of microcalcifications. Publication of the American College of Radiology Imaging Network (ACRIN) trial of full-field digital mammography (6) has shown statistical significance in improved detection of breast cancer in three groups of women: those who are younger than 50 years of age, those who are pre- and perimenopausal, and those with dense breasts. In part, this improvement in detection of cancers may be reflected in the greater detectability of microcalcifications associated with ductal carcinomas.

When a radiologist is interpreting a mammogram, the decision that must be made when calcifications are identified is whether they are clearly benign, probably benign, indeterminate with a suspicion for malignancy, or highly suspicious for breast cancer. Although this assessment can be made on screening views in many cases, diagnostic mammography is often needed for microcalcifications. In particular, magnification views are performed for the complete evaluation of microcalcifications. Once the evaluation of the imaging features of calcifications has been made, a management plan can be recommended, such as routine follow-up annually, early follow-up at 6-month

intervals, or biopsy. For those calcifications that are classified as suspicious and for which biopsy is recommended, the positive predictive value of malignancy is about 25% (7).

In order to accurately analyze small calcifications identified on routine screening mammography, additional evaluation is necessary. Magnification mammography is performed to more clearly depict their morphology, and supplemental views, including mediolateral and tangential views, may be performed to determine the answers to the following questions:

1. Are the microcalcifications real or artifactual?
2. What is the morphology of the calcifications?
3. What is the distribution of the calcifications?
4. Where are the calcifications located?
5. Are the microcalcifications clearly benign, such being dermal or milk of calcium?

Once these questions are answered, a management plan can be better determined.

ARTIFACTS AND PSEUDOCALCIFICATIONS

There are a variety of foreign substances that when present on the skin may have the appearance of microcalcifications on mammography. The technologist must take care to inquire about the presence of such substances, and she should ask the patient to wipe the breast and axilla with a moist cloth if these substances may be present. If the "calcifications" are located very superficially, if they seem to conform to a pattern (such as within skin folds), or if they have a stippled appearance, they may represent pseudocalcifications or artifacts. In this case, the views on which the calcifications are seen should be repeated after skin cleansing.

Substances on the skin (8,9) that can be evident as apparent microcalcifications on mammography include the following: deodorants (Fig. 6.1), bath powders, creams and lotions, ointments such as zinc oxide (Fig. 6.2), and

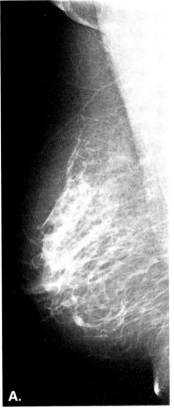

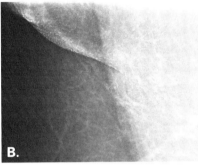

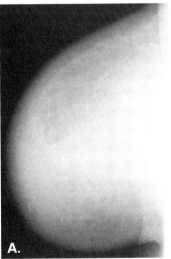

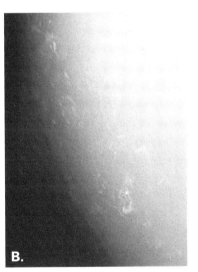

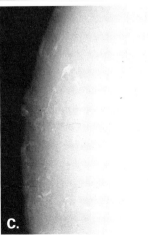

Figure 6.1

HISTORY: Screening mammogram.

MAMMOGRAPHY: Left MLO **(A)** view shows faint calcific densities overlying the skin folds in the axilla better seen on the enlarged image **(B)**. These are uniform and stippled in appearance, typical of deodorant artifact.

IMPRESSION: Deodorant artifact.

Figure 6.2

HISTORY: Elderly patient with Stevens Johnson syndrome and multiple skin excoriations on the breasts. She was treating these with an ointment containing zinc oxide. She had marked enlargement and inflammation of the left breast.

MAMMOGRAPHY: Left ML view **(A)** shows marked increased density of the breast with associated skin thickening. Numerous calcific densities are located anteriorly. On the enlarged images over the subareolar area **(B, C)**, the pseudocalcifications related to the zinc oxide ointment are better seen. The patient was treated with antibiotics for the mastitis, and it resolved.

IMPRESSION: Pseudocalcifications from zinc oxide in skin ulcerations, mastitis.

adhesive tape. Skin lesions, such as seborrheic keratoses, are particularly prone to trap any cosmetics that may be placed on the skin within the crenulations on their surface.

A cause of pseudocalcifications within the patient's breast rather than on the skin surface is the deposition of gold in intramammary and axillary lymph nodes in patients with rheumatoid arthritis treated by chrysotherapy (10,11) (Figs. 6.3 and 6.4). Clinical history is key to confirming the diagnosis when this etiology is suspected. On mammography, the characteristic appearance is that of very fine, stippled "microcalcifications" within one or more intramammary or axillary lymph nodes. Additionally, the nodes may be mildly enlarged as a result of the rheumatoid arthritis.

Bullet fragments that are very small and scattered within the breast may have an appearance suggestive of calcifications, but because of the higher density of the metal, they appear more radiopaque than calcium. Other foreign bodies within the breast are usually not confused with true calcifications because of their defining shapes (i.e., surgical clips and markers, retained wire or hooks from needle localization procedures, sutures) and their overall very high density.

Other types of artifacts that may simulate microcalcifications on mammography are related to technical or non-patient factors, including the following: mammographic equipment artifacts, cassette artifacts, and processing and film-handling artifacts. Most of these are unique to film screen mammography and are related to handling film. With full-field digital mammography, such artifacts do not exist. These artifacts usually have characteristic appearances that aid in differentiating them from true calcifications.

Scratches or "pick-off" from the processor occurs when the film emulsion is damaged as the film makes its transit through the processor, and such artifacts produce white specks on the film. Often these are brighter than true microcalcifications and therefore can be identified as artifactual. The processor must be properly maintained to minimize these.

Debris or dust between the film and screen within the cassette produces a white speck or pseudocalcification and is problematic not only by simulating calcium, but also by

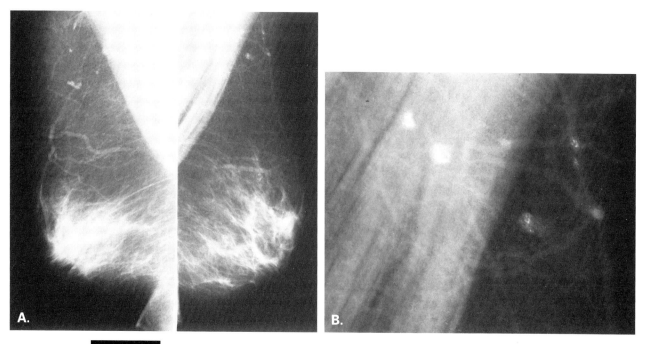

Figure 6.3

HISTORY: A 58-year-old woman with a history of rheumatoid arthritis treated with chrysotherapy.

MAMMOGRAPHY: Bilateral MLO **(A)** views show multiple dense lymph nodes in the axillae. On the magnified view **(B)**, the nodes are noted to contain dense, stippled calcificlike material.

IMPRESSION: Pseudocalcifications: gold deposits secondary to treatment for rheumatoid arthritis.

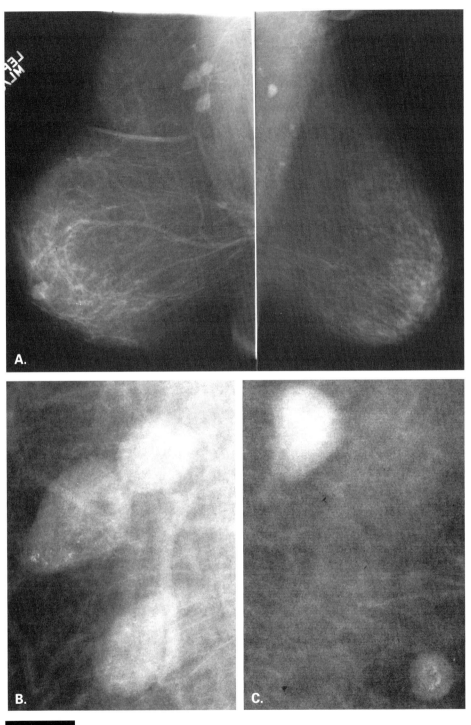

Figure 6.4

HISTORY: A 68-year-old patient with a history of rheumatoid arthritis, for screening mammography.

MAMMOGRAPHY: Bilateral MLO **(A)** views show scattered fibroglandular densities and multiple lymph nodes in the axillae. On close inspection of the nodes **(B, C)**, there are faint, stippled cal-cificlike densities present. These findings represent gold deposits in intramammary nodes, secondary to chrysotherapy for rheumatoid arthritis.

IMPRESSION: Gold deposits in lymph nodes, secondary to chrysotherapy for rheumatoid arthritis.

producing focal blur from poor film screen contact. Cassettes and screens must be cleaned at least weekly according to standards established by the American College of Radiology's (ACR) Mammography Accreditation Program (12), and in darkroom environments where dust control is a problem, more frequent cleaning is necessary to avoid these artifacts. Cassettes must be numbered so that when a film screen artifact is identified, the cassette may be pulled and recleaned.

Other etiologies of white specks or pseudocalcifications relate to improper film handling. Fingerprints on the film occur when the technologist does not handle the film from the corner when loading the cassette. Often the pattern of the whorls in the fingerprint is evident, and the finding is seen on one view only (Figs. 6.5 and 6.6). One can repeat the view to confirm that the abnormality was artifactual without the unnecessary workup of using magnification views.

MAMMOGRAPHIC VIEWS TO EVALUATE MICROCALCIFICATIONS

Once it has been determined that calcifications are real, one must determine where they are located. A clock-face location (one o'clock, etc.) and a position or depth within the breast relative to the nipple (anterior, middle, posterior) is described. If the calcifications are seen on one view only, then additional views are selected to determine their position. If calcifications are seen on one view

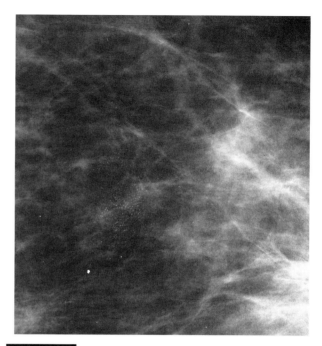

Figure 6.6

HISTORY: Screening mammogram on a 41-year-old woman.

MAMMOGRAPHY: Coned-down MLO view shows fine calcific densities in a regular pattern. These have a stippled appearance and were found to be absent on a repeat film. The finding represents a fingerprint artifact.

IMPRESSION: Fingerprint artifact.

NOTE: This is an artifact unique to film screen mammography and is not found on digital mammography.

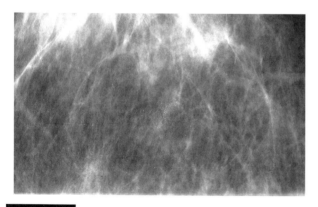

Figure 6.5

HISTORY: Screening mammogram.

MAMMOGRAPHY: Enlarged CC image shows a cluster of bright white calcificlike densities in a pattern. The stippled appearance and pattern are consistent with a fingerprint artifact that occurred during film handling.

IMPRESSION: Fingerprint artifact.

only and are not artifactual, they often are of dermal or milk-of-calcium origin. One should scrutinize the skin thoroughly to see if calcifications that seem to be within the breast on one view are actually on the skin on the other view.

For calcifications that may be dermal, based on their morphology, but that do not project directly within the skin surface on one of the views, two methods of mammographic verification are available. The so-called bead-o-gram can be performed, in which the technologist, using a localization plate as is used in needle localizations, places a BB or radiopaque object over the calcifications on the view on which they are seen (13). The localizer plate is then removed, and a tangential view is performed with the BB in tangent to the beam. If the calcifications are dermal, they will project on the skin with the BB (Fig. 6.7). The second method is to perform stereotactic imaging (14). When dermal calcifications are targeted on a stereotactic pair of images, their z-position or depth will project at the skin surface. Caution should be used to not merely rely on the z-position of the

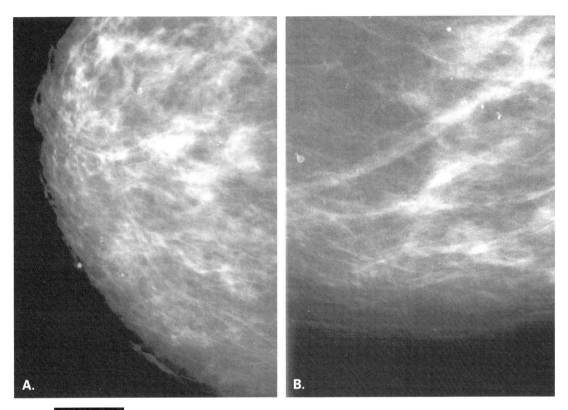

Figure 6.7

HISTORY: A 61-year-old woman for screening mammography.

MAMMOGRAPHY: Left CC view (**A**) shows multiple small round calcifications. On magnification CC view (**B**), the very well-defined, round, and lucent forms are noted.

HISTOPATHOLOGY: Dermal calcifications.

calcifications versus the compressed breast thickness to calculate that the calcifications are at the skin surface. Instead, a needle should be placed through the needle guides with the Δ Z at 0 mm to confirm that the needle tip is at the skin surface.

For parenchymal calcifications located very posteriorly on the mediolateral oblique (MLO) view and not seen on the craniocaudal (CC) view, exaggerated CC views may help to demonstrate their location on the transverse plane. For calcifications seen far medially and posteriorly on the CC view only, the lateromedial projection may demonstrate their position on the sagittal plane.

Once the location of calcifications is confirmed, a careful assessment of their morphology is undertaken. This is best accomplished with the use of magnification mammography (15). Because the assessment of the borders and shapes of individual calcifications is so critical to the determination of the likelihood of malignancy, the value of a high-quality magnification view cannot be overstated.

Magnification mammography requires the use of a microfocal spot (0.1 mm or less), to reduce geometric unsharpness; the breast is elevated on a magnification stand over the cassette, creating an air gap. Spot compression with collimation to the area of interest helps to reduce the scatter radiation and to displace the tissue, enhancing the image. Magnification in two projections, a CC and a mediolateral (ML), is most beneficial in the evaluation of microcalcifications because of the possibility of a diagnosis of milk of calcium.

For calcifications that are better seen, are more dense, or are more linear on the MLO than the CC view, a 90-degree lateral or ML magnification view is performed to determine if they layer and therefore represent milk of calcium in an area of cystic hyperplasia (Figs. 6.8 and 6.9). Because of subtlety of these differences on the MLO and CC views at times, magnification assessment of microcalcifications that are equivocal should include the ML projection.

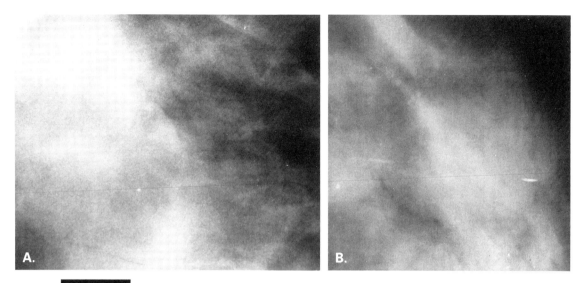

Figure 6.8

HISTORY: A 38-year-old woman with a history of bilateral cysts and new palpable masses.

MAMMOGRAPHY: Right CC (**A**) and ML (**B**) magnification views. On the CC view, the breast tissue is very dense, and there are smudged, punctuate, and round microcalcifications diffusely scattered. On the ML magnification view, some of these appear meniscoid and layer in the base of well-circumscribed masses. A cyst was confirmed on ultrasound and corresponded with the mammographic mass.

IMPRESSION: Fibrocystic changes, cyst containing milk of calcium.

NOTE: Obtaining a cross-table lateral projection (ML view) is key to confirming the diagnosis of cystic hyperplasia with milk of calcium. The calcium salts suspended in the cyst fluid are in the dependent portion of the cyst and layer on the upright view.

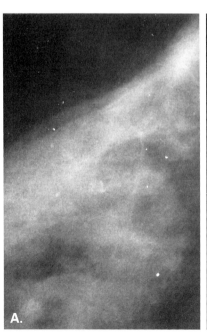
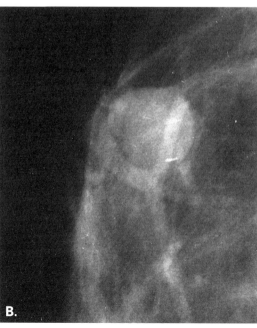

Figure 6.9

HISTORY: Abnormal screening mammogram necessitating magnification views.

MAMMOGRAPHY: Left CC (**A**) and ML (**B**) magnification views show a round mass with circumscribed margins. On the CC view, there are faint smudgy microcalcifications present. On the ML view, these layer in the base of the mass, typical of milk calcium in a cyst.

IMPRESSION: Milk of calcium in a cyst, BI-RADS® 2.

If microcalcifications are assessed as "probably benign" with a likelihood of malignancy of less than 2% and are followed at more frequent intervals (i.e., at 6 months), the magnification views should be repeated at each mammogram in order to optimize comparison with the prior studies.

ANALYSIS OF CALCIFICATIONS: RADIOLOGIC-HISTOLOGIC CORRELATION

The Breast Imaging Reporting and Data System (BI-RADS®) of the American College of Radiology provides a lexicon (16) or nomenclature for the description of calcifications on mammography. The lexicon describes calcifications by morphology, distribution, and location and uses the following structure for overall patient assessment: Category 0: needs additional evaluation, i.e., magnification view; Category 1: normal mammogram; Category 2: benign finding, routine follow-up; Category 3: probably benign finding, early follow-up; Category 4: suspicious findings, recommend biopsy; and Category 5: highly suspicious for malignancy, recommend biopsy. Once the diagnostic evaluation of the patient is complete, calcifications identified on the mammogram are placed in one of the categories 2 to 5.

The assessment of calcifications identified on mammography should include the following points of evaluation: morphology, distribution, number, size, variability, interval stability in comparison with prior exams, and associated findings. Morphology of calcifications is the single most important feature, because it is related so closely to the pathologic or histologic finding. The anatomic location of many types of calcifications, particularly microcalcifications, affects their morphology, and thus their potential etiologies can be suggested.

Patterns of Microcalcifications: Benign Etiologies

The terminal duct lobular unit (TDLU) is the basic histopathologic and physiologic unit (17) of the breast. The TDLU is the site of development of most benign and malignant conditions, including fibrocystic changes, fibroadenomas, and ductal and lobular carcinomas. It is also within the TDLU that microcalcifications are secreted or deposited (Fig. 6.10). The shape and variability of the calcifications relates very much to their location within the TDLU. When microcalcifications are located in the ductules, the blind-ending pouches of the lobule (lobular calcifications), they often appear rounded, punctate, or pearllike, and they are relatively similar or uniform in size and shape. They may be tightly grouped in a floretlike appearance or may be scattered throughout the breast. Because these are associated with fibrocystic conditions, the underlying parenchyma may be relatively dense on mammography.

Fibrocystic changes occur in the TDLU. Fibrocystic changes comprise pathologically a group of benign pro-

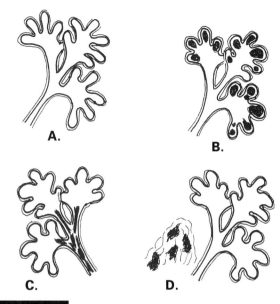

Figure 6.10

HISTOLOGY OF CALCIFICATIONS: (A) Normal terminal duct lobular unit composed of the distal duct and the lobule containing multiple small acini or ductules. **(B)** Formation of lobular calcifications in the terminal ductules within the lobule. Lobular calcifications are smooth and round and similar in morphology. **(C)** Formation of ductal calcifications in the terminal duct. Ductal calcifications often have a variable morphology and may be linear or branching. **(D)** Stromal calcifications occur in the periductal space and are often coarse and variable in shape.

liferative disorders of the breast, including fibrosis, cysts, adenosis, sclerosing adenosis, epithelial hyperplasia, papillomatosis, atypical hyperplasia, apocrine metaplasia, and chronic inflammation. Clinically, the patients are most commonly in the 30- to 50-year-old group and present with lumpy tender breasts that are cyclically symptomatic. Microcalcifications occur frequently in patients who have fibrocystic changes. The differentiation between ductal calcifications of fibrocystic origin and intraductal carcinoma is often not possible (18,19), and many of these clusters will need to be biopsied. About 15% to 30% of microcalcifications that are biopsied in asymptomatic patients are malignant (20–22), and the remainder are benign, mostly representing some form of fibrocystic change (23). Epithelial cells have the potential to secrete calcium actively, and indistinguishable deposits on mammography may be found in benign and malignant conditions. Lobular calcifications can be found in conditions that involve increased activity in the ductules, including adenosis, sclerosing adenosis, cystic hyperplasia, atypical lobular hyperplasia, and lobular carcinoma in situ (LCIS).

Sclerosing adenosis and adenosis often present as a diffuse process involving both breasts, with increased density and fine nodularity. In adenosis there is an increased number of ductules within the lobule. The calcifications that occur in this condition are in the lobule, in the blind-ending ductules; therefore their shapes are punctuate, round, smooth, or granular (24). The process is often diffuse, and the calcifications may be in single or multiple groups, or they may be diffusely scattered and bilateral

(Fig. 6.11). If the process is localized, however, the calcifications may be clustered, and biopsy often is performed to confirm the histology (24).

In sclerosing adenosis, there is lobular proliferation as well as fibrosis or sclerosis in the intralobular zone. The glands may grow haphazardly, producing an appearance

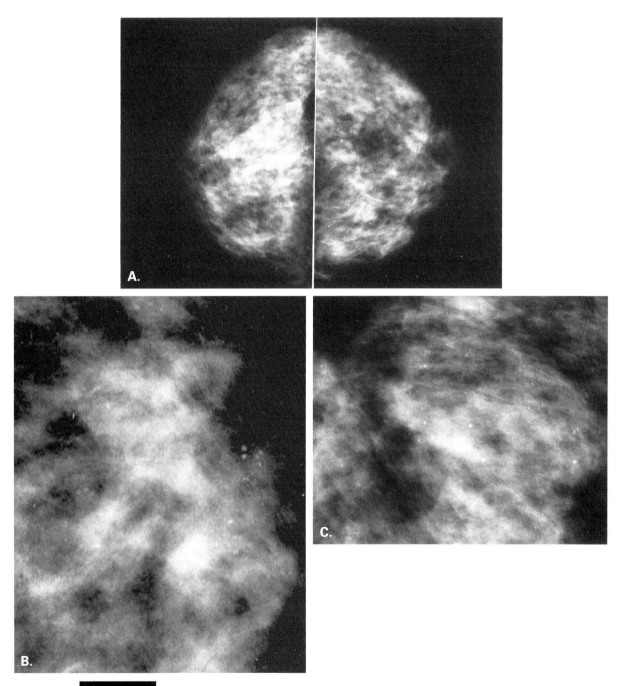

Figure 6.11

HISTORY: A 52-year-old woman for screening.

MAMMOGRAPHY: Bilateral CC **(A)** and left **(B)** and right **(C)** magnification ML views show the breasts to be heterogeneously dense. There are bilateral scattered microcalcifications present. On the magnification views **(B, C)**, the uniform round and punctuate shapes are noted, indicating a lobular origin.

IMPRESSION: Diffuse bilateral lobular microcalcifications, consistent with fibrocystic changes.

similar to that of tubular carcinoma (25,26). Because of the sclerosis, the ductules may be narrowed, and the calcifications may be quite small, appearing somewhat indistinct or amorphous. Like adenosis, sclerosing adenosis is often diffuse and bilateral, but this condition may be focal as well.

In the case of cystic hyperplasia, also a form of fibrocystic change, there is greater unfolding and enlargement of the ductules with the formation of microcysts. Calcium salts may be secreted into the fluid within the microcysts (27), and because the calcium is denser than the fluid, it lies in the dependent portion of the cyst. Therefore, when the patient is imaged in the CC projection, the calcifications lie in the bases of the microcysts and are visualized enface. Their appearance may be round or smudged, or they may not be seen. However, when the patient is imaged in the MLO projection, the calcifications are more dense or more apparent, and they may assume a linear shape. The confirmatory view is the ML magnification view, which is a true cross-table lateral projection. In this view, the calcifications layer in the dependent portion of the cysts and assume linear, crescentic, or the teacup shapes (27). The process may be extensive and bilateral, or it may be focal (28). Occasionally, larger macrocysts may also be associated with milk of calcium and show a dense layer of calcification on the ML view (29). Eventually, there may be complete calcification within the wall of the cysts, creating the appearance of small ringlike calcifications.

Papillomatosis, also known as duct hyperplasia of the common type, produces fine round or punctuate microcalcifications that extend over a large area of the breast (30). A dense prominent ductal pattern may be present and is associated with the fine microcalcifications. Occasionally, papillomatosis is focal or segmental, and biopsy is performed because of the distribution of the calcifications.

In periductal fibrosis, the calcifications occur in the stroma and may be diffuse or grouped. On histology, broad islands of fibrous tissue replace the normal fat of the breast. The calcifications of fibrosis may mimic intraductal calcifications found in ductal carcinoma in situ (DCIS) because they may be clustered, with irregular borders, and variable in size, shape, and density. However, the calcifications of fibrosis tend to be more coarse than is usually found in malignancy. The pattern of periductal fibrosis is that of dystrophic calcifications that develop in the stroma rather than in the ductal lumen.

Columnar cell changes have been more recently described as part of the spectrum of lesions involving the TDLU. The columnar epithelium of the ducts is altered with prominent apical cytoplasm snouts, intraluminal secretions, and varying degrees of nuclear atypia and architectural complexity (31). In a review of 100 breast biopsies performed for microcalcifications, Fraser et al. (31) found that columnar alternation with prominent apical snouts and secretion (CAPSS) was identified in 42% of cases. These lesions ranged from a more benign appearance of the epithelium to atypical lesions bordering on DCIS. Calcifications occurred within the CAPSS in 74% of cases, and these microcalcifications were frequently psammomatous. DCIS occurred with equal frequency with and without CAPSS, and when present with CAPSS was usually of the low-grade micropapillary or cribriform types.

Intraductal microcalcifications occur in epithelial hyperplasia, a proliferative disorder with the ducts. The work of Gallagher and Martin (32,33) with whole-organ specimens in patients with breast cancer showed that there is a spectrum of disease, from epithelial hyperplasia to atypical hyperplasia to carcinoma in situ, which occurs as nonobligate phases in the development of breast cancer.

Depending on the extent of the proliferative fibrocystic process, microcalcifications may be focal or extensive and may be present bilaterally. The calcifications are small (less than 1 mm in diameter) and may be irregular in form and variable in size and density, punctuate, or amorphous in appearance when associated with atypical lobular hyperplasia (ALH) or atypical ductal hyperplasia (ADH). Egan et al. (18) found the calcifications in epithelial hyperplasia to be indistinguishable from those of intraductal carcinoma. Stomper et al. (34) found that a majority of atypical hyperplasias were with or adjacent to another mammographic finding that prompted biopsy—often adenosis. A significant relationship existed between mammographic microcalcifications and ADH in these biopsy specimens that were otherwise benign.

The presence of hyperplastic lesions of the breast places a patient at higher risk for the development of carcinoma (35–37). In particular, atypical lobular hyperplasia increases the risk of developing breast cancer by approximately 6 times (35), and atypical ductal hyperplasia is associated with 4 to 5 times subsequent risk (36). Additionally, the combined factors of a family history of breast cancer and an atypical lesion on biopsy increase the risk of subsequent breast cancer by 11 times that of women with nonproliferative lesions and no family history (37).

Lobular Neoplasia

Lobular carcinoma in situ, or lobular neoplasia, was described by Foote and Stewart (38) as originating in the TDLU. This lesion is associated with other types of cancers and has a high propensity toward multicentricity and bilaterality (39). In a follow-up of 99 patients with LCIS treated by lumpectomy only, Rosen et al. (40) found that there was an equal risk of the patient developing invasive carcinoma in both the ipsilateral and the contralateral breast. Because about one third of patients with LCIS treated with excision alone will develop invasive carcinoma in either breast, the choices for therapy have ranged from lumpectomy only to bilateral mastectomies historically (40,41). Current management of most of these patients is excision only and mammographic surveillance.

The mammographic findings in LCIS are nonspecific and variable. However, grouped, round, lobular microcalcifications have been described in this condition (42). These calcifications are indistinguishable from those of lobular hyperplasia or focal sclerosing adenosis. Occasionally, in biopsies of lesions found on mammography in which the histology reveals LCIS, the calcifications may be located in the abnormal lobules (43), or they may be in adjacent benign lobules or areas of stroma (44,45).

Patterns of Microcalcifications: Malignant Etiologies

Microcalcifications that are of ductal origin are often found in the intralobular or extralobular (Fig. 6.12) terminal ducts, and their morphology and distribution reflect their location. Because the calcifications lie within the duct, which is a tubular structure, their distribution is often linear or segmental. Similarly, the individual microcalcifications may be linear or branching in form. Because the calcifications are deposited with the lumen of a duct

that is lined by hyperplastic or malignant epithelium, their borders are often jagged or irregular, and there tends to be variability in their forms (pleomorphism), although small amorphous or granular calcifications may also occur in pathologic process in small ducts, specifically ductal hyperplasia, atypical ductal hyperplasia, and DCIS.

The formation of breast microcalcifications can occur by two processes: active cellular secretion of calcium salts or calcification of necrotic debris. Ahmed (46) described the concept of breast epithelial cells actively producing and secreting calcifications into the lumen of the ducts. Breast calcifications may be composed of calcium phosphate or calcium oxalate crystals. The calcium phosphate is readily visualized on hematoxylin and eosin (H&E)-stained slides as deeply purple. However, calcium oxalate crystals are not readily observed on H&E-stained slides (47). The use of polarized light microscopy is most helpful for the demonstration of the birefringent calcium oxalate crystals (47). Calcium oxalate, thought to arise as a secretory process in benign breast disease (48), produces colorless birefringent crystals (49). When no calcium is identified

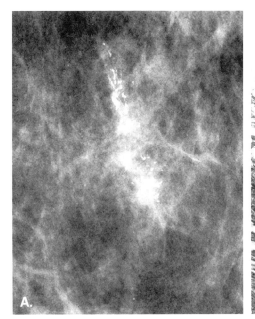 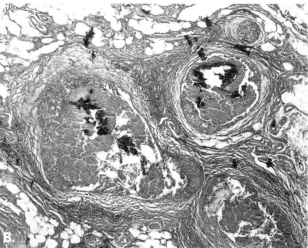

Figure 6.12

HISTORY: A 73-year-old woman for screening mammography.

MAMMOGRAPHY: Right magnified CC image **(A)** and histopathology section **(B)**. There is a cluster of innumerable irregular microcalcifications in the right breast. These calcifications are pleomorphic, linearly arranged, and have jagged irregular margins, all of which are suspicious features for malignancy.

IMPRESSION: Ductal carcinoma, possible comedocarcinoma.

HISTOPATHOLOGY: Comedocarcinoma. The biopsy specimen with comedocarcinoma shows multiple distended ducts filled with intraductal carcinoma and prominent central necrosis. Irregular calcifications are present within the necrotic areas.

NOTE: In comedocarcinoma, there is a thick debris in the ductal lumen that tends to calcify in the characteristic pattern shown here.

on routine H&E staining, pathologists must consider calcium oxalate and use polarized light to evaluate the slides for this type of calcifications (49).

Calcium phosphate crystals are basophilic and nonbirefringent, and they result from cellular degeneration in either benign or malignant disease. Radi (50) found that calcium oxalate accounted for 23% of mammographically detected microcalcifications on biopsy, and none were associated with carcinoma. Others, such as Fondos-Morera et al. (51), found that calcium oxalate may occur in breast cancers, but this type of calcification is more commonly found in benign lesions or associated with LCIS (50,52,53). Calcium oxalate has also been found (54) to be infrequently associated with DCIS.

Stomper et al. (55) found that in 100 cases of intraductal carcinoma, 72% presented as microcalcifications only, and 12% presented as nodules with calcifications. Other less common mammographic features of DCIS include circumscribed nodules, focal asymmetry, dilated ducts, ill-defined nodules, and focal architectural distortion (56). Because the calcifications of DCIS are deposited between crypts formed by irregular projections of epithelial cells, they form casts of the lumina of the ducts and, similarly, have irregular borders. Combinations of forms—including rod-shaped, punctuate, comma-shaped, teardrop–shaped, Y or branching, and lacy calcifications—may be seen together and are considered of high suspicion for malignancy.

In a study of mammographic findings of various subtypes of DCIS, Evans et al. (57) found that calcification was present in 95% of patients with large-cell DCIS (often the comedo subtype) but in only 58% of patients with small-cell DCIS (solid, cribiform, micropapillary subtypes). Calcifications were found in 96% of cases of DCIS with comedonecrosis versus 61% of cases without necrosis. An abnormal mammogram without calcifications and mammograms showing predominately punctuate microcalcifications were seen more frequently in DCIS without necrosis (57).

The calcifications of comedocarcinoma are more likely to be linear, and this pattern is thought to be secondary to dystrophic calcification of intraluminal cellular debris and a high concentration of calcium in necrotic cells (57,58). Stomper et al. (55) found that linear microcalcifications were present in 47% of comedocarcinoma compared with 18% of the cribiform, solid, or papillary subtypes of DCIS. Granular microcalcifications were found in 53% of comedocarcinomas versus in 82% of the noncomedo subtypes. Barreau et al. (59) found a correlation between granular or linear branching calcifications and grade 3 histology with necrosis. These authors also found a correlation between a lesion being associated with greater than 20 calcifications and being grade 3 with comedonecrosis (59). Holland et al. (58) described the calcifications within well-differentiated

DCIS to be small, laminated pearlylike particles in the luminal spaces within the tumorous ducts. Holland et al. (58) found that calcifications in poorly differentiated DCIS were linear, branching, or granular on mammography. The linear calcifications represented the three-dimensional image of the necrotic debris of calcium, which coalesced into casts of the center of the malignant ducts. Although in the majority of cases the calcifications associated with carcinoma are within the malignant ducts, Homer et al. (60) found that in one third of cases, the calcifications were both within the tumor and contiguous to it, and in 5% of cases, the calcifications were not associated with the tumor.

The size of individual calcifications is less important than their morphology for deciding their classification and potential etiology. The assessment of calcifications based on their size can be misleading, because malignancies are usually associated with microcalcifications of 200 μm or less, but this is certainly not always so. Comedocarcinoma, a subtype of DCIS, often manifests mammographically as casting, linear, branching microcalcifications, which can be larger than 200 μm and dense. A pitfall in the mammographic interpretation of microcalcifications is to dismiss somewhat large pleomorphic calcifications as being benign because of their size.

The most common distributions of malignant calcifications are in a focal cluster or group, or in a linear or segmental orientation. If the cancer is more extensive, the malignant calcifications may occur in a larger region of a breast or may even involve an entire breast. Egan et al. (18) found that carcinoma that presented as calcifications only was more often distributed as a cluster (66%); a mixture of scattered and clustered microcalcifications occurred in 34% of cancers. Microcalcifications that are diffusely scattered in all quadrants of both breasts are much more likely to be of benign origin. One should carefully scrutinize diffuse microcalcifications, searching for any cluster or area having a different morphology from the background pattern that might suggest a different etiology. One should also carefully review the mammogram for other clusters of suspicious calcifications when one group has been identified. DCIS has a great tendency to occur in multiple foci. Dershaw et al. (4) found that in 65% of breasts with DCIS, multifocality was present. In 41% of the cases, the maximum tumor expanse was greater than 2.5 cm, and all were multicentric. The detection of multifocal or multicentric carcinoma greatly affects surgical planning and patient management.

Zunzunegui et al. (61) found that in women with small, multifocal breast cancers with extensive casting calcifications and DCIS, the incidence of positive nodes was 33%, and there was a tendency for poor tumor markers. Thurfjell et al. (62) found a worse prognosis when small invasive cancers presented as casting or pleomorphic calcifications. Stomper et al. (63) correlated mammographic features with pathologic findings of breast cancers manifested by calcifications only. In this study, 65% of patients had pure DCIS, 32% had DCIS with a focus of invasion, and 44% had invasive cancer. Invasion was more likely when calcification size was greater than 11 mm or morphology was linear, but invasion was not associated with an extent of calcifications greater than 10 mm.

Tabar et al. (64), in a study of invasive breast cancers less than 15 mm in size, found that the presence of casting calcifications was significantly associated with positive lymph node status, poorer histologic grade, and decreased survival. Twenty-year survival rates for women with 10 to 14 mm tumors were 52% when casting calcifications were present versus 86% to 100% for those women who had mammographic features that did not include casting calcifications.

Variability is size, shape, and density of microcalcifications is a worrisome feature (18), but variability must be assessed in conjunction with morphology. Those calcifications with sharp, jagged margins that are variable in appearance are much more likely to be malignant than are variably sized and shaped but smoothly marginated calcifications. DeLafontan et al. (65) found that vermicular shape, linear branching distribution, and irregularity of size of calcifications were strong predictors of malignancy.

Diffusely scattered, diffuse unilateral calcifications having spherical, hollow, or meniscoid shapes (usually associated with benign lesions) have been described (66) in ductal malignancies with apocrine features. However, in apocrine carcinoma, the pattern of microcalcifications is variable, composed of a mixture of milk of calcium with amorphous and pleomorphic microcalcifications that are unilateral. In cases of intraductal carcinoma in which there is retrograde involvement of the lobule (cancerization of the lobule), the lobular form of microcalcification may also be identified (67).

The greater the number of calcifications in an area, the more suspicious for malignancy (30,68,69). Egan et al. (18) found that 84% of breast cancers containing microcalcifications had more than 10 calcifications in a group. Millis et al. (3) found that in 33 cancers, 6 had less than five calcifications in a cluster. However, one should note that there is no definite distinction between less than versus more than five calcifications in a group and the need for biopsy. If microcalcifications are suspicious morphologically and less than five in number, biopsy should still be performed.

Interval changes from a prior mammogram with the development of new or increasing microcalcifications often warrant investigation with biopsy. However, morphology must be the primary consideration. New benign calcifications of fat necrosis, cystic hyperplasia, and dermal or vascular origin need not be evaluated further. On the other hand, stability of microcalcifications from prior studies of at least 2 years' duration is a helpful indicator that the lesion is probably not malignant. Occasionally, DCIS may be manifested as calcifications that are stable for more than 2 years (70). Because of this, calcifications that are suspicious in morphology but stable on mammography may still need to be biopsied.

The identification of an extensive intraductal component (EIC) associated with an infiltrating cancer may be a predictor of a high risk of finding residual carcinoma on re-excision (71) and a higher local recurrence rate after breast conservation therapy (lumpectomy and breast irradiation) (72). An EIC is defined (73) as the presence of DCIS occupying an area of ≥25% of the area occupied by the infiltrating cancer and the presence of DCIS beyond the edge of the infiltrating tumor. Tumors detected only by mammography or tumors presenting as microcalcifications are more likely to be EIC positive, but this preoperative analysis is not absolute (Figs. 6.13 and 6.14) (74).

The presence of an extensive intraductal component is a major factor for predicting local recurrence after breast conservation and radiotherapy. The presence of malignant-appearing microcalcifications with or without a mass has been found to be associated with an extensive intraductal component, and when the calcifications extend over an area greater than 3 cm, the likelihood of EIC positivity is significantly increased (75).

PATTERNS OF CALCIFICATIONS AS DEFINED BY THE BIRADS LEXICON

The ACR BI-RADS® lexicon (16,76) defines microcalcifications based on morphology and distribution. Those calcifications having a benign morphology include the following patterns: skin, vascular, coarse, dystrophic, large rodlike, eggshell or rimlike, lucent-centered or spherical, sutural, milk of calcium, round, and punctate.

Skin Calcifications

Skin calcifications are typically single or grouped, very-well-demarcated, small, round, spherical, or polygonal calcifications (77). These usually appear to be very superficially located because of their dermal origin, although they may superimpose over the parenchyma on the two standard views. They typically occur in sebaceous glands and are related to chronic inflammation (78). Because of their location within the interconnecting lumina of the sebaceous glands, their pattern may be in the form of a paw print. Another sign that calcifications may be dermal is the "tattoo sign" described by Homer et al. (79). In this case, the calcifications lie in a fixed orientation relative to each other on two different views, indicating a superficial location.

(text continues on page 252)

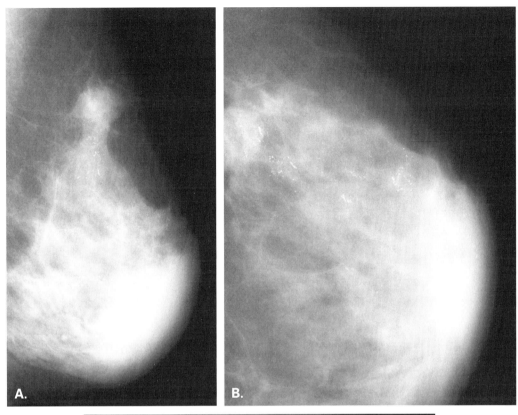

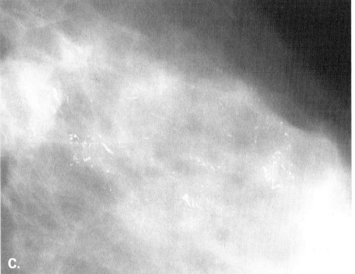

Figure 6.13

HISTORY: A 50-year-old gravida 2, para 1, abortus 1 woman with a firm 2-cm mass in the right upper-outer quadrant.

MAMMOGRAPHY: Right MLO (**A**), CC (**B**), and CC magnification views (**C**). There is a high-density spiculated mass in the outer quadrant, with microcalcifications extending from the mass to the nipple. A magnification of this area (**C**) shows the typically malignant features of the calcifications: linear shapes, irregular margins, variability in size and shape, and extension throughout the ductal system. Irregular microcalcifications are forming casts of the malignant ducts.

IMPRESSION: Ductal carcinoma.

HISTOPATHOLOGY: Infiltrating ductal carcinoma with an extensive intraductal component.

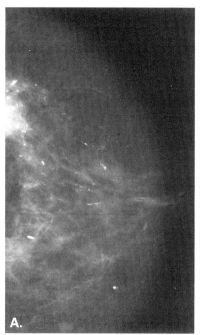
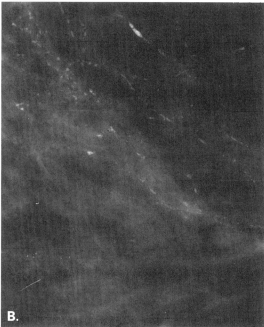

Figure 6.14

HISTORY: A 61-year-old patient with a palpable mass lateral in the right breast.

MAMMOGRAPHY: Right CC **(A)** view shows a high-density indistinct mass located laterally and associated with extensive microcalcifications adjacent to it. On the magnification CC view **(B)**, the fine linear intraductal microcalcifications extending from the mass toward the nipple are seen.

IMPRESSION: Invasive carcinoma with extensive ductal carcinoma in situ.

Dermal calcifications also may occur within or on the surface of skin lesions such as nevi, keratoses, and skin tags. Common locations for dermal calcifications are far medially and posteriorly in the cleavage area, within glands of the areola, and in the axillary region of breast (Figs. 6.15–6.17). Calcifications of dystrophic origin may occur in skin that is scarred, such as at burn sites or within keloids. These calcifications are very well defined and round or spherical in form, and are often more dense than other skin calcifications (Figs. 6.18 and 6.19).

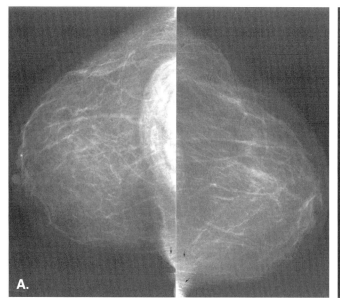
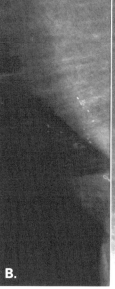
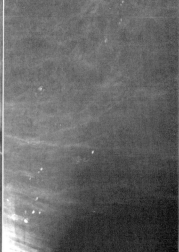

Figure 6.15

HISTORY: A 50-year-old for screening mammography.

MAMMOGRAPHY: Bilateral CC views **(A)** show fatty replaced breasts and small round calcifications medially **(arrows)**. On the enlarged image of the medial aspect of the breasts **(B)**, the morphology of these calcifications is better delineated. These are very well defined, round, and small lucent-centered calcifications in paw-print patterns, characteristic of dermal calcifications.

IMPRESSION: Dermal calcifications.

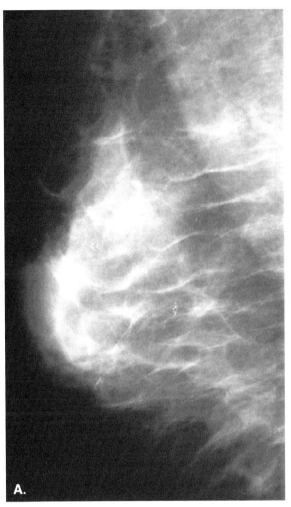

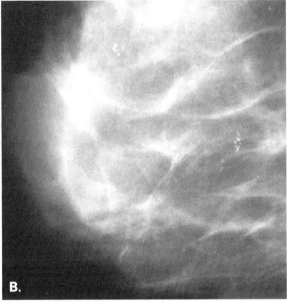

Figure 6.16

HISTORY: Screening mammogram on a 44-year-old woman.

MAMMOGRAPHY: Left MLO view **(A)** shows heterogeneously dense parenchyma and several small groups of calcifications. The enlarged image **(B)** shows the very-well-calcified smooth aspect of these calcifications. The pattern is typical of dermal calcifications in glands in the skin.

IMPRESSION: Skin calcifications.

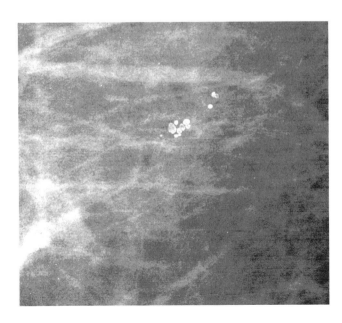

Figure 6.17

Dermal calcifications: small, very-well-defined, round, and lucent shapes.

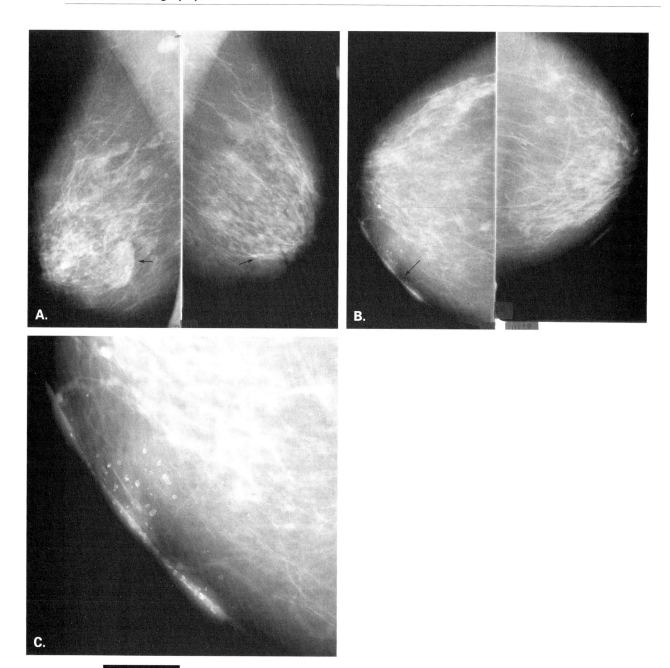

Figure 6.18

HISTORY: A 52-year-old woman with a history of burn injury to the thorax, for screening mammography.

MAMMOGRAPHY: Bilateral MLO views **(A)** show multiple very-well-circumscribed masses in both breasts **(arrows)**, as well as extensive regional calcifications. On the CC views **(B)**, the masses are not identified; however, there is very prominent skin thickening medially **(arrows)**. On an enlarged image **(C)**, the skin thickening with associated lucent-centered calcification is noted.

IMPRESSION: Keloids appearing as pseudomasses with dystrophic calcification in the scars. BI-RADS® 2.

NOTE: The very-well-defined aspect of the "masses" that are seen on one view should suggest the possibility of a skin lesion.

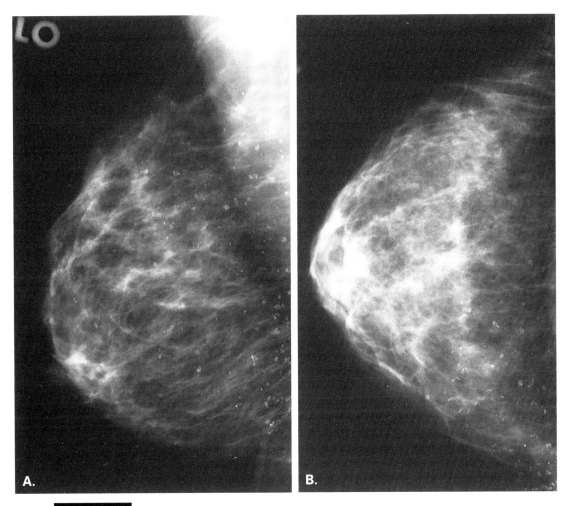

Figure 6.19

HISTORY: Screening mammogram in a patient with a history of burns to the chest wall and keloid formation.

MAMMOGRAPHY: Left MLO (**A**) and CC (**B**) views show extensive small, round, and lucent-centered calcifications over the medial aspect of the breast. This pattern is typical of dystrophic calcifications that occur in the scars on the skin.

IMPRESSION: Keloids with benign dystrophic calcifications in the skin.

Vascular Calcifications

Vascular calcifications occur within arteries of the breast as they do elsewhere in the body. The most common etiologies of vascular calcifications are atherosclerosis and renal disease. Extensive calcification in the small vessels with the breast is usually associated with renal disease (80,81) and secondary hyperparathyroidism. A weak correlation exists between diabetes mellitus and the presence of vascular calcifications (82,83). Kemmeren et al. (84) found that breast arterial calcifications identified on mammography were associated with an increased risk of subsequent cardiovascular death in women older than 50 years and in diabetic women in particular. Moshyedi et al. (85) found that posi-

tive predictive value of breast arterial calcifications for coronary artery disease is 0.88, and the negative predictive value is 0.65, which is statistically significant. For women older than age 59, the correlation between vascular calcifications and coronary artery disease was not strong. Vascular calcifications are typically tramline or parallel lines of calcium corresponding to the calcified intima of the artery. These are usually circuitous and are not oriented in the pattern of the ducts toward the nipple-areolar complex (Figs. 6.20–6.24). Early arterial calcifications may be stippled and fine, and the observation of the vessel corresponding to their path is key in suggesting the proper diagnosis. Magnification

(text continues on page 259)

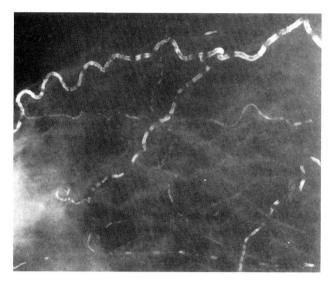

Figure 6.20

HISTORY: A 65-year-old woman for screening.

MAMMOGRAPHY: Magnified image of left breast. Circuitous vessels are associated with calcification in the walls, typical of arterial calcification.

IMPRESSION: Arterial calcifications.

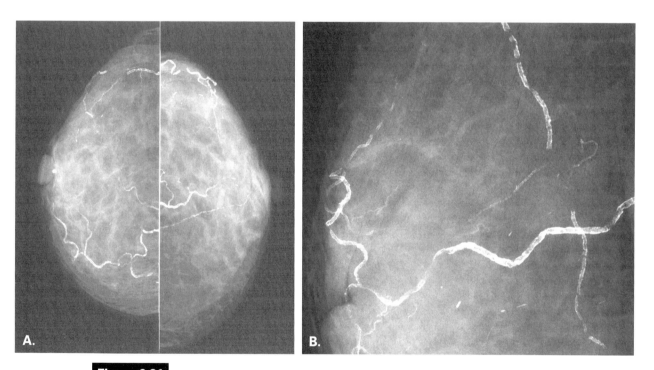

Figure 6.21

HISTORY: A 78-year-old woman for screening.

MAMMOGRAPHY: Bilateral CC views (A) demonstrate extensive vascular calcifications. On the enlarged image (B), the typical tram-line appearance of the calcified intima of the arteries is seen.

IMPRESSION: Arterial calcifications.

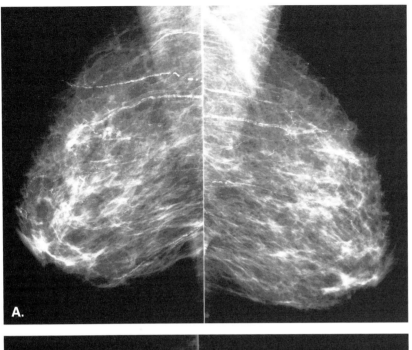

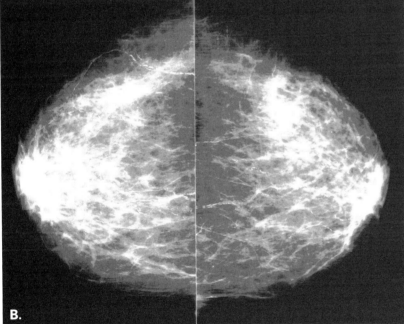

Figure 6.22

HISTORY: A 54-year-old for screening mammography.

MAMMOGRAPHY: Bilateral MLO **(A)** and CC **(B)** views show extensive tramline calcifications in both breasts. These extend toward the axillae, which is a finding typical of arterial calcifications.

IMPRESSION: Arterial calcifications.

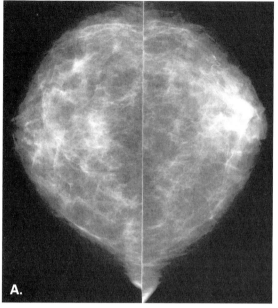

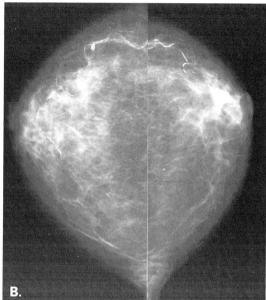

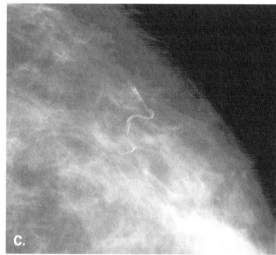

Figure 6.23

HISTORY: A 64-year-old woman for screening with a history of hypertension and diabetes, who was placed on dialysis in the last year.

MAMMOGRAPHY: Bilateral CC views **(A)** 8 years ago and bilateral CC views **(B)** currently show the interval development of bilateral vascular calcifications. Magnified right CC image **(C)** shows extensive arterial calcifications in large and small vessels. The extensive nature of these calcifications suggests chronic renal disease.

IMPRESSION: Diffuse arterial calcifications consistent with renal disease.

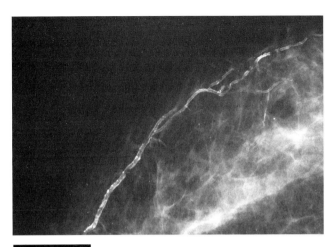

Figure 6.24

HISTORY: Screening mammogram.

MAMMOGRAPHY: Right CC enlarged image shows a densely calcified artery. Typical tramline calcification is seen in the circuitous structure.

IMPRESSION: Vascular calcification.

mammography is often essential in this situation for differentiating early vascular calcifications from clustered fine microcalcifications of ductal or lobular origin (86).

Coarse Calcifications

Coarse calcifications are usually of dystrophic origin and are most commonly associated with fibroadenomas (87).

Fibroadenomas are generally palpated as firm, well-defined breast masses in women younger than 30 years. The lesions tend to involute after menopause, with mucoid degeneration and calcification occurring later in their natural history. The masses may be large and generally well defined, and may contain large, bizarre irregular calcifications that should not be confused with carcinoma. Early in the stage of calcification (Figs. 6.25–6.27), a few punctuate peripheral microcalcifications may develop, and their peripheral location in a circumscribed mass should suggest a fibroadenoma. Occasionally, degenerating fibroadenomas may contain somewhat irregular, mixed-morphology microcalcifications that are indistinguishable from a ductal lesion, and biopsy is necessary (88). Rarely, fibroadenomas can even develop metaplastic bone formation or ossification (89). Later, the calcifications become more dense and coarse and are easily differentiated from malignancy. In the latest stage, the soft tissue masses are no longer apparent and are totally replaced by typical large coarse "popcornlike" calcifications (Figs. 6.28–6.31).

This pattern of coarse calcification is typically benign, although rarely cancers may contain coarse calcifications. Malignancy with associated coarse calcification occurs when a fibroadenoma is immediately adjacent to or is the site of development of a breast cancer or in the unusual case of a breast cancer with central necrosis and the formation of dystrophic central calcification (Fig. 6.32).

Another cause of large coarse calcifications is that of renal disease with secondary hyperparathyroidism

(text continues on page 263)

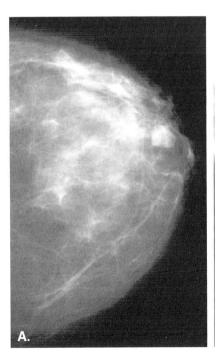

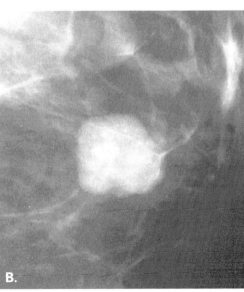

Figure 6.25

HISTORY: A 60-year-old woman with history of a previously excised left breast fibroadenoma.

MAMMOGRAPHY: Right CC **(A)** and magnified CC **(B)** views: There is a circumscribed, lobulated, isodense mass in the subareolar area. A single coarse calcification is eccentrically located in the periphery of mass, most consistent with a calcifying fibroadenoma.

IMPRESSION: Degenerating fibroadenoma.

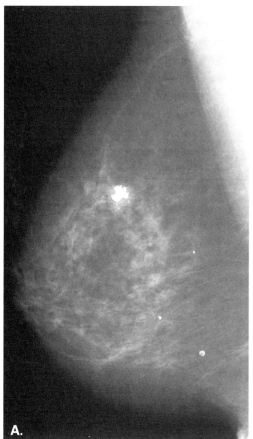

A.

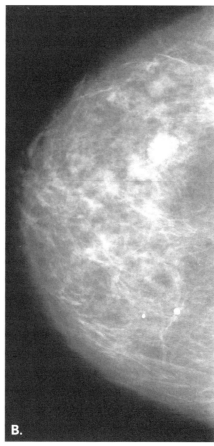

B.

Figure 6.26

HISTORY: A 66-year-old woman for screening mammography.

MAMMOGRAPHY: Left MLO (**A**) and CC (**B**) views show very dense and glandular tissue. In the 12 o'clock position, there is a very-well-defined mass with a fatty halo around most of its margin. Dense popcorn-like calcifications are present in the mass and are typical of a degenerated fibroadenoma. Other scattered benign calcifications are also seen.

IMPRESSION: Degenerated calcified fibroadenoma.

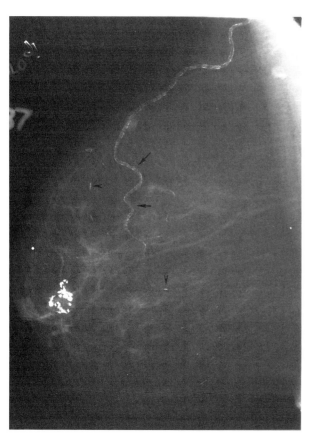

Figure 6.27

HISTORY: A 69-year-old woman for screening mammography.

MAMMOGRAPHY: Left MLO view shows extensive calcifications throughout the breast. There are extensive vascular calcifications (**arrow**) and large rodlike calcifications (**arrowheads**) of secretory disease. In addition, there is a lobulated mass in the subareolar area that contains coarse calcifications, consistent with a degenerated fibroadenoma.

IMPRESSION: Benign calcifications: vascular, secretory disease, and calcified fibroadenoma.

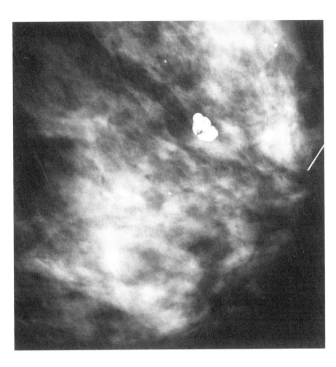

Figure 6.28

HISTORY: Screening mammogram.

MAMMOGRAPHY: Right MLO view shows a dense coarse calcification without an associated mass. The pattern is typical of that of fibroadenoma that has degenerated.

IMPRESSION: Degenerated fibroadenoma with coarse calcification.

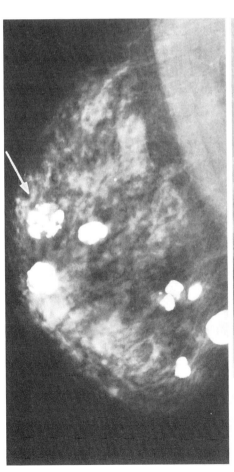
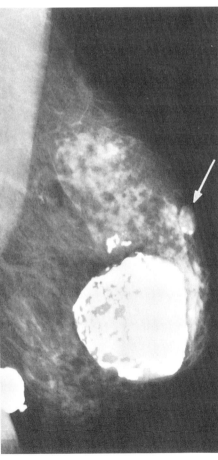

Figure 6.29

HISTORY: A 76-year-old woman who has had multiple palpable breast masses for many years.

MAMMOGRAPHY: Bilateral MLO views. The breasts are glandular for the age of the patient. There are multiple, popcornlike, very coarse, dense calcifications in both breasts. These have almost totally replaced the soft tissue masses from which they originated, except for a few partially calcified nodules **(arrows)**. The appearance of these lesions is characteristic of degenerated fibroadenomas.

IMPRESSION: Degenerated fibroadenomas.

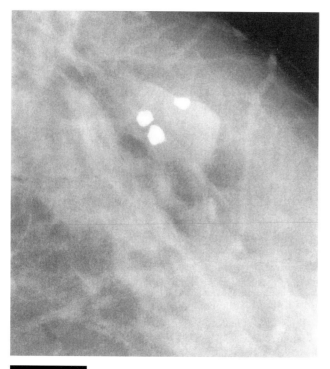

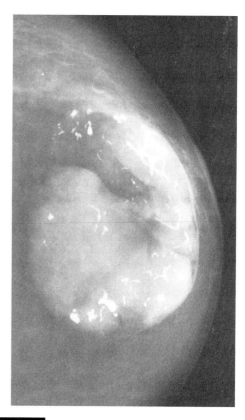

Figure 6.30

HISTORY: A 64-year-old asymptomatic woman.

MAMMOGRAPHY: Right magnification view. There is a 1.5-cm well-defined ovoid mass in the right outer quadrant. This lesion contains coarse peripheral macrocalcifications typical of a degenerating fibroadenoma.

IMPRESSION: Degenerated calcified fibroadenoma.

Figure 6.31

HISTORY: A 72-year-old woman with a long history of a right breast mass unchanged in size.

MAMMOGRAPHY: Right CC view. There is a large well-defined mass in the subareolar area that contains coarse bizarre macrocalcifications. The mass has smooth, lobulated margins. The findings are typical of a fibroadenoma with coarse calcifications.

IMPRESSION: Fibroadenoma.

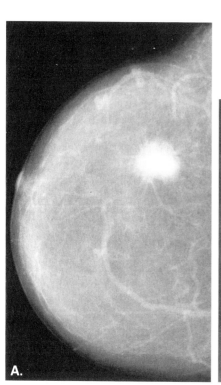

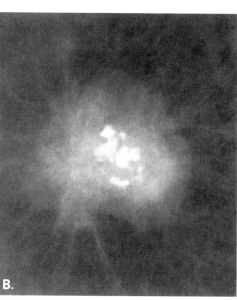

Figure 6.32

HISTORY: A 64-year-old woman with a firm palpable mass in the left breast.

MAMMOGRAPHY: Left CC view (A) and magnified image (B). There is a high-density spiculated mass typical of malignancy. There are relatively coarse dense calcifications, 3–4 mm in diameter, within the mass (B), and larger than are generally considered to be associated with carcinoma. Occasionally, malignancies may contain larger calcifications, and their presence should not alter a diagnosis of carcinoma based on the morphology of the mass.

IMPRESSION: Carcinoma, left breast.

HISTOPATHOLOGY: Infiltrating ductal carcinoma.

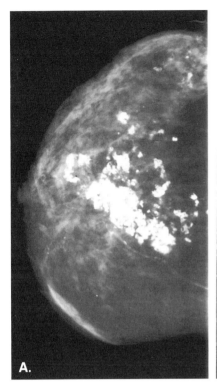
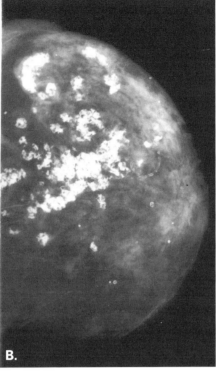

Figure 6.33

HISTORY: Elderly patient with a history of renal failure and hypercalcemia.

MAMMOGRAPHY: Left **(A)** and right **(B)** CC views show dense parenchyma and extensive coarse and vascular calcifications in a bilateral pattern that suggests a systemic etiology. The extensive nature of the calcifications is typical of tumoral calcinosis secondary to hypercalcemia.

IMPRESSION: Tumoral calcinosis, secondary to hypercalcemia.

(90,91). In this condition, the hypercalcemic state is associated with the deposition of coarse, dense diffuse calcifications in both breasts (Fig. 6.33). Because of the systemic nature of this process, the calcifications occur bilaterally (80,90,91) and diffusely. In patients with chronic renal failure and hypercalcemia, the reduction of serum phosphorus levels with hemodialysis, diet, and medication can be associated with disappearance of breast calcifications (90).

In patients who have undergone breast augmentation by injection of silicone or other substances, such as paraffin or talc, calcifications form at the injection sites and are related to a foreign-body reaction. These calcifications may be coarse and dense (Fig. 6.34) or may be ringlike with a pattern more typical of fat necrosis (92). The calcifications associated with a reaction to an injected substance are usually diffuse and bilateral, and they are associated with a very dense and nodular parenchyma. A similar pattern may be seen with extruded silicone from an extracapsular implant rupture and the formation of silicone granulomas except that the dense nodules and calcifications are more localized to the site of rupture.

A rare cause of large coarse calcifications in the breast is osteogenic sarcoma (93). This lesion shows prominent uptake on a radionuclide bone scan as well.

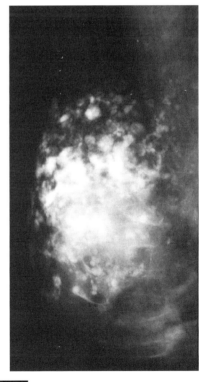

Figure 6.34

HISTORY: Screening mammogram in a patient who has a history of silicone injections for breast augmentation.

MAMMOGRAPHY: Left MLO view shows extensive very-high-density nodules throughout the breast. These represent silicone droplets that have been injected, some of which are calcifying.

IMPRESSION: Silicone granulomas from augmentation mammoplasty.

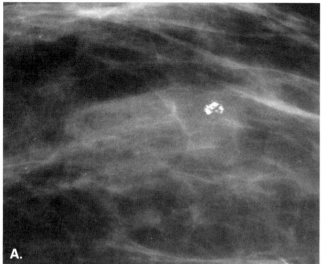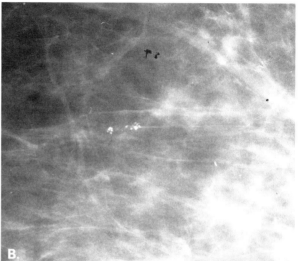

Figure 6.35

HISTORY: A 50-year-old woman for screening.

MAMMOGRAPHY: Left CC magnification views (**A, B**). There are two groups of dystrophic calcifications that are smoothly marginated. The pattern is suggestive of a benign etiology, such as a fibroadenoma, because of the smoothness of the edges of individual calcifications. These had been stable for 4 years.

IMPRESSION: Benign coarse dystrophic calcifications, most consistent with a degenerated fibroadenoma.

Another pattern of calcifications in an osteosarcoma is a more dense, amorphous pattern associated with the osteoid matrix.

Dystrophic Calcifications

Smaller macrocalcifications that have somewhat irregular shapes but relatively smooth edges are classified as dystrophic calcifications. In the newer version of BI-RADS®, these are also termed *coarse pleomorphic*. The pattern may be confused with suspicious calcifications because the shapes are often variable. However, dystrophic calcifications have smooth edges like rock in a river polished by the water, and these calcifications may look crumbled and coalescent. Dystrophic calcifications occur in the same processes that are associated with coarse calcifications, namely in fibroadenomas, fat necrosis, and in areas of fibrosis. Often dystrophic calcifications are grouped because they are related to a focal process (Figs. 6.35–6.37). Focally extensive dystrophic calcifications are typically seen in scars, particularly following reduction mammoplasty (Figs. 6.38 and 6.39).

The presence of extensive bilateral dystrophic calcifications is found in connective tissue disorders, particularly dermatomyositis (94) and systemic lupus erythematosus (Fig. 6.40). The calcifications are located in the subcuta-neous area, are bilateral, and extend up into the axillary region.

Large Rodlike Calcifications

Plasma cells mastitis, or secretory disease, is an aseptic inflammation of the breast thought to be the result of extravasation of intraductal secretions into the periductal connective tissue. As a late phenomenon of secretory disease, calcifications may occur.

In the case of duct ectasia or secretory disease, inspissated secretions within the major lactiferous ducts may calcify in the pattern of large rodlike calcifications (95). Because secretory disease is a process involving the major lactiferous ducts, the pattern of calcification is oriented toward the nipples in the subareolar regions, and the process is usually bilateral. The macrocalcifications have smooth linear shapes, are usually larger and more dense than malignant linear calcifications, and occasionally may be Y-shaped or branching (96,97) (Figs. 6.41–6.47). The calcifications associated with this condition may be intra-ductal, in the wall of the duct, or periductal, and their morphology depends on the location.

(text continues on page 269)

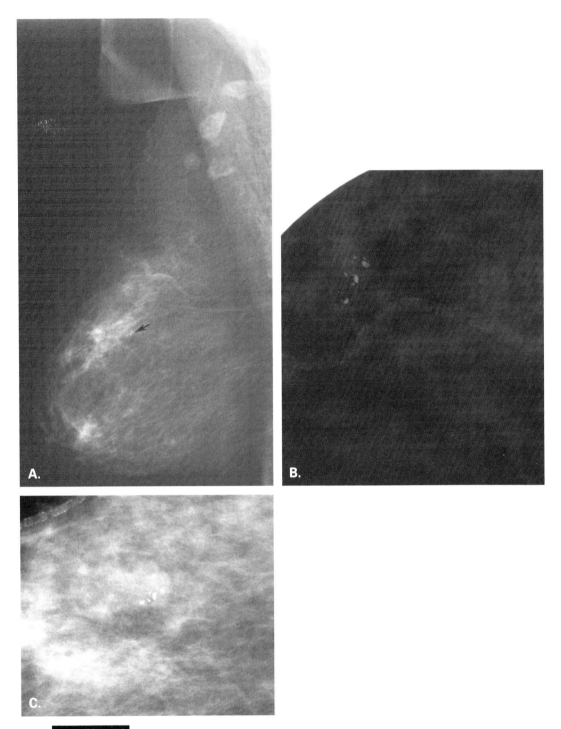

Figure 6.36

HISTORY: A 78-year-old woman referred for biopsy following an abnormal mammogram.

MAMMOGRAPHY: Left MLO (**A**) view shows clustered microcalcifications superiorly (**arrow**). On spot magnification CC (**B**) and ML (**C**) views, the calcifications are noted to be in the periphery of a lobular circumscribed mass. The morphology of the calcifications is punctuate and dystrophic. The pattern of calcifications in the periphery of a mass is typical of early degeneration in a fibroadenoma.

IMPRESSION: Early degeneration in a fibroadenoma.

Figure 6.37

Dystrophic calcifications in a circular configuration: evolving fat necrosis.

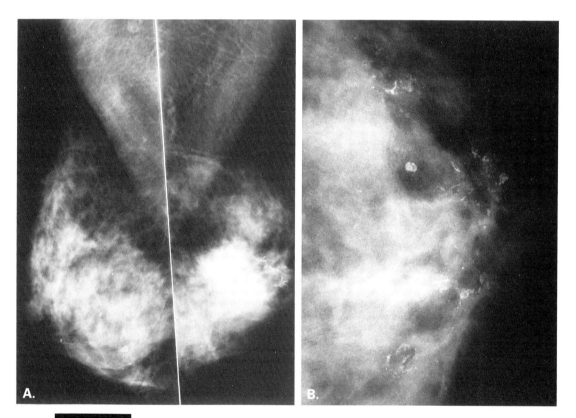

Figure 6.38

HISTORY: A 57-year-old who is status postreduction mammoplasty and who reports diffusely lumpy breasts.

MAMMOGRAPHY: Bilateral MLO views **(A)** show extremely dense tissue. There is overall distortion in the appearance of the parenchyma, consistent with postreduction changes. In the subareolar areas of both breasts, curvilinear calcifications are seen **(arrows)**. On the magnification right CC view **(B)**, the lacy, irregular calcifications are noted. These are varying in shape but are coarse and smoothly marginated, and some of the calcifications have lucent centers, all features of dystrophic calcifications.

IMPRESSION: Extensive dystrophic calcifications related to reduction mammoplasty, BI-RADS® 2.

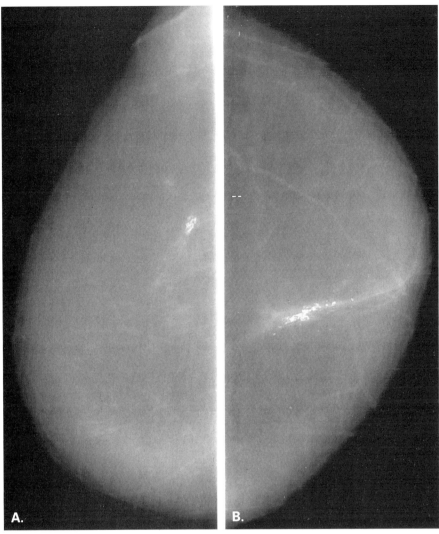

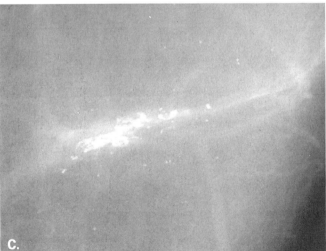

Figure 6.39

HISTORY: A 65-year-old gravida 1, para 1 woman after bilateral reduction mammoplasties, referred for screening mammography.

MAMMOGRAPHY: Left (**A**) and right (**B**) bilateral CC views and magnified right CC image. There are numerous coarse irregular calcifications that are oriented in a linear arrangement and that were situated directly beneath the surgical scars. A right magnified view (**C**) shows the calcifications to be more coarse and pleomorphic. The findings are typical of fat necrosis, and the extent and distribution are seen after reduction mammoplasty.

IMPRESSION: Fat necrosis.

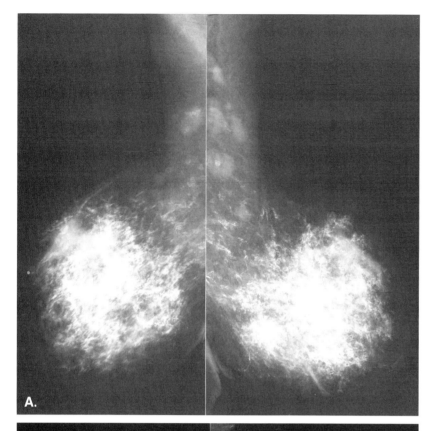

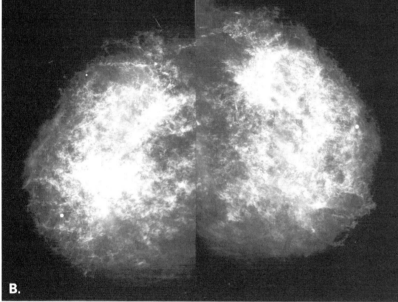

Figure 6.40

HISTORY: A 40-year-old woman with a history of systemic lupus erythematosus and Raynaud disease.

MAMMOGRAPHY: Bilateral MLO (**A**) and CC (**B**) views show extensive, somewhat coarse calcifications bilaterally. (*continued*)

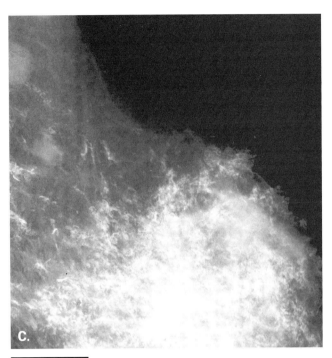

Figure 6.40 *(CONTINUED)*

On the enlarged image **(C)**, the plaquelike appearance of these dystrophic calcification is seen. The calcifications are located superficially in the subcutaneous area and extend beyond the breast toward the axilla. The diffuse, bilateral appearance suggests the possibility of a systemic etiology.

IMPRESSION: Extensive dystrophic calcifications of dermatomyositis.

With secretory disease, the inspissated secretions may leak through the duct wall and produce a plasma cell reaction with periductal fibrosis. Secretory calcifications are large (up to 5 mm in diameter), smooth bordered, and round, ovoid, linear, or needlelike in shape. The centers may be solid or hollow (if periductal). In addition to the large, rodlike calcifications of secretory disease, the periductal inflammation is associated with lucent-centered or tubular periductal macrocalcifications.

Eggshell or Rimlike Calcifications

Trauma to the breast, either surgical or related to blunt trauma and a bruise, may lead to fat necrosis. The evolution of fat necrosis and particularly the formation of an oil cyst can be identified mammographically as an eggshell or rimlike calcification in the edge of a radiolucent mass (98). These calcifications are typically large (Figs. 6.48–6.52), readily visible, and dense, and they were described as liponecrosis macrocystica by Leborgne (99).

Fat necrosis may appear in a variety of ways mammographically, from an irregular mass with overlying skin retraction, to an oil cyst, to a spectrum of forms of calcifications (98). Fat necrosis occurs after trauma and hemorrhage, such as after biopsy, aspiration, or blunt trauma with hematoma formation. Clinically, the patient may be asymptomatic or may appear with an indurated firm mass with or without overlying skin thickening and retraction. On histology, fat necrosis is characterized by anuclear fat cells with giant cells and phagocytic histiocytes. There may be central necrosis and liquefaction with formation of an oil cyst; aspiration of these lesions yields a clear oily fluid.

The calcifications that occur in fat necrosis may be small, smooth, and ringlike (liponecrosis microcystica calcificans) or they may be large circumlinear calcifications in the walls of oil cysts (liponecrosis macrocystica calcificans) that are characteristically benign (99).

Other less frequent causes of eggshell calcifications are duct ectasia with a greatly dilated duct containing periductal calcification and the calcification of the wall of a breast cyst. Eggshell calcification may also occur within a lipoma that contains an area of fat necrosis (Fig. 6.53).

Eggshell or rimlike calcifications indicate a benign process and do not require further work-up.

Lucent-centered or Spherical Calcifications

Liponecrosis microcystica is an area of fat necrosis where a large oil cyst does not form (98). Instead, very small areas of fat necrosis occur, and the associated calcifications are spherical, with lucent centers, but smaller than the eggshell pattern. These may vary from 0.5 mm to 2 or 3 mm in diameter. These calcifications are often multiple, and they are associated with the area of trauma (Figs. 6.54–6.57). The calcifications may eventually disappear as the process of fat necrosis is cleared by macrophages (100,101). When fat necrosis is cleared, the spherical calcifications may begin to crumble and look somewhat irregular—having the appearance of dystrophic or even amorphous or pleomorphic microcalcifications—before they disappear completely (Fig. 6.58).

Sutural Calcifications

Another form of characteristically benign calcification on mammography is that of calcification of sutures in the breast. The characteristic feature of sutural calcification is their morphology, namely smooth linear, curvilinear, and knot shapes (Figs. 6.59 and 6.60). These more commonly occur in patients who have undergone lumpectomy and breast irradiation rather than in patients with prior benign breast biopsies (102). Calcified sutures are thought to be a result of delayed resorption of catgut sutures, which provide a matrix on which calcium can precipitate.

(text continues on page 273)

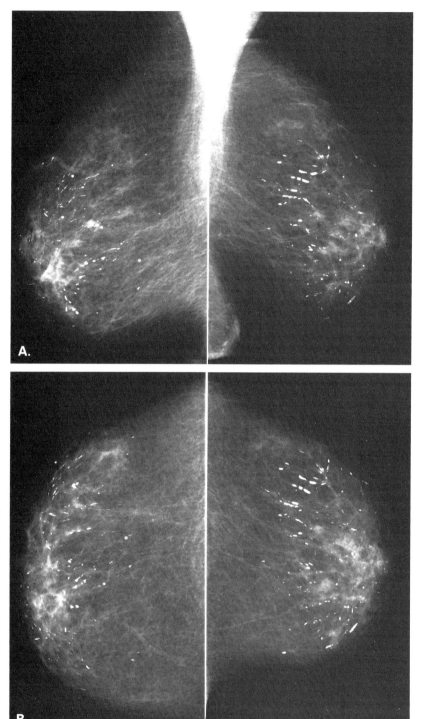

A.

B.

Figure 6.41

HISTORY: A 69-year-old woman for screening.

MAMMOGRAPHY: Bilateral MLO **(A)** and CC **(B)** views show scattered fibroglandular densities. There are extensive rodlike calcifications oriented toward the nipples in both breasts. The pattern and distribution of calcifications is typical of secretory disease or plasma cell mastitis.

IMPRESSION: Secretory disease with large rodlike calcifications.

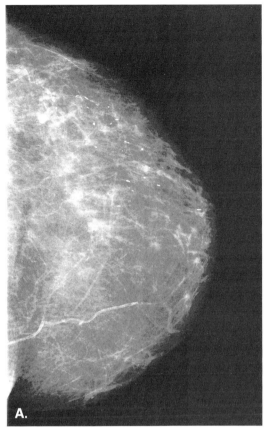
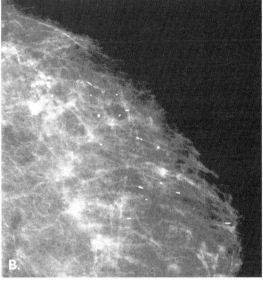

Figure 6.42

HISTORY: An 84-year-old woman for screening mammography.

MAMMOGRAPHY: Right CC **(A)** and enlarged CC **(B)** views show segmentally arranged, large rod-like calcifications on a background of scattered fibroglandular densities.

IMPRESSION: Large rodlike calcifications of secretory disease, BI-RADS® 2.

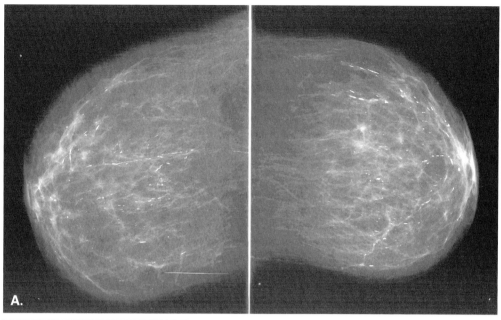

A.

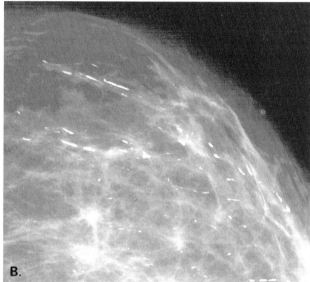

B.

Figure 6.43

HISTORY: A 77-year-old woman for screening mammography.

MAMMOGRAPHY: Bilateral CC **(A)** views show diffuse, scattered, large rodlike calcifications bilaterally. On the enlarged image **(B)**, the smooth, needlelike character of these benign calcifications is seen.

IMPRESSION: Large rodlike calcifications of secretory disease.

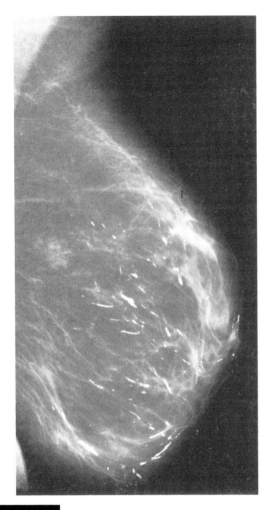

Figure 6.44

HISTORY: Screening mammogram.

MAMMOGRAPHY: Right MLO view shows extensive, large rodlike calcification. These have a smooth needlelike appearance, involve all quadrants, and radiate toward the nipple.

IMPRESSION: Benign calcifications of secretory disease.

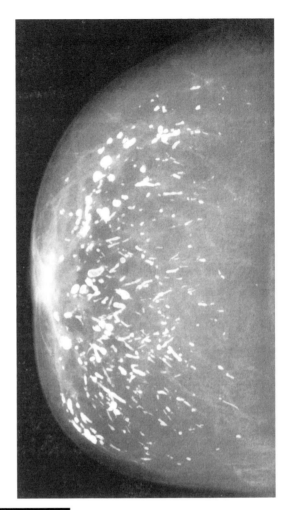

Figure 6.45

Extensive tubular, large rodlike calcifications radiating along the pattern of ducts, typical of secretory disease or plasma cell mastitis.

In a study of 335 women who were treated with lumpectomy and radiation therapy (103), 21 developed calcified sutures, whereas none of 1,140 women who also underwent lumpectomy for benign disease were found to have calcified sutures on mammography.

If sutural calcifications are suspected, the radiologist should correlate the relationship of the position of the surgical scar to the location of the calcifications. Also, care must be taken to not assume that linear calcifications are sutures when they may be associated with a recurrence of cancer.

Milk of Calcium

As discussed earlier, a benign pattern of microcalcifications is that of milk calcium in areas of cystic hyperplasia (27). These are microcalcifications that form within the distended ductules of the lobule, and they represent calcium salts suspended in cyst fluid. When viewed enface (i.e., on the CC view), milk of calcium may be very faint or smudged in appearance or may have a rounded shape. On the cross-table lateral view (ML), the heavier calcifications lie in the dependent aspect of the cyst, taking on the contour of its base (Figs. 6.61–6.63). Therefore, their shape on the ML view is linear, crescentic meniscoid, or cup shaped. Cystic hyperplasia is part of the spectrum of fibrocystic changes and therefore may be extensive or focal (28). It is important to carefully assess areas of milk of calcium for other more suspicious calcifications. The presence of milk

(text continues on page 276)

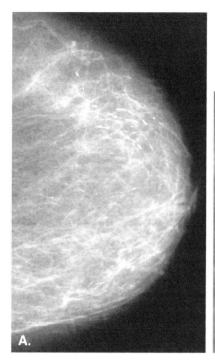

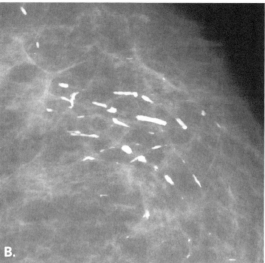

Figure 6.46

HISTORY: Screening mammogram.

MAMMOGRAPHY: Right CC view **(A)** shows extensive, large rodlike calcifications throughout the breast. These calcifications are smooth, regular in margination, and needlelike in configuration on the enlarged image **(B)**.

IMPRESSION: Benign calcifications of secretory disease.

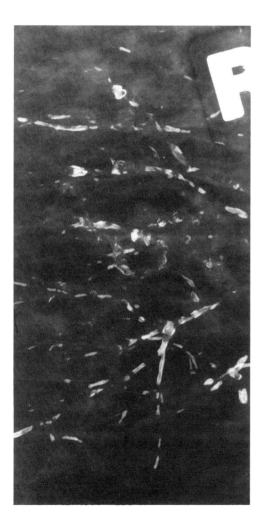

Figure 6.47

HISTORY: Screening mammography.

MAMMOGRAPHY: Enlarged right CC view shows extensive, large rodlike calcifications. The intraductal calcifications are smooth and needlelike, whereas others are lucent centered or tubular and in the periductal area.

IMPRESSION: Large rodlike calcifications of secretory disease.

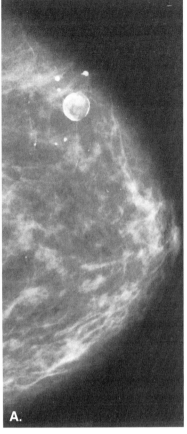

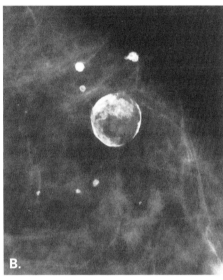

Figure 6.48

HISTORY: A 44-year-old woman who had had previous biopsy of a benign lesion in the right outer quadrant, presenting with a 1-cm smooth mass at the edge of the surgical scar.

MAMMOGRAPHY: Right CC view **(A)** and magnified image **(B)**. There is a well-defined, 1-cm eggshell calcification in the periphery of a radiolucent mass, characteristic of a calcified oil cyst. Other smaller, dense, round, and circular calcifications of fat necrosis (liponecrosis microcystica) are seen. The changes are related to the previous surgery.

IMPRESSION: Fat necrosis, liponecrosis macrocystica and microcystica, BI-RADS® 2.

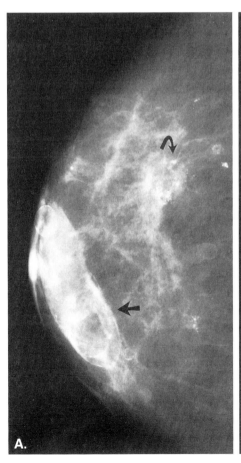

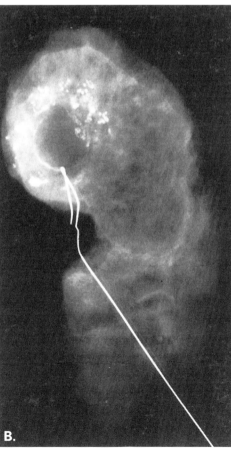

Figure 6.49

HISTORY: A 54-year-old woman with a history of severe trauma to the upper torso and extremities from farm machinery 1 year previously, presenting with multiple palpable masses in the left breast.

MAMMOGRAPHY: Left CC view **(A)** and specimen radiograph **(B)**. There are multiple, relatively lucent, well-defined masses **(straight arrow)** with calcific rims typical of post-traumatic oil cysts and fat necrosis. Clustered pleomorphic microcalcifications are present **(curved arrow)** and had developed since the mammogram 1 year previously.

IMPRESSION: Oil cysts; new clustered calcifications, favoring fat necrosis and fibrosis. Recommend biopsy.

HISTOPATHOLOGY (OF MICROCALCIFICATIONS): Fibrosis, fat necrosis.

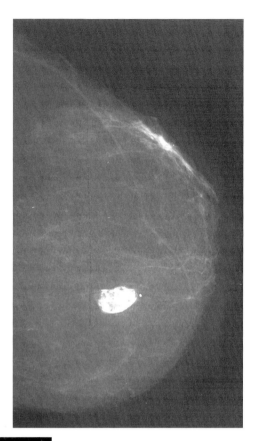

Figure 6.50

HISTORY: Prior car accident with a seat belt injury to the breast.

MAMMOGRAPHY: Right CC magnification view shows regional lucent-centered calcifications typical of fat necrosis. In the same region is a radiolucent mass **(arrow)**, which represents an evolving oil cyst.

IMPRESSION: Calcifications of fat necrosis.

of calcium has been described in apocrine carcinoma (Fig. 6.64) (66); however, in these cases, the pattern of calcifications is very extensive, unilateral, and mixed with pleomorphic microcalcifications as well.

Macrocysts may also contain precipitated calcium salts, creating the appearance of a macroscopic area of milk of calcium. A well-circumscribed isodense mass with meniscoid calcification in its base on the MLO or ML view represents a macrocyst containing milk of calcium and is therefore benign (Fig. 6.65).

Round Calcifications

The ACR lexicon (16) also includes in the benign category calcifications that are round and smooth. These are often multiple and may be 1 to 3 mm in diameter. Round calcifications may occur in multiple conditions, including fat

necrosis, in which the central lucency of the oil cyst is not evident; in secretory disease, in which they are mixed with rodlike calcifications; and in areas of fibrocystic change, in which small cysts are completely calcified (Figs. 6.66 to 6.67). This pattern is usually not problematic in characterizing as clearly benign on mammography. Round calcifications represent one of the patterns that may disappear on subsequent mammography (100). Rarely are round calcifications associated with malignancy, but there are usually other features that raise the suspicious in these cases (Fig. 6.68).

Punctate Calcifications

Small, relatively smooth, pearllike, uniform microcalcifications are classified as punctate. These have well-defined margins and are usually multiple and similar in size, shape, and density. Punctate calcifications usually form within the terminal ductules of the lobule, are associated with fibrocystic conditions, and are sometimes also called lobular microcalcifications. Although they may be grouped, because of their fibrocystic origin, punctate calcifications often are scattered diffusely in both breasts. Etiologies of punctate calcifications include such fibrocystic conditions as adenosis, sclerosing adenosis, and lobular hyperplasia (Figs. 6.69–6.73).

Punctuate microcalcifications may be present in biopsies demonstrating lobular neoplasia or LCIS as well. However, in the case of LCIS, the microcalcifications are a nonspecific finding, sometimes occurring in the lobule involved with LCIS but more often in adjacent benign fibrocystic lobules (44). The identification of microcalcifications as punctuate often requires magnification views to verify their smooth contour. The presence of diffuse or scattered punctate microcalcifications does not generally present diagnostic dilemma. However, grouped punctuate microcalcifications that have developed may prompt biopsy, because these can represent in situ carcinoma (Fig. 6.74). Rarely, DCIS may also present with this pattern.

INTERMEDIATE SUSPICION PATTERNS OF CALCIFICATIONS

The ACR lexicon (16) defines amorphous calcifications within the spectrum of those that are of an intermediate suspicion for malignancy. These are very small microcalcifications (80–200 μm) in diameter) that are not well defined and that have indistinct margins. Magnification views often demonstrate many more calcifications than are obvious on the routine views. Amorphous calcifications, also described as granular, are often numerous

(text continues on page 283)

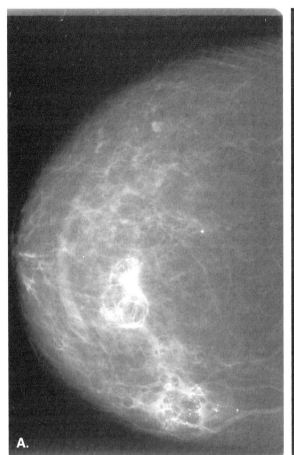

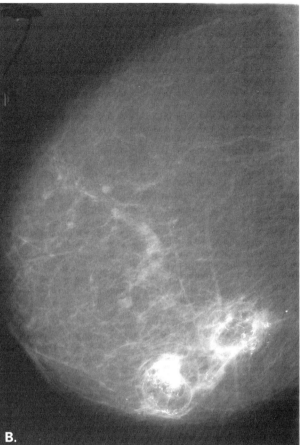

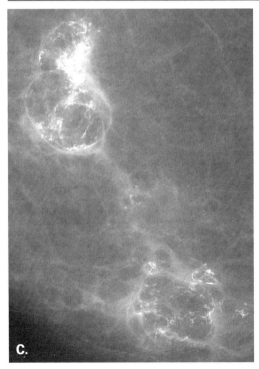

Figure 6.51

HISTORY: Patient with a history of a seat belt injury to the left breast and multiple palpable mass.

MAMMOGRAPHY: Left CC (**A**) and MLO (**B**) views show extensive calcification over the medial and inferior aspect of the breast. These are associated with large radiolucent masses, better seen on the enlarged image (**C**). The pattern of calcification is eggshell and coarse pleomorphic, all consistent with fat necrosis and calcified oil cysts.

IMPRESSION: Extensive calcifications of fat necrosis.

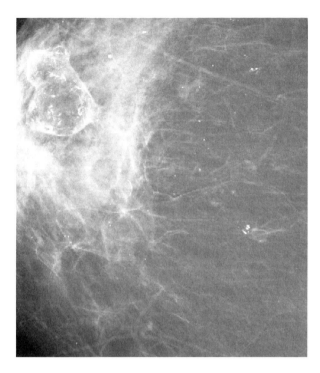

Figure 6.52

HISTORY: An 80-year-old woman with a history of right breast trauma from a car accident.

MAMMOGRAPHY: Right CC enlarged view shows extensive spherical, lucent-centered, and round calcifications consistent with fat necrosis. Large radiolucent masses with eggshell calcifications in their walls are also seen, consistent with oil cysts.

IMPRESSION: Extensive calcifications of fat necrosis, oil cysts.

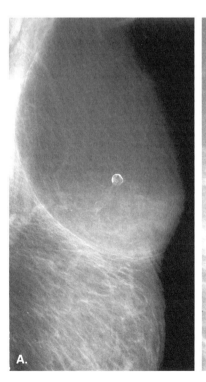

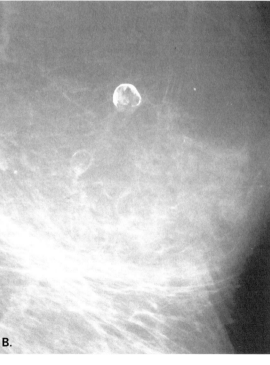

A.

B.

Figure 6.53

HISTORY: A 70-year-old woman with a large palpable mass on the right.

MAMMOGRAPHY: Right MLO **(A)** view shows a large, radiolucent circumscribed mass superiorly, displacing the normal tissue inferiorly. Within the mass are eggshell calcifications of fat necrosis seen on the enlarged view **(B)**.

IMPRESSION: Lipoma with fat necrosis.

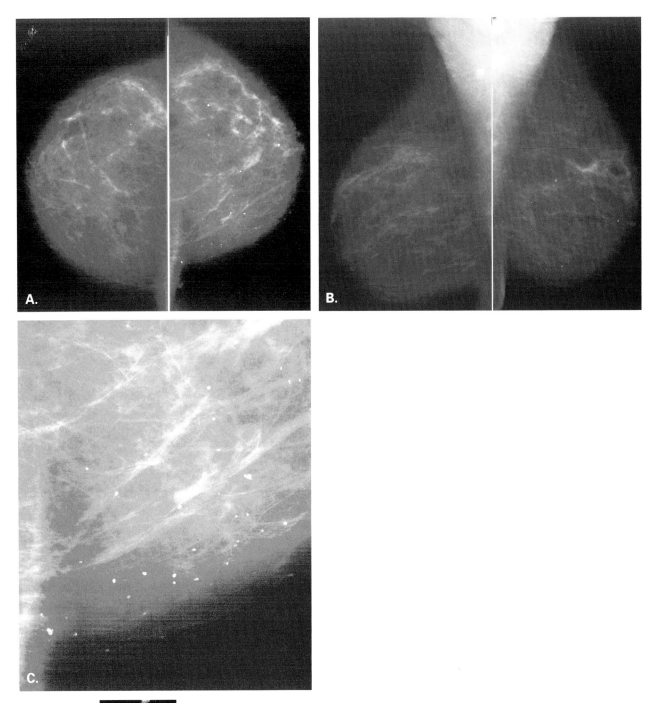

Figure 6.54

HISTORY: A 55-year-old woman with a history of bladder cancer, for screening mammography.

MAMMOGRAPHY: Right CC (**A**) and MLO (**B**) views show scattered, round, lucent-centered calcifications in the right breast. On the enlarged image (**C**), the morphology of these benign calcifications is better seen.

IMPRESSION: Lucent-centered calcifications that are likely secondary to trauma and fat necrosis.

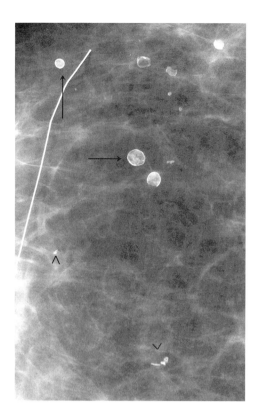

Figure 6.55

HISTORY: A 50-year-old woman status postlumpectomy and radiation therapy for breast cancer.

MAMMOGRAPHY: Left CC magnification view shows multiple eggshell **(arrows)** and lucent-centered calcifications at the lumpectomy site, which is indicated by a wire marker. These are normal posttreatment findings.

IMPRESSION: Eggshell, lucent-centered, and dystrophic calcifications of fat necrosis at the lumpectomy site.

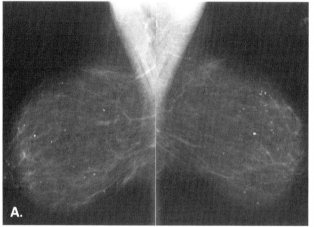

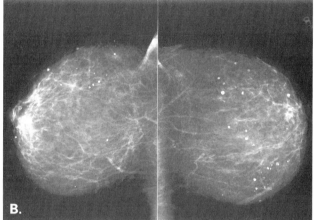

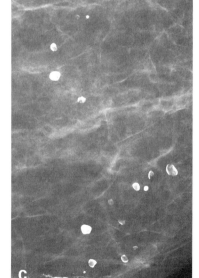

Figure 6.56

HISTORY: A 41-year-old for screening mammography.

MAMMOGRAPHY: Bilateral MLO **(A)** and CC **(B)** views show fatty-replaced breasts. There are extensive lucent-centered calcifications bilaterally. On the enlarged image **(C)**, the calcifications are very well demonstrated and thin rimmed.

IMPRESSION: Lucent-centered calcifications of fat necrosis.

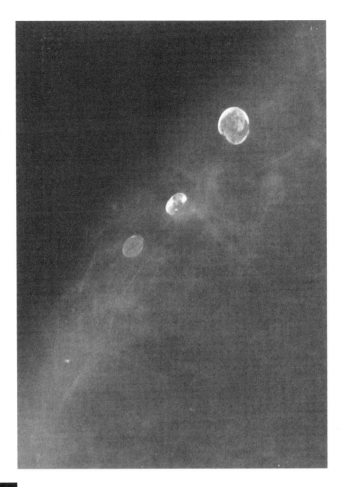

Figure 6.57

HISTORY: A 33-year-old gravida 1, para 1 woman who has had bilateral reduction mammoplasties.

MAMMOGRAPHY: Left magnified MLO view. The breast shows fatty replacement. There are three ringlike eggshell calcifications in the area of a surgical scar. These are typical of oil cysts secondary to reduction mammoplasty.

IMPRESSION: Fat necrosis.

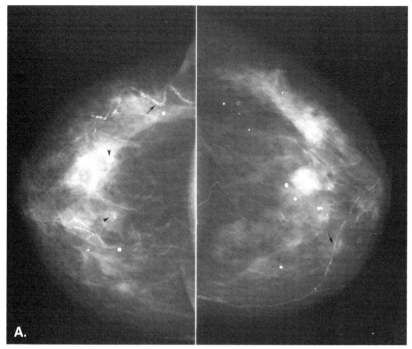

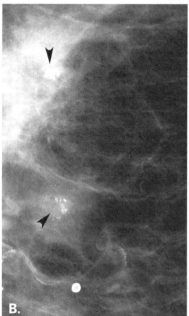

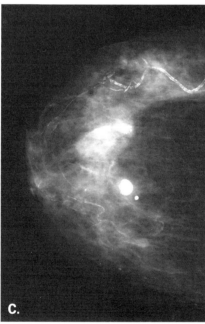

Figure 6.58

HISTORY: A 72-year-old for screening mammography.

MAMMOGRAPHY: Bilateral CC views **(A)** show heterogeneously dense breasts with diffuse vascular **(arrow)** and lucent-centered calcifications. There are two groups of coarse pleomorphic calcifications **(arrowheads)** in the left breast, which are better seen on the enlarged CC view **(B)**. The more medial group of microcalcifications has a more suspicious appearance; however, on the prior mammogram **(C)**, the medial group was a single, round, dense lucent-centered calcification. In the process of disappearance, the calcification has become more fragmented and irregular in appearance.

IMPRESSION: Bilateral benign vascular and lucent calcifications; evolution of a calcified oil cyst to more dystrophic-appearing microcalcifications, BI-RADS® 2.

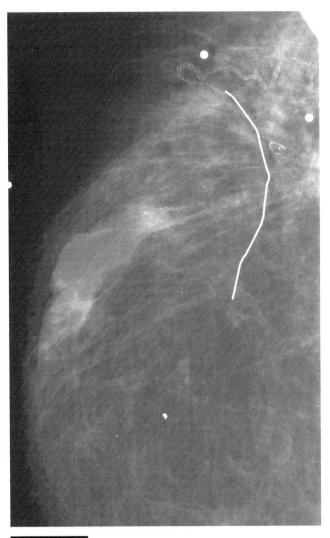

Figure 6.59

SUTURAL CALCIFICATION: Knot-shaped calcification at the site of a prior lumpectomy for breast cancer.

and located in a group or multiple groups (Figs. 6.55–6.61). However, occasionally these may be diffusely scattered in both breasts, mixed with punctate microcalcifications or milk of calcium in cases of fibrocystic changes.

The irregular or indistinct contour of the individual calcifications is related to their location within the terminal duct rather than the lobule in most cases. The calcifications are actively secreted as salts of either calcium phosphate or calcium oxalate by the epithelial cells that line the small ducts. Because the hyperplastic duct lining is associated with the calcifications, their morphology is irregular, reflecting the internal duct lumen. Calcium phosphate stains readily as purple with the routine hematoxylin and eosin stain. However, calcium oxalate is pale pink or invisible on H&E stain and often requires

the use of polarized light to be evident at microscopic analysis.

The etiologies of the amorphous pattern of calcifications include the following: DCIS, atypical ductal hyperplasia, epithelial hyperplasia of the ordinary type, papillomatosis, and sclerosing adenosis (Figs. 6.75–6.86).

Rare causes of amorphous-appearing calcifications are the formation of osteoid in carcinosarcomas or osteosarcoma metastatic to the breast or in the formation of psammomatous calcifications in mucin-producing tumors (Figs. 6.87 and 6.88). The presence of amorphous calcifications usually requires biopsy unless they are diffusely scattered bilaterally or clearly stable for 2 years or more. In a study (104) of 150 cases of biopsied amorphous calcifications, 30 (20%) were malignant, 30 (20%) were high-risk lesions, and the remainder were benign.

SUSPICIOUS PATTERNS OF MICROCALCIFICATIONS

Pleomorphic Calcifications

The presence of pleomorphism in grouped linear, segmental, or regional microcalcifications—particularly when there is variability of size and density as well as shape—is a very worrisome feature. Pleomorphic microcalcifications have a high predictive value of being associated with malignancy.

In the second edition of the BI-RADS® lexicon (105), pleomorphic calcifications have been divided into two groups, namely coarse or fine pleomorphic. The coarse pleomorphic calcifications are those also described as "dystrophic" because they are a bit larger and more smoothly marginated than the fine pleomorphic group. Coarse pleomorphic calcifications are stromal in location and occur primarily in fibrosis and degenerated fibroadenomas and in resolving fat necrosis (Figs. 6.89 and 6.90). The fine pleomorphic microcalcifications are ductal in location and occur in ductal carcinomas and in ductal hyperplasia. The distinction between these two groups on mammography may be difficult, and reliance on other factors, such as distribution and interval stability, are important in the final assessment of the lesion. Biopsy of these two patterns of calcifications is often necessary for confirmation of their etiology.

Like amorphous microcalcifications, those that are pleomorphic are typically located in the terminal ducts. These may be associated with duct hyperplasias or atypical hyperplasias (Fig. 6.91) or with DCIS. Because the malignant cells producing them create a thickening of the duct epithelium in papillary projections, the shape of the calcifications may be quite jagged or irregular. Typically pleomorphic calcifications are larger and more

(text continues on page 287)

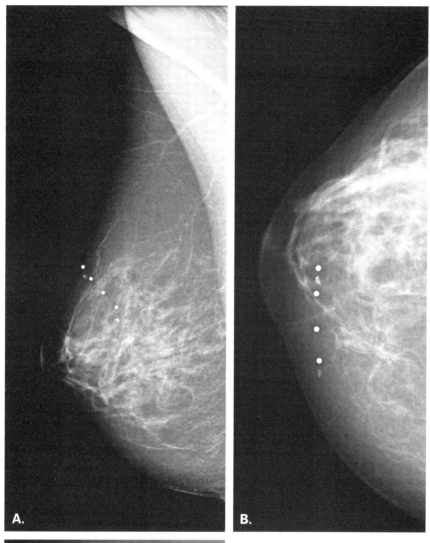

A.

B.

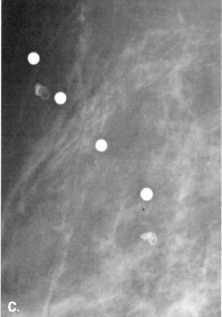

C.

Figure 6.60

HISTORY: A 56-year-old woman with a history of surgical biopsy in left breast for benign disease.

MAMMOGRAPHY: Left MLO (**A**) and BB (**B**) views show a surgical site marked with BBs. There is a somewhat coarse calcification located centrally. On the enlarged MLO image (**C**), the knotlike shape of this sutural calcification is evident.

IMPRESSION: Sutural calcification.

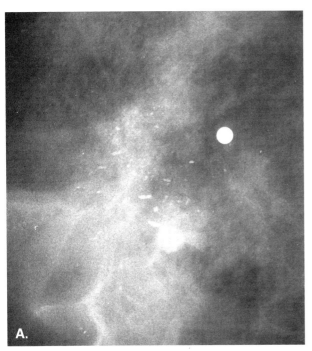

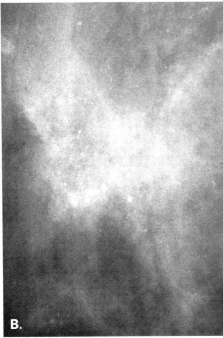

Figure 6.61

HISTORY: A 42-year-old woman recalled from screening mammography.

MAMMOGRAPHY: Left ML **(A)** and left CC **(B)** magnification views show regional microcalcifications. On the CC view **(B)**, the microcalcifications appear rounded and smudged. On the magnification ML view **(A)**, the calcifications appear crescentic, which is typical of milk of calcium.

IMPRESSION: Milk of calcium in areas of cystic hyperplasia.

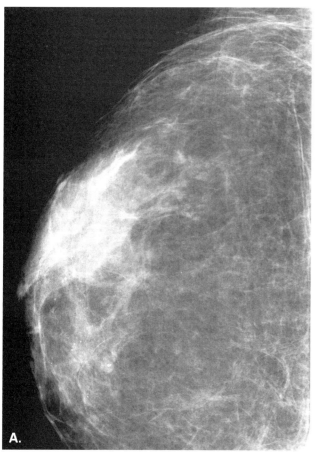

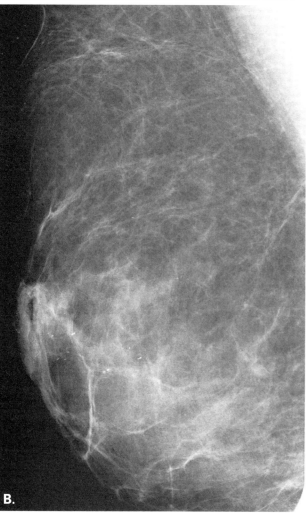

Figure 6.62

HISTORY: A 35-year-old recalled from screening for microcalcification.

MAMMOGRAPHY: Left CC (**A**) and ML (**B**) views. There are regional microcalcifications in the central aspect of the left breast. These appear rounded on the CC view but on the ML are more dense and visible, and many have crescentic shapes.

IMPRESSION: Milk of calcium in microcysts, BI-RADS® 2.

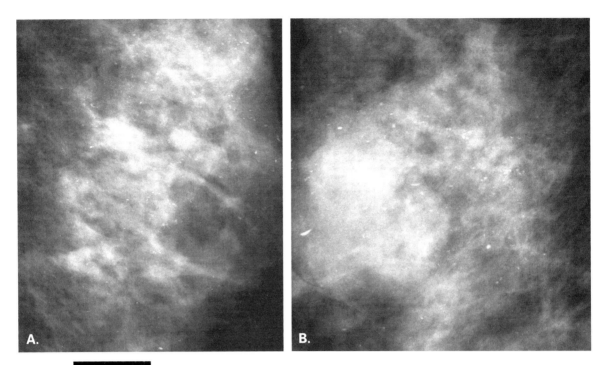

Figure 6.63

HISTORY: A 42-year-old woman for screening mammography.

MAMMOGRAPHY: Magnification CC **(A)** and ML **(B)** views show calcifications that are diffuse, and a mixture of punctate and milk-of-calcium forms are present. On the ML **(B)**, typical meniscoid shapes of layering calcifications in areas of cystic hyperplasia are seen.

IMPRESSION: Diffuse fibrocystic changes, milk of calcium in areas of cystic hyperplasia, BI-RADS® 2.

dense than amorphous calcifications and may be produced by active cellular secretion of calcium salts as well as by the dystrophic calcification of necrotic debris in comedocarcinoma.

A mixture of shapes—including amorphous, punctate, linear, Y-shaped, and teardrop—are seen in groups of pleomorphic calcifications (Figs. 6.92–6.104). The pattern is sometimes described as having the appearance of broken glass or broken stone because of the clean, sharp edges of the individual calcifications (78). The greater the degree of pleomorphism and the sharper the edges of calcifications, the more likely malignant is their etiology.

Fine Linear/Linear Branching

The presence of fine linear or branching microcalcifications is a highly suspicious finding and is associated with a high positive predictive value for malignancy. These calcifications represent casts of the ducts in which they lie. The calcifications are often associated with the comedo subtype of intraductal carcinoma, and they represent the dystrophic calcification of necrotic debris in the duct lumen. Because these microcalcifications are casts of the internal lumen of the duct, their forms reflect their surrounding environment. Clumps and craters created by malignant cells contain the calcium deposits, so the edges of the individual calcifications are irregular, variable, and jagged (Figs. 6.105–6.115). The presence of fine linear microcalcifications, also described as casting calcifications, is often indicative of a high grade or poorly differentiated ductal malignancy. This finding has been associated with a poor prognosis in women with T_1 invasive breast cancer. Tabar et al. (64) found that the 20-year survival for women with 1- to 9-mm invasive cancers and casting type calcifications was 55%; for women with 1- to 9-mm invasive tumors and no calcifications, the 20-year survival was 95%.

Unusual Calcific Densities

The presence of vermiform macrocalcifications, particularly in patients who have lived in endemic areas, may suggest the diagnosis of Loa Loa. Loiasis is an parasitic disease caused by a filaria, Loa Loa, and is a disease seen

(text continues on page 318)

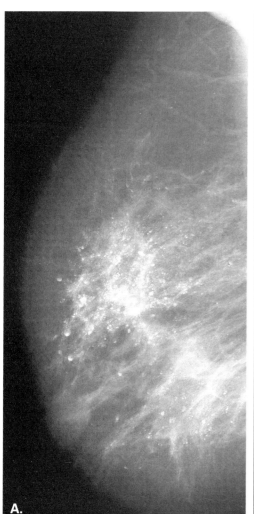

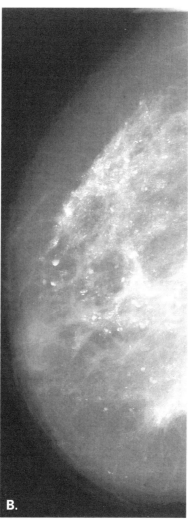

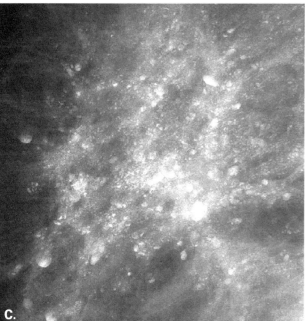

Figure 6.64

HISTORY: Screening mammogram.

MAMMOGRAPHY: Left MLO (**A**) and ML (**B**) views show extensive microcalcifications in the left breast. None were present on the right. The morphology of these is mixed (**C**), with some being crescentic or milk of calcium and others being amorphous and pleomorphic. The unilateral distribution and mixed morphology is suspicious, even though milk of calcium is present.

IMPRESSION: Highly suspicious for malignancy.

HISTOPATHOLOGY: Apocrine carcinoma.

NOTE: This type of malignancy may produce milk of calcium in the cystic spaces around the malignant cells. The pattern, however, is highly pleomorphic and extensive, much different from benign milk of calcium in fibrocystic changes.

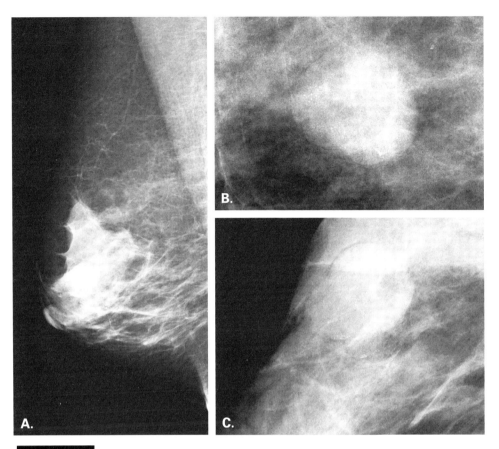

Figure 6.65

HISTORY: A 42-year-old woman for screening.

MAMMOGRAPHY: Left MLO view **(A)** shows heterogeneously dense tissue and an obscured mass in the supra-areolar area. On the magnification CC **(B)** and ML **(C)** views, the mass is found to be circumscribed and round. There are microcalcifications associated with it, which are rounded on the CC view but crescentic on the ML view, typical of milk of calcium in a cyst. Ultrasound confirmed a cyst.

IMPRESSION: Milk of calcium in a cyst.

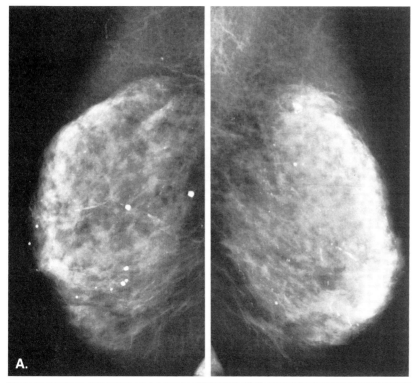

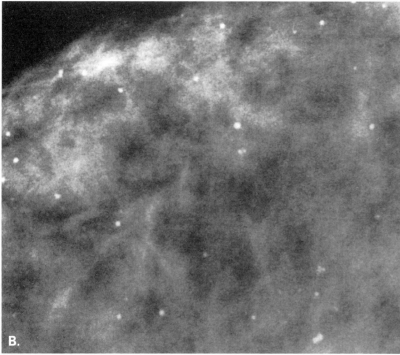

Figure 6.66

HISTORY: An 83-year-old nulliparous woman with a pleural effusion and no palpable breast abnormalities.

MAMMOGRAPHY: Bilateral oblique views **(A)** and magnification image of the right breast **(B)**. The breasts are dense and diffusely nodular, as may be seen in an elderly nulliparous woman. The "snowflake" pattern of nodularity suggests fibrocystic changes with adenosis. There are also innumerable round pearllike microcalcifications distributed evenly throughout both breasts. The smooth-bordered, rounded shapes of the microcalcifications and the similarity in appearance suggest a lobular origin and are consistent with adenosis.

IMPRESSION: Diffuse fibrocystic changes with round lobular calcifications, BI-RADS® 2.

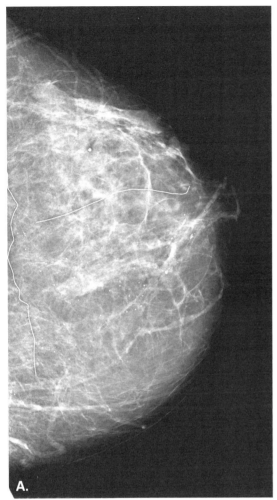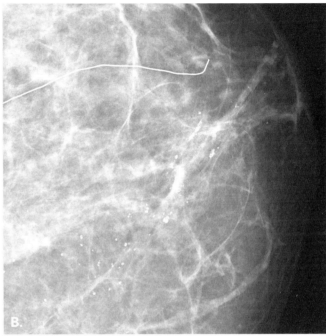

Figure 6.67

HISTORY: A 42-year-old woman status postreduction mammoplasty.

MAMMOGRAPHY: Right CC view **(A)** shows wires marking the surgical scars from the reduction. There are extensive round calcifications distributed primarily over the medial aspect of the breast in the orientation of the scar. On the enlarged image **(B)**, the very-well-defined morphology of these calcifications is seen, indicating a benign etiology.

IMPRESSION: Extensive round and dystrophic calcifications from breast reduction.

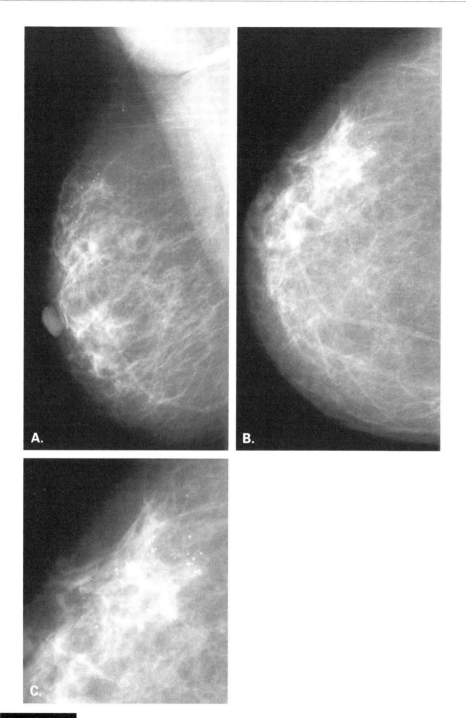

Figure 6.68

HISTORY: Screening mammogram in a patient with no history of trauma to the breast.

MAMMOGRAPHY: Left MLO **(A)** and CC **(B)** views show segmental calcifications in the 2 o'clock position. These are associated with an area of prominent ducts, and they had increased from the prior mammogram. On the enlarged CC image **(C)**, the smooth round morphology of these is seen. Because of their distribution and interval change, they were biopsied.

IMPRESSION: Segmental round microcalcifications, BI-RADS® 4.

HISTOPATHOLOGY: Comedocarcinoma.

NOTE: Morphologically, these are benign. However, the associated dilated ducts, the segmental distribution, and the interval increase were suspicious and therefore should prompt biopsy.

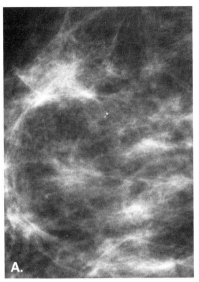

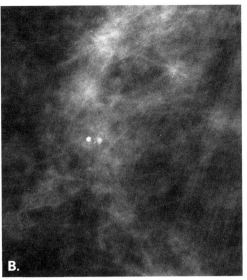

Figure 6.69

HISTORY: A 64-year-old woman for screening.

MAMMOGRAPHY: Left ML **(A)** and magnification ML **(B)** views demonstrate a cluster of punctuate microcalcifications. On the magnification view **(B)**, slight variability in size and shape is noted; however, because of the smooth margins, these are likely benign. The calcifications were new since the prior studies and were therefore biopsied.

IMPRESSION: New microcalcifications likely fibrocystic. Recommend biopsy BI-RADS® 4.

HISTOPATHOLOGY: Adenosis.

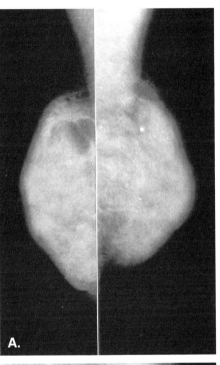

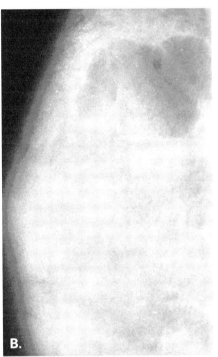

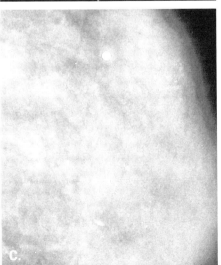

Figure 6.70

HISTORY: Screening mammography.

MAMMOGRAPHY: Bilateral MLO views **(A)** show extremely dense breast tissue and extensive bilateral microcalcifications. On enlarged MLO images **(B, C)**, the microcalcifications are noted to be diffuse, amorphous, and punctuate. These are most consistent with a lobular process, such as adenosis or sclerosing adenosis.

HISTOPATHOLOGY: Diffuse lobular microcalcifications consistent with fibrocystic changes.

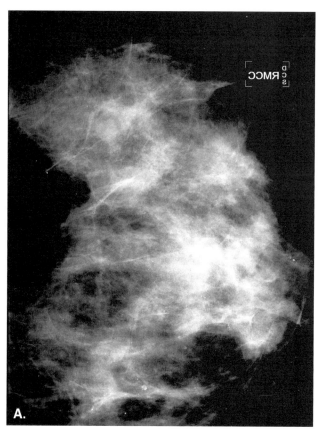

A.

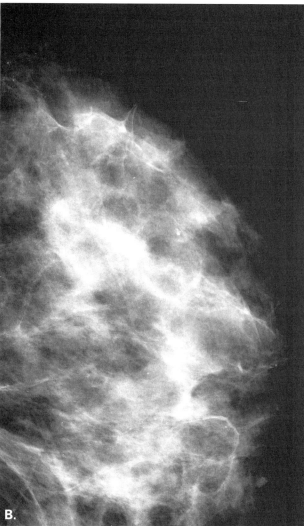

B.

Figure 6.71

HISTORY: A 43-year-old woman for screening mammography.

MAMMOGRAPHY: Right CC **(A)** and ML **(B)** views show diffuse punctuate, round, and amorphous microcalcifications. The pattern of calcifications was bilateral, as was the dense breast parenchyma.

IMPRESSION: Diffusely scattered punctuate microcalcifications of fibrocystic change, BI-RADS® 2.

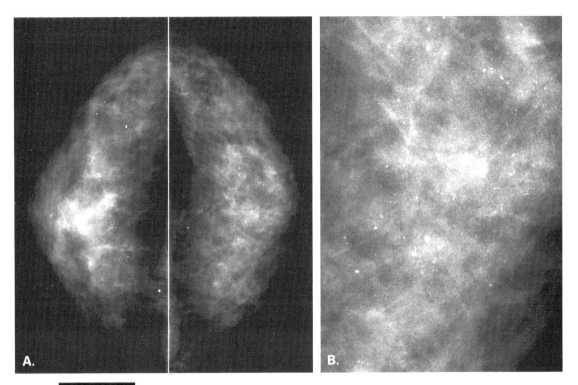

HISTORY: A 54-year-old woman for screening mammography.

MAMMOGRAPHY: Bilateral CC views **(A)** show diffuse bilateral microcalcifications. On an enlarged image **(B)**, these are uniform and punctuate, suggesting a benign lobular etiology. This pattern of calcifications is usually associated with fibrocystic changes or adenosis because of their lobular origin.

IMPRESSION: Diffuse punctuate microcalcifications of fibrocystic change.

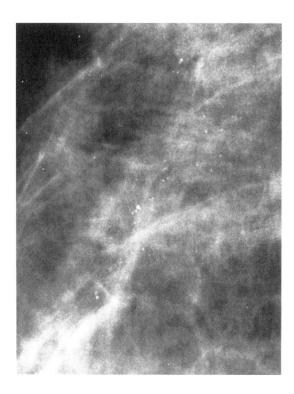

Figure 6.73

HISTORY: A 49-year-old woman with a positive family history of breast cancer, for routine screening.

MAMMOGRAPHY: Left CC magnification view. There are punctuate, smooth, and round microcalcifications with little variability, suggesting a lobular origin. The findings are nonspecific and may be seen in adenosis, lobular hyperplasia, and LCIS. A needle localization–directed biopsy was performed.

HISTOPATHOLOGY: Fibrocystic changes with epithelial hyperplasia.

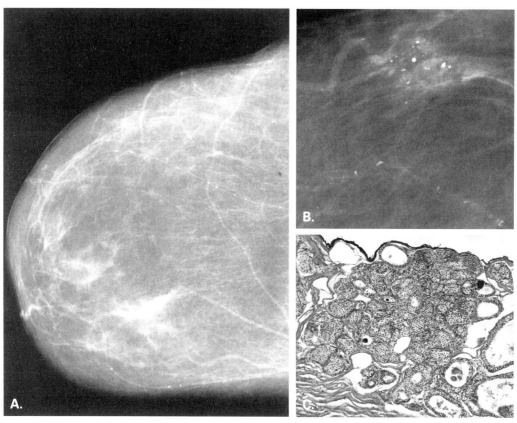

Figure 6.74

HISTORY: An 80-year-old woman with a history of lymphoma, for screening mammography.

MAMMOGRAPHY: Left ML **(A)** and magnification **(B)** views and histopathology **(C)**. There is focal asymmetry in the lower inner quadrant, containing variably shaped microcalcifications and macrocalcifications. Many of these are smooth and round, suggesting a lobular origin, but histologic examination is necessary to confirm the diagnosis.

IMPRESSION: Microcalcification, BI-RADS® 4. Recommend biopsy.

HISTOPATHOLOGY: Sclerosing adenosis with focal LCIS. On histology **(C)**, the distended lobules are filled by a monomorphic cell population diagnostic of LCIS. Rounded microcalcifications are present within the abnormal lobules.

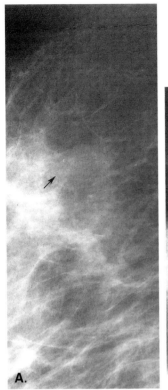

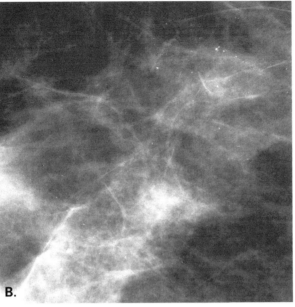

Figure 6.75

HISTORY: A 40-year-old woman with an abnormal screening mammogram.

MAMMOGRAPHY: Left CC **(A)** and ML **(B)** spot magnification views show clustered microcalcifications within dense parenchyma. The morphology of the calcifications is punctuate and somewhat amorphous, suggesting most likely a lobular origin.

IMPRESSION: Punctuate and amorphous microcalcification. Recommend biopsy.

HISTOPATHOLOGY: Nonproliferative fibrocystic change.

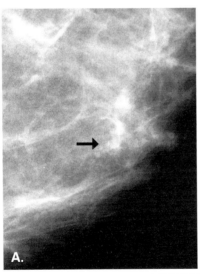

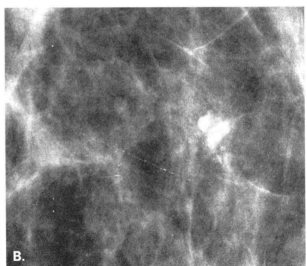

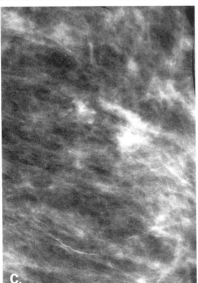

Figure 6.76

HISTORY: A 60-year-old woman with a history of benign right breast biopsy, for routine screening.

MAMMOGRAPHY: Right CC view **(A)** shows a faint cluster of microcalcifications located anteriorly at 2 o'clock **(arrow)**. Magnification CC **(B)** and MLO **(C)** views show the microcalcifications to be clustered and amorphous.

IMPRESSION: Suspicious microcalcifications. Recommend biopsy.

HISTOPATHOLOGY: Benign breast tissue, intraductal hyperplasia, adenosis, apocrine metaplasia with microcalcifications.

NOTE: The morphology of the calcifications suggests a lobular origin, and fibrocystic etiology most likely. However, biopsy is necessary to confirm this.

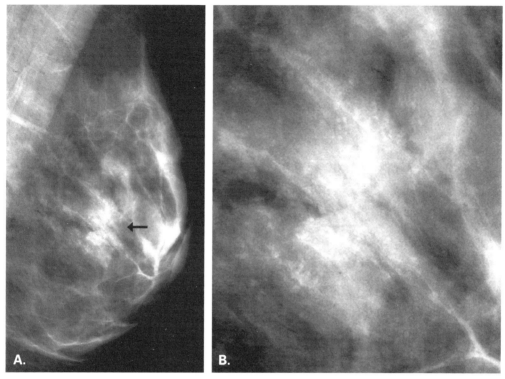

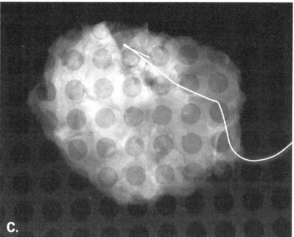

Figure 6.77

HISTORY: A 41-year-old for screening mammography.

MAMMOGRAPHY: Right MLO view **(A)** shows dense parenchyma and a region of faint amorphous microcalcifications **(arrow)** centrally. On the magnified view **(B)**, the fine amorphous pattern is seen. Core needle biopsy was performed showing radial scar. Excision was performed, and the specimen radiography **(C)** shows the extent of calcifications.

IMPRESSION: Amorphous microcalcifications, BI-RADS® 4.

HISTOPATHOLOGY: Radial scar.

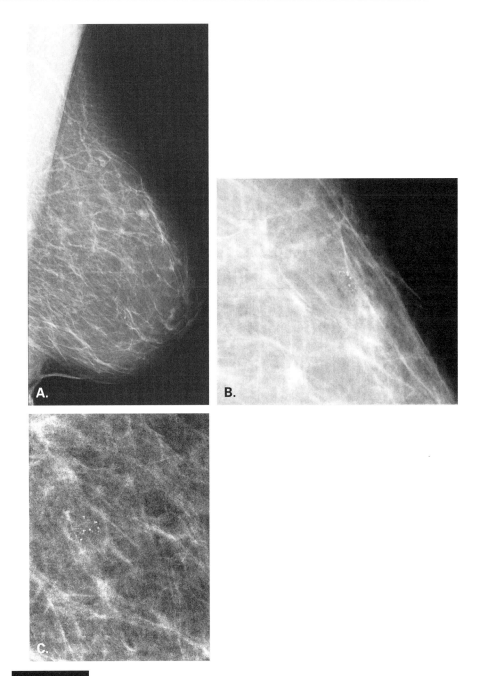

Figure 6.78

HISTORY: A 62-year-old woman for screening mammography.

MAMMOGRAPHY: Right MLO view **(A)** shows scattered fibroglandular densities and a small cluster of microcalcifications located superiorly **(arrow)**. On the magnification ML **(B)** and CC **(C)** views, the amorphous grouped microcalcifications are evident. Core needle biopsy was performed.

IMPRESSION: Amorphous microcalcifications, BI-RADS® 4.

HISTOPATHOLOGY: Fibrocystic change with calcifications.

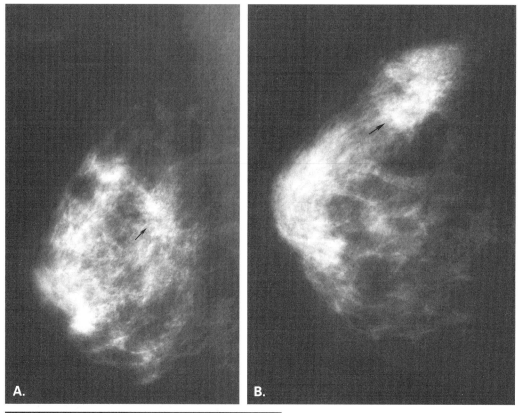

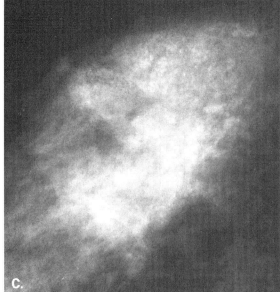

Figure 6.79

HISTORY: A 35-year-old woman for screening mammography.

MAMMOGRAPHY: Left ML **(A)** and CC **(B)** views show a focal asymmetric density with associated faint calcifications in the 3 o'clock position **(arrows)**. On the enlarged image **(C)**, the calcifications are better visualized as being uniform and punctuate, suggesting a lobular location.

IMPRESSION: Asymmetry with microcalcifications, probably of fibrocystic origin. Recommend biopsy.

HISTOPATHOLOGY: Sclerosing adenosis, hyperplasia, micropapillomas, LCIS, radial scars.

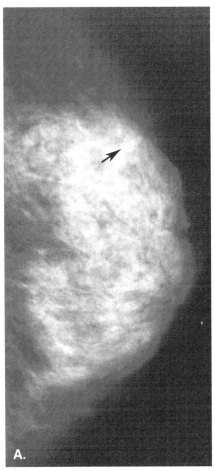

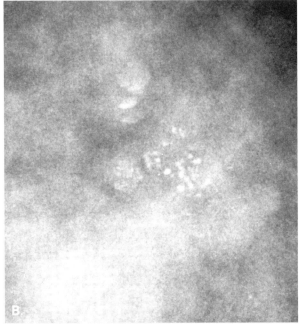

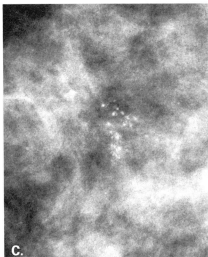

Figure 6.80

HISTORY: A 58-year-old woman for screening mammography.

MAMMOGRAPHY: Right ML **(A)** shows dense parenchymal clustered microcalcifications **(arrow)** superiorly. On the ML **(B)** and CC **(C)** magnification views, the microcalcifications are clustered and amorphous, and somewhat uniform in size and shape. This pattern suggests a lobular origin.

IMPRESSION: BI-RADS® 4 microcalcifications. Recommend biopsy.

HISTOPATHOLOGY: Atypical lobular hyperplastica on core biopsy and LCIS on excision.

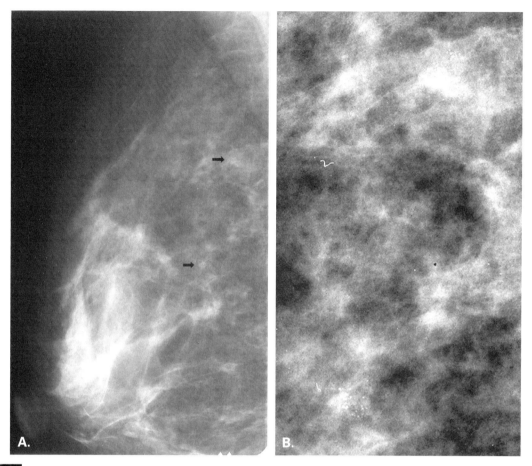

Figure 6.81

HISTORY: A 61-year-old woman for screening.

MAMMOGRAPHY: Left MLO view **(A)** shows two clusters of microcalcification located posteriorly *(arrows)*. On the magnified view **(B)**, the microcalcifications appear to be punctuate, amorphous, and tightly clustered, suggesting most likely a lobular origin.

IMPRESSION: Suspicious microcalcifications, BI-RADS® 4, most likely fibrocystic change.

HISTOPATHOLOGY: LCIS.

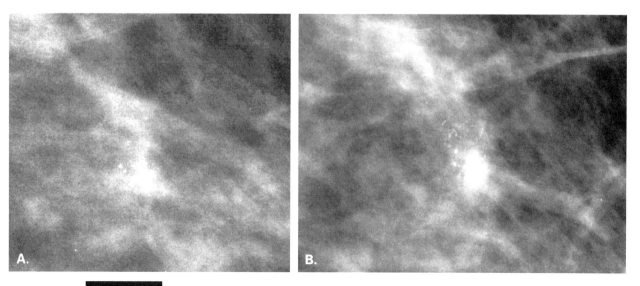

Figure 6.82

Clustered amorphous and slightly pleomorphic microcalcifications **(A, B)**; DCIS with invasion.

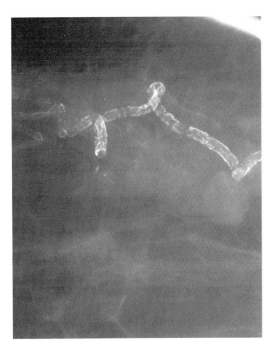

Figure 6.83

HISTORY: A 79-year-old woman for screening mammography.

MAMMOGRAPHY: Left CC magnification view shows amorphous grouped microcalcifications adjacent to benign vascular calcifications.

IMPRESSION: Amorphous microcalcifications, suspicious. Recommend biopsy.

HISTOPATHOLOGY: Invasive ductal carcinoma, with DCIS.

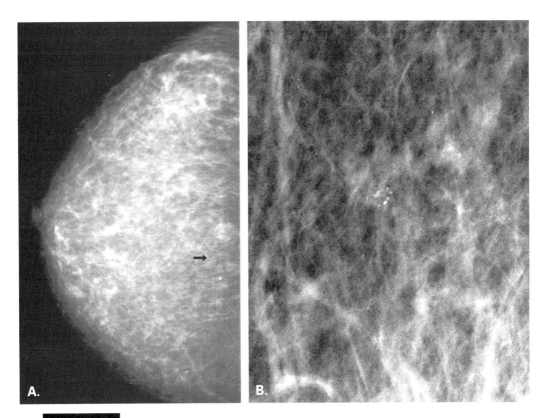

Figure 6.84

HISTORY: Screening mammogram.

MAMMOGRAPHY: Left CC view **(A)** shows a cluster of very faint microcalcifications **(arrow)** located far posteriorly. On the CC magnification view **(B)**, the clustered microcalcifications are amorphous and slightly variable in size. The most likely diagnosis is fibrocystic change.

IMPRESSION: Clustered amorphous microcalcifications, BI-RADS® 4.

HISTOPATHOLOGY: DCIS.

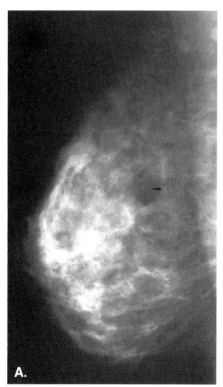

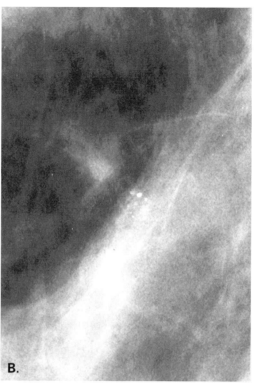

Figure 6.85

HISTORY: Screening mammogram.

MAMMOGRAPHY: Left MLO view **(A)** shows dense parenchyma and a faint cluster of microcalcifications posteriorly. On the CC magnification view **(B)**, the few, faint, amorphous microcalcifications are present.

IMPRESSION: Amorphous microcalcifications, BI-RADS® 4.

HISTOPATHOLOGY: DCIS, intermediate grade with comedonecrosis.

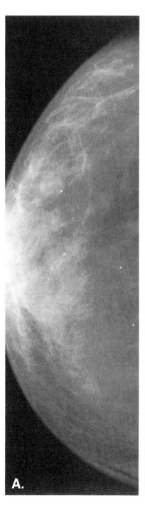

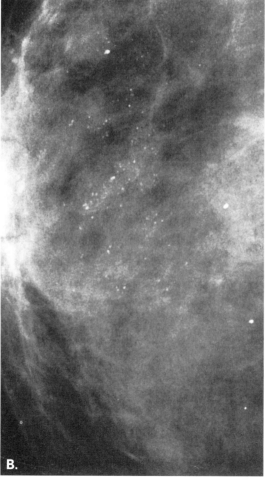

Figure 6.86

HISTORY: A 76-year-old woman with a palpable carcinoma in the right breast.

MAMMOGRAPHY: Left CC **(A)** and magnification **(B)** views. There are fine granular microcalcifications extending throughout the subareolar ducts of the left breast. These are of variable morphology, suggesting a suspicious etiology.

IMPRESSION: Microcalcifications suspicious for ductal carcinoma.

HISTOPATHOLOGY: Extensive intraductal carcinoma.

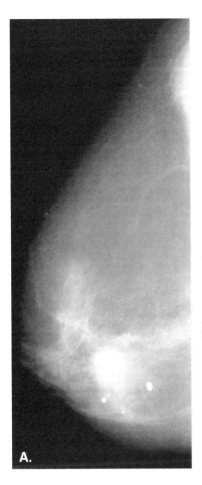

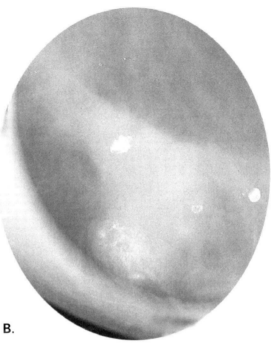

A.

B.

Figure 6.87

HISTORY: Elderly patient with a palpable left breast mass.

MAMMOGRAPHY: Left ML view **(A)** shows an indistinct, high-density round mass with associated microcalcifications. The magnification CC **(B)** shows that the mass contains unusual dense amorphous calcifications.

IMPRESSION: Highly suspicious for malignancy.

HISTOPATHOLOGY: Carcinosarcoma with osteoid matrix.

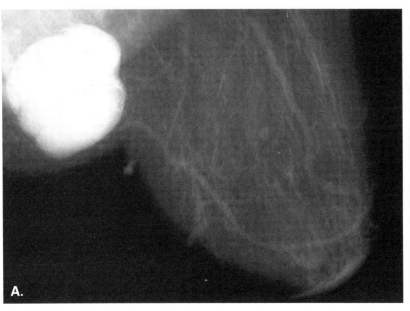

A.

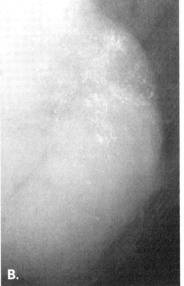

B.

Figure 6.88

HISTORY: An 80-year-old with a palpable right axillary mass.

MAMMOGRAPHY: Right MLO view **(A)** shows a large, lobulated, high-density mass in the axilla. Faint microcalcifications having a powdery appearance are within the mass on the magnified image **(B)**. The differential includes a primary breast cancer versus one metastatic node.

IMPRESSION: Axillary mass, highly suspicious for neoplasm.

HISTOPATHOLOGY: Metastatic mucinous carcinoma from the umbilicus.

NOTE: The psammomatous calcifications are amorphous and are associated with mucin-producing tumors.

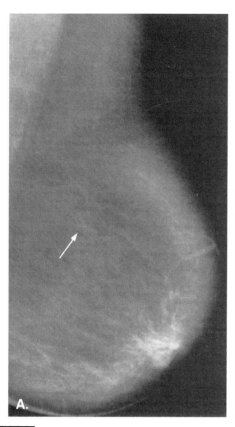

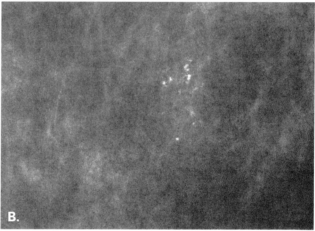

Figure 6.89

HISTORY: A 68-year-old woman for screening mammography.

MAMMOGRAPHY: Right MLO view **(A)** and magnified image **(B)**. In the upper outer quadrant of the right breast, showing otherwise fatty replacement, are clustered amorphous microcalcifications **(arrow)** in an area of low-density soft tissue **(A)**. The magnified image **(B)** shows the irregularity of borders of the calcifications, but no branching or linear forms are noted.

IMPRESSION: Cluster of calcifications of mild to moderate suspicion, favoring fibrocystic changes.

HISTOPATHOLOGY: Fibroadenoma with calcifications.

NOTE: Occasionally, a small fibroadenoma may degenerate, and the soft tissue mass decreases in size, leaving only calcifications visible. Although calcifications in fibroadenomas are generally coarse, microcalcifications may be seen, particularly early in the degenerative process.

Figure 6.90

HISTORY: A 57-year-old woman for screening mammography.

MAMMOGRAPHY: Right CC view **(A)** shows scattered fibroglandular densities and clustered microcalcifications medially **(arrow)**. On the magnification and CC view **(B)**, the somewhat pleomorphic, faint microcalcifications are evident.

IMPRESSION: Microcalcifications, BI-RADS® 4. Recommend biopsy.

PATHOLOGY: Periductal and stromal fibrosis with microcalcifications.

NOTE: Fibrosis with associated microcalcifications is a striking mimicker of DCIS.

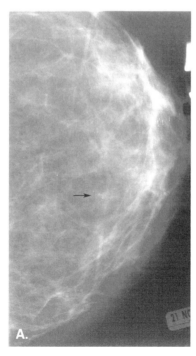

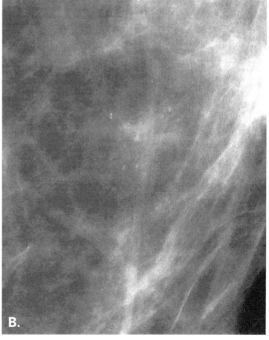

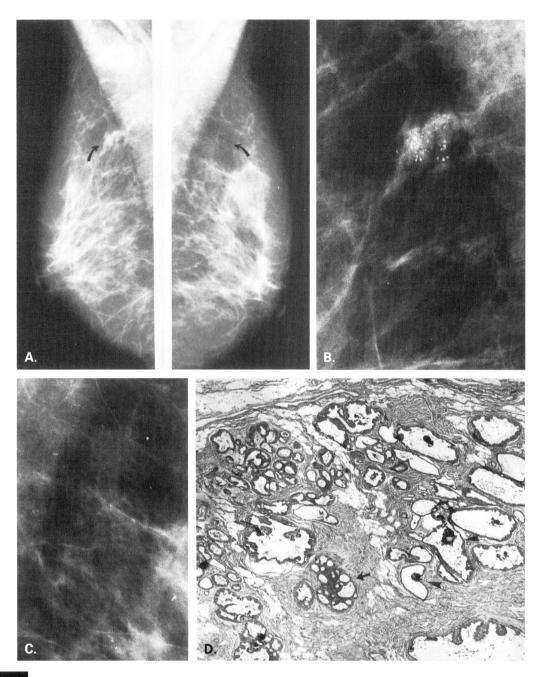

Figure 6.91

HISTORY: A 58-year-old woman with a strong family history of breast cancer, for routine screening.

MAMMOGRAPHY: Bilateral MLO views **(A)** and magnification images of the left **(B)** and right **(C)** upper outer quadrants and histopathology section **(D)**. There are areas of focally clustered microcalcifications in the right upper-outer quadrant **(A** and **C)** that are punctuate, relatively smooth bordered, and similar is size and shape. These have an appearance suggesting a lobular origin, such as is found in adenosis or sclerosing adenosis. In the left upper-outer quadrant, there is a cluster of pleomorphic microcalcifications **(A** and **B)** associated with a soft tissue density. Because of the jagged edges of these calcifications, they are of moderate suspicion for malignancy, particularly an intraductal lesion.

IMPRESSION: Right: Lobular type of calcifications, favoring fibrocystic changes. Left: Moderately suspicious calcifications, possible intraductal carcinoma. Recommend bilateral biopsy.

HISTOPATHOLOGY: Right: Adenosis, fibrocystic changes. Left: severely atypical intraductal hyperplasia. An enlarged duct **(D)** is filled with hyperplasia with architectural atypia, forming cribriform structures **(arrow)**. Irregular intraductal calcifications **(arrowhead)** are present in the adjacent ducts.

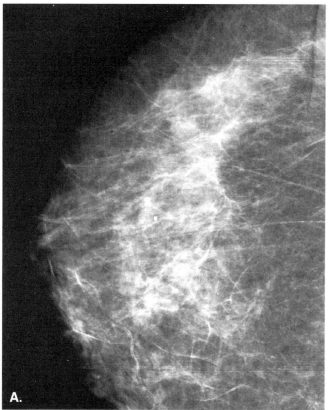

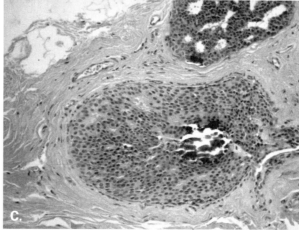

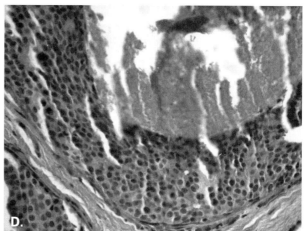

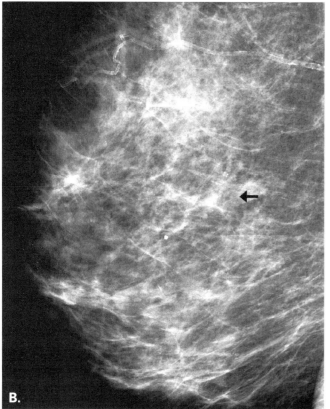

Figure 6.92

HISTORY: A 63-year-old woman recalled from screening mammography for microcalcifications.

MAMMOGRAPHY: Left CC magnification **(A)** and ML magnification **(B)** views show segmental pleomorphic microcalcifications in the central aspect of the breast. The ductal distribution is very suspicious for malignancy.

IMPRESSION: Highly suspicious for carcinoma (BI-RADS® 5).

HISTOPATHOLOGY: DCIS with comedonecrosis. This is shown on the histologic section **(C)**, where the duct is filled with a malignant cell population. There is central calcification of the necrotic material, better seen on the high-power image **(D)**.

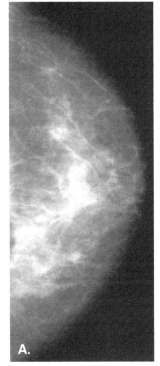

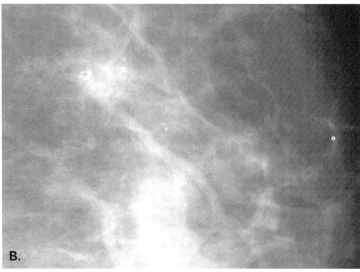

Figure 6.93

HISTORY: Screening mammogram.

MAMMOGRAPHY: Right CC view **(A)** and enlarged CC image **(B)** show two clusters of fine pleomorphic and linear microcalcifications in the central aspect of the breast. The morphology is highly suspicious for malignancy.

IMPRESSION: Multifocal carcinoma.

HISTOPATHOLOGY: Invasive ductal carcinoma and DCIS, multifocal.

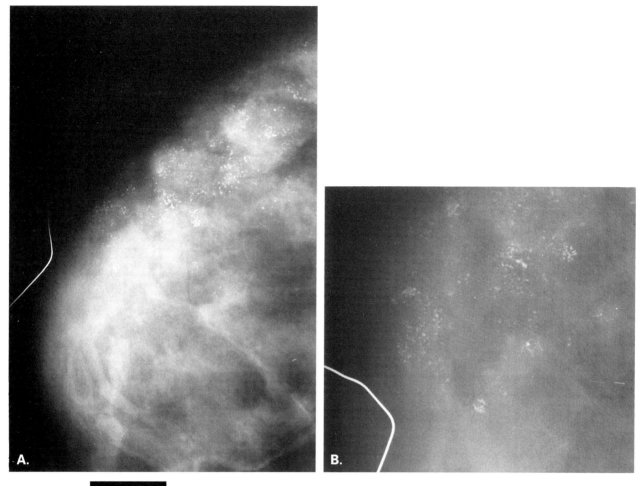

Figure 6.94

HISTORY: A 40-year-old with thickening in the left breast.

MAMMOGRAPHY: Left CC view (A) shows extremely dense parenchyma with regional microcalcifications located laterally. On the magnified CC view (B), the highly pleomorphic, jagged irregular pattern of these microcalcifications is better seen.

IMPRESSION: Highly suspicious for carcinoma, BI-RADS® 5.

HISTOPATHOLOGY: DCIS with foci of invasion.

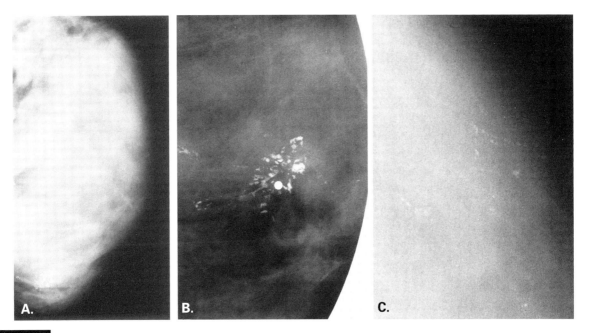

Figure 6.95

HISTORY: A 27-year-old woman with a history of surgical excision of a left breast fibroadenoma, who now presents with a new palpable mass on the right.

MAMMOGRAPHY: Right MLO view **(A)** shows extremely dense breast tissue. There are clustered microcalcifications inferiorly at the site of the palpable lump **(arrow)**. There are also faint microcalcifications located in the supra-areolar and posterior central areas **(arrowheads)**. Magnification **(B)** of the palpable lump **(B)** shows the highly pleomorphic nature of the calcifications, some of which extend into the ducts in a more linear pattern. Magnification **(C)** of the superior microcalcifications shows that they are fine and linear and distributed segmentally.

IMPRESSION: Highly suspicious for multicentric ductal carcinoma, BI-RADS® 5.

HISTOPATHOLOGY: Multicentric DCIS with comedonecrosis and foci of invasion.

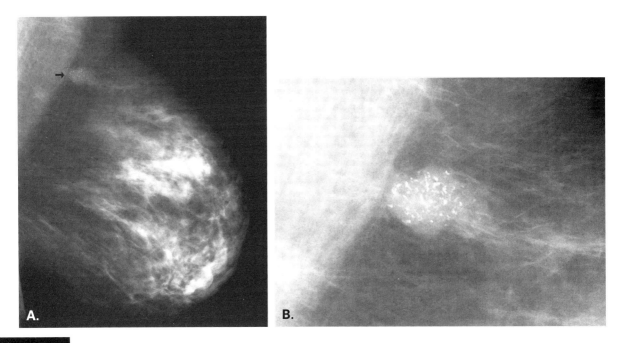

Figure 6.96

HISTORY: A 47-year-old woman for screening.

MAMMOGRAPHY: Right MLO **(A)** shows dense parenchyma and a lobulated circumscribed calcified mass located posteriorly **(arrow)**. On the magnification MLO view **(B)**, the highly pleomorphic nature of the microcalcification is noted.

IMPRESSION: Highly suspicious for malignancy, BI-RADS® 5.

HISTOPATHOLOGY: Invasive ductal carcinoma and DCIS.

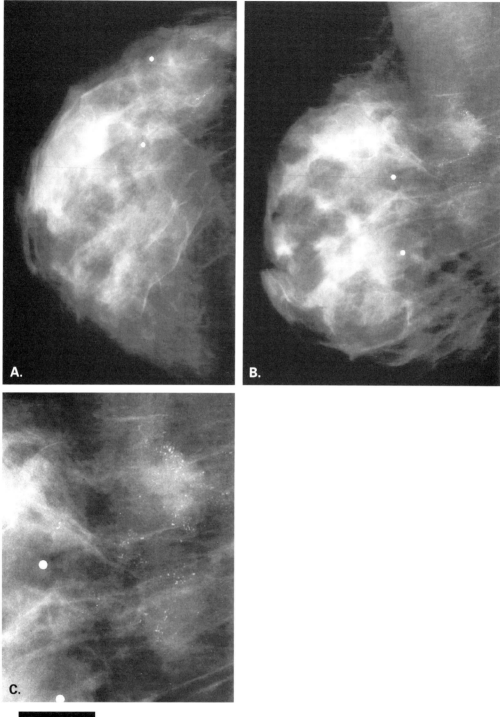

Figure 6.97

HISTORY: A 48-year-old woman with a palpable left breast mass.

MAMMOGRAPHY: Left CC **(A)** and MLO **(B)** views show dense parenchyma and regional micro-calcifications within focal asymmetry posteriorly and marked by BBs. On the magnified MLO view **(C)**, the highly pleomorphic, granular appearance of the microcalcifications is noted.

IMPRESSION: Highly suspicious for ductal carcinoma.

HISTOPATHOLOGY: Invasive ductal carcinoma and DCIS.

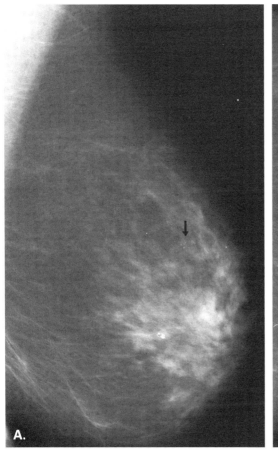

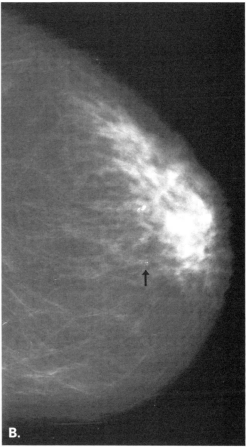

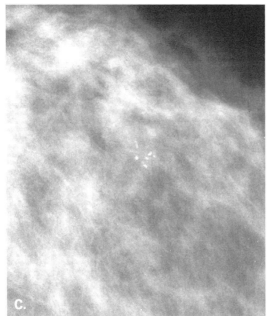

Figure 6.98

HISTORY: A 78-year-old woman for screening mammography.

MAMMOGRAPHY: Right MLO **(A)** and CC **(B)** views show two clusters of microcalcifications. The more lateral group is coarse and dystrophic, suggesting a fibroadenoma. The more medial group **(arrow) (C)** is fine and pleomorphic, therefore suspicious in nature. Core needle biopsy of the medial group was performed.

IMPRESSION: Clustered benign and clustered suspicious microcalcifications.

HISTOPATHOLOGY: DCIS low grade (medial group).

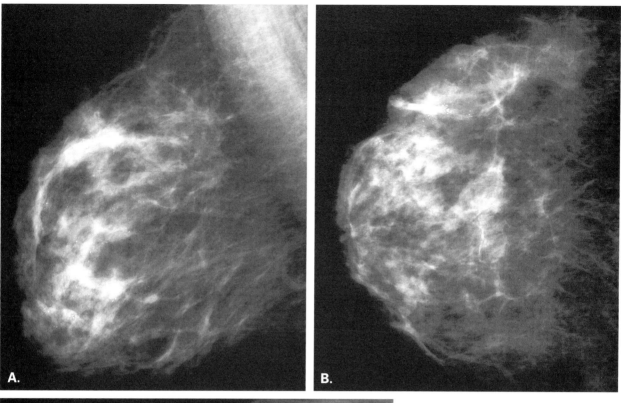

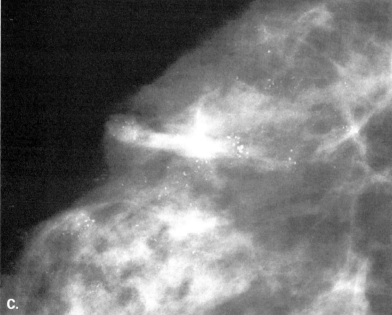

Figure 6.99

HISTORY: A 33-year-old woman who presents with palpable thickening and a serous nipple discharge.

MAMMOGRAPHY: Left MLO **(A)** and CC **(B)** views show dense parenchyma and regional microcalcifications laterally. On the magnified CC **(C)** view, the highly pleomorphic nature of the microcalcifications in a segmental distribution is seen.

IMPRESSION: Segmental microcalcification, highly suspicious for malignancy.

HISTOPATHOLOGY: DCIS with comedonecrosis, intermediate nuclear grade, solid and cribiform type.

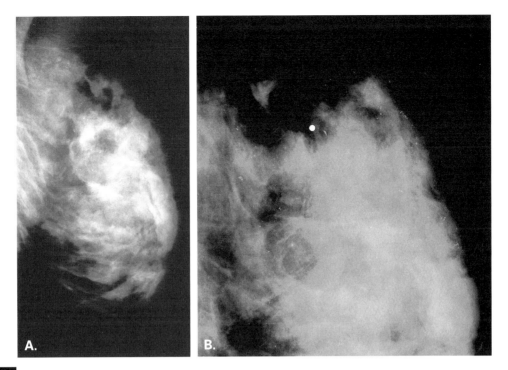

Figure 6.100

HISTORY: A 38-year-old woman who is 1 year postpartum and who presents with diffuse heaviness of the right breast. She was not lactating.

MAMMOGRAPHY: Right MLO view **(A)** shows extremely dense parenchyma with diffuse scattered microcalcifications. No calcifications were present on the left. On the magnification ML view **(B)**, the calcifications are fine and pleomorphic but diffusely scattered.

IMPRESSION: Suspicious microcalcifications, BI-RADS® 4. Recommend biopsy.

HISTOPATHOLOGY: DCIS with comedonecrosis, diffusely involving the breast.

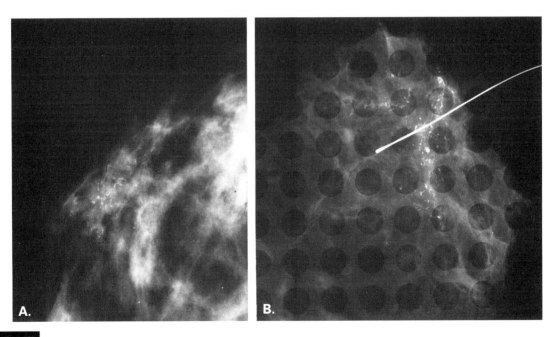

Figure 6.101

HISTORY: A 54-year-old woman with an abnormal screening mammogram.

MAMMOGRAPHY: Left CC magnification view **(A)** and specimen radiograph **(B)**. There are markedly pleomorphic, heterogeneous microcalcifications in a segmental distribution in the left breast. The calcifications are jagged, simulating the appearance of slivers of broken glass. The appearance is highly consistent with that of DCIS.

IMPRESSION: Highly suspicious microcalcifications.

HISTOPATHOLOGY: Intraductal carcinoma, comedo subtype.

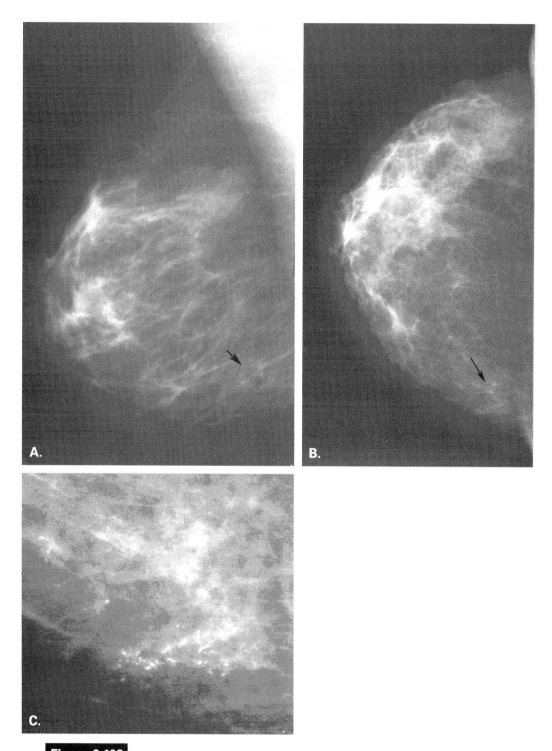

Figure 6.102

HISTORY: A 48-year-old woman for screening mammography.

MAMMOGRAPHY: Left MLO **(A)** and CC **(B)** views show segmental microcalcifications in the 8 o'clock position **(arrow)**. On the enlarged image **(C)**, the pleomorphic nature of the calcifications is evident.

IMPRESSION: Highly suspicious for carcinoma, BI-RADS® 5.

HISTOPATHOLOGY: Infiltrating ductal carcinoma and DCIS.

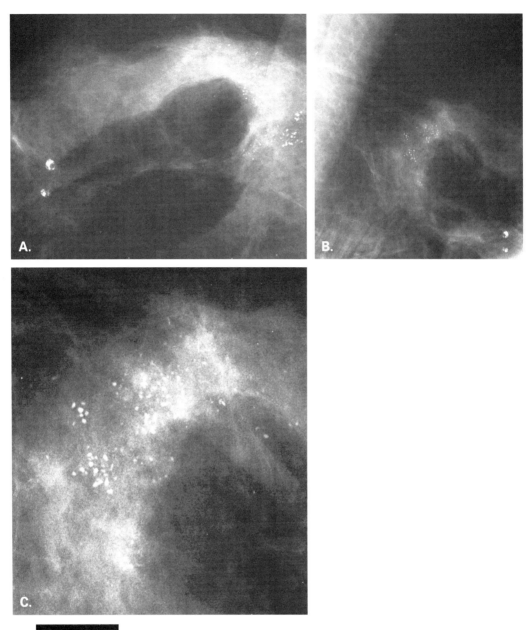

Figure 6.103

HISTORY: A 50-year-old woman with microcalcifications identified on screening, for additional views.

MAMMOGRAPHY: Right CC magnification **(A)** and MLO magnification **(B)** views demonstrate grouped pleomorphic microcalcifications within dense tissue located in the axillary tail. On the enlarged image **(C)**, the variable morphology and sharp edges of the microcalcifications are seen, which are highly malignant features.

IMPRESSION: Highly suspicious for ductal carcinoma.

HISTOPATHOLOGY: DCIS, intermediate grade, solid type with comedonecrosis extending into the adjacent lobules.

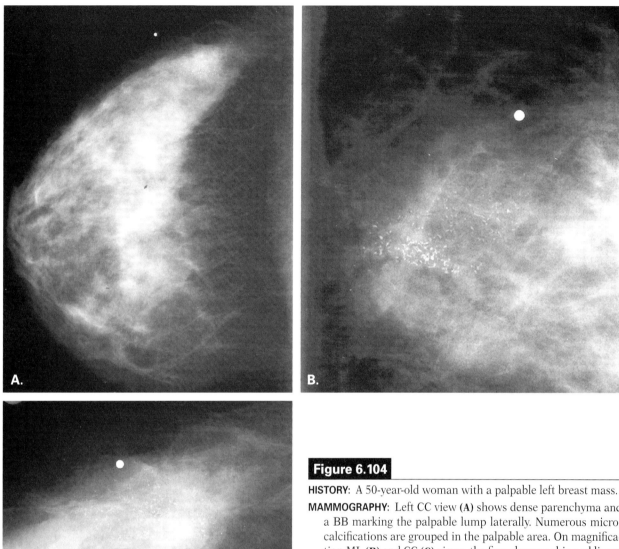

Figure 6.104

HISTORY: A 50-year-old woman with a palpable left breast mass.

MAMMOGRAPHY: Left CC view **(A)** shows dense parenchyma and a BB marking the palpable lump laterally. Numerous microcalcifications are grouped in the palpable area. On magnification ML **(B)** and CC **(C)** views, the fine pleomorphic and linear calcifications are noted.

IMPRESSION: Highly suspicious for ductal carcinoma, BI-RADS® 5.

HISTOPATHOLOGY: DCIS with invasion.

in subtropical Africa. The adult parasite is found preferentially in the subcutaneous tissues. Because this is a systemic infestation, the calcified parasites may be present bilaterally on mammography (106,107) (Fig. 6.116).

In patients infected with *Trichinella spiralis*, fine microcalcifications may be evident in the pectoralis major muscle. These appear finely stippled and diffuse (108) and represent calcified parasite larvae within the muscle (Fig. 6.117).

Calcifications Following Breast Conservation Therapy

Following lumpectomy and breast irradiation, mammography may reveal various types of calcifications. Normal changes following breast conservation therapy include the formation of dystrophic, lucent-centered, eggshell, and sutural calcifications (Fig. 6.118). The dystrophic and lucent-centered calcifications are secondary to fat necrosis and often appear at least a year or more following treatment (Fig. 6.119). Dershaw et al. (109) found that benign coarse calcifications formed in about one fourth of women treated conservatively.

The development of pleomorphic amorphous or linear microcalcifications is of concern for recurrence of carcinoma (Figs. 6.120–6.123) . These may occur at the tumor bed or elsewhere in the treated breast, and their presence

(text continues on page 328)

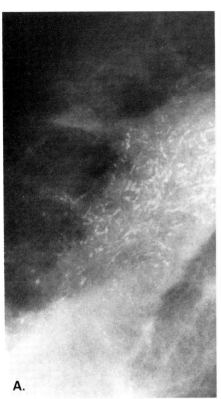
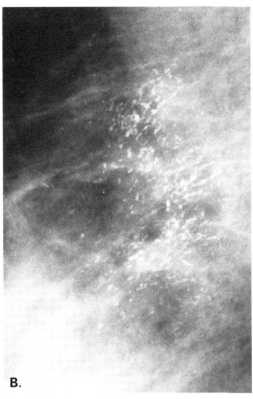

A.

B.

Figure 6.105

HISTORY: A 57-year-old woman with an abnormal screening mammogram.

MAMMOGRAPHY: Left CC **(A)** and ML **(B)** magnified views demonstrate segmental fine linear and branching microcalcifications. The morphology and distribution are highly suspicious for DCIS.

IMPRESSION: Microcalcifications highly suspicious for malignancy, BI-RADS® 5.

HISTOPATHOLOGY: DCIS, comedo subtype.

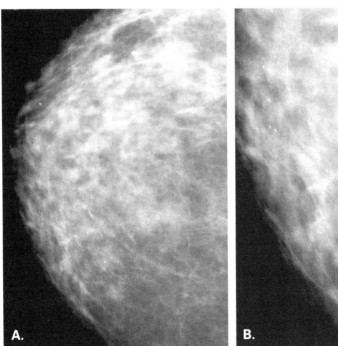
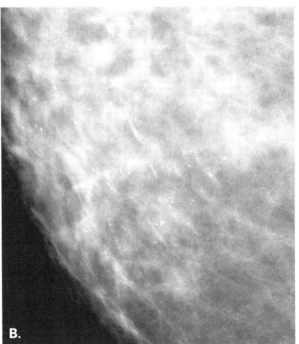

A.

B.

Figure 6.106

HISTORY: Screening mammogram.

MAMMOGRAPHY: Left CC view **(A)** shows dense parenchyma. There are extensive granular and fine linear calcifications throughout the medial and central aspect of the breast. Many of the calcifications appear to be in linear structures, as they fill the abnormal ducts on the magnified CC view **(B)**.

IMPRESSION: BI-RADS® 5, highly suspicious for malignancy.

HISTOPATHOLOGY: DCIS, with comedonecrosis.

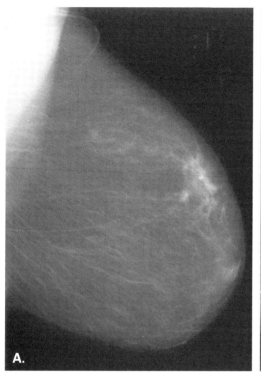

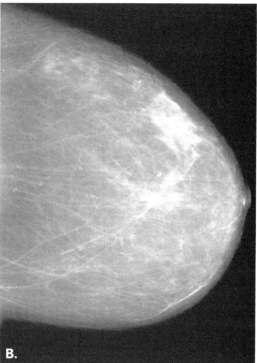

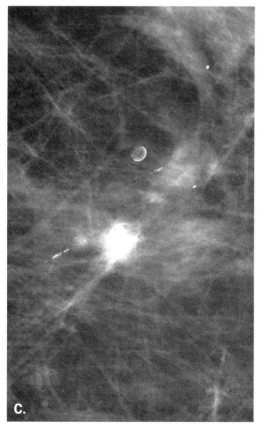

Figure 6.107

HISTORY: Screening mammogram on a 75-year-old woman.

MAMMOGRAPHY: Right MLO **(A)** and CC **(B)** views show a small, dense indistinct mass with adjacent linear microcalcifications. The microcalcifications are better demonstrated on the enlarged image **(C)**. The finding suggests the appearance of an invasive cancer with intraductal extension.

IMPRESSION: Highly suspicious for carcinoma.

HISTOPATHOLOGY: Invasive ductal carcinoma with DCIS.

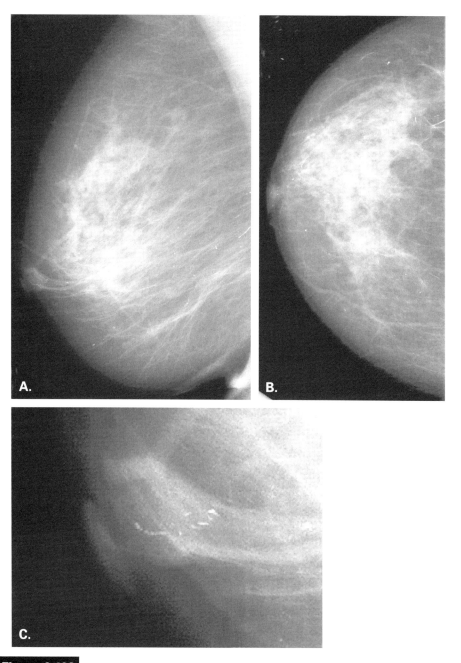

Figure 6.108

HISTORY: An 85-year-old woman who presents with a scaling nipple.

MAMMOGRAPHY: Left MLO **(A)** and CC **(B)** views show multiple clusters of pleomorphic and linear microcalcifications. In particular, there are fine linear microcalcifications **(C)** in the left subareolar area, extending to the nipple. This spectrum of clinical and mammographic findings is consistent with Paget disease with intraductal extension.

IMPRESSION: Paget disease.

HISTOPATHOLOGY: Paget carcinoma with multicentric DCIS on mastectomy.

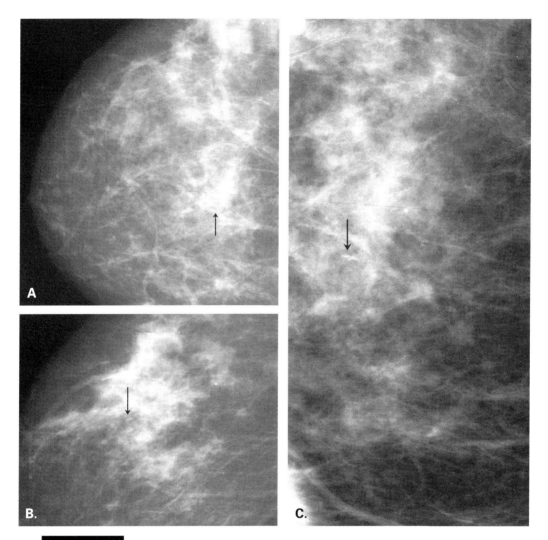

Figure 6.109

HISTORY: A 68-year-old woman for screening mammography.

MAMMOGRAPHY: Left CC **(A)** and coned-down MLO **(B)** views show a small cluster of microcalcifications centrally **(arrow)**. On spot-compression magnification **(C)**, the calcifications **(arrow)** are fine, linear in shape, and are located in a linear distribution. Just posterior to these is a small indistinct mass with associated amorphous calcifications.

IMPRESSION: Calcifications suspicious for ductal carcinoma.

HISTOPATHOLOGY: DCIS and invasive ductal carcinoma.

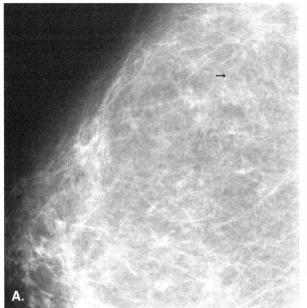

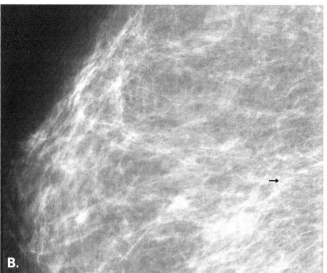

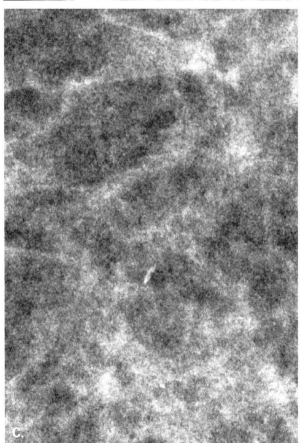

Figure 6.110

HISTORY: A 45-year-old woman with an abnormal screening mammogram.

MAMMOGRAPHY: Left CC magnification **(A)** and ML **(B)** views show scattered fibroglandular densities and a single microcalcification **(arrows)**. On the enlarged image **(C)**, the single fine linear microcalcification is seen. This was new in comparison with the prior mammogram and was biopsied.

IMPRESSION: New linear microcalcification, suspicious for DCIS, BI-RADS® 4.

HISTOPATHOLOGY: Invasive ductal carcinoma and DCIS.

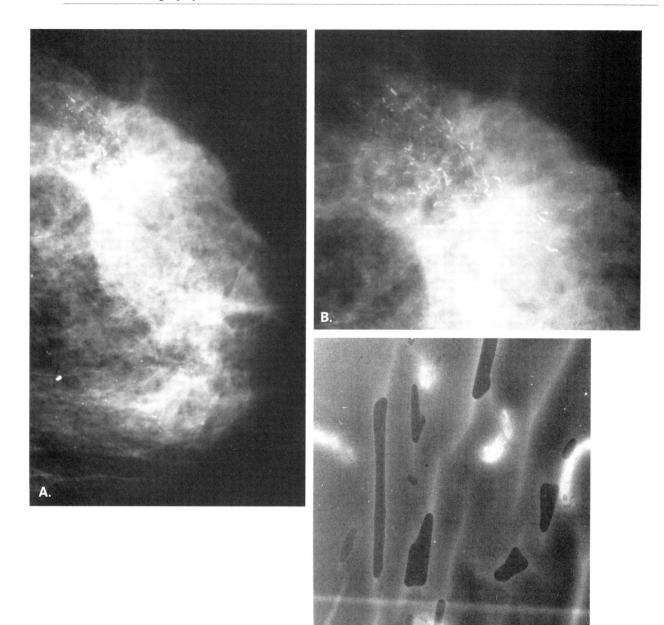

Figure 6.111

HISTORY: A 55-year-old woman for screening mammography.

MAMMOGRAPHY: Right MLO view **(A)** and enlarged ML **(B)** show segmentally distributed, fine linear microcalcifications in the upper aspect of the breast. The pattern is highly suggestive of malignancy. Core needle biopsy was performed, and specimen radiography **(C)** demonstrates numerous microcalcifications to be included in the cores. Pathology of the cores showed atypical ductal hyperplasia. Because of the presence of atypia, surgical excision was recommend and performed.

IMPRESSION: Microcalcifications, highly suspicious for malignancy, BI-RADS® 5.

HISTOPATHOLOGY: A typical ductal hyperplasia on core. Ductal carcinoma in situ on excision.

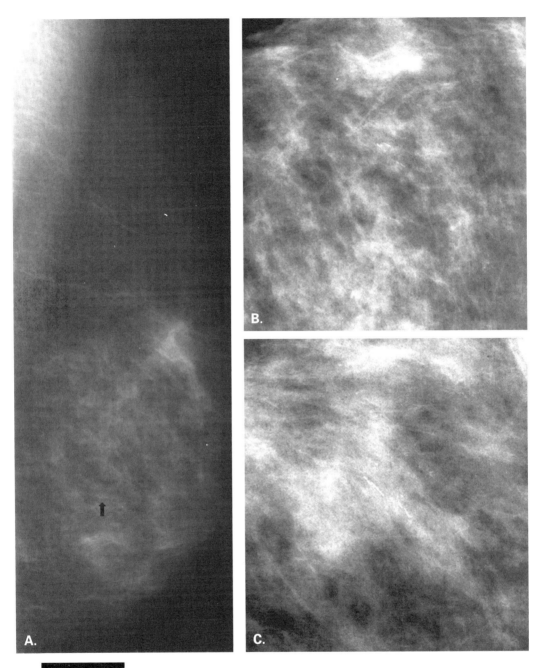

Figure 6.112

HISTORY: A 56-year-old woman who is status post–left breast cancer, for screening of the right breast.

MAMMOGRAPHY: Right MLO view **(A)** shows a small cluster of fine microcalcifications centrally **(arrow)**. On the enlarged MLO **(B)**, the linear calcifications are better seen. The magnification view **(C)** demonstrates the malignant appearance of these microcalcifications that are in a linear distribution.

IMPRESSION: Highly suspicious calcifications.

HISTOPATHOLOGY: DCIS, comedo type.

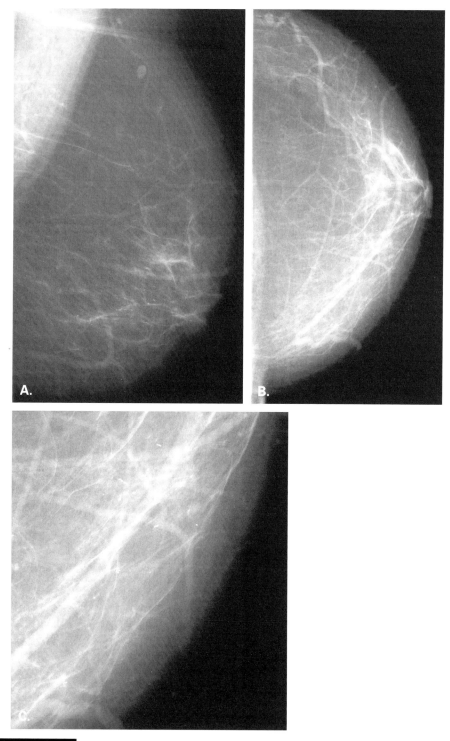

Figure 6.113

HISTORY: A 58-year-old woman for screening mammography.

MAMMOGRAPHY: Right MLO (**A**) and CC (**B**) views show segmental microcalcification in the right breast at 5 o'clock. An enlarged image (**C**) shows the calcifications to be fine, linear, and branching.

IMPRESSION: Linear microcalcifications, highly suspicious for malignancy.

HISTOPATHOLOGY: DCIS, with comedonecrosis.

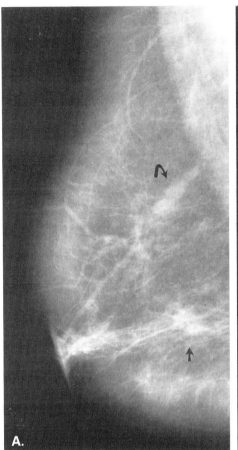

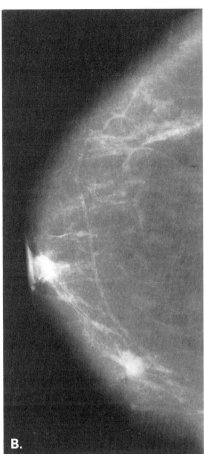

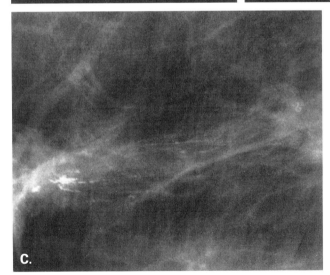

Figure 6.114

HISTORY: A 61-year-old woman with a palpable mass in the left subareolar area.

MAMMOGRAPHY: Left MLO **(A)** and CC **(B)** views and magnified image **(C)**. There are linear ductal calcifications of varying sizes extending back from a retracted nipple-areolar complex to a spiculated mass **(straight arrow)**. A second mass **(curved arrow)** is present in the upper outer quadrant **(A)**. A magnified image **(C)** of the subareolar area shows the pleomorphism of the linear casting calcifications that have a highly malignant appearance.

IMPRESSION: Multicentric carcinoma with intraductal extension to the nipple.

HISTOPATHOLOGY: Infiltrating ductal and intraductal carcinoma in two sites, with 2 of 25 lymph nodes positive for tumor.

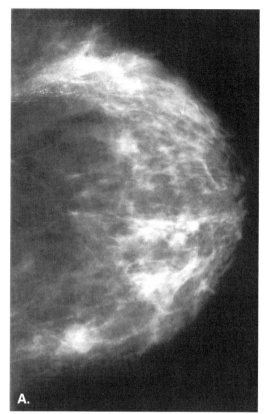

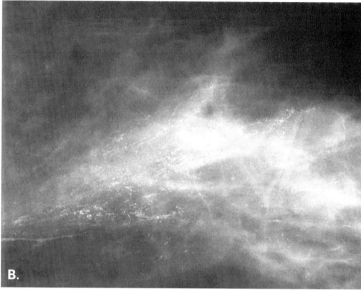

Figure 6.115

HISTORY: A 48-year-old woman with a palpable mass in the medial aspect of the right breast.

MAMMOGRAPHY: Right CC view **(A)** shows a lobular, slightly indistinct, dense mass in the inner aspect of the breast, corresponding to the palpable finding. In addition, there are extensive segmentally distributed microcalcifications located laterally. On the enlarged CC image **(B)**, the fine pleomorphic and fine linear microcalcifications are better seen.

IMPRESSION: Multicentric carcinoma.

HISTOPATHOLOGY: Invasive ductal carcinoma (medial mass) and invasive ductal with comedo-carcinoma (lateral calcifications).

necessitates biopsy. In a study of patients treated with breast conservation therapy, Rebner et al. (110) found that 10 of 152 (7%) developed suspicious microcalcifications in the tumor bed and that 4 of 10 (40%) of these had recurrent malignancies. The mammographic features of the microcalcifications were not specific enough to differentiate benign disease from recurrent carcinoma (110). Vora et al. (111) found that various types of benign-appearing calcifications, including punctuate microcalcifications, developed at the lumpectomy sites. The authors recommended conservative management with follow-up mammography of patients with the benign-appearing calcifica-

tions. Dershaw et al. (112) found that recurrent tumors were associated with >10 calcifications in 77% of cases. Recurrences presented as linear calcifications in 68% and pleomorphic calcifications in 77% (111).

In summary, patients who have undergone breast conservation therapy often develop calcifications. Many of these are clearly benign and are posttraumatic or sutural in origin. Careful attention to the mammogram is important to detect amorphous or pleomorphic microcalcifications that may indicate recurrent carcinoma.

(References continue on page 336)

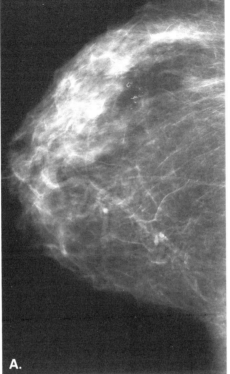

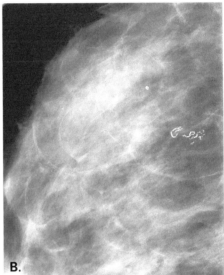

Figure 6.116

HISTORY: A 50-year-old Nigerian woman who presents for screening mammography.

MAMMOGRAPHY: Left CC view **(A)** shows a group of serpiginous calcifications in the lateral aspect of the breast. On magnification **(B)**, these are dense, curvilinear calcifications not corresponding to a vessel or duct. The pattern is typical of parasitic calcification.

IMPRESSION: Calcified worms, likely Loiasis. (Case courtesy of Dr. Lindsay Cheng, Sacramento, California.)

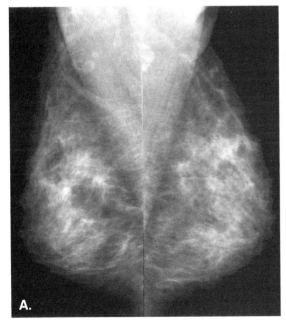

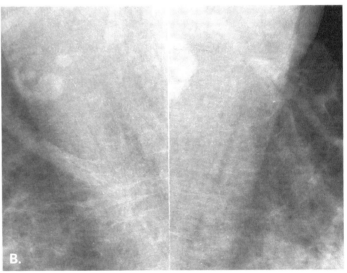

Figure 6.117

HISTORY: Screening mammography performed on an immigrant from Central America.

MAMMOGRAPHY: Bilateral MLO views **(A)** and magnified MLO views **(B)** of the axillary region show innumerable stippled calcifications overlying the pectoralis major muscles bilaterally. The pattern is associated with calcified intramuscular parasites in Trichinella.

IMPRESSION: Trichinosis with calcified parasites in the pectoralis muscle. (Case courtesy of Dr. Jan Walecki, Washington, DC.)

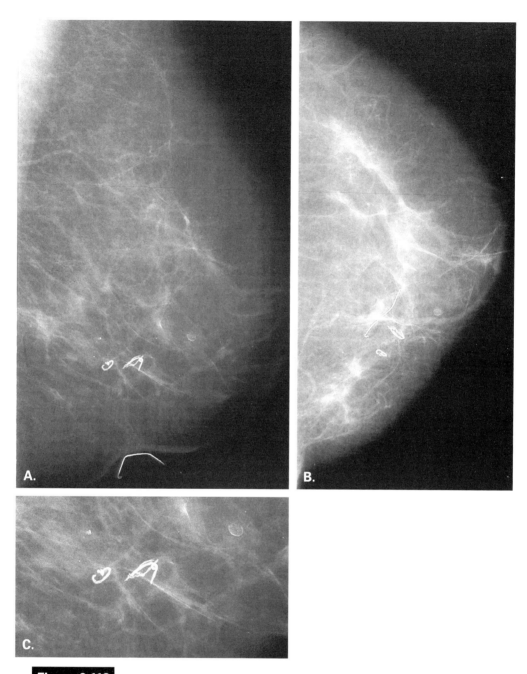

Figure 6.118

HISTORY: Patient is status posttreatment of right breast cancer with lumpectomy and radiation therapy.

MAMMOGRAPHY: Right MLO **(A)** and CC **(B)** views show a wire marking the lumpectomy site inferiorly. In this area are somewhat coarse curvilinear calcifications. On the MLO magnification view **(C)**, the knot-shaped calcifications are seen.

IMPRESSION: Sutural calcifications at the lumpectomy site, BI-RADS® 2.

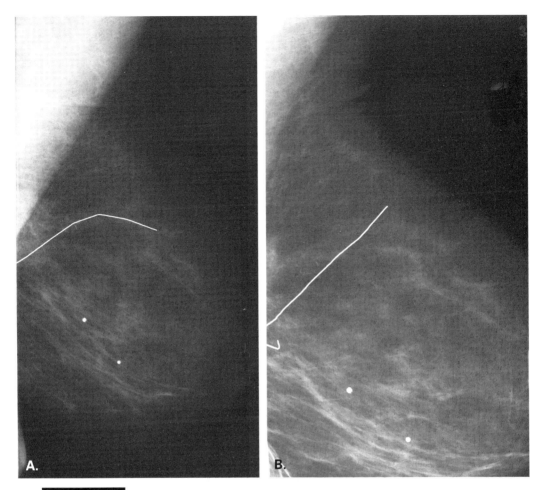

Figure 6.119

HISTORY: Patient is status postlumpectomy and radiation therapy for right breast cancer.

MAMMOGRAPHY: Right MLO **(A)** view shows a scar mark the lumpectomy site. There are round and lucent calcifications present both centrally in the breast as well as at the tumor bed, seen on the magnification view **(B)**.

IMPRESSION: Normal posttreatment changes with dystrophic calcifications of fat necrosis.

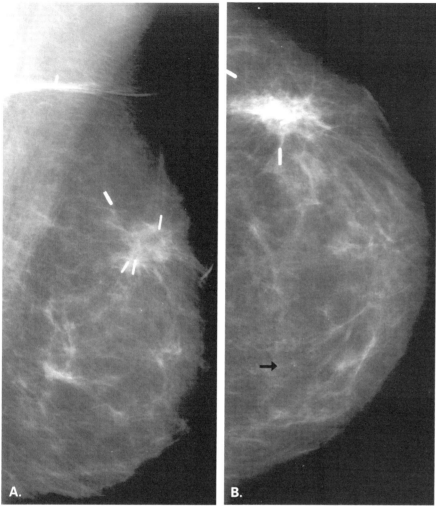

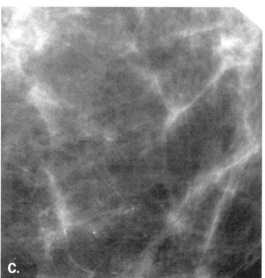

Figure 6.120

HISTORY: A 44-year-old woman who was 3 years status posttreatment of right breast cancer with lumpectomy and radiation therapy.

MAMMOGRAPHY: Right MLO **(A)** and CC **(B)** views show distortion at the lumpectomy site consistent with postsurgical scar. In the medial aspect of the breast are faint microcalcifications **(arrow)**. On spot CC magnification **(C)**, the microcalcifications are amorphous and linearly arranged, which is a suspicious distribution pattern.

IMPRESSION: Microcalcifications, suspicious for recurrence of carcinoma.

HISTOPATHOLOGY: DCIS, high grade, cribriform and solid types with comedonecrosis.

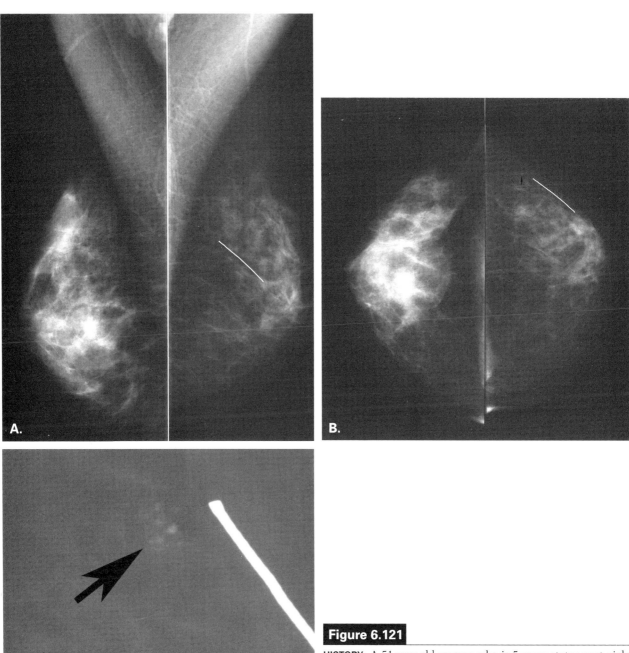

Figure 6.121

HISTORY: A 51-year-old woman who is 5 years status post–right lumpectomy and radiation therapy for DCIS.

MAMMOGRAPHY: Bilateral MLO **(A)** and CC **(B)** views show the paucity of parenchyma in the right upper-outer quadrant, secondary to the lumpectomy, as indicated by the wire marker. At the posterior margin of the lumpectomy site on the right CC view **(arrow)** is a small cluster of microcalcifications. On magnification exaggerated CC lateral view **(C)**, the calcifications are pleomorphic and suspicious for malignancy. (*continued*)

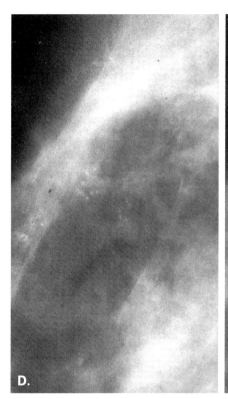

D.

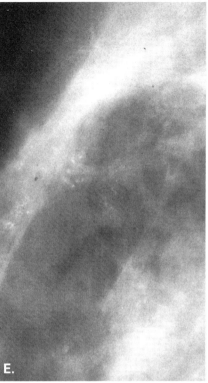

E.

Figure 6.121 *(CONTINUED)*

On the left MLO view **(D)**, two groups of amorphous calcifications are seen. On the magnification view **(E)**, these faint amorphous microcalcifications are also suspicious for malignancy.

IMPRESSION: Highly suspicious for recurrent right breast carcinoma and possible carcinoma in the left breast.

HISTOPATHOLOGY: DCIS, multifocal in the left breast; DCIS recurrent, right breast.

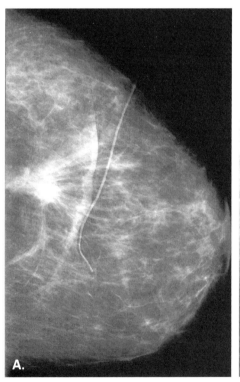

A.

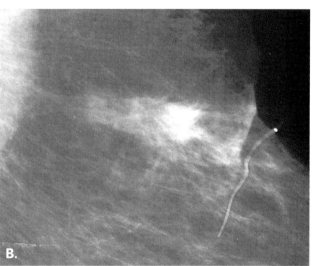

B.

Figure 6.122

HISTORY: A 76-year-old woman with prior history of right breast cancer treated with lumpectomy and radiation therapy.

MAMMOGRAPHY: Right CC view **(A)** and enlarged MLO view **(B)** demonstrate an irregular mass at the lumpectomy site consistent with the postsurgical scar. Within the scar are faint amorphous microcalcifications that had developed from an earlier postoperative study.

IMPRESSION: New microcalcifications in the tumor bed suspicious for recurrence of carcinoma.

HISTOPATHOLOGY: DCIS.

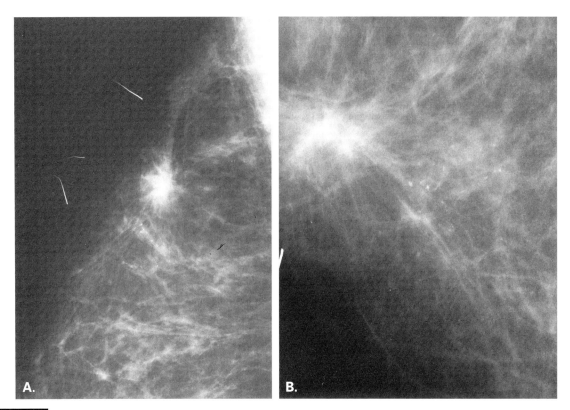

Figure 6.123

HISTORY: A 61-year-old woman who is status posttreatment of left breast cancer with lumpectomy and radiation therapy.

MAMMOGRAPHY: Left ML (**A**) and magnification (**B**) views show the lumpectomy site indicated by wire markers. The scar was stable in comparison with prior examinations. However, faint amorphous microcalcifications are in the inferior aspect of the tumor bed and are suspicious in appearance.

IMPRESSION: Postsurgical changes with adjacent microcalcifications, suspicious for malignancy, BI-RADS® 4.

HISTOPATHOLOGY: Recurrent DCIS.

REFERENCES

1. Leborgne R. Diagnosis of tumors of the breast by simple roentgenography: calcifications in carcinoma. *AJR Am J Roentgenol* 1951;65:1–11.
2. Gershon-Cohen J, Yiu LS, Berger SM. The diagnostic importance of calcareous patterns in roentgenography of breast cancer. *AJR Am J Roentgenol* 1962;88:1117–1125.
3. Millis RR, Davis R, Stacey AJ. The detection and significance of calcifications in the breast: a radiological and pathological study. *Br J Radiol* 1976;49:12–26.
4. Dershaw DD, Abramson A, Kinne DW. Ductal carcinoma in situ: mammographic findings and clinical implications. *Radiology* 1989;170:411–415.
5. Herman E, Janus C, Schwartz IS, et al. Occult malignant breast lesions in 114 patients: relationship to age and presence of calcifications. *Radiology* 1988;17:321–324.
6. Pisano ED, Gatsonis C, Hendrick E, et al. Diagnostic performance of digital versus film mammography for breast-cancer screening. *N Engl J Med* 2005;353(17):1773–1783.
7. Franceschi D, Crowe J, Zollinger R, et al. Breast biopsy for calcifications in nonpalpable breast lesions. *Arch Surg* 1990;125:170–173.
8. Barton JW, Kornguth PJ. Mammographic deodorant and powder artifact: is there confusion with malignant microcalcifications? *Breast Dis* 1990;3:121–126.
9. Pamilo M, Soiva M, Suramo I. New artifacts simulating malignant microcalcifications on mammography. *Breast Dis* 1989;1:321–322.
10. Bruwer A, Nelson GW, Spark RP. Punctate intranodal gold deposits simulating microcalcifications on mammograms. *Radiology* 1987;163:87–88.
11. Bolen JW, Shaw de Paredes E, Carter T. Intranodal gold deposits: simulating malignant microcalcifications. *Breast Dis* 1988;2:105–107.
12. American College of Radiology. *ACR Mammography Quality Control Manual.* Reston, VA: American College of Radiology, 1999.
13. Berkowitz JE, Gatewood MB, Donovan GB, et al. Dermal breast calcifications: localization with template-guided placement of skin marker. *Radiology* 1987;163:282.
14. Linden SS, Sullivan DC. Breast skin calcifications: localization with a stereotactic device. *Radiology* 1989;171:570–571.
15. Sickles EA. Microfocal spot magnification mammography using xeroradiologic and screen-film recording systems. *Radiology* 1979;131:599–607.
16. American College of Radiology. *Breast Imaging Reporting and Data System (BI-RADS®).* Reston, VA: American College of Radiology, 1993.
17. Wellings SR, Jensen HM, Marcum RG. An atlas of subgross pathology of the human breast cancer. *Am J Obstet Gynecol* 1986;154:1280–1284.
18. Egan RL, McSweeney MB, Sewell CW. Intramammary calcifications without an associated mass in benign and malignant disease. *Radiology* 1980;137:1–7.
19. Shaw de Paredes E, Abbitt PL, Tabbarah S, et al. Mammographic and histologic correlations of microcalcifications. *RadioGraphics* 1990;10:577–589.
20. Powell RW, McSweeney MB, Wilson CE. X-ray calcifications as the only basis for breast biopsy. *Ann Surg* 1983;197:555–559.
21. Wilhelm MC, Shaw de Paredes E, Pope TL, et al. The changing mammogram: a primary indication for needle localization biopsy. *Arch Surg* 1986;121:1311–1314.
22. Feig SA, Shaber GS, Patchefsky A, et al. Analysis of clinically occult and mammographically occult breast tumors. *AJR Am J Roentgenol* 1977;128:403–408.
23. Homer MJ. Nonpalpable breast abnormalities: a realistic view of the accuracy of mammography in detecting malignancies. *Radiology* 1984;153:831–832.
24. MacErlean DP, Nathan BE. Case reports: calcification in sclerosing adenosis simulating malignant breast calcification. *Br J Radiol* 1972;45:944–945.
25. Rosen PP. Microglandular adenosis: a benign lesion simulating invasive mammary carcinoma. *Am J Surg Pathol* 1983;7:137–144.
26. Clement PB, Azzopardi JG. Microglandular adenosis of the breast: a lesion simulating tubular carcinoma. *Histopathology* 1983;7:169–180.
27. Sickles EA, Abele JS. Milk of calcium within tiny benign breast cysts. *Radiology* 1981;141:655–658.
28. Homer MJ, Cooper AG, Pile-Spellman ER. Milk of calcium in breast microcysts: manifestation as a solitary focal disease. *AJR Am J Roentgenol* 1988;150:789–790.
29. Pennes DR, Rebner M. Layering granular calcifications in macroscopic breast cysts. *Breast Dis* 1988;1:109–112.
30. Wolfe JN. *Xeroradiography: Breast Calcifications.* Springfield, IL: Charles C. Thomas, 1977.
31. Fraser JL, Raza S, Chorny K, et al. Columnar alteration with prominent apical snouts and secretions: a spectrum of changes frequently present in breast biopsies performed for microcalcifications. *Am J Surg Pathol* 1998;22(12):1521–1527.
32. Gallager HS, Martin JE. Early phases in the development of breast cancer. *Cancer* 1969;24:1170–1178.
33. Gallager HS, Martin JE. The study of mammary carcinoma by mammography and whole organ sectioning: early observations. *Cancer* 1969;23:855–873.
34. Stomper PC, Cholewinski BS, Penetrante RB, et al. Atypical hyperplasia: frequency and mammographic and pathologic relationships in excisional biopsies guided with mammography and clinical examination. *Radiology* 1993;189:667–671.
35. Page DL, Zwaag RV, Rogers LW, et al. Relation between component parts of fibrocystic disease complex and breast cancer. *J Natl Cancer Inst* 1978;61:1055–1063.
36. Page DL, Dupont WD, Rogers LW, et al. Atypical hyperplasia lesions of the female breast: a long-term follow-up study. *Cancer* 1985;55:2698–2708.
37. Dupont WD, Page DL. Risk factors for breast cancer in women with proliferative breast disease. *N Engl J Med* 1985;312:146–151.
38. Foote FW, Stewart FW. Lobular carcinoma in situ: a rare form of mammary cancer. *Am J Pathol* 1941;17:491–495.
39. Urban JA. Bilaterality of cancer of the breast: biopsy of the opposite breast. *Cancer* 1967;20:1867–1870.
40. Rosen PP, Lieberman PH, Braun DW. Lobular carcinoma in situ of breast: detailed analysis of 99 patients with average follow-up of 24 years. *Am J Surg Pathol* 1978;2:225–251.
41. Hutter RV. The management of patients with lobular carcinoma in situ of the breast. *Cancer* 1984;53:798–802.
42. Synder RE. Mammography and lobular carcinoma in situ. *Surg Obstet Gynecol* 1966;122:255–260.
43. Georgian-Smith D, Lawton TJ. Calcifications of lobular carcinoma in situ of the breast: radiologic-pathologic correlation. *AJR Am J Roentgenol* 2001;176(5):1255–1259.
44. Pope TL Jr, Fechner RE, Wilhelm MC, et al. Lobular carcinoma in situ of the breast: mammographic features. *Radiology* 1988;168:63–66.
45. Sonnenfeld MR, Frenna TH, Weidner N, et al. Lobular carcinoma in situ: mammographic-pathologic correlation of results of needle-directed biopsy. *Radiology* 1991;181:363–367.
46. Ahmed A. Calcification in human breast carcinomas: ultrastructural observations. *J Pathol* 1975;117:247–251.
47. Tornos C, Silva E, El-Naggar A, et al. Calcium oxalate crystals in breast biopsies. *Am J Surg Pathol* 1990;14(10):961–968.
48. Winston JS, Yeh I-T, Evers K, Friedman AK. Calcium oxalate is associated with benign breast tissue: can we avoid biopsy? *Am J Clin Pathol* 1993;100:488–492.
49. Dondalski M, Bernstein JR. Disappearing breast calcifications: mammographic-pathologic discrepancy due to calcium oxalate. *South Med J* 1992;85(12):1252–1254.
50. Radi MJ. Calcium oxalate crystals in breast biopsies. *Arch Pathol Lab Med* 1989;113:1367–136,.
51. Fondos-Morera A, Prats-Esteve M, Tura-Soteras JM, et al. Breast tumors: composition of microcalcifications. *Radiology* 1988;169:325–327.

52. Busing CM, Keppler U, Manges V. Differences in microcalcification in breast tumors. *Virchows Arch* 1981;393: 307–313.

53. Frappart L, Remy I, Chilin H, et al. Different types of microcalcifications observed in breast pathology. *Virchows Arch* 1986;410:179–187.

54. D'Orsi CJ, Reale FR, Davis MA, et al. Is calcium oxalate an adequate explanation for nonvisualization of breast specimen calcifications? *Radiology* 1992;182:801–803.

55. Stomper PC, Connolly JL, Meyer JE, et al. Clinically occult ductal carcinoma in situ detected with mammography: analysis of 100 cases with radiologic-pathologic correlation. *Radiology* 1989;172:235–241.

56. Ikeda DM, Anderson I. Ductal carcinoma in situ: atypical mammographic appearances. *Radiology* 1989;172:661–666.

57. Evans A, Pinder S, Wilson R, et al. Ductal carcinoma in situ of the breast: correlation between mammographic and pathologic findings. *AJR Am J Roentgenol* 1994;162: 1307–1311.

58. Holland R, Hendricks JHCL, Verbeek ALM, et al. Extent, distribution, and mammographic/histological correlations of breast ductal carcinoma in situ. *Lancet* 1990;335: 519–522.

59. Barreau B, de Mascarel I, Feuga C, et al. Mammography of ductal carcinoma in situ of the breast: review of 909 cases with radiographic-pathologic correlations. *Eur J Radiol* 2005;54(1):55–61.

60. Homer MJ, Safaii H, Smith TJ, et al. The relationship of mammographic microcalcification to histologic malignancy: radiologic-pathologic correlation. *AJR Am J Roentgenol* 1989; 153:1187–1189.

61. Zunzunegui RG, Chung MA, Oruwari J, et al. Casting-type calcifications with invasion and high-grade ductal carcinoma in situ. *Arch Surg* 2003;138:537–540.

62. Thurfjell E, Thurfjell MG, Lindgren A. Mammographic finding as predictor of survival in 1–9 mm invasive breast cancers: worse prognosis for cases presenting as calcifications alone. *Breast Cancer Res Treat* 2001;67:177–180.

63. Stomper PC, Geradts J, Edge SB, et al. Mammographic predictors of the presence and size of invasive carcinomas associated with malignant microcalcification lesion without a mass. *AJR Am J Roentgenol* 2003;181(6): 1679–1684.

64. Tabar L, Chen HHT, Yen MFA, et al. Mammographic tumor features can predict long-term outcomes reliably in women with 1–14-mm invasive breast carcinoma. *Cancer* 2004;101(8): 1745–1759.

65. deLafontan B, Daures JP, Salicru B, et al. Isolated clustered microcalcifications: diagnostic value of mammography— series of 400 cases with surgical verification. *Radiology* 1994;190:479–483.

66. Kopans DB, Nguyen PL, Koerner FC, et al. Mixed form diffusely scattered calcifications in breast cancer with apocrine features. *Radiology* 1990;177:807–811.

67. Homer MJ, Safaii H. Cancerization of the lobule: implication regarding analysis of microcalcification shape. *Breast Dis* 1990;3:131–133.

68. Hassler O. Microradiographic investigations of calcifications of the female breast. *Cancer* 1969;23:1103–1109.

69. Muir BB, Lamb J, Anderson TJ, et al. Microcalcifications and its relationship to cancer of the breast: experience in a screening clinic. *Clin Radiol* 1983;34:193–200.

70. Lev-Toaff AS, Feig SA, Saitas VL, et al. Stability of malignant breast microcalcifications. *Radiology* 1994;192:153–156.

71. Schnitt SJ, Connolly JL, Khettry U, et al. Pathologic findings on re-excision of the primary site in breast cancer patients considered for treatment by primary radiation therapy. *Cancer* 1987;59:675–681.

72. Harris JR, Connolly JL, Schnitt SJ, et al. The use of pathologic features in selecting the extent of surgical resection necessary for breast cancer patients treated by primary radiation therapy. *Ann Surg* 1985;201:164–169.

73. Osteen RT, Connolly JL, Recht A, et al. Identification of patients at high risk for local recurrence after conservative surgery and radiation therapy for stage I or II breast cancer. *Arch Surg* 1987;122:1248–1252.

74. Wazer DE, Schmidt-Ullrich R, Homer MJ, et al. The utility of preoperative physical examination and mammography for detecting an extensive intraductal component in early stage breast carcinoma. *Breast Dis* 1990;3: 181–185.

75. Stomper PC, Connolly JL. Mammographic features predicting an extensive intraductal component in early-stage infiltrating ductal carcinoma. *AJR Am J Roentgenol* 1992;158: 269–272.

76. D'Orsi CJ, Kopans DB. Mammographic feature analysis. *Semin Roentgenol* 1983;28(3):204–230.

77. Kopans DB, Meyer JE, Homer MJ, et al. Dermal deposits mistaken for breast calcifications. *Radiology* 1983;149: 592–594.

78. Tabar L, Dean PB. *Teaching Atlas of Mammography.* Stuttgart: George Thieme Verlag, 1985.

79. Homer MJ, D'Orsi CJ, Sitzman SB. Dermal calcifications in fixed orientation: the tattoo sign. *Radiology* 1994;192:161–163.

80. Sommer G, Kopsa H, Zazgornik J, et al. Breast calcifications in renal hyperparathyroidism. *AJR Am J Roentgenol* 1987;148:855–857.

81. Evans AJ, Cohen MEL, Cohen GF. Patterns of breast calcification in patients on renal dialysis. *Clin Radiol* 1992;45: 343–344.

82. Sickles EA, Galvin HB. Breast arterial calcifications in association with diabetes mellitus: too weak a correlation to have clinical utility. *Radiology* 1985;55:577–579.

83. Braun JK, Comstock CH, Joseph L. Intramammary arterial calcifications associated with diabetes. *Radiology* 1980;136: 61–62.

84. Kemmeren JM, Beijerinck D, van Noord PAH, et al. Breast arterial calcifications: association with diabetes mellitus and cardiovascular mortality. *Radiology* 1996; 201:75–78.

85. Moshyedi AC, Puthawala AH, Kurland RJ, et al. Breast arterial calcification: association with coronary artery disease. *Radiology* 1995;194:181–183.

86. Meybehm M, Pfeifer U. Vascular calcifications mimicking grouped microcalcifications on mammography. *Breast Dis* 1990;3:81–86.

87. Gershon-Cohen J, Ingleby H. Roentgenography of fibroadenoma of the breast. *Radiology* 1952;59:77–87.

88. Meyer JE, Lester SC, DiPiro PJ, et al. Occult calcified fibroadenomas. *Breast Dis* 1995;8:29–38.

89. Spagnolo DV, Shilkin KB. Breast neoplasms containing bones and cartilage. *Virchows Arch* 1983;400:287–295.

90. Cooper RA, Berman S. Extensive breast calcification in renal failure. *J Thorac Imaging* 1988;3(2):81–82.

91. Han SY, Witten DM. Diffuse calcification of the breast in chronic renal failure. *AJR Am J Roentgenol* 1977;129: 341–342.

92. Koide T, Katayama H. Calcification in augmentation mammoplasty. *Radiology* 1979;130:337–340.

93. Harvey JA, Fondriest JE, Smith MM. Densely calcified breast mass. *Invest Radiol* 1994;29:516–518.

94. Kim SM, Park JM, Moon WK. Dystrophic breast calcifications in patients with collagen diseases. *Clin Imaging* 2004;28(1):6–9.

95. Gershon-Cohen J III, Ingleby H, Hermel MB. Calcification in secretory disease of the breast. *AJR Am J Roentgenol* 1956;76:132–135.

96. Levitan LH, Witten DM, Harrison EG. Calcifications in breast disease: mammographic pathologic correlation. *AJR Am J Roentgenol Radium Ther Nucl Med* 1964;92: 29–39.

97. Asch T, Fry C. Radiographic appearance of mammary duct ectasia with calcification. *N Engl J Med* 1962;266: 86–87.

98. Bassett LW, Gold RT, Cove HC. Mammographic spectrum of traumatic fat necrosis: the fallibility of "pathognomonic" signs of carcinoma. *AJR Am J Roentgenol* 1978;130:119–122.

99. Leborgne R. Esteatonecrosis quistica calcificata de la mama. *Torace* 1967;16:172.

100. Fewins HE, Whitehouse GH, Leinster SJ. The spontaneous disappearance of breast calcification. *Clin Radiol* 1988;39:257–261.

101. Parker MD, Clark RL, McLelland R, et al. Disappearing breast calcifications. *Radiology* 1989;172:677–680.

102. Davis SP, Stomper PC, Weidner N, et al. Suture calcification mimicking recurrence in the irradiated breast: a potential pitfall in mammographic evaluation. *Radiology* 1989;172:247–248.

103. Stacey-Clear A, McCarthy KA, Hall DA, et al. Calcified suture material in the breast after radiation therapy. *Radiology* 1992;183:207–208.

104. Berg WA, Arnoldus CL, Teferra E, et al. Biopsy of amorphous breast calcifications: pathologic outcome and yield at stereotactic biopsy. *Radiology* 2001;221:495–503.

105. ACR BI-RADS® Breast Imaging Atlas. 4th ed. Reston, VA: American College of Radiology, 2003.

106. Carme B, Paraiso D, Gombe-Mbalawa C. Calcifications of the breast probably due to Loa Loa. *Am J Trop Med Hyg* 1990;42(1):65–66.

107. Novak R. Calcifications in the breast in filaria Loa infection. *Acta Radiol* 1989;30:507–508.

108. Ikeda DM, Sickles EA. Mammographic demonstration of pectoral muscle calcifications. *AJR Am J Roentgenol* 1988;151:475–479.

109. Dershaw DD, Shank B. Reisinger S. Mammographic findings after breast cancer treatment with local excision and definitive irradiation. *Radiology* 1987;164:455–461.

110. Rebner M, Pennes DR, Adler DD, et al. Breast microcalcifications after lumpectomy and radiation therapy. *Radiology* 1989;170:691–693.

111. Vora SA, Wazer DE, Homer MJ. Management of microcalcifications that develop at the lumpectomy site after breast-conserving therapy. *Radiology* 1997;203:667–671.

112. Dershaw DD, Giess CS, McCormick B, et al. Patterns of mammographically detected calcifications after breast-conserving therapy associated with tumor recurrence. *Cancer* 1997;79(7):1355–1361.

Chapter 7

Prominent Ductal Patterns

Linear densities on the mammogram may represent arteries, veins, and lactiferous ducts. There should be no confusion between vascular shadows and ducts.

Lactiferous ducts are linear, slightly nodular densities that radiate back from the nipple into the breast. The normal lactiferous ducts are thin, measuring 1 to 2 mm in diameter, and often are not evident as separate structures on mammography. Enlarged ducts may occur in benign and malignant conditions. When ducts are enlarged, correlation with clinical examination as to the presence of discharge is important. Galactography is of help in providing further information in the evaluation of a nipple discharge, with or without dilated ducts being seen on mammography.

A diffusely prominent ductal pattern bilaterally (Fig. 7.1), associated with small nodular densities, has been described by Wolfe et al (1,2) as placing the patient at higher-than-average risk for developing breast cancer. According to Wolfe, the breast parenchyma was classified into four patterns: N1 or fatty replaced, and P1, P2, or DY with increasing amounts of ductal or glandular tissue. Because of surrounding collagen, individual ducts may not be identified; instead, a dense, triangular fan-shaped density is present beneath the areola (3). The association between a prominent ductal pattern and breast cancer incidence has been debated, with some authors (4,5) agreeing with the association and others (6–8) finding no reliable indicator of risk by mammographic pattern. Ernster et al. (9) suggested that nulliparous women and women with a family history of breast cancer are more likely to have dense breasts and a prominent ductal pattern and that breast parenchymal pattern may be related to other risk factors. Funkhouser et al. (10) found a twofold increase in breast cancer risk in women with a P2 or DY Wolfe pattern in comparison with an N1 pattern (fatty breasts). Andersson et al. (11) also found an increased frequency of the dense ductal patterns with advancing age at first pregnancy and with nulliparity. Brisson et al. (12) assessed breast cancer risk as related to parenchymal pattern in a study of 3,412 women and found that parenchymal pattern was strongly correlated with risk. The authors found that the risk of breast cancer was five- to sixfold greater in women who had breasts that were composed of 85% or more dense tissue than in women who had no density on mammography.

DUCT ECTASIA

Another cause of bilateral ductal prominence is duct ectasia (Figs. 7.2–7.5). Haagenson (13) described the condition as beginning with bilateral dilation of the main lactiferous ducts in postmenopausal women. Amorphous debris within the ducts is irritating and causes periductal inflammation and fibrosis without epithelial proliferation. Retraction of the nipple may occur secondary to fibrosis in the periductal space. In a more recent study, Dixon et al. (14) found that periductal inflammation around nondilated ducts occurred in younger patients and that older patients had ductal dilatation as the main feature. Neither parity nor breastfeeding was found to be an important etiologic factor in this condition (14).

Dilated ductal structures may also be associated with inflammatory or infectious etiologies (Fig. 7.6). In a patient with a breast abscess or with chronic mastitis, there may be intraductal extension of the infection. This may appear as dilated ducts around an indistinct mass or as dilated subareolar ducts with overlying skin thickening. Sonography may depict the abscess cavity and the extension of fluid into ducts surrounding the cavity.

PAPILLOMATOSIS

Intraductal papillomatosis is a benign lesion characterized by a papillary proliferation of the epithelium that may fill and distend the duct (15). This lesion is distinguished from a solitary intraductal papilloma. Papillomatosis tends to be scattered throughout the parenchyma and is within the

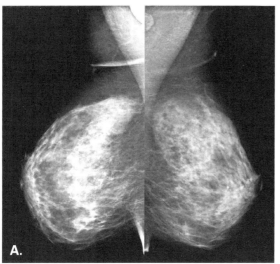
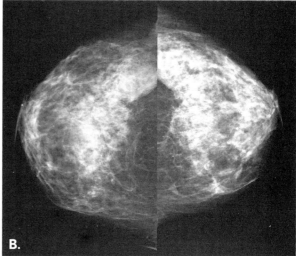

Figure 7.1

HISTORY: A 74-year-old gravida 4, para 4 patient for screening.

MAMMOGRAPHY: Bilateral MLO **(A)** and CC **(B)** views show heterogeneously dense breasts. These are diffuse small areas of nodularity and linear structures consistent with a prominent ductal pattern.

IMPRESSION: Prominent ductal pattern bilaterally, within normal limits.

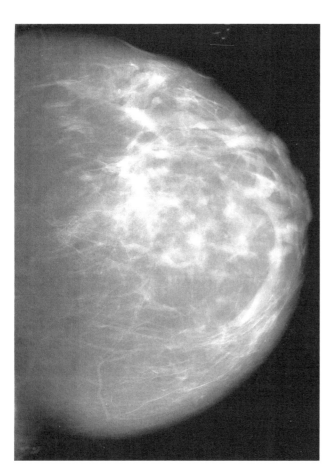

Figure 7.2

HISTORY: A 64-year-old patient who is status post–right breast biopsy, for routine screening of the right breast.

MAMMOGRAPHY: Right CC view shows extensive ductal dilatation extending from the subareolar area centrally and medially. Architectural distortion is present in the area of surgical scar. This pattern had been stable for many years and is consistent with duct ectasia.

IMPRESSION: Duct ectasia.

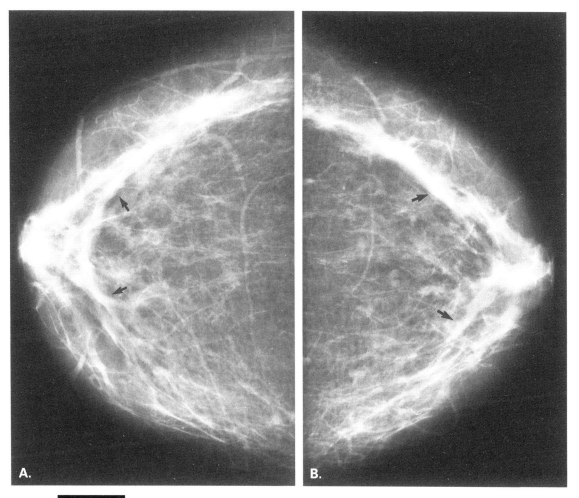

Figure 7.3

HISTORY: A 58-year-old gravida 8, para 8 woman for screening mammography.

MAMMOGRAPHY: Left **(A)** and right **(B)** CC views show the breasts to contain scattered fibroglandular densities. There are prominent ducts present bilaterally **(arrows)**, appearing as tubular nodular structures extending back from the nipples.

IMPRESSION: Bilateral ductal ectasia.

spectrum of fibrocystic change. Sometimes papillomatosis is also called intraductal hyperplasia of the common type. On mammography, the finding of a prominent ductal pattern may be evident, and fine microcalcifications are sometimes seen. On galactography, an irregular filling defect or multiple filling defects are found (Fig. 7.7).

Papillary duct hyperplasia is an unusual lesion that occurs in children and young adults (16). Three patterns have been described: a solitary papilloma, papillomatosis, and sclerosing papillomatosis. The condition causes a distention of the duct or ducts.

Solitary or Focally Dilated Ducts

When asymmetrically dilated ducts or a solitary duct are found on mammography, the possibility of ductal malignancy must be considered. Huynh et al. (17), in a review of 46 women with asymmetrically dilated ducts, found that 24% had ductal carcinoma. Factors associated with malignancy in dilated duct patterns were the presence of associated microcalcifications, a nonsubareolar location, and interval change. The benign causes for the appearance of dilated ducts include a solitary papilloma, multiple papillomas, papillomatosis, ductal hyperplasia, and ductal adenoma.

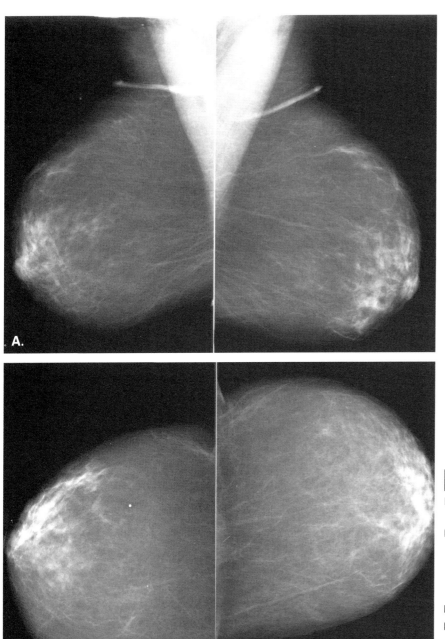

A.

B.

Figure 7.4

HISTORY: A 62-year-old woman for screening.

MAMMOGRAPHY: Bilateral MLO (**A**) and CC (**B**) views show scattered fibroglandular densities. There are prominent tubular densities in both subareolar areas, radiating back from the nipple.

IMPRESSION: Bilateral duct ectasia.

NOTE: Because the ducts are evident as discrete tubular structures, and because of their widened diameter, the finding represents dilated ducts or duct ectasia.

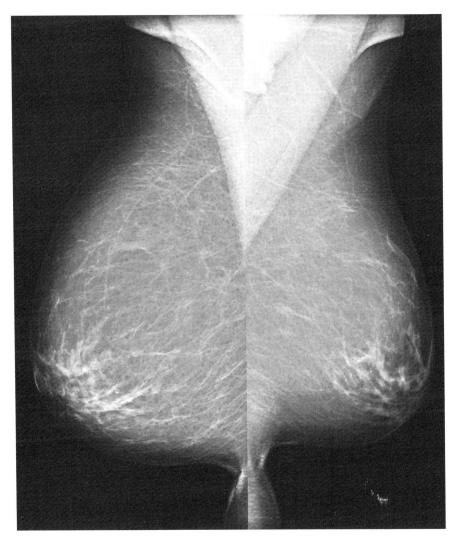

Figure 7.5

HISTORY: A 56-year-old woman for screening.

MAMMOGRAPHY: Bilateral MLO views show relatively fatty-replaced breasts. There are enlarged subareolar ducts bilaterally in a symmetrical distribution. The ducts can be observed as individual structures, and they radiate back from the nipple in a typical pattern of duct ectasia.

IMPRESSION: Duct ectasia.

Dilated ducts are an uncommon presentation of carcinoma but occasionally may be the only sign of this disease. A unilateral dilated duct or ducts, especially those with associated microcalcifications, are suspicious for the possibility of malignancy (18). Dilated ducts located deeper in the breast may be of greater concern for a hyperplastic or malignant lesion; a subareolar duct is more commonly seen in an intraductal papilloma (18).

Intraductal Papilloma

A solitary intraductal papilloma often presents when small and nonpalpable with a serosanguineous or bloody nipple discharge. Papillomas are usually situated beneath the nipple in a major duct; in 90% of cases, they arise within 1 cm of the nipple (19). The papilloma is connected to the duct by a thin connective tissue stalk that contains the blood supply, and it is covered by a frondlike epithelium. Because of the tenuous blood supply, these lesions tend to undergo infarction and sclerosis (20,21). When a papilloma infarcts, it may produce a bloody discharge, identified on clinical examination, and it may calcify.

Depending on the size of the papilloma, it may not be seen on mammography, and a galactogram may be necessary to identify the location of the lesion. When papillomas are identified on the mammogram, they appear as a dilated duct or as a well-defined mass (20) (Figs. 7.8–7.13). In a study of 51 patients with solitary papillomas, Cardenosa and Eklund (22) found that 37 were symptomatic; 36 presented with spontaneous nipple discharge, and 1 had a palpable mass. Ductography was performed in 35 patients and was positive in 32. In some patients, prominent asymmetric ducts were noted at mammography, yet galactography was more useful in diagnosis by

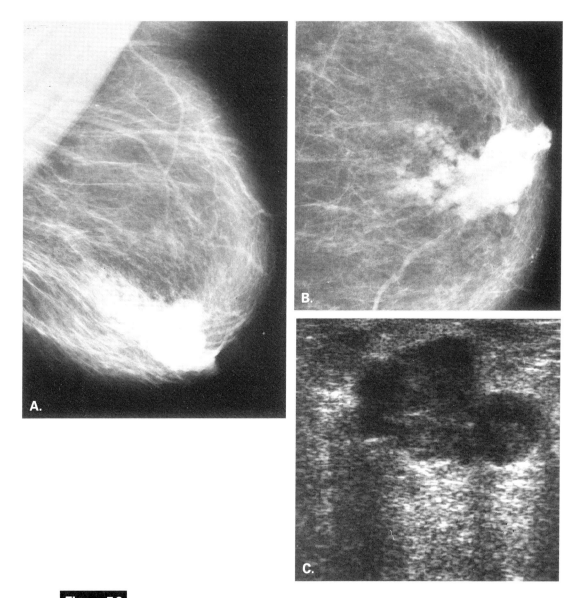

Figure 7.6

HISTORY: Patient presents with a very tender, red right breast with a palpable subareolar mass.

MAMMOGRAPHY: Right MLO **(A)** and CC **(B)** views show a dense microlobulated mass in the immediate subareolar area. There are numerous tubular structures extending from the mass posteriorly into the breast. Ultrasound **(C)** shows a markedly hypoechoic mass with microlobulated borders.

IMPRESSION: Large mass with intraductal extension: carcinoma versus abscess.

NOTE: The lesion was drained and represented on large breast abscess. Follow-up mammography was negative.

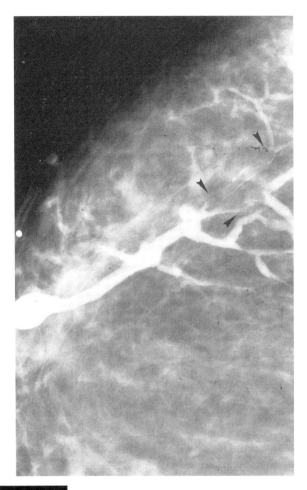

Figure 7.7

HISTORY: A 46-year-old woman with a bloody left nipple discharge.

MAMMOGRAPHY: Left galactogram magnification view. The cannulated duct is dilated. There is a smooth filling defect **(arrowheads)** involving two branches of the lactiferous duct, without evidence for distortion of architecture or encasement of the ducts. The finding suggests intraductal papilloma or papillomatosis, although a papillary carcinoma cannot be excluded.

HISTOPATHOLOGY: Intraductal papillomatosis. (Case courtesy of Dr. George Oliff, Richmond, VA.)

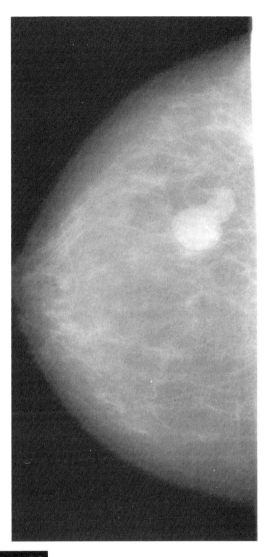

Figure 7.8

HISTORY: A 52-year-old woman for screening.

MAMMOGRAPHY: Left CC view shows a lobular mass with relatively circumscribed margins located laterally. There is a tubular extension from the mass posteriorly, suggesting that this could be a dilated duct. Excisional biopsy was performed.

IMPRESSION: Suspicious mass, possibly an intraductal lesion.

HISTOPATHOLOGY: Papilloma.

showing a dilated duct with an intraluminal filling defect. Woods et al. (23) reviewed the clinical and imaging findings in 24 women with solitary intraductal papillomas and found that 88% presented with nipple discharge. In 42% of patients, mammography was abnormal, including showing dilated ducts in 26% of women. Galactography was successfully performed in 13 patients and showed an intraluminal defect in 12 (92%) and a duct obstruction in 1 patient.

On ultrasound, a papilloma may be observed as a small hypoechoic solid mass. Often the dilated duct containing fluid is seen, and a solid component representing the papilloma is evident. The sonographic distinction between benign or malignant papillary lesions is not reliable (24). Women who are diagnosed with solitary intraductal papilloma are thought to have a 1.5 to 2 times relative risk of developing breast cancer (25). However, women who have multiple small papillomas, a condition

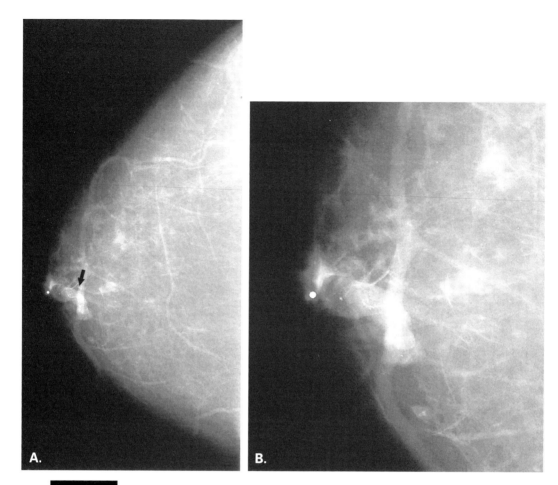

Figure 7.9

HISTORY: A 48-year-old woman with a small palpable left breast mass.

MAMMOGRAPHY: Left CC view **(A)** shows a fatty-replaced breast. There is a markedly dilated duct containing microcalcifications **(arrow)** in the immediate subareolar area, at the site of palpable abnormality. On the magnified image **(B)**, the somewhat pleomorphic appearance of these intraductal calcifications is noted.

IMPRESSION: Dilated duct, suspicious for DCIS.

HISTOPATHOLOGY: Intraductal papilloma.

often involving several ducts, have a 7.4 times relative risk of developing breast cancer (26).

Ductal Carcinoma In Situ

Unilateral dilated ducts, with or without microcalcifications (27), or a solitary dilated duct (28,29) may be the only mammographic indication of a malignancy (Figs. 7.14–7.25). Usually, no mass is palpable (29); however, in an extensive area of ductal dilatation associated with ductal carcinoma in situ (DCIS), palpable thickening may be noted. In some patients, a uniorificial serous or

bloody nipple discharge is observed. The solitary duct has a tubular, slightly nodular shape that tapers as it proceeds into the parenchyma (29). When the lesion is associated with microcalcifications, the level of suspicion is greater. Although the presentation of a nonpalpable cancer as a solitary dilated duct is not common (30,31), this finding should not be overlooked. In a series of 73 women with intraductal carcinoma in whom no microcalcifications were present on mammography, Ikeda and Andersson (32) found that 12 presented with focal ductal-nodular patterns, and 2 had dilated retroareolar ducts.

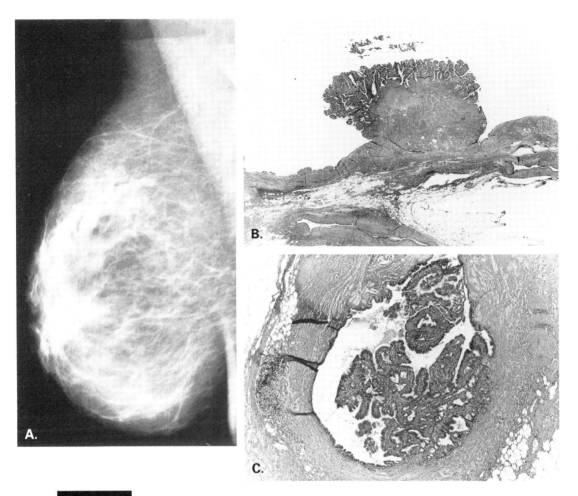

Figure 7.10

HISTORY: A 47-year-old asymptomatic woman for screening mammography.

MAMMOGRAPHY: Left MLO view **(A)** and histopathology **(B** and **C)**. The breast is heterogeneously dense. In the upper aspect of the breast, there is a linear, slightly nodular density representing a solitary duct. A solitary dilated duct is one of the least common signs of nonpalpable breast cancer. Other possible diagnoses in this case are a papilloma, papillomatosis, or duct ectasia.

IMPRESSION: Solitary dilated duct: intraductal carcinoma versus papilloma.

HISTOPATHOLOGY: Intraductal papilloma.

NOTE: The papilloma projects into the ductal lumen; its dense, central, connective-tissue core is covered by the papillary epithelium (12.5×) **(B)**. A cross section through the duct **(C)** shows a less sclerotic portion of the papilloma with complex branching and prominent fibrovascular stalks (50×).

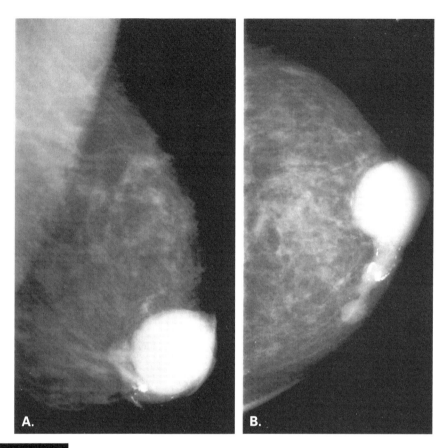

Figure 7.11

HISTORY: A 65-year-old gravida 3, para 3 woman with a family history of breast cancer, presenting with a right nipple discharge and a subareolar mass of at least 10 years' duration.

MAMMOGRAPHY: Right MLO **(A)** and CC **(B)** views. The breast is mildly glandular. There is a large, high-density circumscribed mass in the immediate subareolar area. The posterior margin of the lesion is contiguous with a tubular density containing coarse calcifications **(B)**. The shape of the lesion suggests that this is a dilated duct, obstructed and mostly fluid filled. The calcification may be related to chronic hemorrhage. The chronicity of findings is more consistent with a benign lesion, such as an intraductal papilloma, although a neoplasm cannot be entirely excluded.

IMPRESSION: Massive duct dilatation secondary to an obstructing lesion.

HISTOPATHOLOGY: Intraductal papilloma, cystic dilatation of duct.

Ductal dilatation may also be evident on sonography in some cases of DCIS. In a study of 60 patients with symptomatic DCIS, Yang and Tse (33) found that 22% of patients had ductal dilatation and/or extension on ultrasound. Sonography may also demonstrate as intraductal solid component within a distended, fluid-filled duct. This finding has the appearance of a complex cyst when observed in cross section. On magnetic resonance imaging, DCIS may have an appearance of segmental, linear clumped enhancement, which represents the involved dilated ducts.

Papillary carcinoma constitutes 1% to 2% of breast cancers in women (34) and presents with bloody nipple discharge in 22% to 34% of cases (34,35). On histology, papillary cancers are characterized by a frondlike growth pattern on a fibrovascular core that lacks a

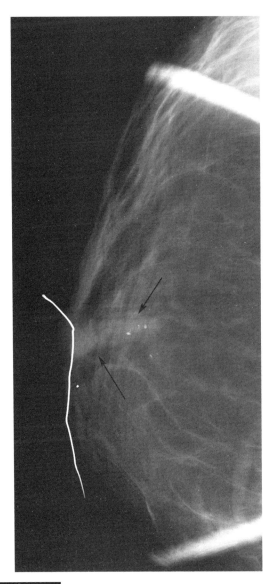

Figure 7.12

HISTORY: A 58-year-old woman with left bloody nipple discharge.

MAMMOGRAPHY: Left spot ML view shows a dilated duct **(arrow)** in the left subareolar area. There are punctuate and dystrophic calcifications within the duct, a finding that may be present in an infarcted papilloma or DCIS.

IMPRESSION: Dilated duct, papilloma versus DCIS.

HISTOPATHOLOGY: Intraductal papilloma.

myoepithelial layer. Intraductal papillary carcinoma may be multifocal and present as dilated ducts or as multiple clusters of microcalcifications (35). An appreciation of the indirect and subtle signs of malignancy is key in making the diagnosis of breast cancer at an early stage.

Ductal Adenoma

Another cause of focally dilated ducts or a solitary dilated duct is ductal adenoma (Fig. 7.26). These are benign glandular tumors that fill and distend the ductal lumen (36). The lesion may present as a palpable mass and is not associated with a nipple discharge. It can simulate malignancy both radiographically and macroscopically. Microcalcifications may occur and may be irregular in a linear orientation (37). Pathologically, two forms have been described: a solitary adenomatous nodule within a ductal lumen and a more complex form with apparent encroachment on the ductal wall (36).

Adenoma of the nipple is a rare benign tumor also called *florid papillomatosis of the nipple ducts* (38). Clinical presentation in nipple discharge is uncommonly associated with a crusted or ulcerated nipple. On pathology, the lesion is composed of a proliferation of ducts varying in size and shape with prominent fibrosis (38). A papillary growth pattern of intraductal hyperplasia is present as well (38).

OTHER LINEAR DENSITIES

Vascular structures also appear as linear densities on mammography and should not be confused with a prominent ductal pattern (Fig. 7.27). Vessels are smooth and undulating. Arteries are smaller than veins and may be seen extending into the upper aspect of the breast and the axillary area. Tramline calcifications occur often in the arteries of elderly women. Prominence of venous structures has been described as a secondary sign of malignancy (39), but this is not common and is nonspecific. Other causes of dilated veins include (a) obstruction of the subclavian vein with development of venous collaterals over the breast (40) (Fig. 7.28) and (b) superior vena cava obstruction causing development of bilateral collaterals over the breasts.

Mondor disease or superficial thrombophlebitis of the breast and upper abdominal wall (41) (Figs. 7.29 and 7.30) may cause a mildly prominent-appearing vein on mammography, but often the mammogram is normal. Patients with Mondor disease may report a history of trauma, surgery, or excessive lifting or exercise. The vein most commonly involved is the lateral thoracoepigastric vein, which crosses over the upper abdominal wall and the lateral aspect of the breast. The findings are most characteristic on clinical examination: namely, a firm cordlike structure beneath the skin, having a reddened appearance. The thrombosed vein is tender to palpation; the disease is treated with aspirin or nonsteroidal anti-inflammatory medications.

(References begin on page 362.)

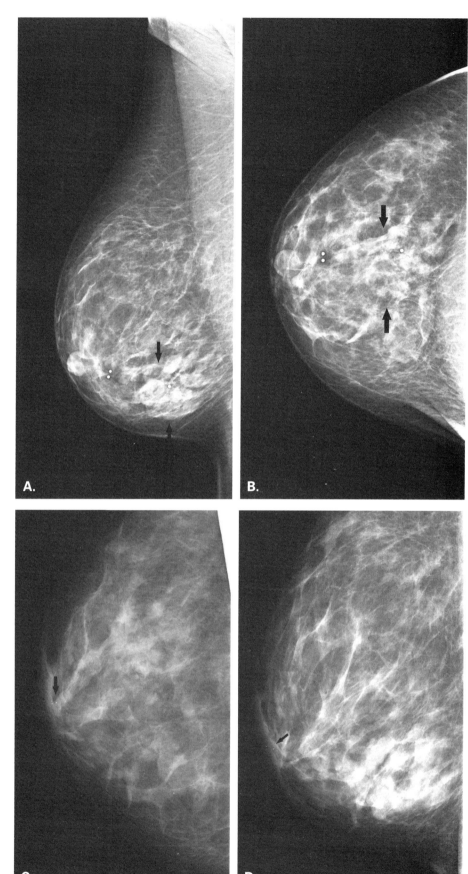

A.   B.   C.   D.

Figure 7.13

HISTORY: A 54-year-old woman for screening mammography.

MAMMOGRAPHY: Left MLO (**A**) and CC (**B**) views show focally dilated ducts (**arrows**) in the 6 o'clock position of the left breast. These were markedly asymmetric in comparison with the contralateral breast. There are some associated ductal pleomorphic calcifications at the proximal end of the duct seen best on the magnification CC (**C**) and ML (**D**) views (**arrow**).

IMPRESSION: Dilated ducts, suspicious for DCIS. Recommend excision.

HISTOPATHOLOGY: Atypical ductal hyperplasia, intraductal papilloma.

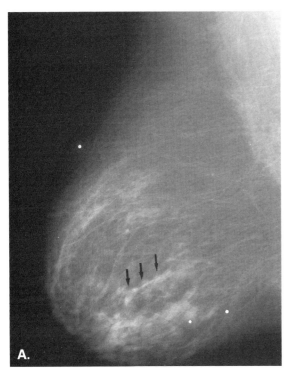

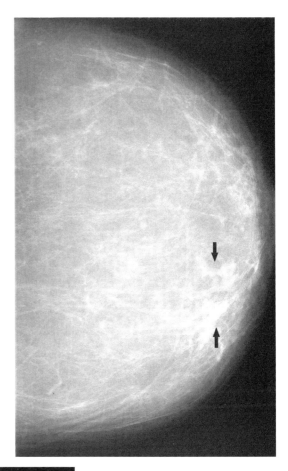

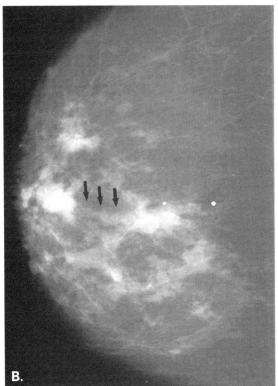

Figure 7.15

HISTORY: Elderly woman for screening.

MAMMOGRAPHY: Right CC view shows a fatty-replaced breast. In the medial aspect of the subareolar area is a focal area of branching ductal dilatation **(arrow)**. No similar finding was present on the left.

IMPRESSION: Focally dilated ducts. Recommend biopsy.

HISTOPATHOLOGY: DCIS.

Figure 7.14

HISTORY: A 67-year-old woman with bloody nipple discharge.

MAMMOGRAPHY: Left MLO **(A)** and CC **(B)** views show a segment of dilated ducts in the 6 o'clock position of the left breast. Tubular-nodular densities extend from the nipple posteriorly into the breast **(arrows)** and are suspicious for an intraductal filling process.

HISTOPATHOLOGY: DCIS.

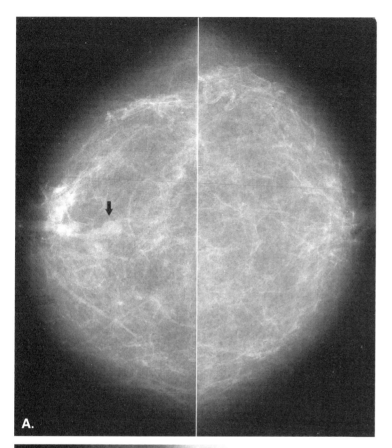

A.

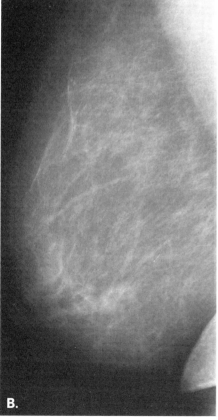

B.

Figure 7.16

HISTORY: A 56-year-old woman for screening mammography.

MAMMOGRAPHY: Bilateral CC views **(A)** show asymmetrically dilated ducts in the left subareolar area. The duct bifurcates centrally **(arrow)** in the breast. On the MLO view **(B)**, the unilateral duct is located at 6 o'clock.

IMPRESSION: Solitary dilated duct, papilloma versus DCIS. Recommend excision.

HISTOPATHOLOGY: DCIS.

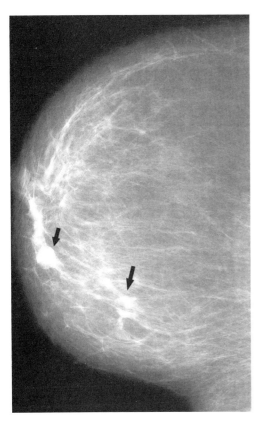

Figure 7.17

HISTORY: An 81-year-old woman for screening.

MAMMOGRAPHY: Left ML view shows a prominent segment of dilated ducts in the inferior aspect of the breast **(arrows)**. These have a tubulonodular appearance, and a small mass is present within this region of abnormality. The findings were unilateral.

IMPRESSION: Focally dilated ducts. Recommend excision.

HISTOPATHOLOGY: DCIS and invasive ductal carcinoma.

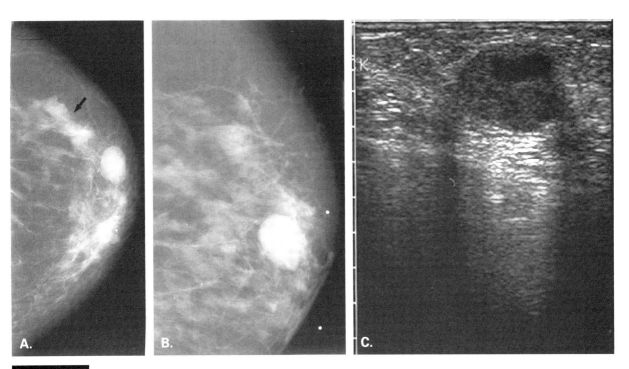

Figure 7.18

HISTORY: A 74-year-old patient with a palpable right breast marked with a BB.

MAMMOGRAPHY: Right CC view **(A)** shows two round isodense masses, one of which is marked with a BB. Extending into the lateral aspect of the breast are tubular structures **(arrow)** with associated microcalcifications, seen best on the magnification CC view **(B)**. On ultrasound **(C)**, the masses are complex with a solid component, raising the possibility of a papillary lesion or DCIS.

IMPRESSION: Dilated ducts with intracystic solid components, suspicious for papillary carcinoma.

HISTOPATHOLOGY: DCIS, micropapillary type.

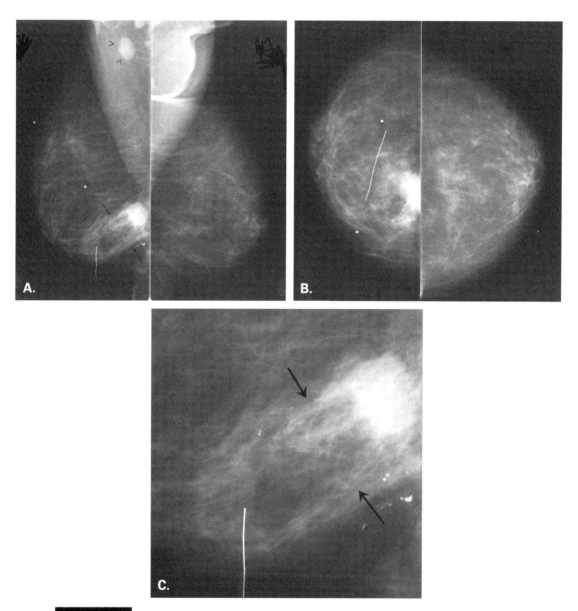

Figure 7.19

HISTORY: A 55-year-old woman with a palpable mass in the left breast.

MAMMOGRAPHY: Bilateral MLO **(A)** and CC **(B)** views show a high-density, indistinct lobular mass in the left breast at 6 o'clock with associated dilated ducts **(B) (arrow)**. On the coned-down MLO view **(C)**, the lesion is associated with adjacent dystrophic calcifications and linear extensions anteriorly **(arrows)**, suggesting intraductal extension of tumor. A prominent lymph node **(arrowheads)** is present in the left axilla.

IMPRESSION: Invasive carcinoma with DCIS.

HISTOPATHOLOGY: Invasive duct carcinoma and micropapillary DCIS, with no metastatic carcinoma in the axillary nodes.

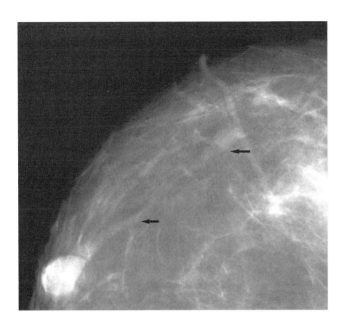

Figure 7.20

HISTORY: A 42-year-old woman for screening.

MAMMOGRAPHY: Left coned-down CC view shows a branching dilated duct **(arrows)** in the left breast. This finding was unilateral and asymmetric. Needle localization with excision was performed.

IMPRESSION: Dilated duct, DCIS versus papilloma.

HISTOPATHOLOGY: DCIS cribriform type, and intraductal papilloma.

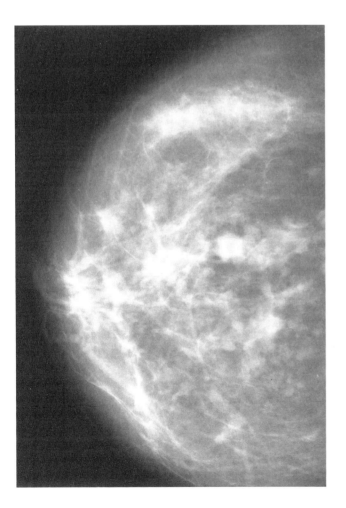

Figure 7.21

HISTORY: A 65-year-old woman for screening mammography.

MAMMOGRAPHY: Left CC view shows moderate glandularity present. In the central posterior aspect of the breast, there are well-defined tubular nodular densities that represent focally dilated ducts. The focal nature of these ducts—particularly the location, apart from the main ducts at the nipple—suggests an area of localized intraductal activity. The differential includes multiple papillomas, papillomatosis, intraductal carcinoma, and ductal hyperplasia.

IMPRESSION: Focally dilated ducts, moderately suspicious for carcinoma.

HISTOPATHOLOGY: Extensive multifocal intraductal carcinoma with papillomatosis.

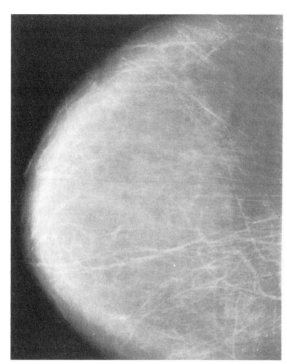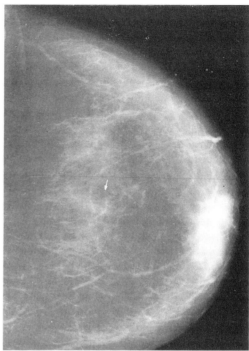

Figure 7.22

HISTORY: A 65-year-old woman with a scaling, ulcerating lesion of the right nipple.

MAMMOGRAPHY: Bilateral CC views. The breasts show fatty replacement. There is a fan-shaped asymmetric density radiating back from the right nipple, corresponding to the location of the subareolar lactiferous ducts. The asymmetric ductal dilatation should be regarded with suspicion, and particularly with the nipple lesion, this finding is highly compatible with that of Paget disease and intraductal carcinoma. There are also two groups of microcalcification deeper in the right breast that are suspicious for other foci of intraductal carcinoma **(arrow)**.

IMPRESSION: Paget disease, ductal carcinoma.

HISTOPATHOLOGY: Intraductal papillary small cell carcinoma and large cell carcinoma with pagetoid spread.

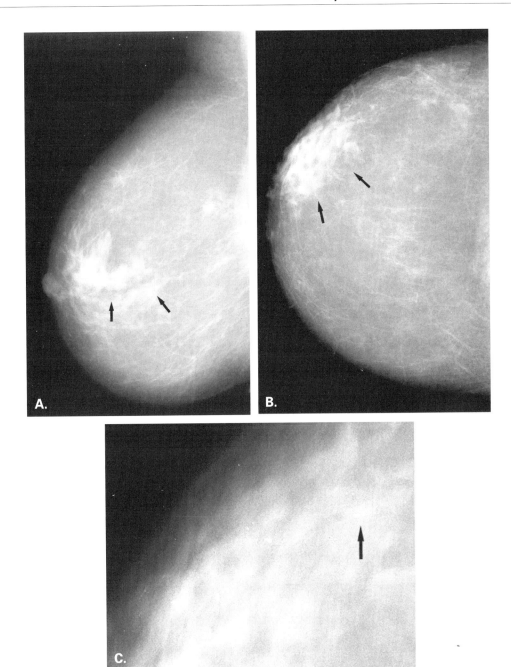

Figure 7.23

HISTORY: A 70-year-old woman for screening mammography.

MAMMOGRAPHY: Left MLO **(A)**, left CC **(B)**, and magnification CC **(C)** views. There are several dilated ducts **(arrows)** in the left subareolar area **(A, B)**. Within these ducts are fine linear and punctate microcalcifications **(arrow) (C)**. No similar findings were noted in the opposite breast. Focal ductal dilatation is one of the less common signs of breast cancer. With the associated ductal calcifications in this case, the degree of suspicion that this was a malignant lesion was increased.

IMPRESSION: Ductal carcinoma.

HISTOPATHOLOGY: Intraductal small cell carcinoma.

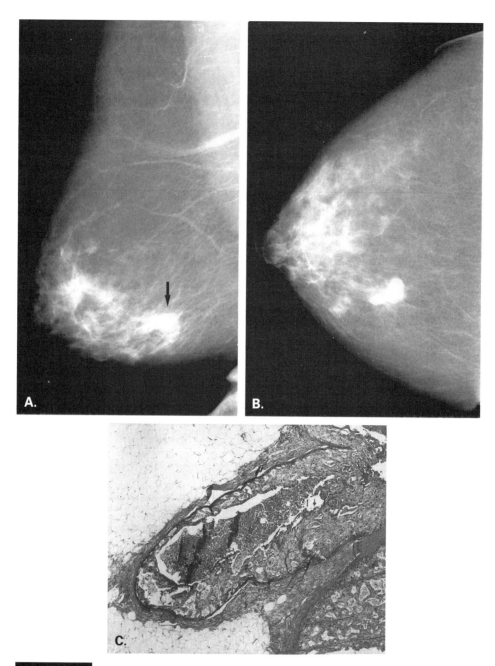

Figure 7.24

HISTORY: A 78-year-old woman with family history of breast cancer, for screening mammography.

MAMMOGRAPHY: Left MLO view **(A)**, magnified CC view **(B)**, and histopathology **(C)**. There is a relatively well-defined, high-density tubular structure **(A, arrow)** in the lower aspect of the breast. The lobulated fusiform shape of the lesion is also demonstrated on the CC view **(B)**. Sonography of the lesion showed it to be solid and hypoechoic. The shape of the lesion suggests a dilated duct. The lesion had appeared since a previous mammogram 6 years earlier. Because of this, a fibroadenoma would not be likely, and primary considerations are carcinoma, possibly localized within a dilated duct, or focal fibrocystic disease.

IMPRESSION: Solitary dilated duct in the left breast, highly suspicious for carcinoma.

HISTOPATHOLOGY: Intraductal carcinoma.

NOTE: The histopathologic section shows the dilated duct filled with intraductal carcinoma **(C)**.

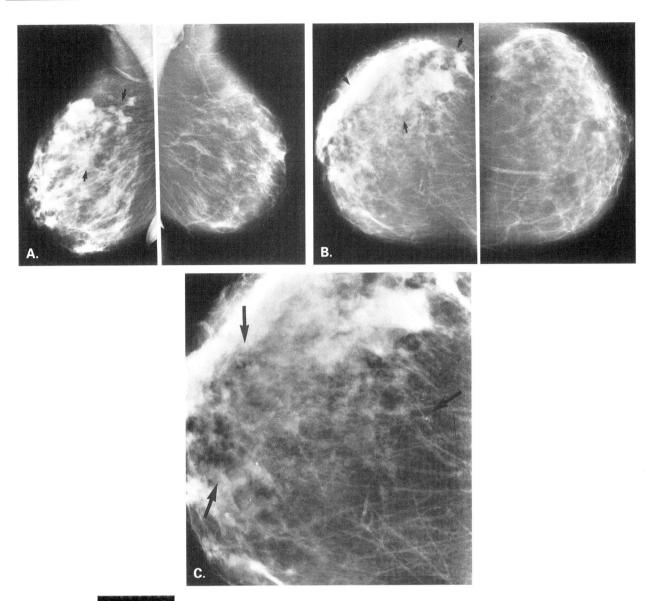

Figure 7.25

HISTORY: A 44-year-old gravida 4, para 4 woman with a positive family history of breast cancer, presenting with a "heavy" sensation in the left breast. Clinical examination showed a thicker left breast, without a dominant palpable mass.

MAMMOGRAPHY: Bilateral MLO **(A)**, CC **(B)**, and enlarged (1.5×) left CC **(C)** views. There is marked asymmetry in the appearance of the breasts **(A** and **B)**. In the left upper quadrant, there are numerous tubular and rounded densities **(arrows)** radiating back from the nipple. This pattern of tubular structures represents markedly dilated ducts. In addition, within these ducts and extending more medially into the central aspect of the left breast **(C)** are extensive granular irregular microcalcifications **(arrows)**. This finding alone is highly suspicious for carcinoma and, in combination with the prominent duct pattern, is even more so.

IMPRESSION: Highly suspicious for extensive ductal carcinoma, left breast.

HISTOPATHOLOGY: Intraductal and infiltrating ductal carcinoma.

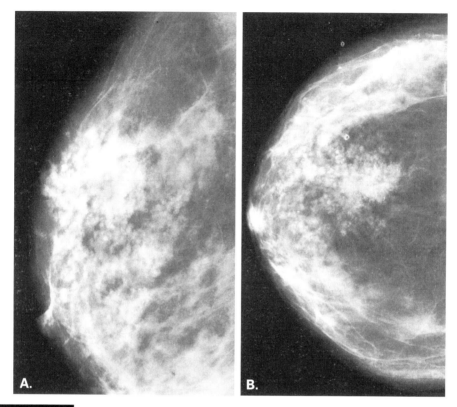

Figure 7.26

HISTORY: A 52-year-old woman for screening mammography.

MAMMOGRAPHY: Left MLO **(A)** and CC **(B)** views. In the 12 o'clock position of the left breast, there is a 5-cm area of focal ductal dilatation and proliferation in a bizarre shape. Fine granular microcalcifications are associated with this lesion. The differential was thought to include ductal carcinoma, papillomatosis, or other epithelial proliferation.

HISTOPATHOLOGY: Ductal adenoma, complex form. (Case courtesy of Alexander Girevendulis, Richmond, VA.)

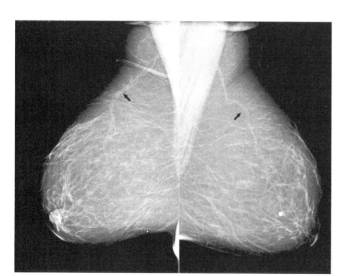

Figure 7.27

HISTORY: Screening mammogram on a 34-year-old woman.

MAMMOGRAPHY: Bilateral MLO show essentially fatty-replaced breasts. There are circuitous tubular structures that extend over the breast and are oriented toward the axilla, typical of normal vascular structures **(arrows)**.

IMPRESSION: Normal arteries and veins.

Figure 7.28

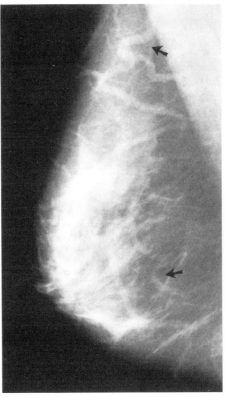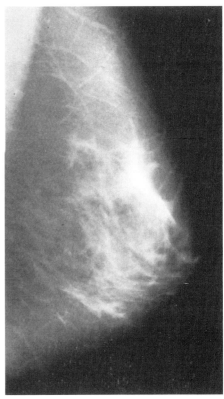

HISTORY: A 38-year-old woman with a tender swollen left breast and axilla.

MAMMOGRAPHY: Bilateral MLO views. There are asymmetric circuitous linear densities **(arrows)** in the left breast, extending into the left axilla. These represent asymmetrically dilated veins. The patient was sent for venography of the left upper extremity, which showed thrombosis in the left subclavian vein and dilated venous collaterals over the left breast.

IMPRESSION: Dilated venous collaterals secondary to subclavian vein thrombosis.

Figure 7.29

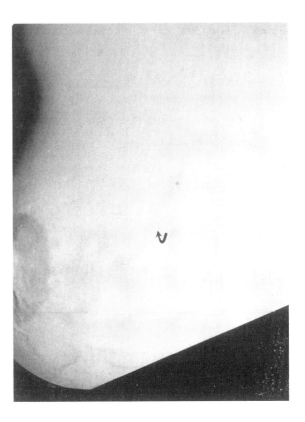

HISTORY: A 35-year-old nurse who, after excessive lifting, developed severe pain, tenderness, and swelling of the upper aspect of the left breast.

IMAGE: A palpable cord **(curved arrow)** extended from the nipple toward the upper outer quadrant. The vein was focally tender. The mammogram showed a normal vein and no other abnormalities.

IMPRESSION: Mondor disease (superficial thrombophlebitis).

NOTE: On this mammogram, the pertinent finding is the lack of abnormalities with the exception of the vein in the area of palpable thickening. This condition may occur after trauma or repeated exercise and regresses on anticoagulants and anti-inflammatory medications.

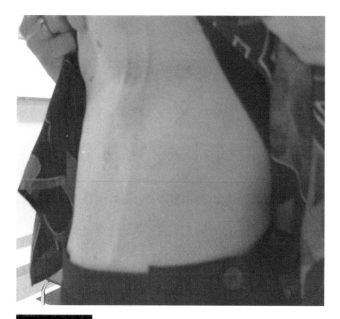

Figure 7.30

HISTORY: A 57-year-old woman who is 3 months status postlumpectomy and -brachytherapy for left breast cancer. She presents with a tender, hard palpable cord extending from the periumbilical area up over the lateral aspect of the thorax on the left side.

IMAGE: The photograph of the left anterior thoracoabdominal wall shows a linear structure extending up along the lateral aspect of the abdomen toward the axilla. The structure appears to bifurcate and is located very superficially. Clinical examination showed this to be quite firm on palpation and tender.

IMPRESSION: Mondor disease.

REFERENCES

1. Wolfe JN. The prominent duct pattern as an indicator of cancer risk. *Oncology* 1968;23:149–158.
2. Wolfe JN, Albert S, Belle S, et al. Breast parenchymal patterns: analysis of 332 incident breast carcinomas. *AJR Am J Roentgenol* 1982;138:113–118.
3. Wolfe JN, Albert S, Belle S, et al. Breast parenchymal patterns and their relationship to risk for having or developing carcinoma. *Radiol Clin North Am* 1983;21(1):127–136.
4. Janzon L, Andersson I, Petersson H. Mammographic patterns as indicators of risk of breast cancer. *Radiology* 1982;143:417–419.
5. Threatt B, Norbeck JM, Ullmann NAS, et al. Association between mammographic parenchymal pattern classification and incidence of breast cancer. *Cancer* 1980;45:2250–2256.
6. Egan RL, McSweeney MB. Mammographic parenchymal patterns and risk of breast cancer. *Radiology* 1979;133:65–70.
7. Egan RL, Mosteller RC. Breast cancer mammography patterns. *Cancer* 1977;40:2087–2090.
8. Moskowitz M, Gartside P, McLaughlin C. Mammographic patterns as markers for high-risk benign breast disease and incident cancers. *Radiology* 1980;134:293–295.
9. Ernster VL, Sacks ST, Peterson CA, et al. Mammographic parenchymal patterns for risk factors for breast cancer. *Radiology* 1980;134:617–620.
10. Funkhouser E, Waterson JW, Cole P. Mammographic patterns and breast cancer risk: a meta-analysis. *Breast Dis* 1993;6:277–284.
11. Andersson I, Janzon L, Petersson H. Radiographic patterns of mammary parenchyma. *Radiology* 1981;138:59–62.
12. Brisson J, Diorio C, Masse B. Wolfe's parenchymal pattern and percentage of the breast with mammographic densities. *Cancer Epidemiol Biomarkers Prev* 2003;12:728–732.
13. Haagenson CD. Mammary-duct ectasia: a disease that may simulate carcinoma. *Cancer* 1951;4:749–761.
14. Dixon JM, Anderson TJ, Lumsden AB, et al. Mammary duct ectasia. *Br J Surg* 1983;70:601–603.
15. Haagenson CD. Papillomatosis. In: *Diseases of the Breast.* Philadelphia: WB Saunders, 1971.
16. Rosen PP. Papillary duct hyperplasia of the breast in children and young adults. *Cancer* 1985;56:1611–1617.
17. Huynh PT, Parellada JA, Shaw de Paredes E, et al. Dilated duct patterns at mammography. *Radiology* 1997;204(1):137–141.
18. Shaw de Paredes E. Pitfalls in mammography. *Imaging* 1994;6:157–170.
19. Paulus DD. Benign disease of the breast. *Radiol Clin North Am* 1983;21:27–50.
20. D'Orsi CJ, Weissman BNW, Berkowitz DM. Correlation of xeroradiology and histology of breast disease. *CRC Crit Rev Diagn Imaging* 1978;11(1):75–119.
21. Haagenson CD. Solitary intraductal papilloma. In: *Diseases of the Breast.* Philadelphia: WB Saunders, 1971.
22. Cardenosa G, Eklund GW. Benign papillary neoplasms of the breast: mammographic findings. *Radiology* 1997;187:751–755.
23. Woods ER, Helvie MA, Ikeda DM, et al. Solitary breast papilloma: comparison of mammographic, galactographic and pathologic findings. *AJR Am J Roentgenol* 1992;159:487–491.
24. Pisano ED, Braeuning MP, Burke E. Case 8: solitary intraductal papilloma. *Radiology* 1999;210:795–798.
25. Cancer Committee of the College of American Pathologists. Is "fibrocystic disease" of the breast precancerous? *Arch Pathol Lab Med* 1986;110:171–173.
26. Pellettiere EV. The clinical and pathologic aspects of papillomatous disease of the breast: a follow-up of 97 patients treated by local excision. *Am J Clin Pathol* 1971;55:740–748.
27. Wolfe JN. Mammography: ducts as a sole indicator of breast carcinoma. *Radiology* 1967;89:206–210.
28. Martin JE. Mammographic diagnosis of minimal breast cancer and treatment. In: Feig SA, McLelland R. eds. *Breast carcinoma: current diagnosis.* New York: Masson Publishing, 1983, pp. 257–264.
29. Sickles EA. Mammographic features of early breast cancer. *AJR Am J Roentgenol* 1984;143:461–464.
30. Moskowitz M. The predictive value of certain mammographic signs in screening for breast cancer. *Cancer* 1983;51:1007–1011.
31. Sickles EA. Mammographic features of 300 consecutive nonpalpable breast cancers. *AJR Am J Roentgenol* 1986;146:661–663.
32. Ikeda DM, Andersson I. Ductal carcinoma in situ: atypical mammographic appearance. *Radiology* 1989;172:661–666.
33. Yang WT, Tse GMK. Sonographic, mammographic, and histopathologic correlation of symptomatic ductal carcinoma. *AJR Am J Roentgenol* 2004;182:101–110.
34. Rosen PP. The pathology of invasive breast carcinoma. In: Harris J, Hellman S, Henderson IC, et al., eds. *Breast Diseases.* Philadelphia: Lippincott, 1991:261–263.
35. Soo MS, Williford ME, Walsh R, et al. Papillary carcinoma of the breast: imaging findings. *AJR Am J Roentgenol* 1995;164:321–326.
36. Azzopardi JG, Salm R. Ductal adenoma of the breast: a lesion which can mimic carcinoma. *J Pathol* 1984;144:15–23.
37. Moskovic E, Ramachandra S. Ductal adenoma of the breast: mammographic appearances and pathological correlation. *Br J Radiol* 1989;62:1021–1023.
38. Santini D, Taffurelei M, Gelli MC, et al. Adenoma of the nipple: a clinico-pathological study and is relation with carcinoma. *Breast Dis* 1990;3:153–163.
39. Dodd GD, Wallace JD. The venous diameter ratio in the radiographic diagnosis of breast cancer. *Radiology* 1968;90:900–904.
40. Carter MM, McCook BM, Shoff MI, et al. Case report: dilated mammary veins as a sign of superior vena cava obstruction. *Appl Radiol* 1987;16:100–102.
41. Grow JL, Lewison EF. Superficial thrombophlebitis of the breast. *Surg Gynecol Obstet* 1963;53:180–182.

Chapter 8

Asymmetry and Architectural Distortion

Asymmetry of the parenchyma is a common finding on mammography, and it is observed when the same mammographic views are visualized together as mirror images. The observation of asymmetry may be related to a greater degree of parenchyma in one breast, loss of parenchyma through surgery, superimposition of parenchyma, or a true lesion that may be benign or malignant. In the current *Breast Imaging Reporting and Data System* (BI-RADS®) lexicon (1), three terms are used to describe nonmass densities: focal asymmetry, global asymmetry, and architectural distortion. A previously used term for a potential abnormality on a screening study was *a density on one view*. In this chapter, the etiologies and management of these findings will be described.

A DENSITY SEEN ON ONE VIEW

Overlying glandular tissue can be visualized on one projection as a focal density, but on the orthogonal view, it is seen to disperse. Such density may be a pseudolesion that is related to superimposition of the parenchyma, creating the appearance of an asymmetry or mass on one view. A density seen on one view also may be caused by a true lesion that is obscured by dense parenchyma on the other view (Fig. 8.1). In many cases, a single additional image provides sufficient information to differentiate overlapping tissue from a true lesion (2–5). Spot compression views of the area may be of help in its evaluation and in displacing the surrounding glandular tissue. In addition, off-angle views such as rolled craniocaudal (CC), 90-degree lateral, or step-obliques are used to confirm that a density is a real finding and to verify its location.

The step-oblique mammography technique is used to determine with confidence whether a mammographic finding visible on one projection only represents a summation artifact or if it is a true mass. Pearson et al. (6) described this technique, in which serial images are obtained at 15-degree intervals from the view on which

the finding is seen, moving toward the view in which it is not seen. Based on the persistence of the finding or its disappearance on the additional views, the nature of the density can be elucidated (6).

ASYMMETRY

The BI-RADS® lexicon (1) describes a global asymmetry as asymmetric breast tissue or a greater volume of breast tissue in comparison with the corresponding region of the opposite breast. Global asymmetry is usually a normal variant, but when it is palpable or associated with other suspicious findings, it may be significant. For global asymmetry to be considered benign based on mammography, it should not be associated with a mass, architectural distortion, or suspicious microcalcifications. Global asymmetry may be related to a greater volume of parenchyma in one breast, a hypoplastic breast, or the removal of parenchyma in one breast (Figs. 8.2–8.4).

Asymmetric breast tissue has been reported to occur on 3% of mammograms and is most often benign (7). However, asymmetric breast tissue that is new, enlarging, or more dense than on prior mammograms may prompt further evaluation. Piccoli et al. (8) found that a common histopathologic finding in cases of developing asymmetric breast tissue that was biopsied was pseudoangiomatous stromal hyperplasia (PASH). In 13 biopsied cases of an enlarging asymmetry, the authors (8) found that PASH was extensive in 12 cases, and in 9%, it was the predominant feature.

A focal asymmetry, also sometimes called an asymmetric density, refers to an area of tissue that is visible on two views. A focal asymmetry has a similar shape on two views, but it does not have the conspicuity or the borders of a mass (1). A focal asymmetry can represent an island of normal breast tissue, or it can be caused by a variety of benign and malignant conditions. A focal asymmetry that is new or enlarging, palpable,

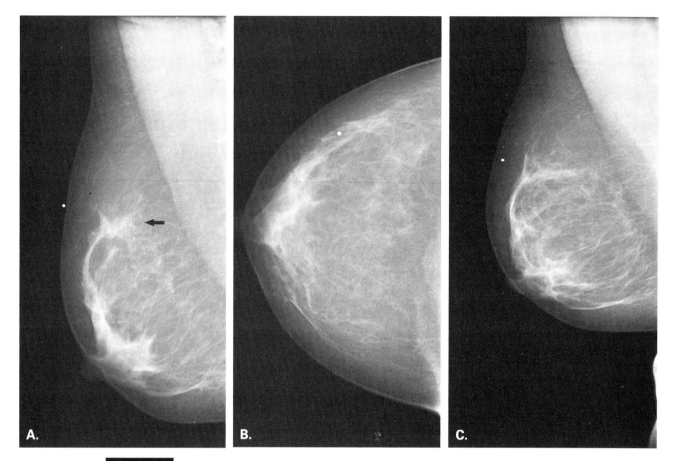

Figure 8.1

HISTORY: A 35-year-old woman for baseline mammogram.

MAMMOGRAPHY: Left MLO **(A)** and CC **(B)** views show a focal density in the superior aspect of the breast seen only on the MLO view **(arrow)**. The finding is not seen on a similar configuration on the CC view and therefore represents superimposition of parenchyma. An ML view **(C)** confirms that the density does not remain in a similar configuration.

IMPRESSION: Pseudolesion: superimposition of tissue creating a focal density.

associated with suspicious microcalcifications or architectural distortion, or that is evident on ultrasound as a solid mass necessitates further evaluation with biopsy. The types of focal asymmetries that may require biopsy are shown in Table 8.1.

▶ TABLE 8.1 Suspicious Asymmetries

- New or enlarging from prior mammography
- Palpable
- Associated with architectural distortion
- Associated with suspicious microcalcifications
- Associated with skin or nipple retraction
- A solid mass on ultrasound

The mammographic evaluation of a focal asymmetry is to determine if it has a similar appearance on two views, where it is located, and if it has associated findings (Figs. 8.5 and 8.6). If the asymmetry is most evident on the CC view, rolled lateral and medial CC views are most helpful in addition to the spot compression to determine whether a focal asymmetry is real or not. In addition, the rolled view helps to establish the location of an asymmetry (9). Spot compression magnification helps to identify suspicious microcalcifications associated with the asymmetry as well as the margins of the abnormality.

In addition to the diagnostic mammographic evaluation of a focal asymmetry, ultrasound is also important. Sonography may reveal a solid or cystic mass that accounts for the asymmetric density. The presence of a solid mass that is associated with a focal asymmetry

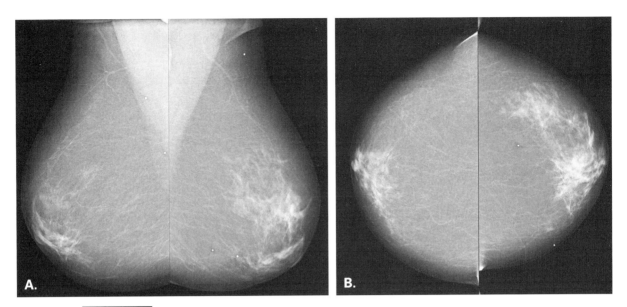

Figure 8.2

HISTORY: A 41-year-old woman for baseline screening mammography.

MAMMOGRAPHY: Bilateral MLO **(A)** and CC **(B)** views show an asymmetric appearance of the breasts. There is generally more volume of breast parenchyma on the right, located superiorly and laterally.

IMPRESSION: Global asymmetry, a normal variant.

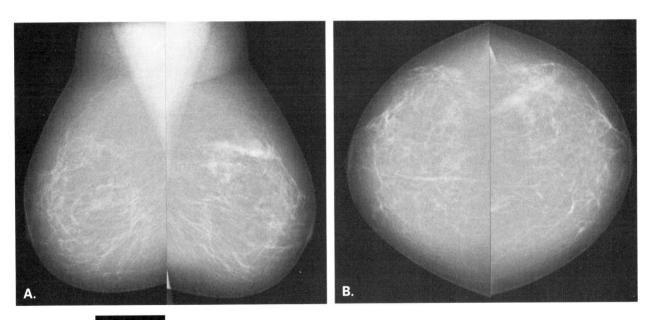

Figure 8.3

HISTORY: A 37-year-old woman for baseline screening mammography.

MAMMOGRAPHY: Bilateral MLO **(A)** and CC **(B)** views show a greater region of parenchyma in the right upper-outer quadrant in comparison with the left breast. There are no suspicious associated findings.

IMPRESSION: Global asymmetry, right breast.

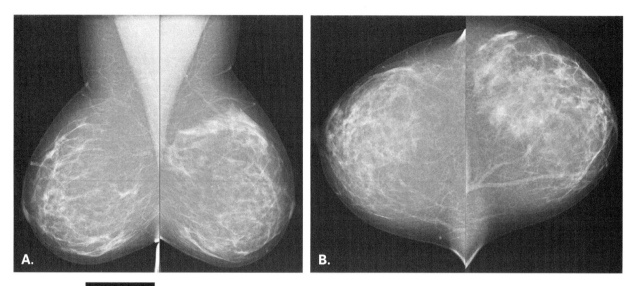

Figure 8.4

HISTORY: A 38-year-old woman for a baseline mammogram.

MAMMOGRAPHY: Bilateral MLO **(A)** and CC **(B)** views show an asymmetric appearance of the breasts. There is generalized increased parenchymal density in the right breast, consistent with global asymmetry.

IMPRESSION: Global asymmetry, a normal variant.

should be viewed with suspicion. A negative ultrasound may also be helpful to confirm that a focal asymmetry thought to be breast tissue on mammography is benign.

The etiologies of focal asymmetries range from normal glandular tissue to benign and malignant entities (Table 8.2). Normal fibroglandular tissue may be the cause of a focal asymmetry on mammography. Normal fibroglandular tissue should not be palpable or associated with distortion or microcalcifications (Table 8.3). Such asymmetries are sensitive to hormonal stimulation and may occur in women on oral contraceptives or on hormone replacement therapy (10). Because of this, a follow-up mammogram in 3 to 4 weeks after discontinuation of hormones may be performed for a questionable asymmetry. Normal fibroglandular tissue usually regresses and

may be followed with mammography rather than evaluated further. A persistent new focal asymmetry that developed when the patient was placed on hormones, but that does not diminish with discontinuation of hormonal therapy, should be biopsied.

Benign Causes of Asymmetry

Benign etiologies of focal asymmetries are the same as the causes of indistinct masses. Fibrocystic changes (Figs. 8.7 and 8.8), particularly focal fibrosis, and sclerosing adenosis often appear as a focal asymmetry. Sclerosing adenosis is a proliferation of ductules and lobular glands (adenosis) with intralobular and perilobular sclerosis that constricts and distorts the lobular structures. Often lobular-type punctate and round microcalcifications are associated

(text continues on page 370)

▌**TABLE 8.2 Etiologies of a Focal Asymmetry**

- Normal fibroglandular tissue
- Ectopic breast tissue
- Focal fibrocystic change
- Hematoma
- Diabetic fibrous mastopathy
- Pseudoangiomatous stromal hyperplasia
- Carcinoma (invasive lobular, invasive ductal)
- Lymphoma

▌**TABLE 8.3 Etiologies of Architectural Distortion**

- Postsurgical scar
- Radial scar
- Sclerosing adenosis, fibrocystic change
- Carcinoma (invasive lobular, tubular, invasive ductal)
- Fibromatosis
- Plasma cell mastitis

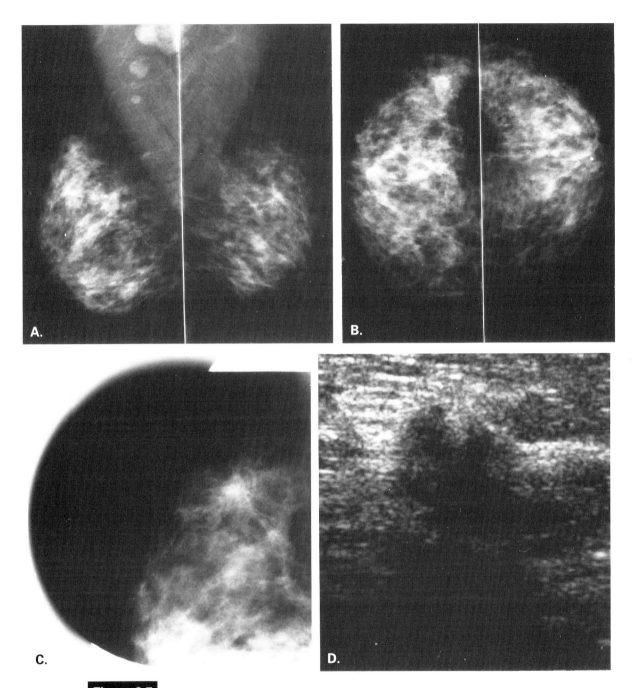

Figure 8.5

HISTORY: A 51-year-old woman for screening mammography.

MAMMOGRAPHY: Bilateral MLO **(A)** and CC **(B)** views show dense breast tissue. There is focal asymmetry laterally in the left breast on the CC view **(B)**, not clearly seen on the MLO. On spot compression **(C)**, the area appears to be distorted and spiculated. Ultrasound **(D)** of the lateral aspect of the breast was performed and demonstrated dense shadowing at 4 o'clock. Ultrasound-guided core needle biopsy of this abnormality was performed.

IMPRESSION: Highly suspicious for malignancy.

HISTOPATHOLOGY: Invasive ductal carcinoma, with multiple positive axillary nodes.

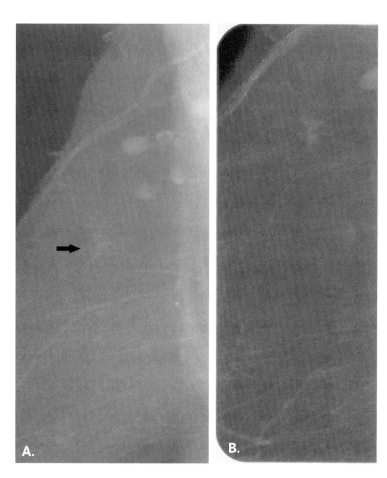

HISTORY: A 76-year-old woman for screening mammography.

MAMMOGRAPHY: Left enlarged MLO **(A)** and magnified exaggerated CC lateral **(B)** views of the upper outer quadrant demonstrate a fatty-replaced breast. There is a small focal density **(arrows)** in the upper outer quadrant. The lesion appears more dense and masslike with indistinct edges on the spot-magnification view.

IMPRESSION: Focal asymmetry, suspicious for malignancy.

HISTOPATHOLOGY: Invasive lobular carcinoma.

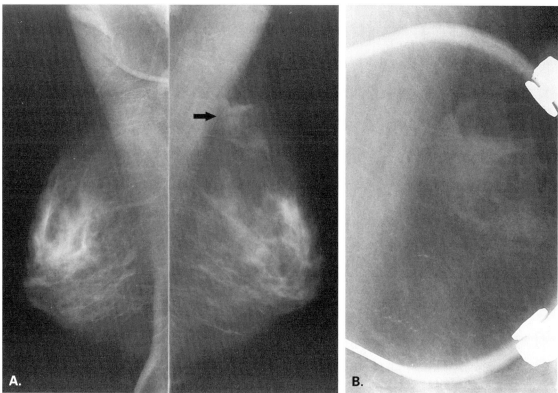

HISTORY: A 42-year-old woman for screening mammography.

MAMMOGRAPHY: Bilateral MLO views **(A)** demonstrate a focal asymmetry posteriorly in the right axillary tail **(arrow)**, not seen on the CC view. On the spot-compression MLO view **(B)**, the density persists and is somewhat more suspicious. Stereotactic biopsy was performed.

HISTOPATHOLOGY: Focal fibrosis.

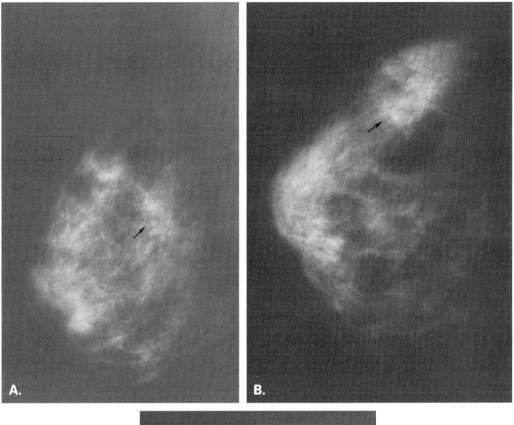

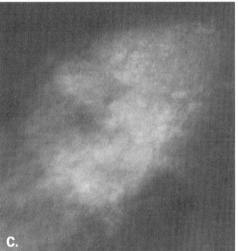

Figure 8.8

HISTORY: A 35-year-old woman for screening mammography.

MAMMOGRAPHY: Left ML **(A)** and CC **(B)** views show a focal asymmetric density with associated faint calcifications in the 3 o'clock position **(arrow)**. On the enlarged image **(C)**, the calcifications are better visualized as being uniform and punctuate, which suggests a lobular location.

IMPRESSION: Asymmetry with microcalcifications, probably of fibrocystic origin. Recommend biopsy.

HISTOPATHOLOGY: Sclerosing adenosis, hyperplasia, micropapillomas, lobular carcinoma in situ, radial scar.

with this condition. Sometimes, because of the constriction of the ductules of the lobule, the microcalcifications contained within these spaces are very small and amorphous.

Another benign etiology of focal asymmetry is diabetic fibrous mastopathy (Fig. 8.9). This condition occurs in patients with insulin-resistant type 1 diabetes, who usually present with a palpable breast mass several decades after their diagnosis of diabetes. These patients have impaired breakdown of collagen (11,12), which is thought to be related to the mammographic finding. On mammography, the breast tissue is very dense, and a focal asymmetry may correspond to the palpable mass. Sonography shows dense shadowing that has an appearance suspicious for carcinoma. Needle biopsy confirms the benign nature of the lesion.

In patients who have sustained trauma, a hematoma may be visualized on mammography. Although more commonly presenting as a round mass or indistinct mass, some hematomas may dissipate and have the appearance of a focal or global asymmetry. Clinical correlation is key in suggesting the diagnosis.

Malignant Causes of Asymmetry

Malignant causes of a focal asymmetry include carcinoma and lymphoma, with lymphoma less likely. Although breast cancer most often presents as a discrete mass with spiculated, indistinct, or microlobulated margins, or as microcalcifications, carcinoma occasionally is evident on mammography as a focal asymmetry (Figs. 8.10–8.14). In a study of 300 patients with mammographically detected clinically occult breast cancers, Sickles (13) found that about two thirds presented with nonclassical findings of breast cancer. Included in these nontypical presentations were a focal asymmetric density and a developing density (13). Because invasive lobular carcinoma (ILC) has a diffusely invading pattern of involvement in the tissue, the mammographic manifestations are often subtle and may include an area of focal asymmetry or distortion (14). In addition, invasive ductal carcinoma (IDC) or even ductal carcinoma in situ (DCIS) may be diagnosed based on a focal asymmetry on mammography. Of particular concern for malignancy are those asymmetries that are new or associated with a palpable or a sonographic mass, or those with associated suspicious microcalcifications.

ARCHITECTURAL DISTORTION

Architectural distortion is spiculation without a central dense mass (1). This finding is visualized in dense parenchyma as a tethering, indentation, or straightening of the breast tissue. In very dense breasts, architectural distortion may appear almost lucent as fat is trapped within the spiculations. In architectural distortion, the spiculation is usually fine and surrounds the center of the lesion. The disruption of the architecture and the spiculation are the findings that allow observation of the distortion in dense breasts.

The imaging evaluation of an area of architectural distortion often includes the use of spot compression with magnification (Fig. 8.15). If the distortion is not as clearly evident on one of the routine views as the other, additional off-angle views are important to elucidate the lesion and to help identify its exact location. These views may include rolled CC views if the distortion is best seen on the CC and the mediolateral (ML) view or step-obliques if the lesion is best seen on the mediolateral oblique (MLO) view.

In addition to mammographic evaluation, ultrasound (Fig. 8.16) and clinical examination are important in the assessment of an area of architectural distortion. The finding of an associated palpable mass or palpable thickening is suspicious for malignancy. The observation of a scar on the skin under the area of distortion suggests that it might be a surgical scar. In cases of ILC, a palpable mass may not be present even when the tumor is large. However, subtle dimpling of the skin, retraction of the nipple, or deviation of the nipple-areolar complex may occur when the ILC involves the Cooper's ligaments. On ultrasound, the presence of a solid mass or shadowing is suspicious for malignancy. When this is observed, ultrasound guidance is often used for needle biopsy of the lesion.

Postsurgical Scar

A common benign cause of architectural distortion is a postsurgical scar (Figs. 8.17 and 8.18). Initially after lumpectomy, mammography often demonstrates a hematoma or seroma at the surgical site. Subsequently, as the fluid collection resolves, scarring occurs. The scar may be nearly imperceptible on mammography, or it may be evident as a spiculated mass or as an area of architectural distortion (15). Postsurgical scars usually have a different appearance on the standard mammographic views. On one view, the scar may appear dense and spiculated, but on the other view, it has a more longitudinal shape, and the center appears more radiolucent. The placement of a wire or radiopaque markers on the skin over the surgical scar is helpful to correlate the position of an area of architectural distortion with the prior surgical site.

Comparison with prior images is also helpful to verify that a distortion represents a scar. Importantly, a scar should remain stable or decrease in size on subsequent mammography. An increase in the size of an area of distortion should be regarded as suspicious for malignancy.

(text continues on page 374)

Figure 8.9

HISTORY: A 32-year-old patient with insulin-resistant type I diabetes who presents with a firm mass in the left breast.

MAMMOGRAPHY: Left ML (**A**) and right MLO (**B**) views show very dense parenchyma bilaterally. In the left breast, corresponding to the palpable mass is a focal area of asymmetric density superimposed on the dense parenchyma. Ultrasound (**C**) of the mass shows dense shadowing. Sonography of the contralateral breast (**D**) shows similar findings. The history of the patient and the sonographic findings were most compatible with diabetic fibrous mastopathy. Biopsy was performed on the palpable mass for confirmation.

IMPRESSION: Diabetic fibrous mastopathy.

HISTOPATHOLOGY: Dense fibrosis consistent with diabetic mastopathy.

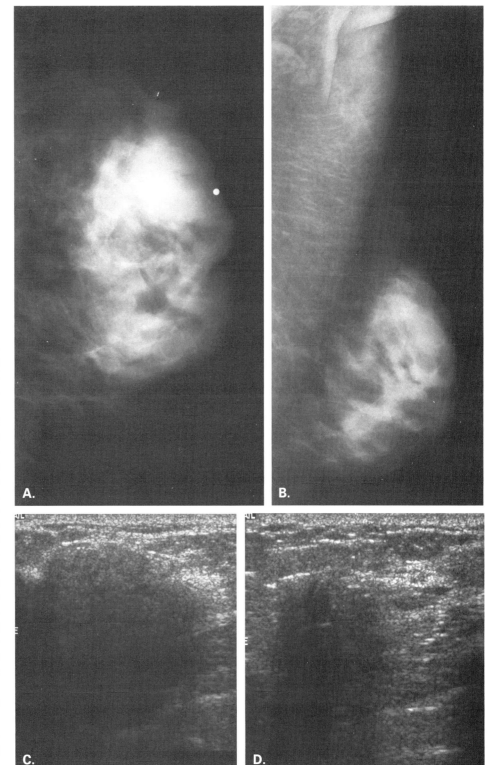

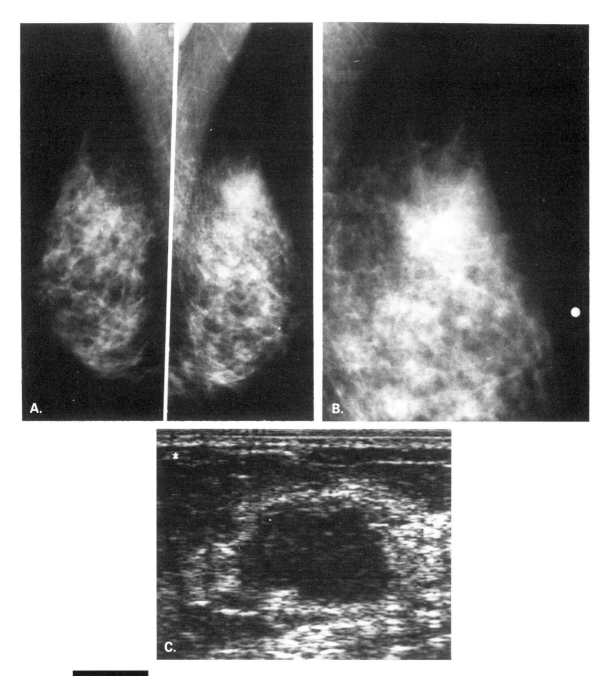

Figure 8.10

HISTORY: A 52-year-old woman with a new palpable mass in the right breast at 10 o'clock.

MAMMOGRAPHY: Bilateral MLO views **(A)** demonstrate a focal asymmetry in the right breast superiorly. On the right ML view **(B)**, the area is better seen and is associated with some distortion of the architecture. Ultrasound **(C)** shows the area to be a solid mass that is hypoechoic and somewhat irregular in margination. The associated palpable mass that is a solid mass on ultrasound and architectural distortion are features that warrant biopsy of the asymmetry.

IMPRESSION: Focal asymmetry, solid on ultrasound, suspicious for carcinoma.

HISTOPATHOLOGY: Invasive ductal carcinoma.

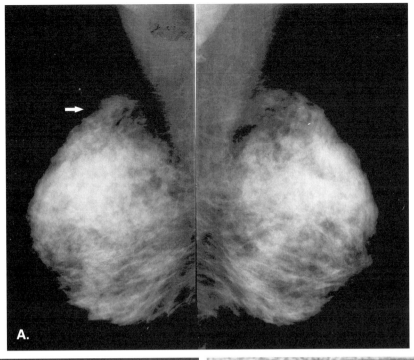

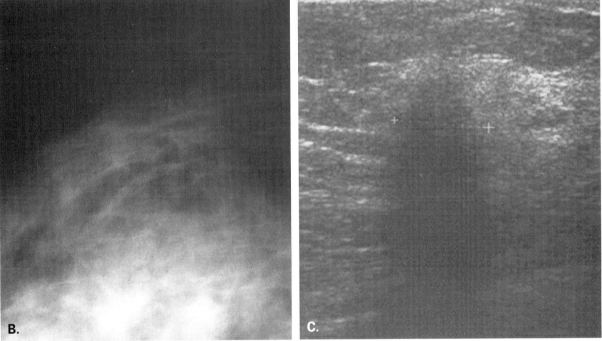

Figure 8.11

HISTORY: A 50-year-old woman who presents with subtle palpable thickening in the left axillary tail.

MAMMOGRAPHY: Bilateral MLO views **(A)** show heterogeneously dense breasts. There is slight focal asymmetry in the left axillary tail **(arrow)** and corresponding to the area of palpable concern. On spot compression **(B)**, the density appears slightly distorted. Ultrasound **(C)** was performed and demonstrates a dense area of shadowing that is suspicious for malignancy.

IMPRESSION: Suspicious for carcinoma.

HISTOPATHOLOGY: Invasive lobular carcinoma.

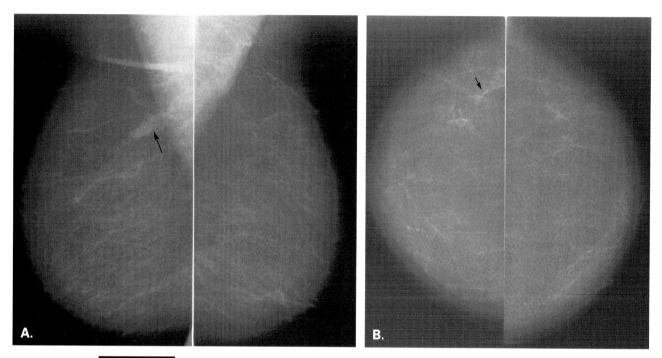

Figure 8.12

HISTORY: A 65-year-old woman for screening.

MAMMOGRAPHY: Bilateral MLO **(A)** and CC **(B)** views show fatty-replaced breasts. There is an oval density seen on the left MLO view posteriorly **(arrow)**. This is partially visible on the CC view laterally **(arrow)**, but it is much less distinct than it is on the MLO view. The MLO demonstrates best the axillary tail region, and it may show lesions that are not evident on the CC view.

HISTOPATHOLOGY: Papillary carcinoma.

In postlumpectomy patients, serial mammography usually allows for the diagnosis of a normal postsurgical scar because of the lack of increase in size of the distortion. However, in questionable cases, magnetic resonance imaging is most helpful to differentiate scar from recurrent tumor.

Other Benign Causes of Architectural Distortion

Sclerosing adenosis is a benign lesion that is a form of fibrocystic change, and it has a pathologic appearance somewhat similar to that of a radial scar. Sclerosing adenosis is a proliferative lesion containing increased ductules and sclerosis that distorts the glands. Microcalcifications are commonly present. The mammographic appearance of sclerosing adenosis may be architectural distortion or a focal asymmetry.

Other forms of fibrocystic change may be identified on biopsy of an area of architectural distortion. Hyperplasias of the common and atypical types, as well as focal fibrosis,

may be identified on biopsy of a distortion. Most often, these lesions are smaller, more subtle areas of distortion and not the larger, highly spiculated lesions seen in malignant etiologies (Figs. 8.19–8.21).

Plasma cell mastitis, which is part of the spectrum of duct ectasia, may occasionally present as an area of architectural distortion or focal asymmetry. This is usually located in the immediate subareolar area, where the ducts are ectatic. Like fibrocystic change, plasma cell mastitis is not highly spiculated (Fig. 8.22). In this condition, the inspissated secretions in the ectatic ducts may leak and cause a periductal inflammatory response with fibrosis. Nipple retraction occurs secondary to this response in about 20% of patients.

Radial Scar

Radial scar is a rosettelike proliferative breast lesion (16) that has also been described as sclerosing papillary

(text continues on page 377)

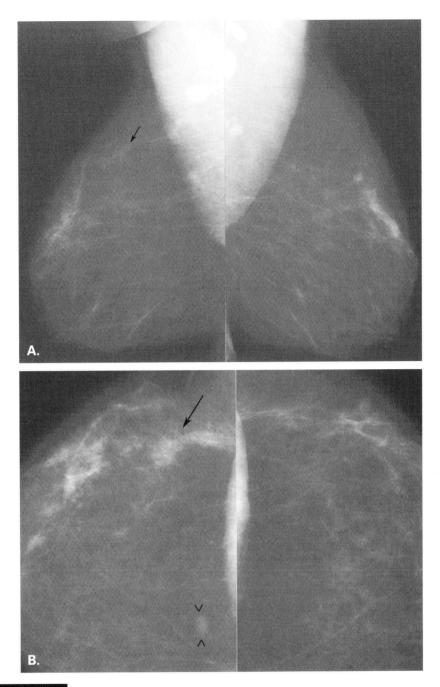

Figure 8.13

HISTORY: A 40-year-old woman who presented with metastatic carcinoma of unknown primary in a vertebral body.

MAMMOGRAPHY: Bilateral MLO (**A**) and CC (**B**) views show asymmetric density in the left upper-outer quadrant (**arrow**). There is also an oval isodense circumscribed mass (**arrowhead**) posteromedially on the left CC view. (*continued*)

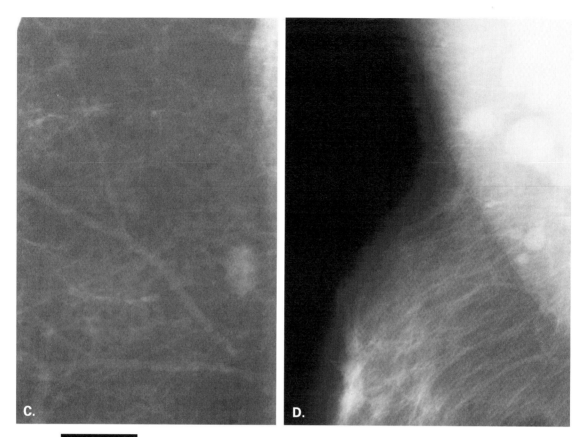

Figure 8.13 (*CONTINUED*)

On spot compression (**C**), the edges of the medial mass are relatively well defined. A left axillary view (**D**) shows multiple enlarged indistinct nodes, highly suggestive of metastatic carcinoma. Biopsies of the lateral asymmetry and the medial mass were performed.

IMPRESSION: Findings highly suggestive of multicentric carcinoma with positive axillary nodes.

HISTOPATHOLOGY: Asymmetric density: Infiltrating ductal carcinoma with angiolymphatic invasion DCIS, comedotype. Mass: Infiltrating ductal carcinoma. Axillary nodes were positive for metastatic carcinoma.

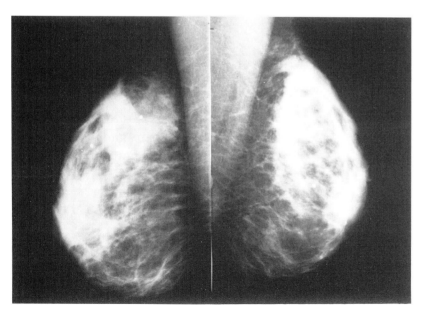

Figure 8.14

HISTORY: A 48-year-old woman with palpable thickening in the left upper-outer quadrant.

MAMMOGRAPHY: Bilateral MLO views show the breasts to be heterogeneously dense. In the left breast superiorly and posteriorly is a focal asymmetry at the site of the BB marking the palpable finding. In comparison with the opposite breast, this region is asymmetric and is occupying the retroglandular fat, findings that are suspicious for malignancy. Importantly, the asymmetry is also palpable, which prompts biopsy.

IMPRESSION: Palpable focal asymmetry suspicious for malignancy.

HISTOPATHOLOGY: Invasive lobular carcinoma.

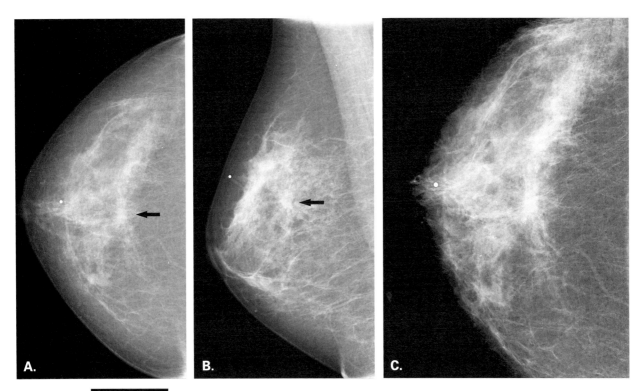

Figure 8.15

HISTORY: A 48-year-old woman who presents with a palpable left breast mass of 4 months duration.

MAMMOGRAPHY: Left CC **(A)** and MLO **(B)** views show heterogeneously dense tissue. There is architectural distortion **(arrows)** at 12 o'clock corresponding to the palpable mass that is marked with a BB. On the magnified CC view **(C)**, the central area of architectural distortion is better seen, and there are extensive pleomorphic microcalcifications throughout the breast. The palpable nature of the distortion and the microcalcifications increase the likelihood of malignancy.

IMPRESSION: Highly suspicious for malignancy.

HISTOPATHOLOGY: Invasive ductal carcinoma and DCIS.

proliferation (17), benign sclerosing ductal proliferation (18), nonencapsulated sclerosing lesion (19), infiltrating epitheliosis, and indurative mastopathy (20). The lesion has been confused with cancer by mammographers (21) and pathologists. Most radial scars are microscopic, but some are larger and at gross examination may appear as fine gray to white irregular lesions with central chalky streaks (22).

Radial scar or complex sclerosing lesion of the breast is a pathologic entity characterized by a fibroelastic core surrounded by a spoke-wheel pattern of proliferative ducts. The ducts that are trapped in the radial scar often appear sclerosed, and varying degrees of sclerosing adenosis and cyst formation may be seen in the periphery of the lesion (23). Radial scars are also called radial sclerosing lesions, because they contain a sclerosing papillary ductal proliferation (11). Occasionally carcinoma (especially DCIS) or atypical ductal hyperplasia may occur

within the ducts of the radial scar. Because of this, most radiologists recommend excision of a radial scar identified on core needle biopsy of the breast.

In a study of 32 cases of radial scars, Andersen and Gram (16) found most lesions to be small (mean diameter of 7 mm) and in a stellate configuration. In 93% of the cases, either papillomatosis or a benign epithelial proliferation was present with the radial scar. Small round microcalcifications were seen in 63% of cases (16). Because of the presence of elastosis with sclerosis and ductal distortion, a pseudoinfiltrative pattern occurs, and the lesion may be confused with carcinoma histologically (20).

The frequency of radial scars is not known. In a study from female autopsies, Nielson et al. (23) found radial scars in 23 of 83 autopsies. In this study, the frequency of

(text continues on page 380)

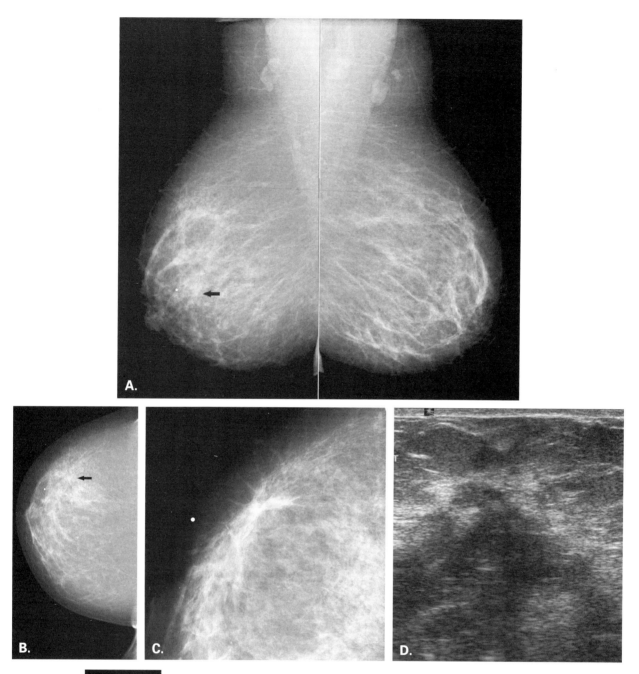

Figure 8.16

HISTORY: A 50-year-old woman with a palpable left subareolar mass and nipple retraction.

MAMMOGRAPHY: Bilateral MLO views **(A)** show asymmetry in the left breast subareolar area **(arrow)**. On the CC view **(B)**, the area appears slightly distorted **(arrow)**. On the spot CC view **(C)**, the architectural distortion is evident and corresponds to the palpable abnormality. Ultrasound **(D)** was performed and demonstrates a solid irregular mass with posterior shadowing. Because the distortion was palpable and associated with the clinical finding of nipple retraction, it is most likely related to malignancy.

IMPRESSION: Architectural distortion highly suspicious for malignancy.

HISTOPATHOLOGY: Invasive ductal carcinoma.

Figure 8.17

HISTORY: A 77-year-old woman who is status post-treatment of right breast cancer with lumpectomy and radiation therapy. Studies from 1995 and 1997 are presented.

MAMMOGRAPHY: Right MLO view **(A)** in 1995, 1 year after lumpectomy and radiation therapy, shows a dense area of distortion at the surgical site, consistent with posttreatment changes and scar. Two years later **(B)**, the area is much smaller, and it remains spiculated, consistent with postsurgical scar.

IMPRESSION: Normal evolution of postsurgical scar.

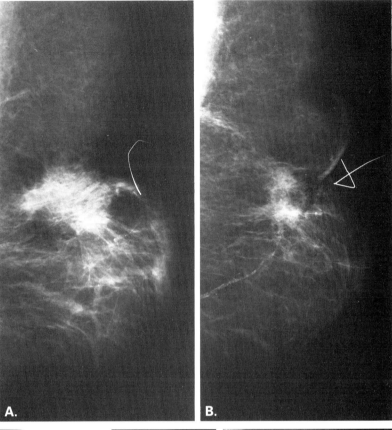

Figure 8.18

HISTORY: A 64-year-old woman who is 12 years status post-treatment of right breast cancer with lumpectomy and radiation therapy.

MAMMOGRAPHY: Bilateral MLO views **(A)** show heterogeneously dense tissue and the right breast appearing smaller and more dense than the left, consistent with posttreatment changes. There is focal asymmetry in the right axillary tail corresponding to the surgical site. On the magnified right MLO view **(B)**, the distortion related to the postsurgical scar is noted.

IMPRESSION: Normal postlumpectomy scar.

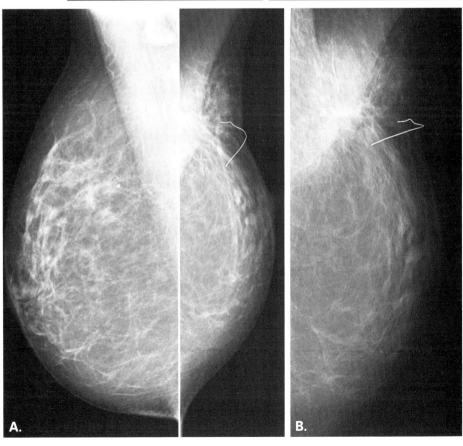

radial scars was significantly increased among women with fibrocystic disease (43%) compared with women without this entity (17%). In this study (23), no association between radial scar and breast cancer was found.

There is debate as to whether radial scars represent a premalignant lesion (19) or not (16–18, 20, 23–25). Fisher et al. (19) raised the concern that the lesion may represent an incipient form of tubular carcinoma. Vega and Garijo (26) found that 4 of 17 patients with radial scars had associated tubular carcinomas. However, in an average follow-up of 19.5 years of 32 patients treated with local excision of radial scar, Andersen and Gram (16) found no significant increase in the incidence of breast cancer.

On mammography, a radial scar is often an ill-defined lesion that produces retraction and distortion of surrounding structures (27) (Figs. 8.23–8.30). These lesions may be microscopic and may sometimes present on mammography as clustered punctuate or amorphous microcalcifications (28). The larger radial scars present on mammography as the so-called black star described by Tabar

and Dean (29). The radial scar is seen on two views but may vary in appearance on the two projections. A radial scar has a radiolucent center with long, fine radiating spicules that may bunch; it is not palpable and it is not associated with skin changes (29). Wallis et al. (22), however, described six patients in whom a radial scar produced a palpable mass on clinical examination. In this series of 24 radial scars (22), 88% were described as stellate lesions on mammography, and 62% had a lucent center. Orel et al. (28) described four cases of radial scar that presented with varying degrees of architectural distortion and associated microcalcifications from a series of 10 patients.

Of importance in the interpretation of an area of architectural distortion on mammography is the understanding that radial scar and carcinoma cannot be reliably differentiated based on the mammographic findings. Mitnick et al. (30) found in a study of 255 consecutive stellate lesions, of which 73 were cancers, that 19% of the cancers had mammographic features of radial scars. Calcifications were more commonly associated with carcinoma than

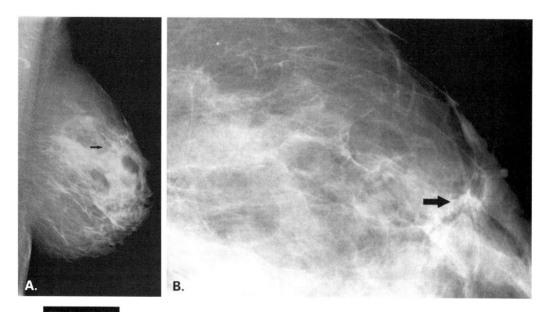

Figure 8.19

HISTORY: A 60-year-old woman for screening.

MAMMOGRAPHY: Right MLO (**A**) and spot CC (**B**) views show an area of architectural distortion (**arrow**) in the 10 o'clock position. This distortion has a central lucency, which suggests the possibility of radial scar.

IMPRESSION: Architectural distortion, question radial scar.

HISTOPATHOLOGY: Sclerosing adenosis, papillomatosis.

NOTE: Sclerosing adenosis and papillomatosis are part of the spectrum of pathologic changes associated with radial scar.

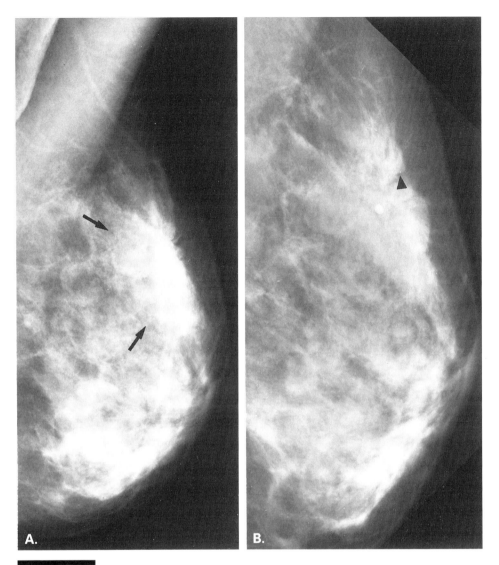

Figure 8.20

HISTORY: A 52-year-old woman for screening mammography.

MAMMOGRAPHY: Right MLO view **(A)** shows heterogeneously dense parenchyma. There is a subtle area of architectural distortion located superiorly **(arrow)**. On the spot ML magnification view **(B)**, the spiculation **(arrow)** has an appearance of a black star, suggesting the possibility of a radial scar.

IMPRESSION: Distortion, possible radial scar. Recommend biopsy.

HISTOPATHOLOGY: Atypical lobular hyperplasia.

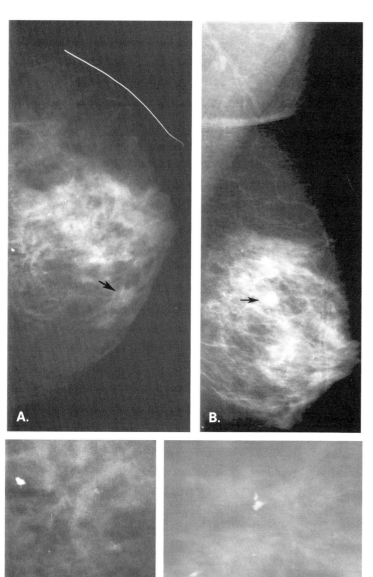

Figure 8.21

HISTORY: A 68-year-old woman with a history of benign right breast biopsy for screening mammography.

MAMMOGRAPHY: Right CC **(A)** and MLO **(B)** views show heterogeneously dense parenchyma with scattered calcifications. In the 1 o'clock position is an area of architectural distortion, associated with amorphous microcalcifications **(arrows)**. On the coned-down image **(C)**, the area is better seen. Magnification MLO **(D)** shows the prominent distortion and numerous microcalcifications.

IMPRESSION: Architectural distortion with microcalcifications of suspicious nature. Recommend biopsy.

HISTOPATHOLOGY: Sclerosing adenosis, periductal fibrosis.

radial scars. In addition, four of nine radial scars had a dense central region suggestive of carcinoma. The presence of small radiolucencies within the lesion are more in favor of a radial scar than of malignancy (29), but histologic examination is necessary to confirm the diagnosis (27,30). In a study of 40 patients with a preoperative diagnosis of radial scar, Frouge et al. (31) found that pathologic examination revealed 20 pure radial scars, 12 carcinomas, and 8 malignant lesions associated with radial scars.

Sonography has been found to be helpful in the evaluation of radial scars (31a). In a study of 12 mammographically detected radial scars, ultrasound also demonstrated 8 of the lesions. Sonographic findings were an irregular hypoechoic mass with ill-defined borders and posterior shadowing. Sonographic demonstration of a mass for a questionable mammographic finding is certainly important in prompting biopsy. However, like mammography,

(text continues on page 386)

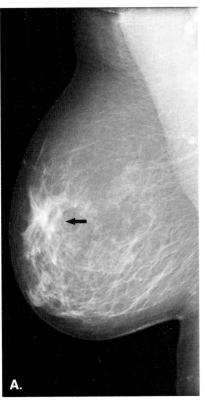

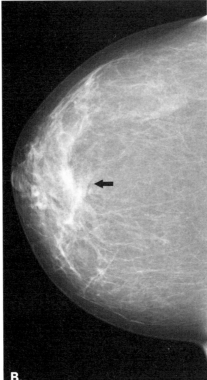

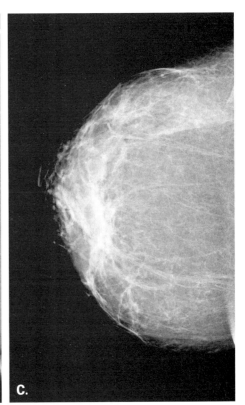

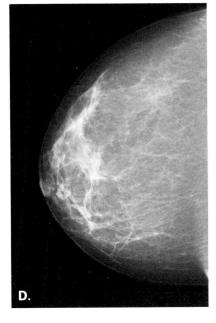

Figure 8.22

HISTORY: Screening mammography for a 48-year-old woman. She had no history of prior surgery.

MAMMOGRAPHY: Left MLO **(A)** and CC **(B)** views show a focal area of increased density in the left subareolar area **(arrow)** with associated subtle architectural distortion. On the rolled CC views medial **(C)** and lateral **(D)**, the distortion persists and moves with the superior aspect of the breast. Also noted is ductal ectasia in the subareolar region.

IMPRESSION: Architectural distortion. Recommend biopsy.

HISTOPATHOLOGY: Chronic mastitis, periductal inflammation, and fibrosis.

NOTE: These findings are consistent with duct ectasia and secretory disease.

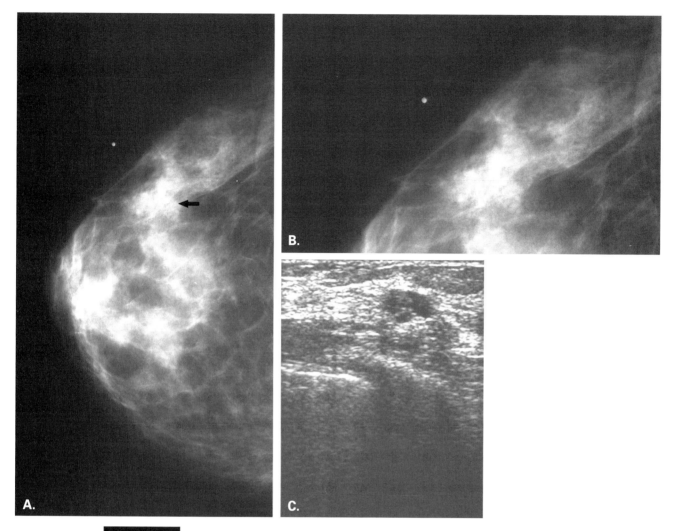

Figure 8.23

HISTORY: A 58-year-old patient who reports palpable thickening in the left upper-outer quadrant.

MAMMOGRAPHY: Left CC **(A)** and enlarged CC **(B)** views show a focal density **(arrow)** in the left upper-outer quadrant. The lesion is associated with some distortion of the architecture, which is more apparent on the enlarged CC view. On ultrasound **(C)**, a lobulated heterogeneous lesion with somewhat angular margins is seen.

IMPRESSION: Asymmetry with distortion, suspicious for malignancy.

HISTOPATHOLOGY: Radial scar.

NOTE: The lesion is more dense centrally than is usually seen in a radial scar.

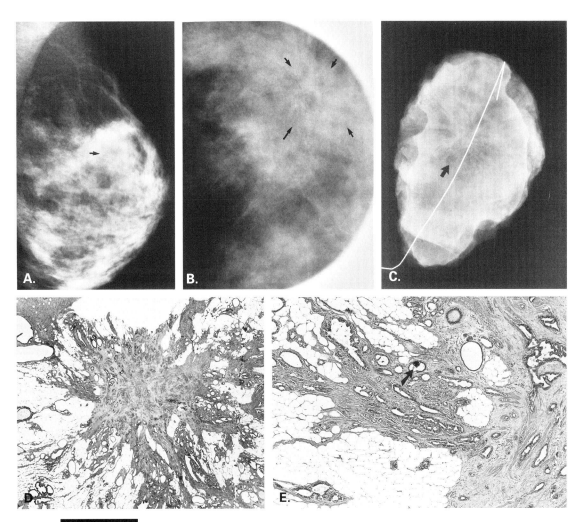

Figure 8.24

HISTORY: A 45-year-old gravida 2, para 2 woman with a history of nodular breasts for routine mammography. She had no history of breast biopsy.

MAMMOGRAPHY: Right MLO view **(A)**, spot compression CC view **(B)**, specimen film **(C)**, and histopathology at 10X **(D)** and at 60X **(E)**. The breast is very dense for the patient's age and parity. In the upper aspect on the MLO view **(A)**, there is focal area of architectural distortion **(arrow)**. On spot compression **(B)**, the lesion persists and is found to have a central lucency surrounded by dense spicules **(arrows)**. The finding suggests a radial scar as the most likely diagnosis. However, carcinomas may occasionally have this appearance; therefore, a biopsy was recommended. The specimen film **(C)** from the needle localization demonstrates well the spiculated lesion **(arrow)**. On the specimen film, the lesion appears more dense, and the central lucency is not evident.

IMPRESSION: Spiculated lesion, favoring radial scar.

HISTOPATHOLOGY: Radial scar, sclerosing adenosis. At 10X magnification, the stellate appearance of the lesion is evident. There is a spokewheel pattern of central fibrosis interposed with epithelial proliferation. At high power (60X), there are haphazardly arranged ductules within bands of fibrous tissue. Focal calcification is present in a ductule **(arrow)**.

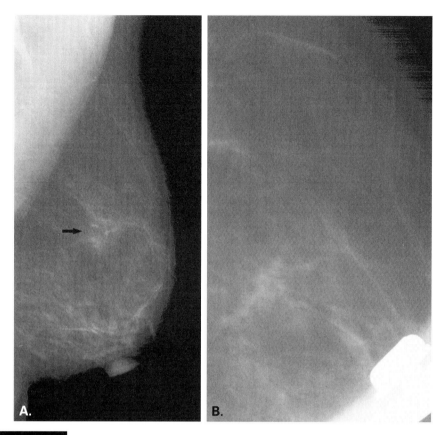

Figure 8.25

HISTORY: A 39-year-old gravida 1, para 1 patient with a clinical history of fibrocystic breasts for screening.

MAMMOGRAPHY: Right MLO **(A)** and ML magnification (1.5×) **(B)** views. The breast is dense, compatible with the age of the patient. In the upper outer quadrant, there is 3-cm area of architectural distortion (**B, arrowhead**). The lesion is of similar density to the background but has an irregular spiculated margin. The lack of a palpable finding corresponding to a lesion of this size on mammography would decrease the level of suspicion for malignancy from high to moderate. The differential includes radial scar, carcinoma, and sclerosing adenosis.

IMPRESSION: Distortion, moderately suspicious for malignancy.

HISTOPATHOLOGY: Radial scar, fibrocystic change with focal severe atypia.

sonography does not reliably differentiate radial scar from cancer (32).

Fibromatosis

Fibromatosis or extra-abdominal desmoid tumor may appear as a focal area of architectural distortion or as an indistinct or spiculated mass (Fig. 8.31). Fibromatosis is made up of a uniform population of fibroblasts arranged in interlocking bundles and entrapping mammary ducts (33). Clinically, these patients present with a painless hard mass that is clinically suggestive of carcinoma. Dimpling of the skin and fixation to the pectoralis muscle are common and are related to the extension of the lesion from the pectoralis fascia. The lesion has been described on mam-

mography as an area of spiculation near the chest wall (34). Fibromatosis may be associated with a prior history of trauma or surgery (35). Although histologically benign, fibromatosis recurs locally, and it is therefore treated with wide local excision.

Malignant Causes of Architectural Distortion

Tubular Carcinoma

One of the specialized subtypes of IDC is tubular carcinoma. Tubular carcinoma is a very-well-differentiated form of invasive carcinoma and is characterized by a

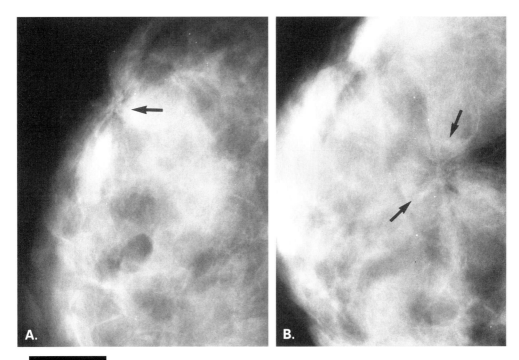

Figure 8.26

HISTORY: A 30-year-old woman with a positive family history of breast cancer and no palpable findings.

MAMMOGRAPHY: Left enlarged (2×) ML **(A)** and CC **(B)** views. The background parenchymal pattern is dense and glandular. There is a focal area of architectural distortion **(arrows)** in the 12 o'clock position of the breast, having the appearance of a spiculated lesion. This lesion has a radiolucent center and is associated with some adjacent lobular-type microcalcifications. The differential includes radial scar versus carcinoma; radial scar is favored because of the central lucency.

HISTOPATHOLOGY: Radial scar.

single layer of malignant cells forming small tubular structures. Tubular carcinomas are very slow growing, and therefore they may be present on mammography without significant change for several years. Peters et al. (36) found that in cases of pure tubular or almost pure tubular carcinomas, the tumor size was small, no metastases or recurrences occurred, and there were no deaths related to the cancer. However, in a study of 50 patients diagnosed with tubular carcinoma between 1944 and 1992, Winchester et al. (37) found that 20% had axillary metastases and four developed recurrences. Contralateral cancer was identified in 26% of these patients. In this study, however, the patient database included those with tumors that were at least 80% tubular histology and not just pure tubular cancers.

Tubular carcinoma and radial scars have similar histologic features and can be confused on histopathology (16,39). The two lesions also share some cytologic features (40), because the tubular angular structures that are characteristic of tubular carcinoma may also occur in radial scar. The important feature of a radial scar or of benign lesions is the presence of myoepithelial cells, which are lacking in tubular cancer. Some authors believe that radial scar is the precursor lesion to tubular cancer (19,41), whereas others disagree (16,23).

The mammographic features of tubular carcinoma include masses, masses with calcifications, architectural distortion, or asymmetry with or without microcalcifications (Figs. 8.32–8.34). Elson et al. (42) found that 73% of lesions were spiculated, and the median size was 8 mm. The majority were nonpalpable lesions that were detected on screening mammography. Because tubular cancers are well differentiated, the rate of growth is slow. Therefore, these are often visible in retrospect and change little from year to year.

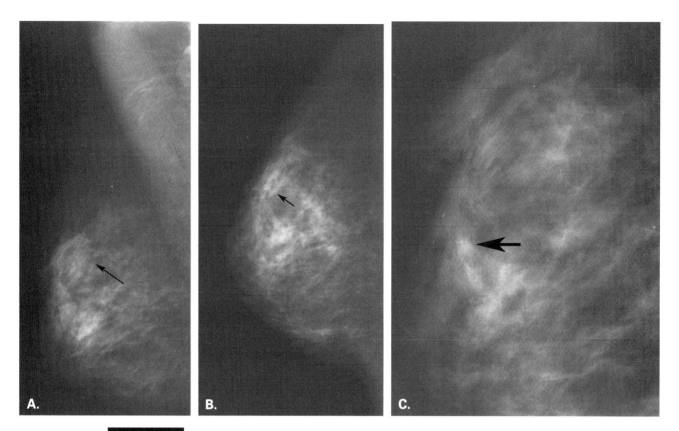

Figure 8.27

HISTORY: A 56-year-old woman for screening.

MAMMOGRAPHY: Left MLO **(A)** and ML **(B)** views show a focal area of architectural distortion **(arrow)** in the breast superiorly. On spot compression **(C)**, the distortion is noted and is associated with a distended duct and microcalcifications.

IMPRESSION: Architectural distortion, possible radial scar. Recommend biopsy.

HISTOPATHOLOGY: Proliferative fibrocystic change with focal microcalcifications of left breast, intraductal papilloma, and focal lymphohistiocytic tissue reaction.

Invasive Lobular Carcinoma

ILC was first described by Cornil (43) in 1865 as a diffusely infiltrative tumor that was composed of small monomorphic cells that formed single lines throughout a desmoplastic stroma. From 1987 to 1999, cases of ILC increased from 9.5% of all breast cancers to 15.6% according to an analysis of more than 190,000 women with breast cancer (44). ILC accounts for about 10% of all breast cancers (45,46).

In comparison with IDC, ILC is more likely to occur in older patients, to be larger in size, and to be estrogen and progesterone receptor positive. The incidence of contralateral cancer has been found to be higher (20% versus 11.2%) in patients with ILC compared with those with

IDC (47). In addition, ILC has a substantially increased propensity for multifocal and multicentric extent in comparison with IDC (48–50). Although the biologic phenotype of ILC is favorable, the overall 7-year survival is the same as that of IDC (47).

ILC typically is subtle on mammography and is easily missed (13,51–53). ILC histologically is composed of malignant cells invading the breast tissue in a single file pattern, often extending over a large area without having a central dense tumor nidus. Because of this, the mammographic findings are often a subtle area of focal asymmetry or an architectural distortion. False-negative rates for ILC have been reported to range from 8% (54) to 19% (55). Clinical examination may be normal, or the patient

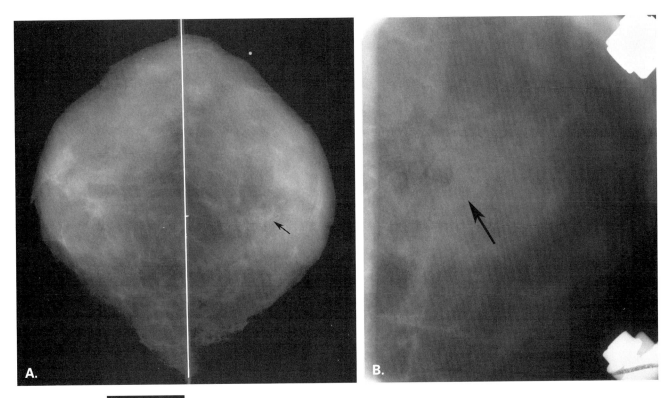

Figure 8.28

HISTORY: A 34-year-old woman for screening mammography, positive family history.

MAMMOGRAPHY: Bilateral CC views **(A)** show very dense parenchyma bilaterally. There is focal architectural distortion in the right breast medially **(arrow)**. On spot compression magnification **(B)**, the distortion is better seen. The lesion has central lucency and spiculation having an appearance of a black star.

IMPRESSION: Probable radial scar. Recommend biopsy.

HISTOPATHOLOGY: Radial scar.

NOTE: Although a black star is most suggestive of radial scar, carcinoma can have a similar appearance, and biopsy is necessary for diagnosis.

may present with palpable thickening or deviation of the nipple-areolar complex.

In a review of 37 patients with ILC, Newstead et al (56) found that 57% of patients presented with asymmetric opacities or architectural distortions on mammography. None of the patients in this series (56) had microcalcifications associated with the tumor on mammography. In the same study, the authors found that IDC presented as a focal asymmetry or distortion in only 13.6% of cases. There is little connective tissue reaction to the diffusely invading tumor, so a discrete mass is not commonly seen. In other series, the presentations of ILC included a focal asymmetry in 3% to 25% of cases or architectural distortion in 10% to 25% (54,55) (Figs. 8.35–8.44).

On mammography, ILC is often as dense as or less dense than the normal fibroglandular tissue and commonly is seen on one view only, most often the CC view (51,53,56). In a study of the use of computer-aided detection (CAD) for ILC, Evans et al. (57) found that the sensitivity of the CAD was 91% and that 77% of the retrospectively visible tumors were also marked by the CAD. In order to detect ILC, the radiologist must be vigilant for the subtle distortions and asymmetries that are hallmarks of this disease.

Because ILC is often diffusely invading the tissue, patients with ILC have a high risk of having tumor-positive margins at initial resection. Moore et al. (58) found that 51% of patients with ILC had positive margins at lumpectomy and that the mammographic finding that was of higher risk for margin positivity was architectural

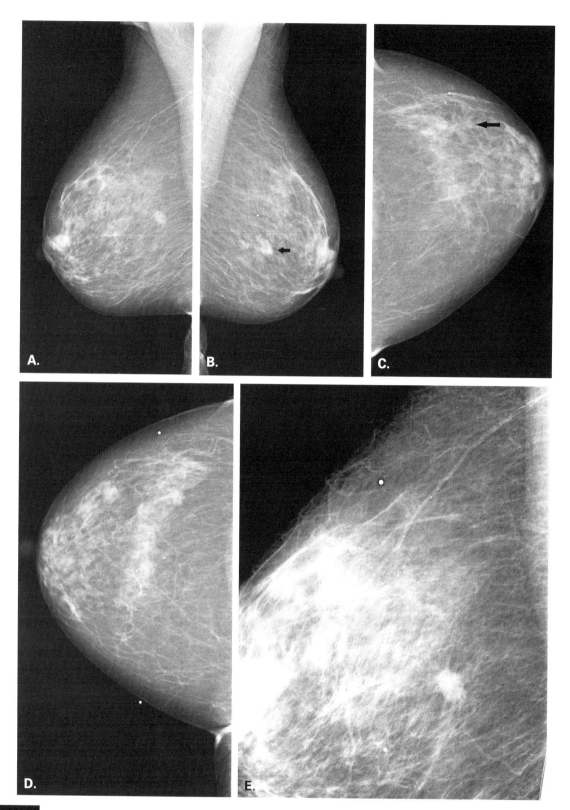

Figure 8.29

HISTORY: A 74-year-old woman for screening mammography.

MAMMOGRAPHY: Left MLO **(A)** and right MLO **(B)** views show areas of spiculation bilaterally. On the right MLO **(B)** and CC **(C)** views, in the lower outer quadrant **(arrows)**, there is an area of architectural distortion with the central lucency. On the left MLO **(A)** and CC **(D)** views, there is a high-density, spiculated mass. Associated pleomorphic microcalcifications are seen on the spot CC magnification **(E)** of the left breast mass.

IMPRESSION: Bilateral spiculated lesions suspicious, BI-RADS® 5 left breast, BI-RADS® 4 right breast.

HISTOPATHOLOGY: Right radial scar, left invasive ductal carcinoma with DCIS.

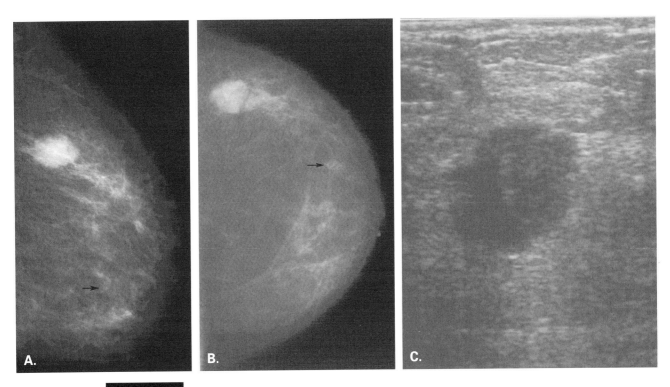

Figure 8.30

HISTORY: A 48-year-old woman with a palpable mass in the right upper-outer quadrant.

MAMMOGRAPHY: Right MLO **(A)** and CC **(B)** views show a high-density lobulated mass with indistinct margins. Anterior to this lesion is a small area of architectural distortion **(arrow)**. Multiple punctuate microcalcifications are also present. Sonography of the palpable mass **(C)** shows a hypoechoic lobular mass with slightly irregular margins.

IMPRESSION: Palpable mass, highly suspicious for carcinoma; architectural distortion anteriorly. Recommend biopsy of both lesions.

HISTOPATHOLOGY: Posterior mass: infiltrating ductal carcinoma, with negative nodes. Anterior lesion: radial scar.

distortion. Even so, the rate of use of breast conservation therapy for ILC increased almost threefold from 1989 to 2001 (59).

Ductal Carcinoma

IDC most commonly presents as a mass with indistinct or spiculated margins. Pleomorphic intraductal microcalcifications are often associated with IDC. Other presentations for IDC include a relatively circumscribed mass, areas of architectural distortion, or even focal asymmetry (Figs. 8.45–8.53). The association of architectural distor-

tion and of intraductal microcalcifications is very suspicious for IDC.

DCIS usually presents as clustered or linear/segmentally arranged microcalcifications. However, occasionally DCIS presents as a noncalcified lesion, either as a small mass or focal asymmetry or architectural distortion. Reiff et al. (60) described a stellate noncalcified lesion as the presentation of 7 of 86 (8%) cases of DCIS. Of these seven lesions, four were caused by a complex sclerosing lesion with associated DCIS, and three were DCIS alone.

(References begin on page 416)

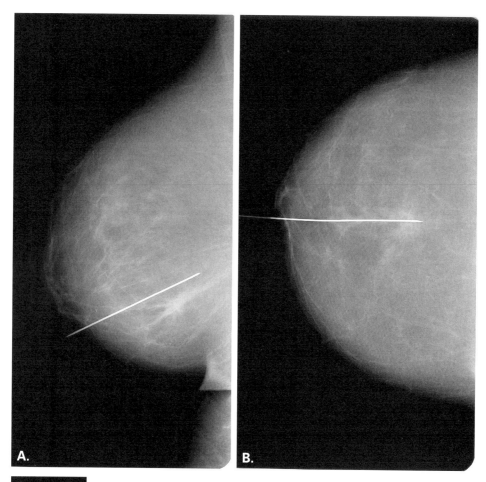

Figure 8.31

HISTORY: Screening mammography.

MAMMOGRAPHY: Left ML (**A**) and CC (**B**) views from a needle localization procedure. There is an ill-defined, somewhat-spiculated mass of medium density in the deep central portion of the left breast. The lesion is of moderate suspicion for malignancy.

HISTOPATHOLOGY: Fibromatosis.

NOTE: Fibromatosis is a fibroblastic lesion that is nonmetastasizing but locally invasive. This lesion can occur in the soft tissues of the trunk and limbs as a "desmoid tumor." In the breast, the lesion usually represents an extension from the pectoralis fascia. (Case courtesy of Dr. Gary Lichtenstein, South Boston, VA.)

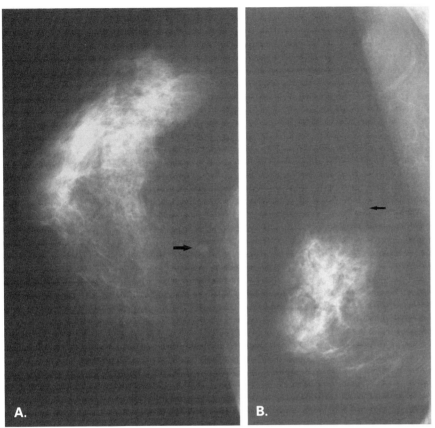

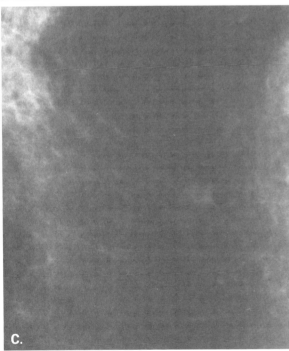

Figure 8.32

HISTORY: A 73-year-old woman recalled from an abnormal screening mammogram.

MAMMOGRAPHY: Left CC (**A**) and ML (**B**) views show a small area of architectural distortion located posteriorly at 12 o'clock (**arrows**). The density is better seen on the CC spot magnification view (**C**) and is noted to be spiculated and somewhat dense for its size.

IMPRESSION: Suspicious for carcinoma.

HISTOPATHOLOGY: Tubular carcinoma.

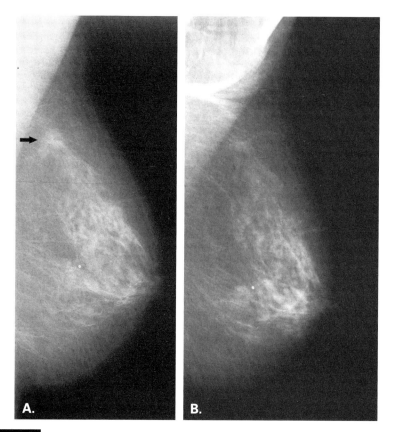

Figure 8.33

HISTORY: Postmenopausal patient for screening mammography. Prior films from 6 years earlier are available for comparison.

MAMMOGRAPHY: Right MLO view **(A)** shows a focal density superiorly **(arrow)** with indistinct margins. This area was not seen on the CC view. On the prior study 6 years earlier **(B)**, the finding was present, but it was smaller and somewhat less dense. Because of the slow change in this lesion, it is suspicious for a malignancy that is most likely well differentiated.

IMPRESSION: Suspicious for carcinoma.

HISTOPATHOLOGY: Tubular carcinoma. *Note:* Tubular carcinoma is a specialized type of invasive ductal carcinoma that is well differentiated and has a favorable prognosis. The slow change on mammography is typical of these lesions because of their low mitotic rate.

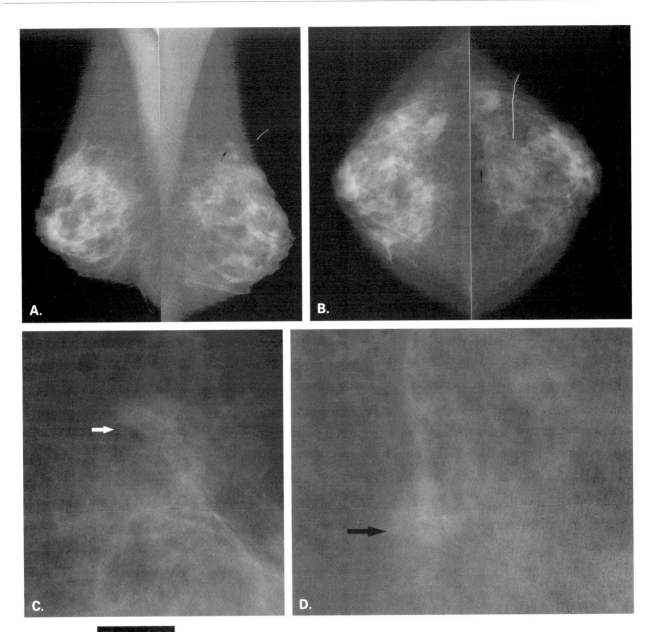

Figure 8.34

HISTORY: A 59-year-old for screening.

MAMMOGRAPHY: Bilateral MLO **(A)** and CC **(B)** views show heterogeneously dense breasts. There is a small indistinct density in the superior aspect of the right breast at the 11 o'clock position **(arrows)**. On spot-magnification MLO **(C)** and CC **(D)** views, the density **(arrows)** persists, and it has slightly spiculated margins.

IMPRESSION: Small right breast mass, suspicious for carcinoma.

HISTOPATHOLOGY: Tubular carcinoma.

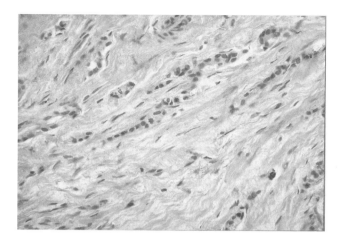

Figure 8.35

Pathology of invasive lobular carcinoma: High-power histopathologic section shows features of invasive lobular carcinoma. A monomorphic cell population is forming single lines and invading normal fibrofatty stroma.

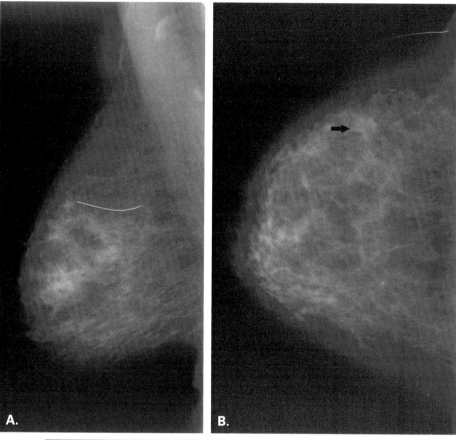

A.

B.

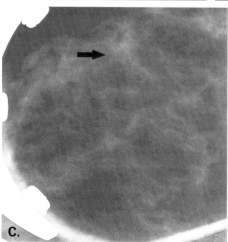

C.

Figure 8.36

HISTORY: A 55-year-old woman with a history of prior benign left breast biopsy for routine screening.

MAMMOGRAPHY: Left MLO (**A**) and CC (**B**) views demonstrate scattered fibroglandular densities, and a radiopaque wire marks the surgical scar. On the CC view only (**B**), there is a focal asymmetry (**arrow**) that had developed from the prior study. On spot-compression CC (**C**) view, the density (**arrow**) persists and appears somewhat distorted.

IMPRESSION: Focal asymmetry, suspicious, BI-RADS® 4.

HISTOPATHOLOGY: Infiltrating lobular carcinoma.

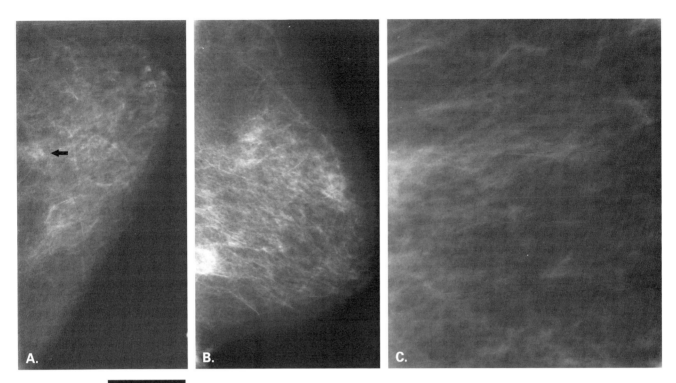

Figure 8.37

HISTORY: A 49-year-old woman recalled for additional evaluation from a screening mammogram.

MAMMOGRAPHY: Right exaggerated CC medial (**A**) and ML (**B**) views show a focal density located at the chest wall. On the spot compression magnification MLO view (**C**), the distortion associated with the focal density is seen. Because the lesion is located far posteriorly, the possibility of malignancy is increased.

IMPRESSION: Suspicious for carcinoma.

HISTOPATHOLOGY: Invasive lobular carcinoma.

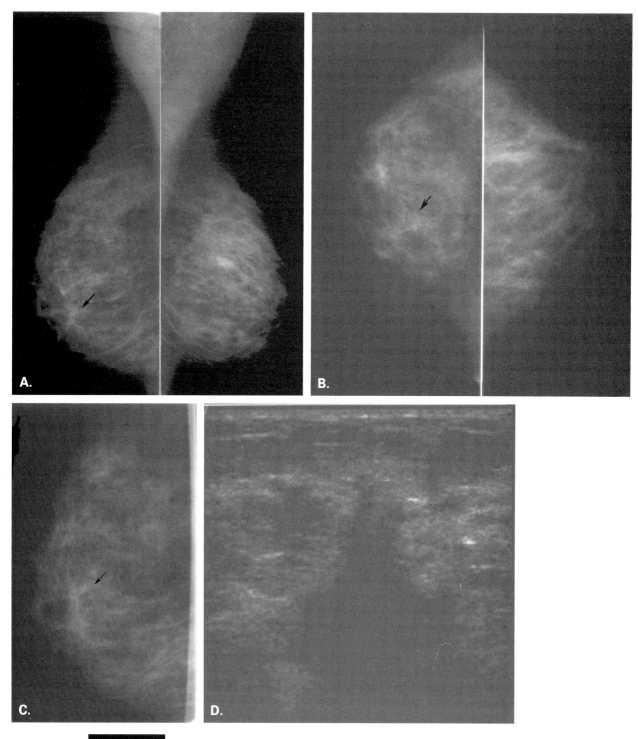

Figure 8.38

HISTORY: A 52-year-old woman for screening mammography.

MAMMOGRAPHY: Bilateral MLO **(A)** and CC **(B)** views show heterogeneously dense breasts. In the left subareolar area, there is a focal density with associated architectural distortion **(arrow)**. On the left MLO magnification view **(C)**, the spiculation is better seen. Sonography **(D)** demonstrates an irregular mass with dense shadowing, highly suspicious for malignancy.

IMPRESSION: Highly suspicious for carcinoma.

HISTOPATHOLOGY: Infiltrating lobular carcinoma.

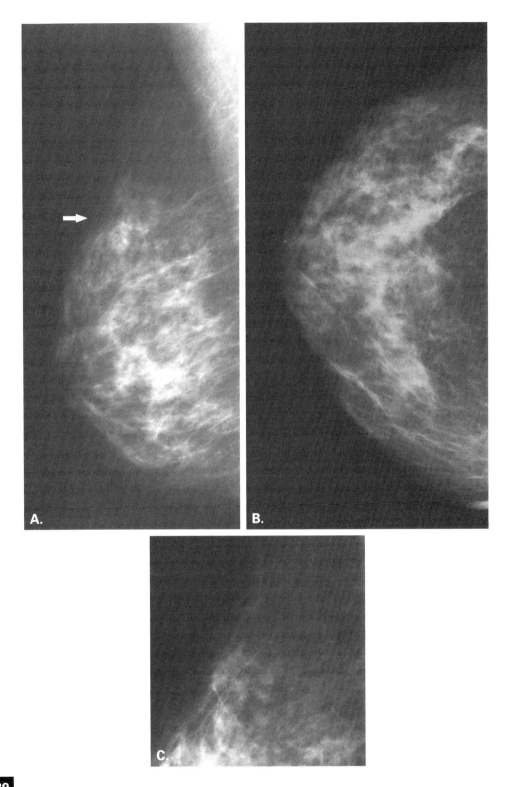

Figure 8.39

HISTORY: Left screening mammogram on a 60-year-old patient who is status post–right mastectomy.

MAMMOGRAPHY: Left MLO (**A**) and CC (**B**) views show a heterogeneously dense breast. There is a focal area of architectural distortion (**arrow**) seen on the MLO view only that is causing an indentation of the parenchyma superiorly. The area persists and appears more spiculated on spot compression (**C**).

IMPRESSION: Architectural distortion, suspicious, BI-RADS® 4.

HISTOPATHOLOGY: Invasive lobular carcinoma.

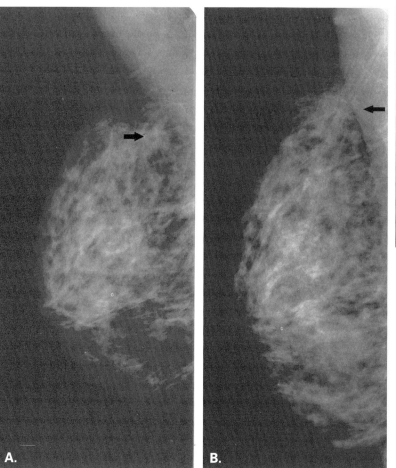
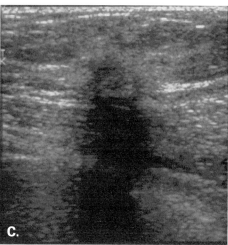

Figure 8.40

HISTORY: A 53-year-old woman for screening mammography.

MAMMOGRAPHY: Left MLO view **(A)** shows a heterogeneously dense left breast and a focal area of architectural distortion superiorly **(arrow)**. The distortion appears to tether the breast tissue around it. The area was not seen on the CC view. However, on an ML view **(B)**, the distortion **(arrow)** appears to be located higher than on the MLO view, indicating that it is located medially. Ultrasound **(C)** shows a shadowing lesion in the upper inner quadrant, highly suspicious for malignancy.

IMPRESSION: Distortion highly suspicious for malignancy.

HISTOPATHOLOGY: Invasive lobular carcinoma.

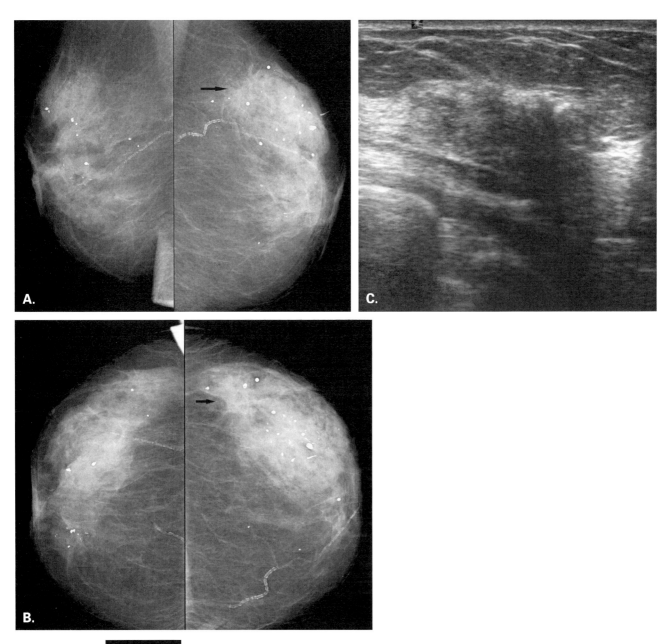

Figure 8.41

HISTORY: A 74-year-old woman with palpable thickening in the right breast. She was referred with a recent mammogram interpreted as negative. Bilateral magnification views were performed.

MAMMOGRAPHY: Bilateral ML magnification **(A)** and CC magnification **(B)** views show dense parenchyma with bilateral round, rodlike, and dystrophic calcifications, all of which have a benign appearance. On the right, in the upper outer quadrant, in the area of palpable concern is an area of architectural distortion **(arrows)**. The patient had no history of surgery, but did have palpable thickening that corresponded to the distortion. Ultrasound **(C)** of this area shows an irregular solid mass with angular margins.

IMPRESSION: Highly suspicious for malignancy.

HISTOPATHOLOGY: Invasive lobular carcinoma.

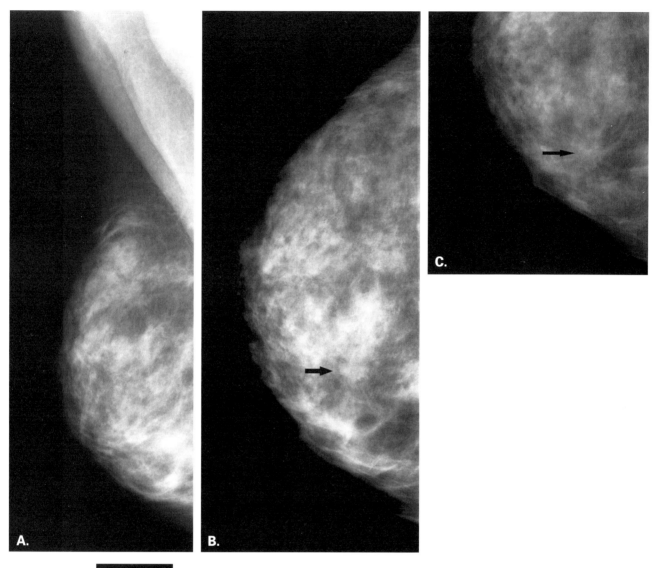

Figure 8.42

HISTORY: A 56-year-old woman who is status post–right mastectomy for invasive lobular carcinoma.

MAMMOGRAPHY: Left MLO **(A)** and CC **(B)** views show a dense left breast. In the medial aspect of the CC view, there is a questionable area of architectural distortion **(arrow)**. On spot-compression magnification CC **(C)**, the distortion is much more apparent, and it is associated with some punctuate microcalcifications.

IMPRESSION: Architectural distortion, radial scar versus carcinoma.

HISTOPATHOLOGY: Invasive lobular carcinoma.

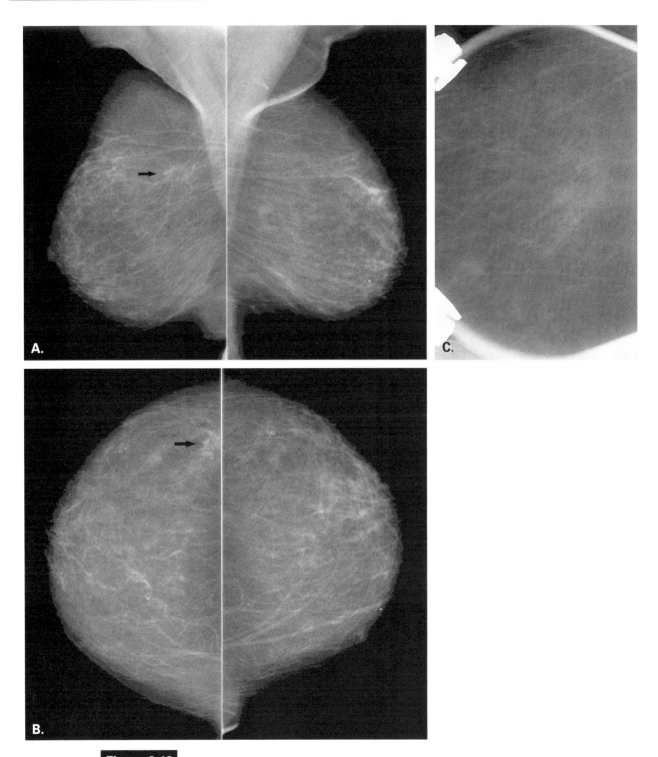

Figure 8.43

HISTORY: Screening mammogram on a 67-year-old woman.

MAMMOGRAPHY: Bilateral MLO (**A**) and CC (**B**) views show the breasts to be nearly fatty replaced. There is a focal area of architectural distortion (**arrows**) in the left upper-outer quadrant. On spot compression (**C**), the distortion persists and appears slightly more dense. The very posterior location and the lack of fibrocystic changes otherwise would suggest a malignant etiology rather than a radial scar.

IMPRESSION: Suspicious for malignancy.

HISTOPATHOLOGY: Infiltrating lobular carcinoma.

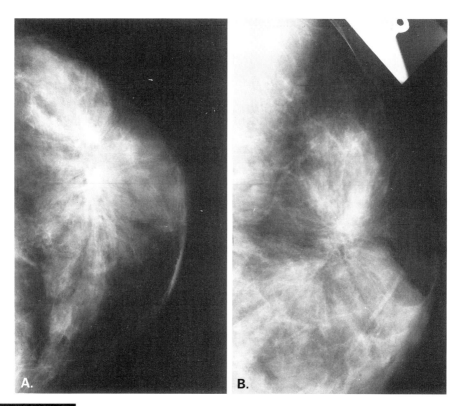

Figure 8.44

HISTORY: Patient who presents with palpable thickening in the right breast superiorly.

MAMMOGRAPHY: Right CC **(A)** and spot compression ML **(B)** views show the breast to be heterogeneously dense. There is a marked area of architectural distortion in the central aspect at 12 o'clock. The area produces an indented, tethered appearance of the parenchyma. Because of the clinical finding and the large size of the distortion, radial scar is much less likely than carcinoma.

IMPRESSION: Suspicious for carcinoma.

HISTOPATHOLOGY: Invasive lobular carcinoma.

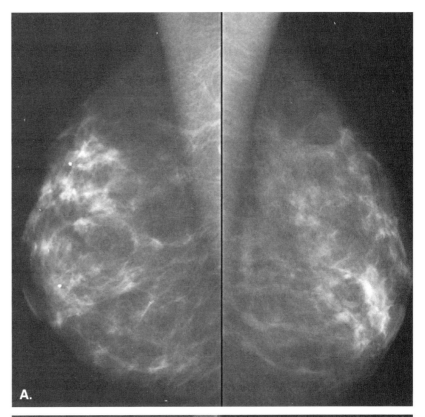

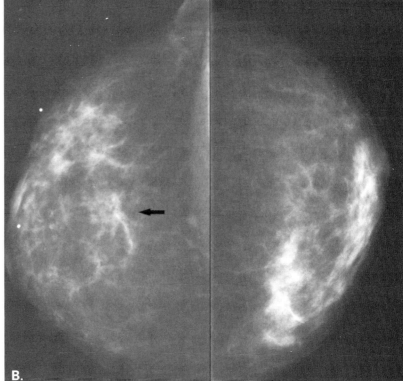

Figure 8.45

HISTORY: A 46-year-old gravida 2, para 2 woman who presents with a small palpable mass in the left breast at 2 o'clock.

MAMMOGRAPHY: Bilateral MLO **(A)** and CC **(B)** views show scattered parenchymal densities. A BB marks the palpable left breast mass, which is an area of focal asymmetry. In addition, there is an area of architectural distortion **(arrow)** at 12 o'clock, separate from the palpable lesion. The spiculation of this lesion **(arrow)** is better seen on the enlarged left CC view **(C)**. (*continued*)

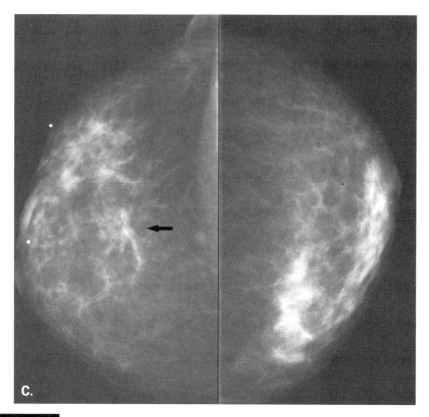

Figure 8.45 (CONTINUED)

Enlarged left CC view **(C)**.

IMPRESSION: Palpable asymmetry and nonpalpable architectural distortion. Recommend biopsy of each area.

HISTOPATHOLOGY: Invasive ductal carcinoma, multicentric, with negative axillary nodes.

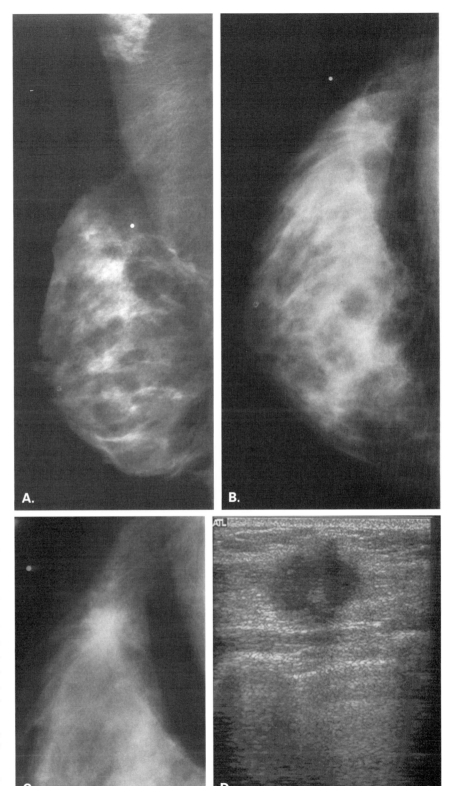

Figure 8.46

HISTORY: A 44-year-old woman with a small palpable mass in the left axillary tail.

MAMMOGRAPHY: Left MLO (**A**) and CC (**B**) views show heterogeneously dense tissue. A BB marks the palpable lesion, which is an area of architectural distortion. The lesion appears more dense and masslike on the CC view, and on the spot CC (**C**) view, it is very dense and spiculated. Ultrasound (**D**) demonstrates an irregular, hypoechoic mass.

IMPRESSION: Palpable area of distortion that is a mass on ultrasound, highly suspicious for malignancy.

HISTOPATHOLOGY: Invasive ductal carcinoma.

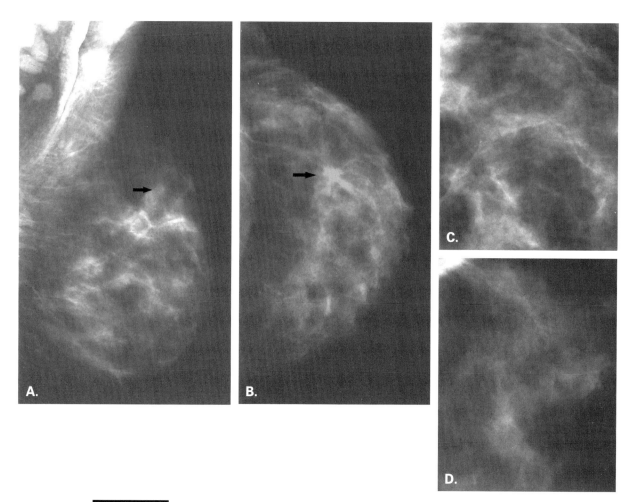

Figure 8.47

HISTORY: A 43-year-old woman for a baseline mammography.

MAMMOGRAPHY: Right MLO **(A)** and CC **(B)** views show the parenchyma to be heterogeneously dense. There is a focal area of distortion **(arrow)** located laterally on the CC view and questionably located superiorly on the MLO view. On spot MLO **(C)** and CC **(D)** views, the area remains somewhat distorted, but it is much less dense. Biopsy was performed using stereotactic guidance via a superior approach.

IMPRESSION: Suspicious for malignancy, BI-RADS® 4.

HISTOPATHOLOGY: Invasive ductal carcinoma.

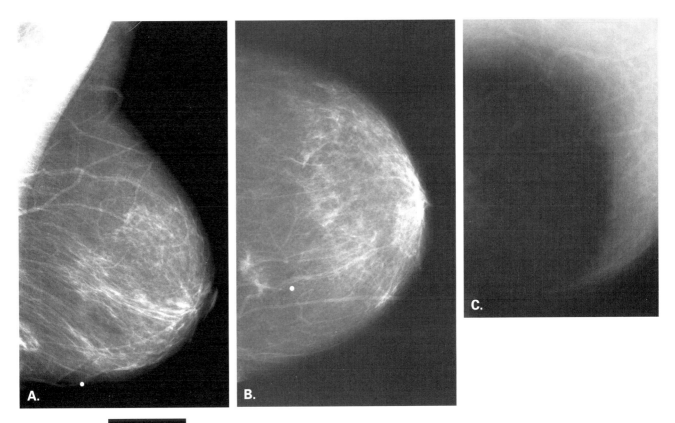

Figure 8.48

HISTORY: A 69-year-old gravida 4, para 4 woman who presents with a soft mass in the inferior aspect of the right breast.

MAMMOGRAPHY: Right MLO (**A**) and CC (**B**) views show a focal asymmetry with distortion in the far posterior aspect of the breast at 5 o'clock. On spot compression (**C**), the area appears less dense, but it persists. Because of the location of the lesion and its appearance, it is very suspicious for malignancy. Also considered in the differential is an inflammatory process, such as a skin infection extending into the parenchyma.

IMPRESSION: Suspicious for carcinoma.

HISTOPATHOLOGY: Invasive ductal carcinoma.

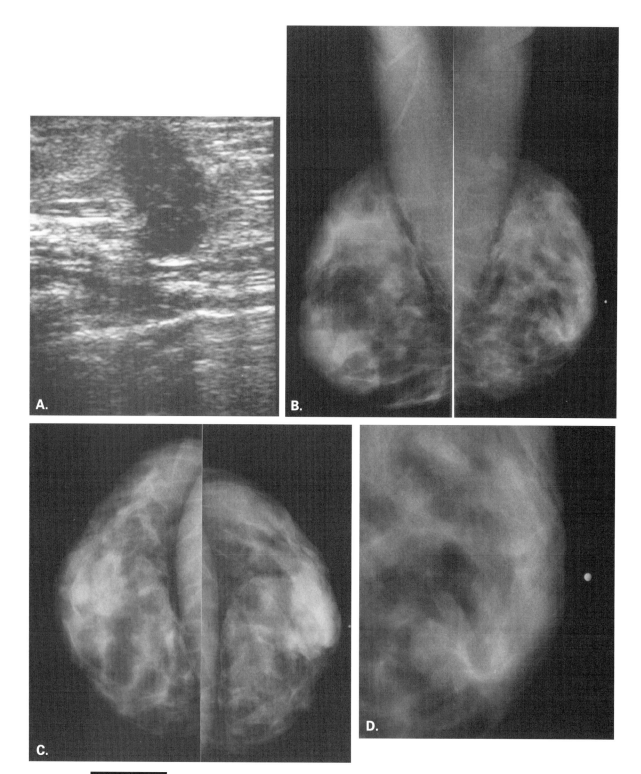

Figure 8.49

HISTORY: A 22-year-old woman with a palpable mass in the right subareolar area.

MAMMOGRAPHY: Right breast ultrasound (**A**) was performed first because of the patient's age. Sonography demonstrates a solid hypoechoic mass that is taller than wide. Sonographic findings of the palpable mass are suspicious for carcinoma. Because of this, bilateral mammography was performed. There is an area of distortion in the right subareolar area seen on MLO (**B**) and CC (**C**) views marked by a BB. The architectural distortion associated with the lesion is evident on the enlarged ML spot image (**D**).

IMPRESSION: Highly suspicious for carcinoma.

HISTOPATHOLOGY: Infiltrating ductal carcinoma.

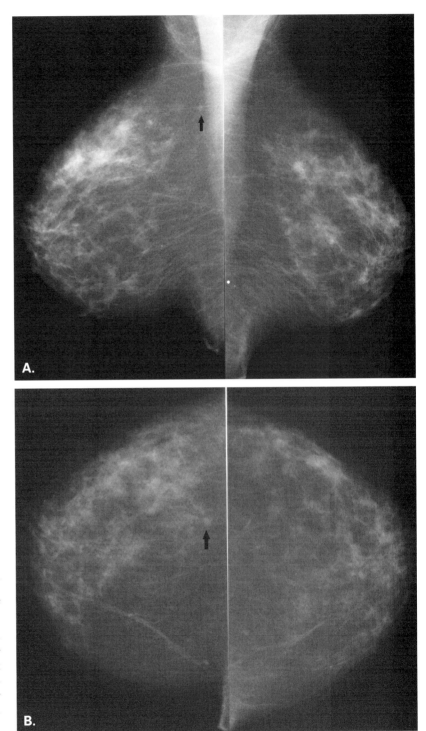

Figure 8.50

HISTORY: A 69-year-old gravida 0, para 0 woman with a positive family history of breast cancer for routine screening.

MAMMOGRAPHY: Bilateral MLO **(A)** and CC **(B)** views show scattered fibroglandular densities. In the posterior aspect of the left breast on the CC view **(B)** is a small indistinct density **(arrow)** that was possibly located superiorly on the MLO **(A, arrow)**. *(continued)*

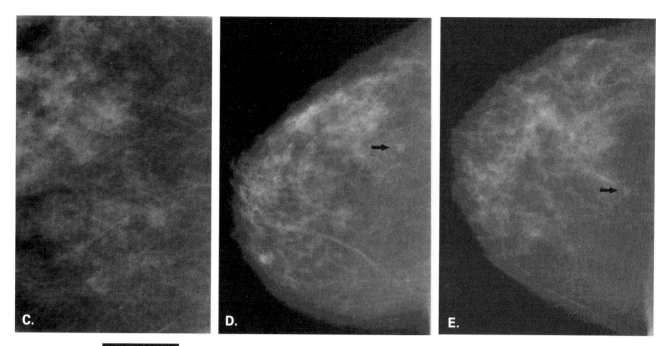

Figure 8.50 *(CONTINUED)*

Spot compression **(C)** shows the spiculation associated with the lesion. Rolled lateral **(D)** and medial **(E)** CC views show that the lesion displaces with the top of the breast, confirming that it is located superiorly.

IMPRESSION: Small density with spiculation, suspicious for malignancy.

HISTOPATHOLOGY: Invasive ductal carcinoma with tubular features.

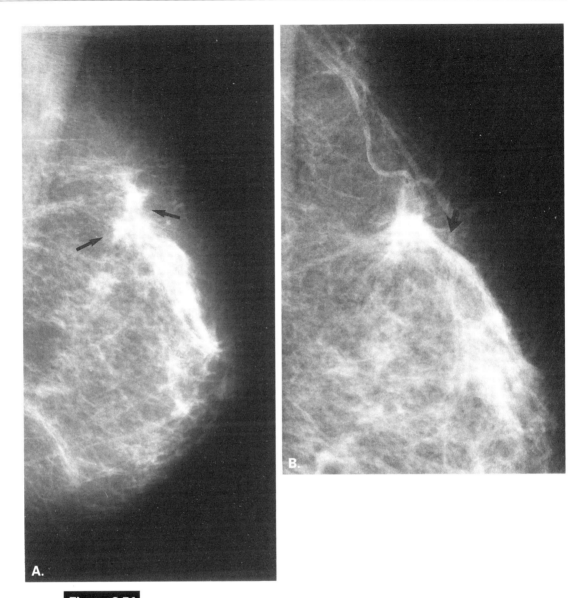

Figure 8.51

HISTORY: A 70-year-old gravida 4, para 4 woman for screening.

MAMMOGRAPHY: Right MLO **(A)** and enlarged (2X) CC **(B)** views. There is minimal residual glandularity present. In the upper outer quadrant, there is an irregular area of increased density that is producing architectural distortion **(A, arrows)**. Fine spicules surround this high-density lesion, and linear stranding appears to pucker **(B, arrow)** the normal fibroglandular tissue inferiorly. The high density of the lesion and its secondary features are consistent with carcinoma.

IMPRESSION: Carcinoma.

HISTOPATHOLOGY: Infiltrating ductal carcinoma, with 18 nodes negative.

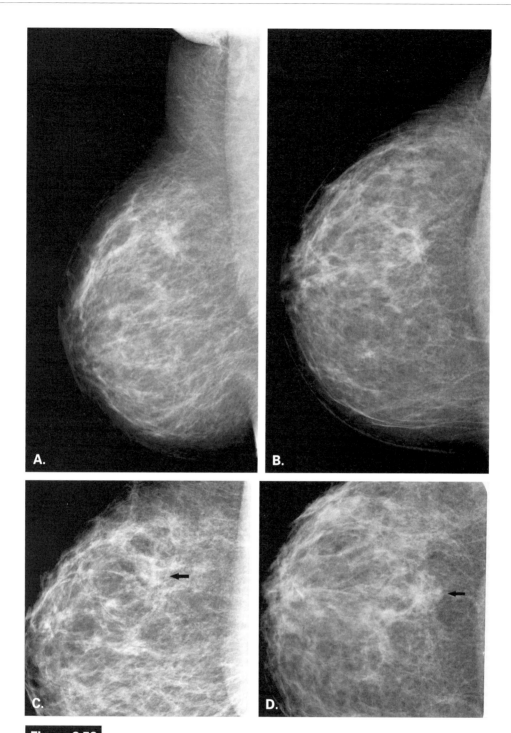

Figure 8.52

HISTORY: A 42-year-old patient for screening mammography.

MAMMOGRAPHY: Left MLO (**A**) and CC (**B**) views show a focal density in the 12 o'clock position. On spot MLO (**C**) and CC (**D**) views, the spiculation and distortion associated with the asymmetry is visible (**arrow**).

IMPRESSION: Suspicious for malignancy.

HISTOPATHOLOGY: Invasive ductal carcinoma.

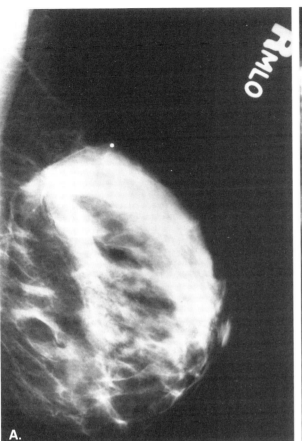

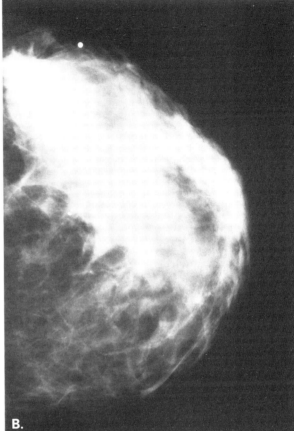

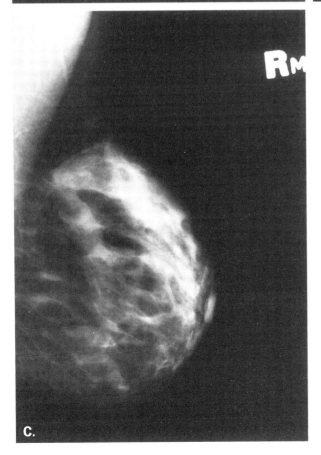

Figure 8.53

HISTORY: Postmenopausal patient who presents with a palpable mass in the right upper-outer quadrant. Prior films from 3 years earlier are available for comparison.

MAMMOGRAPHY: Right MLO (**A**) and CC (**B**) views show architectural distortion in the upper outer quadrant, corresponding to the palpable mass indicated by the BB. On the prior MLO view from 3 years earlier (**C**), the distortion was present (**arrow**) and was less prominent. It was not identified on this earlier study, but it has suspicious features on this study as well as the later one.

IMPRESSION: Right architectural distortion that is palpable and enlarging, highly suspicious for malignancy.

HISTOPATHOLOGY: Invasive ductal carcinoma.

REFERENCES

1. American College of Radiology. *Breast imaging reporting and data system (BI-RADS®).* Reston, VA: ACR, 2003.
2. Logan WW, Janus J. Use of special mammographic views to maximize radiographic information. *Radiol Clin North Am* 1987;25:953–959.
3. Sickles EA. Practical solutions to common mammographic problems: tailoring the examination. *AJR Am J Roentgenol* 1988;151:31–39.
4. Feig SA. Importance of mammographic views to diagnostic accuracy. *AJR Am J Roentgenol* 1988;151:40–41.
5. Sickles SA. Findings at mammographic screening on only one standard projection: outcomes analysis. *Radiology* 1998;208:471–475.
6. Pearson KL, Sickles EA, Frankel SD, et al. Efficacy of step-oblique mammography for confirmation and localization of densities seen on only one standard mammographic view. *AJR Am J Roentgenol* 2000;174:745–752.
7. Kopans DB, Swann CA, White G, et al. Asymmetric breast tissue. *Radiology* 1998;171:639–643.
8. Piccoli CW, Feig SA, Palazzo JP. Developing asymmetric breast tissue. *Radiology* 1999;211:111–117.
9. Brenner RJ. Strategies in the evaluation of breast asymmetries: extended use of rolled view. Appl Radiol 1998;15–22.
10. Stomper PC, Vanvoorhis BJ, Ravnikar VA, et al. Mammographic changes associated with postmenopausal hormone replacement therapy: a longitudinal study. *Radiology* 1990;174:487–490.
11. Rosen PP. *Rosen's breast pathology.* Philadelphia, PA: Lippincott, 2001.
12. Seidman JD, Schnaper LA, Phillips LE. Mastopathy in insulin requiring diabetes mellitus. *Hum Pathol* 1994;25:819–824.
13. Sickles E. Mammographic features of 300 consecutive non-palpable breast cancers. *AJR Am J Roentgenol* 1986;146:661–663.
14. Mendelson EB, Harris KM, Doshi N, et al. Infiltrating lobular carcinoma: mammographic patterns with pathologic correlation. *AJR Am J Roentgenol* 1989;153:265–271.
15. Mendelson EB. Imaging the post-surgical breast. *Semin Ultrasound CT MR* 1989;10(2):154–170.
16. Andersen JA, Gram JB. Radial scar in the female breast: a long-term follow-up study of 32 cases. *Cancer* 1984;53:2557–2560.
17. Fenoglic C, Lattes R. Sclerosing papillary proliferations in the female breast. *Cancer* 1974;33:691–700.
18. Tremblay G, Buell RH, Seemayer TA. Elastosis in benign sclerosing ductal proliferation of the female breast. *Am J Surg Pathol* 1977;1:155–159.
19. Fisher ER, Palekar AS, Kotwal N, et al. A nonencapsulated sclerosing lesion of the breast. *Am J Clin Pathol* 1979;71:240–246.
20. Rickert RR, Kalisher L, Hutter RVP. Indurative mastopathy: a benign sclerosing lesion of breast with elastosis which may simulate carcinoma. *Cancer* 1981;47:561–571.
21. Cohen MI, Matthies HJ, Mintzer RA, et al. Indurative mastopathy: a cause of false positive mammograms. *Radiology* 1985;155:69–71.
22. Wallis MG, Devakumar R, Hosie KB, et al. Complex sclerosing lesions (radial scar) of the breast can be palpable. *Clin Radiol* 1993;48:319–320.
23. Nielsen M, Jensen J, Andersen JA. An autopsy study of radial scar in the female breast. *Histopathology* 1985;9:287–295.
24. Fisher ER, Palekar AS, Kotwal N, et al. A nonencapsulated sclerosing lesion of the breast. *Am J Clin Pathol* 1979;71:240–246.
25. Andersen JA, Gram JB. Radial scar in the female breast: a long-term follow-up study of 32 cases. *Cancer* 1984;53:2557–2560.
26. Vega A, Garijo F. Radial scar and tubular carcinoma: mammographic and sonographic findings. *Acta Radiol* 1993;34:43–47.
27. Andersson I. Mammography in clinical practice. *Med Radiogr Photogr* 1986;62.
28. Orel SG, Evers K, Yeh IT, et al. Radial scar with microcalcifications: radiologic-pathologic correlation. *Radiology* 1992;183:479–482.
29. Tabar L, Dean PB. *Teaching atlas of mammography.* New York: Thieme-Stratton, 1985.
30. Mitnick JS, Vazquez MF, Harris MN, et al. Differentiation of radial scar from scirrhous carcinoma of the breast: mammographic-pathologic correlation. *Radiology* 1989;173:697–700.
31. Frouge C, Tristant H, Guinebretière JM, et al. Mammographic lesions suggestive of radial scars: Microscopic findings in 40 cases. *Radiology* 1995;195:623–625.
31a. Cohen MA, Sferlazza SJ. Role of sonography in evaluation of radial scars of the breast. *AJR Am J Roentgenol* 2000;174:1075–1078.
32. Finlay ME, Liston JE, Lunt LG, et al. Assessment of the role of ultrasound in the differentiation of radial scars and stellate carcinomas of the breast. *Clin Radiol* 1994;49:52–55.
33. Wargotz ES, Norris HJ, Austin RM, et al. Fibromatosis of the breast: a clinical and pathological study of 28 cases. *Am J Surg Pathol* 1987:11(1):38–45.
34. Cederlund CG, Gustavsson S, Linell F, et al. Fibromatosis of the breast mimicking carcinoma at mammography. *Br J Radiol* 1984;57:98–101.
35. Rosen PP, Ernsberger D. Mammary fibromatosis: a benign spindle-cell tumor with significant risk for local recurrence. *Cancer* 1989;63:1363–1369.
36. Peters GN, Wolff M, Haagensen CD. Tubular carcinoma of the breast: clinical pathologic correlations based on 100 cases. *Ann Surg* 1981;193(2):138–149.
37. Winchester DJ, Sahin AA, Tucker SL, et al. Tubular carcinoma of the breast: predicting axillary nodal metastases and recurrence. *Ann Surg* 1996;223(3):342–347.
39. Oberman HA, Fidler WJ Jr. Tubular carcinoma of the breast. *Am J Surg Pathol* 1979;3:386–395.
40. de la Torre M, Lindholm K, Lindgren A. Fine needle aspiration cytology of tubular breast carcinoma and radial scar. Acta Cytol 1994;38(6):884–890.
41. Linell F, Ljungberg O, Anderson I. Breast carcinoma: aspects of early stages, progression and mammographic presentations. *Acta Pathol Microbiol* [A] 1980;272(suppl):1–133.
42. Elson BC, Helvie MA, Frank TS, et al. Tubular carcinoma of the breast: mode of presentation, mammographic appearance, and frequency of nodal metastases. *AJR Am J Roentgenol* 1993;161:1173–1176.
43. Cornil A. Contributions a l'histoire du development histologique des tumeur epitheliale. *Journal de l'anatomie et de la physiologie* 1865;2:226–276.
44. Li CI, Anderson BO, Daling JR, et al. Trends in incidence rates of invasive lobular and ductal breast carcinoma. *JAMA* 2003;289:1421–1424.
45. McDivitt RW, Stewart FW, Berg JW. Tumors of the breast: carcinoma of the mammary lobules. Washington, DC: Armed Forces Institute of Pathology, 1968:63–86.
46. Fisher ER, Gregorio RM, Fisher B. The pathology of invasive breast cancer. *Cancer* 1973;36:1–84.
47. Arpino G, Bardou VJ, Clark GM, et al. Infiltrating lobular carcinoma of the breast: tumor characteristics and clinical outcomes. *Breast Cancer Res* 2004;6:R149–R156.
48. Cornford EJ, Wilson AR, Athanassiou E, et al. Mammographic features of invasive lobular and invasive ductal carcinoma of the breast: a comparative analysis. *Br J Radiol* 1995;68:450–453.
49. Dixon JM, Anderson TJ, Page DL, et al. Infiltrating lobular carcinoma of the breast: an evaluation of the incidence and consequence of bilateral disease. *Br J Surg* 1983;70:513–516.
50. Lesser ML, Rosen PP, Kinne DW. Multicentricity and bilaterality in invasive breast carcinoma. *Surgery* 1982;91:234–240.
51. Hilleren DJ, Andersen IT, Lindholm K, et al. Invasive lobular carcinoma: mammographic findings in a 10-year experience. *Radiology* 1991;178:149–151.

52. Adler OB, Engel A. Invasive lobular carcinoma: mammographic pattern. *Rofo* 1990;152:460–462.
53. Sickles EA. The subtle and atypical mammographic features of invasive lobular carcinoma. *Radiology* 1991;178:25–26.
54. Helvie MA, Paramagul C, Oberman HA, et al. Invasive lobular carcinoma: imaging features and clinical detection. *Invest Radiol* 1993;28:202–207.
55. Krecke KN, Gisvold JJ. Invasive lobular carcinoma of the breast: mammographic findings and extent of disease at diagnosis in 184 patients. *AJR Am J Roentgenol* 1993;161: 957–960.
56. Newstead GM, Baute PB, Toth HK. Invasive lobular and ductal carcinoma: mammographic findings and stage at diagnosis. *Radiology* 1992;184:623–627.
57. Evans WP, Warren Burhenne LJ, Laurie L, et al. Invasive lobular carcinoma of the breast: mammographic characteristics and computer-aided detection. *Radiology* 2002;225:182–189.
58. Moore MM, Borossa G, Imbrie JZ, et al. Association of infiltrating lobular carcinoma with positive surgical margins after breast-conservation therapy. *Ann Surg* 2000;231(6):877–882.
59. Singletary SE, Patel-Parekh L, Bland KI. Treatment trends in early-stage invasive lobular carcinoma: a report from the National Cancer Data Base. *Ann Surg* 2005;242:281–289.
60. Reiff DB, Cooke J, Griffin M, et al. Ductal carcinoma in situ presenting as a stellate lesion on mammography. *Clin Radiol* 1994;49:396–399

Chapter 9

The Thickened Skin Pattern

Thickening of the skin over the surface of the breast may occur in primary inflammatory carcinoma, other malignancies, and several benign conditions. It is important for the radiologist to be aware of ranges for normal thickness and to evaluate the skin carefully on the mammogram to detect an alteration that may be associated with an underlying disease process.

Although the normal skin thickness of the breast has been described as generally less than 1.5 mm (1), a study by Wilson et al. (2) of 150 normal patients showed the range to vary from 0.8 to 3 mm in thickness. In 92% of patients, the medial skin thickness was greater than the lateral skin thickness, and in 91% of patients, the skin was thicker inferiorly than superiorly. The mean thickness of the skin was greater in smaller breasts. In a study of skin thickness in 250 asymptomatic women, Pope et al. (3) found that the medial and inferior aspects of the breast skin were thickest and that the maximum thickness was 2.7 mm. Table 9.1 shows the ranges of skin thickness for different sizes of breasts as determined by Wilson et al. (2).

Edema of the breast is characterized by an increase in skin thickness and prominence of the interstitial or trabecular markings. A thickened skin pattern may occur with primary breast cancers, with metastatic carcinoma to the breast, or in a number of benign conditions (4) (Table 9.2) that cause the interstitium to be distended or edematous.

MALIGNANT CAUSES OF THE THICKENED SKIN PATTERN

Locally Advanced Breast Cancer

Breast cancer may extend locally into the subcutaneous fat and produce focal skin thickening and/or retraction, indicating locally advanced disease (Figs. 9.1–9.3). Dunkley et al. (5) found skin thickening on mammography in 24% of breast cancer patients; in 68% of these patients, the skin thickening seen on mammography was not evident on clinical examination. This thickening of skin is focal and is much less generalized than the skin edema associated with inflammatory carcinoma. In addition, the erythematous pitting edema of inflammatory breast cancer is not usually present in these cases.

Inflammatory breast cancer was described in Bell's surgery text of 1816 (6,7) as "a purple color on the skin over the tumor accompanied by shooting pains." Because of the involvement of the dermis, a diffuse edema pattern with skin thickening is seen in inflammatory carcinoma. Inflammatory cancer can account for 1% to 4% of breast cancers (8), with an average age at onset of 52 years (7). Inflammatory breast cancer is a stage IIIB, locally advanced lesion and has a poor prognosis.

In inflammatory breast cancer, the patient presents clinically with a tender, firm, heavy breast with purplish discoloration and a *peau d'orange* thickening of the skin. The clinical presentation is often indistinguishable from mastitis. A focal mass may be palpable, or the entire breast may be hardened. Biopsy of the skin is used to diagnose this entity; the hallmark pathologic feature is involvement of the dermal lymphatics with tumor emboli.

Mammographically, skin thickening and a marked increase in the density of the breast are seen (Figs. 9.4–9.8). Much of this density is caused by edematous changes in the trabeculae or interstitium of the breast. The breast affected by inflammatory carcinoma is less compressible on positioning for mammography, and the overall size of the breast on the mammogram may appear to be less than the normal breast because of its hardness and lack of compressibility. The underlying tumor mass may be evident on mammography, or the density may be so great because of the edema and the decreased compression of the thickened breast that evaluation of the underlying parenchyma is unsatisfactory.

In a review of 142 cases of pathology-proven inflammatory breast cancer, Günhan-Bilgen et al. (10) found the following manifestations on mammography: skin thickening in 84%, trabecular thickening in 81%, a mass in 16%, an asymmetric focal density in 61%, and microcal-

▌ TABLE 9.1 **Range of Normal Skin Thickness**

Breast Size	Skin Thickness (mm)
Small Breast	
Medial	1.3–2.5
Lateral	1.0–2.2
Superior	1.0–2.0
Inferior	1.4–3.0
Medium Breast	
Medial	1.2–2.7
Lateral	0.8–2.5
Superior	0.9–2.0
Inferior	1.1–3.0
Large Breast	
Medial	1.0–2.8
Lateral	0.9–2.0
Superior	0.8–2.1
Inferior	1.0–3.0

See Reference (2).

cification in 56%. Sonography showed skin thickening in 96% and a solid mass in 80%. Ultrasound was helpful in the depiction of masses that were obscured by the edema pattern as well as in the demonstration of skin and pectoral muscle invasion and axillary involvement. In another series, Kushwala et al. (11) found that mammographic findings of skin and trabecular thickening were common (92% and 62%, respectively) and that masses

▌ TABLE 9.2 **Causes of Skin Thickening**

Benign Causes

Common
Small breasts
Postirradiated breast
Mastitis—acute
Obstruction to lymphatic drainage after axillary node dissection or
    excisional biopsy in the axillary tail of the breast
Hematoma and fat necrosis
Cardiac failure
Renal failure
Hypoalbuminemia

Uncommon
Complication of Coumadin therapy
Unintentional subcutaneous infusion of fluid (5)
Central venous stenosis (9)

Malignant Causes

Locally advanced primary breast cancer—focal thickening
Inflammatory breast cancer—diffuse thickening
Recurrent carcinoma after lumpectomy and radiation therapy
Lymphatic obstruction secondary to metastatic axillary nodes
Metastatic disease to the breast (to breast from nonbreast primaries)
Lymphoma

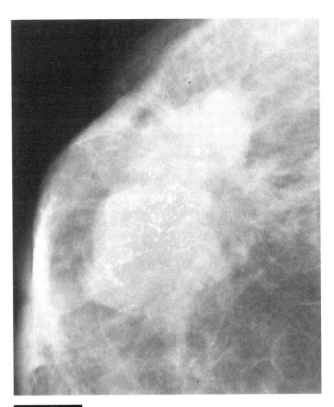

Figure 9.1

HISTORY: A 58-year-old woman with a palpable breast mass and overlying skin retraction.

MAMMOGRAPHY: Left spot CC view shows a large lobular mass with spiculated margins and associated pleomorphic microcalcifications. Overlying skin thickening and retraction are noted, as well as edema surrounding the mass.

IMPRESSION: Carcinoma, locally advanced.

HISTOPATHOLOGY: Invasive ductal carcinoma.

and microcalcifications were uncommon manifestations of inflammatory breast cancer. Dershaw et al. (12), however, found that a vast majority of patients with inflammatory breast cancer had an edema pattern as well as an associated mass or malignant microcalcifications on mammography.

Sonography is often more helpful than mammography in identifying malignant masses in patients with inflammatory breast cancer. Sonography is also useful in defining the extent of inflammatory carcinoma, including the involvement of lymph nodes in the axillary and supraclavicular areas (13). The skin thickness can be measured on sonography, and a decrease in skin thickening can be used to quantify the response to chemotherapy (Figs. 9.9 and 9.10).

(text continues on page 424)

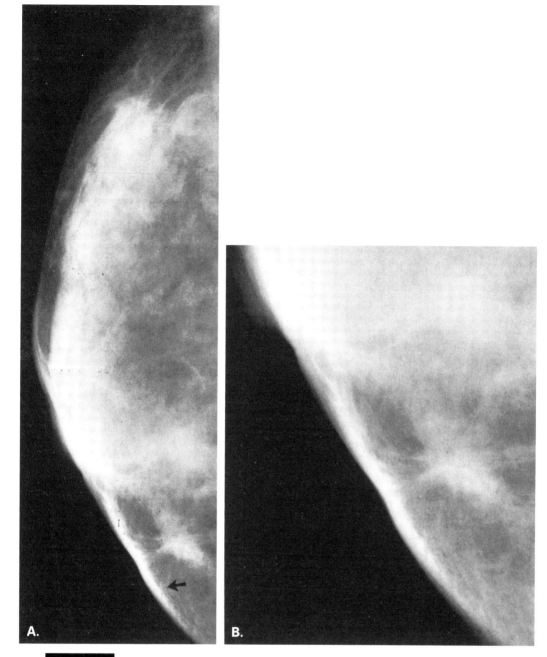

Figure 9.2

HISTORY: A 46-year-old woman for screening.

MAMMOGRAPHY: Left MLO view **(A)** and magnified image **(B)**. The breast is quite dense and glandular. There is focal skin thickening **(arrow)** on the lower aspect of the breast. Beneath the thickening is a 1-cm spiculated mass that is tethering the skin by fine spicules **(B)**.

IMPRESSION: Focal skin thickening associated with underlying carcinoma.

HISTOPATHOLOGY: Infiltrating ductal carcinoma.

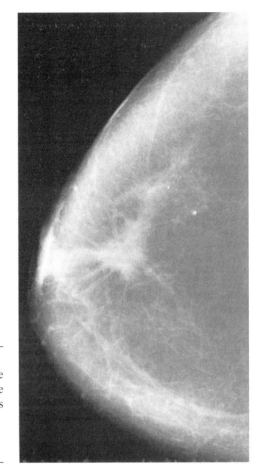

Figure 9.3

HISTORY: A 64-year-old woman with a left breast mass and dimpling of the skin.

MAMMOGRAPHY: Left CC view. A high-density spiculated mass is present in the subareolar area. Long spicules surround the mass and extend anteriorly to the periareolar area, where they tether the skin. Focal prominent skin thickening is seen. The findings are typical of malignancy.

IMPRESSION: Highly suspicious for locally advanced breast cancer.

HISTOPATHOLOGY: Infiltrating lobular carcinoma, with 1 of 16 nodes positive.

Figure 9.4

HISTORY: A 49-year-old woman with swelling of the left breast.

MAMMOGRAPHY: Left CC views **(A)** show generalized increase in density of the left breast with abnormal skin thickening in the periareolar area. The right breast **(B)** has a normal appearance. There is also a spiculated mass **(arrow)** in the medial aspect of the left breast highly suspicious for carcinoma. A prominent asymmetric density is noted laterally, probably also representing malignancy.

IMPRESSION: Inflammatory breast cancer, left breast.

HISTOPATHOLOGY: Multicentric invasive ductal carcinoma with involvement of dermal lymphatics.

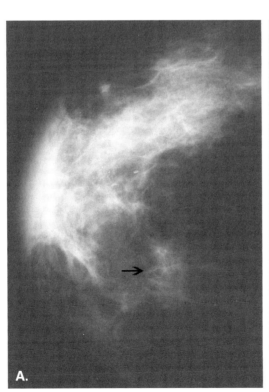

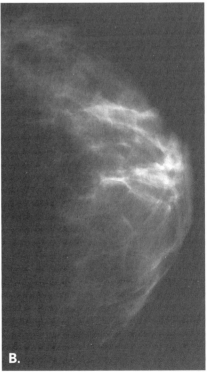

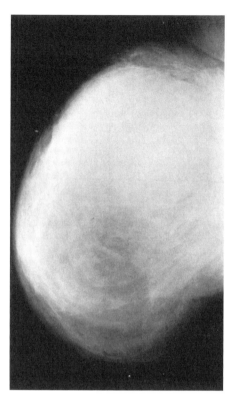
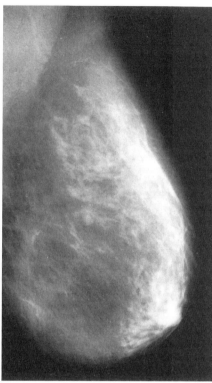

Figure 9.5

HISTORY: A 60-year-old woman who presented with a red, tender, very firm left breast with a 15-cm palpable mass in the upper outer quadrant.

MAMMOGRAPHY: Bilateral MLO views. There is markedly increased density of the left breast relative to the right. Diffuse increase in density of the stroma is noted with marked thickening of the skin diffusely. A large rounded mass is noted in the left upper-outer quadrant.

IMPRESSION: Inflammatory carcinoma.

HISTOPATHOLOGY: Infiltrating ductal carcinoma, with tumor in lymphatics (inflammatory).

NOTE: The concurrent finding of a mass with the marked skin thickening in older patients makes the level of suspicion for carcinoma extremely high.

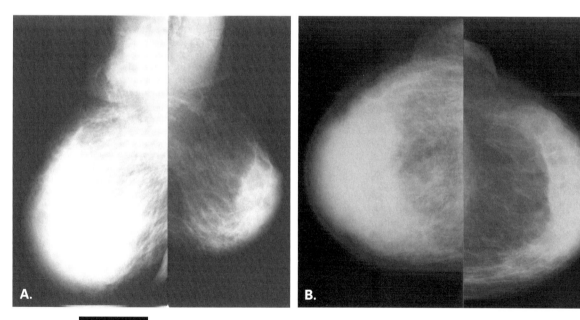

A.   B.

Figure 9.6

HISTORY: A 55-year-old woman reporting swelling and pain in the left breast.

MAMMOGRAPHY: Bilateral MLO **(A)** and CC **(B)** views show marked increase in size and density of the left breast. There is marked skin and trabecular thickening present. Multiple enlarged nodes are also noted in the left axilla.

IMPRESSION: Inflammatory breast cancer with metastatic nodes in the axilla.

HISTOPATHOLOGY: Invasive ductal carcinoma, high nuclear grade, with involvement of dermal lymphatics.

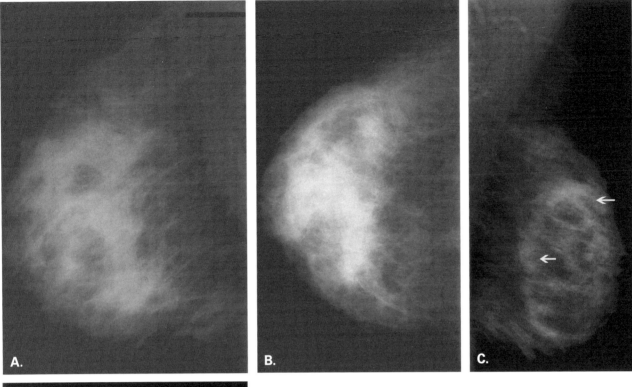

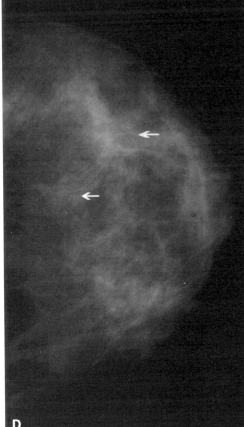

Figure 9.7

HISTORY: A 66-year-old with heaviness of the left breast.

MAMMOGRAPHY: Left MLO **(A)** and CC **(B)** views show marked increase in density with trabecular thickening of the left breast. In addition, in the right breast on the MLO **(C)** and CC **(D)** views are two areas of architectural distortion located laterally **(arrows)**.

IMPRESSION: Edema pattern of the left breast, suspicious for inflammatory carcinoma. Two suspicious lesions right breast. Recommend biopsy.

HISTOPATHOLOGY: Carcinoma left breast involving dermal lymphatics; multicentric invasive lobular carcinoma of the right breast.

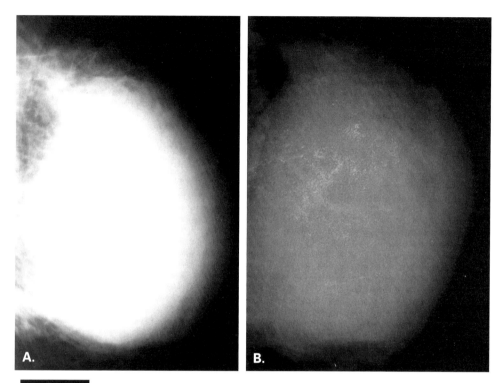

Figure 9.8

HISTORY: Elderly woman with a large palpable mass in the right breast and overlying skin thickening and erythema.

MAMMOGRAPHY: On right MLO **(A)** and CC **(B)** views, there is a large, very-high-density mass that is occupying the breast. The mass contains extensive pleomorphic microcalcifications, and there is marked overlying skin thickening as well.

IMPRESSION: Highly suspicious for inflammatory carcinoma.

HISTOPATHOLOGY: Poorly differentiated carcinoma involving dermal lymphatics.

The mammographic finding of diffuse skin thickening and increase in density of the breast may be present several weeks before the clinically inflammatory signs appear (14). Keller and Herman (15) found that patients with inflammatory cancers had an average skin thickness of 6 mm and diffuse increase in density on mammography, compared with a skin thickness of 9 mm and a prominent reticular pattern in patients with a benign cause of a breast edema pattern. Patients with locally advanced breast cancer and secondary inflammatory changes may have a similar clinical presentation to those patients with inflammatory breast cancer (7)—namely, edema of the breast.

Pathologically, the two are different. In inflammatory breast cancer, tumor emboli are present within dermal lymphatics and cause edema of the skin (Fig. 9.11). In locally advanced breast cancer with skin involvement focally, the dermal lymphatics are not involved with tumor.

On magnetic resonance imaging (MRI), inflammatory breast cancer has been found (16) to have a strong signal on the T_2-weighted images in the retromammary and the subcutaneous area. Rieber et al. (17), however, found that it may be difficult to distinguish inflammatory carcinoma from mastitis based on the presence of edema alone. MRI is helpful in demonstrating other findings in the patient with an edematous breast. Subtracted images will demonstrate the underlying tumor that may not be evident on mammography because of the marked overlying edema and breast density. In addition, the thickened skin will show enhancement on the T_1-weighted postcontrast and subtraction images (Fig. 9.12).

(text continues on page 427)

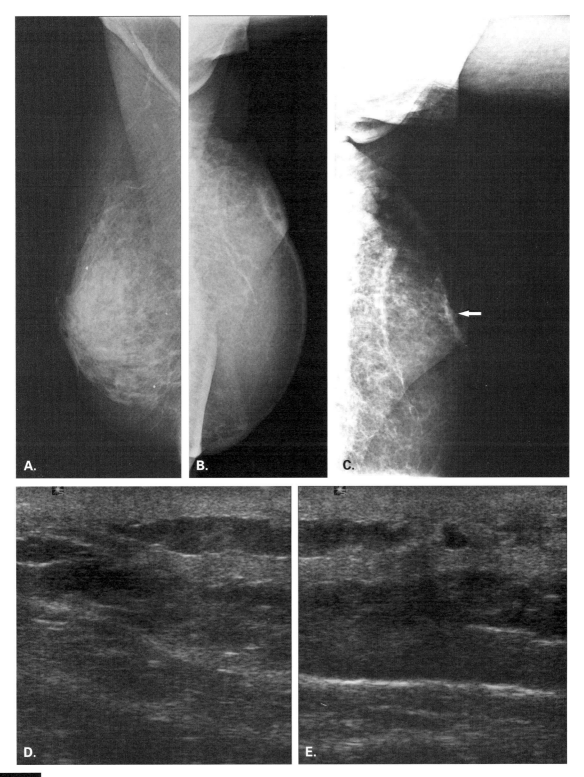

Figure 9.9

HISTORY: A 58-year-old woman who is status post–right mastectomy and breast reconstruction with a transverse rectus abdominis myocutaneous (TRAM) flap. She now presents with a painful, heavy, reconstructed right breast.

MAMMOGRAPHY: Left **(A)** and right **(B)** MLO views show asymmetry of the appearance of the breasts consistent with the history of mastectomy and reconstruction on the right. In the right breast, there is no parenchyma present. The skin appears thickened on the right, and this edema is better demonstrated **(arrow)** on a spot view of the axillary tail **(C)**. Clinical examination demonstrated erythema of the native skin of the breast extending down to the suture line of the TRAM flap. Ultrasound **(D, E)** shows marked edema of the skin. The thickness was greater than 4 mm throughout the area of erythema, suggesting an inflammatory recurrence of carcinoma.

IMPRESSION: Inflammatory carcinoma, recurrent.

HISTOPATHOLOGY: Poorly differentiated carcinoma in dermal lymphatics.

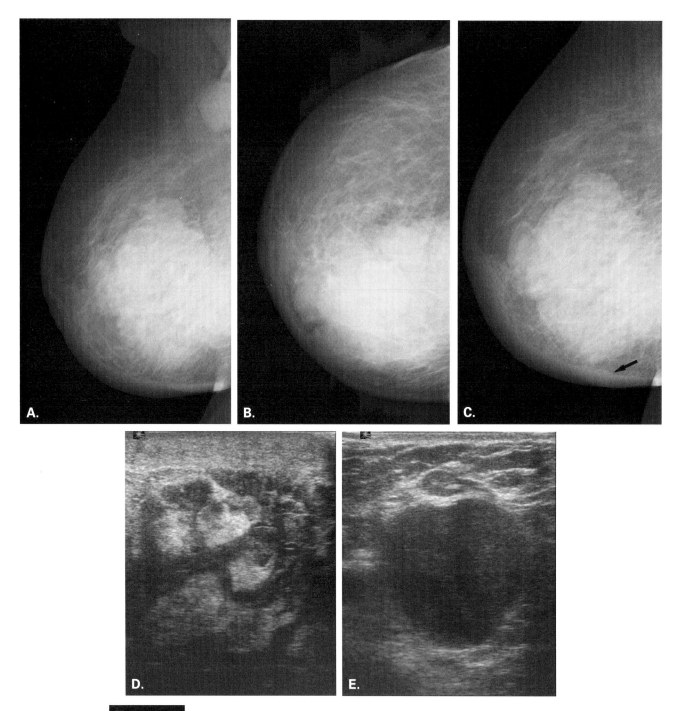

Figure 9.10

HISTORY: A 70-year-old woman who presents with a palpable left breast mass.

MAMMOGRAPHY: Left MLO **(A)** and CC **(B)** views show a large lobulated mass occupying the lower central aspect of the left breast. There is marked skin thickening **(arrow)** associated with the mass **(C)**, as well as diffuse trabecular thickening. The mass is highly malignant in appearance on ultrasound **(D)**. An enlarged, abnormal-appearing lymph node is present in the left axilla on mammography, and the node is also demonstrated on ultrasound **(E)**.

IMPRESSION: Inflammatory carcinoma with axillary nodal metastases.

HISTOPATHOLOGY: Invasive ductal carcinoma poorly differentiated with metastatic disease in the nodes.

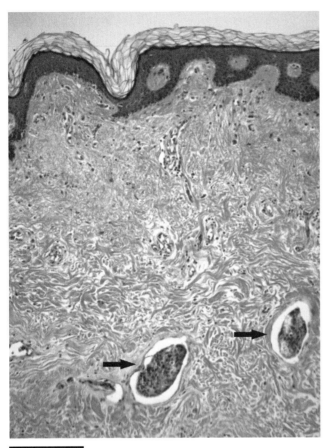

Figure 9.11

Low power histologic section of the skin and subcutaneous tissue showing plugs of malignant cells within dermal lymphatics **(arrows)**. This is the hallmark pathologic feature of inflammatory breast cancer.

Metastatic Disease

Another malignant cause of diffuse skin edema is metastatic disease to the breast from a nonbreast primary carcinoma. Metastatic disease may manifest itself as skin thickening (18) by diffusely invading the dermal lymphatics or by producing impaired lymphatic drainage of the breast by involving the axillary nodes. Lymphangitic metastases to the breast may occur from contralateral breast cancer (19), as well as from other malignancies, including ovarian and endometrial cancers and melanoma (Figs. 9.13 and 9.14).

Lymphomas and pseudolymphomas may produce an appearance of edema secondary to either infiltration of the breast or lymphatic obstruction from malignant axillary nodes. Primary lymphoma of the breast tends to infiltrate the lobules, surrounding and compressing the ducts (20), and mammographically presents as a mass with minimal spiculation (21). Secondary lymphomatous involvement of the breast may produce a focal mass or may present as diffuse increase in density with skin thickening (21). Sabaté et al. (22), in a review of 28 patients with lymphoma, found that unilateral diffuse involvement of the breast occurred in 25% and bilateral diffuse involvement occurred in 8.3% of the cases of primary lymphoma. In secondary lymphoma, diffuse breast involvement occurred in 31.2% of cases. The authors observed an association between high-grade types of malignancy and the diffuse pattern of breast involvement. In a study of 32 cases of non-Hodgkin lymphoma of the breast, Liberman et al. (23) found that mammographic findings of diffuse increased density with skin thickening occurred in 9% of patients.

Pseudolymphoma is a benign pathologic process that resembles malignant lymphoma. In a series of five patients, the presentation of pseudolymphoma was of an enlarging breast mass that was composed of mature lymphoid cells on histologic examination (24). The mammographic manifestations of pseudolymphoma may be a thickened skin pattern (Fig. 9.15).

BENIGN CAUSES OF A THICKENED SKIN PATTERN

Radiotherapy

After therapeutic irradiation of the breast, skin thickening and edema are generally seen (Figs. 9.16–9.18). The findings are most prominent during the first 6 months after treatment and gradually decline, approaching a normal appearance in a variable time period (25–27). Libshitz et al. (25) found that 60% of patients treated with tylectomy and radiation therapy had returned to a normal skin thickness by 2 years and that 80% had returned by 3 years.

If a patient who has been treated with radiation develops a new onset of breast edema with skin thickening after the initial edema has resolved or decreased, the radiologist must be alerted to the possible development of recurrent carcinoma (Fig. 9.19). It is therefore very important in evaluating the mammogram of a treated patient to compare it with the series of pretreatment and posttreatment films. The clinical examination of these patients may, at times, be difficult if the breast becomes firm and fibrotic; therefore, the radiologist must be aware of any changes that may suggest recurrent disease.

Infection

Mastitis may produce focal or diffuse skin edema (Figs. 9.20 and 9.21). Typically, acute mastitis occurs in young

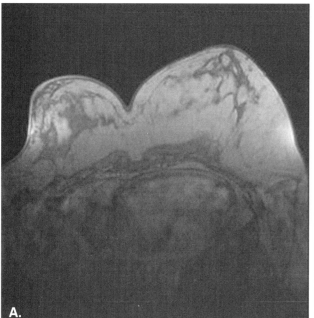 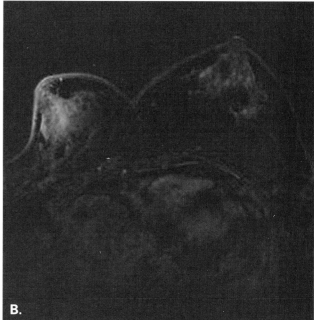

A.   B.

Figure 9.12

HISTORY: A 56-year-old woman who is status postlumpectomy for a small invasive ductal carcinoma of the right breast. She had completed chemotherapy but had not yet begun radiation. Mammography had shown extremely dense breast tissue with no focal abnormalities.

MRI: T_1-weighted postcontrast axial image (**A**) and subtraction image (**B**) show a focal irregular region of enhancement in the lateral aspect of the right breast. This lesion showed rapid washing and washout of contrast on the kinetics curves. There is also skin thickening that enhances in the right breast, particularly laterally.

IMPRESSION: Highly suspicious for residual carcinoma with possible skin involvement.

HISTOPATHOLOGY: Punch biopsy of the skin was performed showing tumor in dermal lymphatics. Subsequent mastectomy showed invasive ductal carcinoma with lymphatic involvement.

---

women and is related to lactation. Common organisms are staphylococcus and treptococcus. Other causes of mastitis are skin or nipple infections with extension into the breast or hematogenous spread of infection. The patient often has a fever and elevated white count.

Diffuse mastitis may be associated with a breast abscess that appears as an ill-defined mass mammographically. In a review of 21 patients with a breast infection, Crowe et al. (28) found that 21% had skin thickening on mammography. Ultrasound may demonstrate a complex mass; aspiration of purulent fluid and positive cultures confirm the diagnosis. The dermal manifestations on biopsy in acute mastitis generally are prominent perivascular and periductal inflammation with or without dilated dermal lymphatics (1). Mastitis should improve soon after implementation of antibiotic therapy. If the symptoms do not clear, one should exclude inflammatory breast cancer and perform a punch biopsy of the skin.

Impaired Lymphatic Drainage

In patients with obstructed lymphatic drainage of the breast from node removal or nodal involvement with neoplasm, skin edema occurs (5). Prominence of the interstitium and thickening of the skin without an underlying mass are present mammographically (Fig. 9.22). Enlarged axillary nodes may be present when neoplastic involvement obstructs lymphatic drainage. After node removal or dissection, edema of the breast may persist mammographically and may be less obvious clinically. If an axillary node dissection is performed for

(text continues on page 437)

Figure 9.13

HISTORY: A 70-year-old woman with a history of endometrial carcinoma, presenting with a painful swollen left breast.

MAMMOGRAPHY: Left ML (**A**) and CC (**B**) views. The left breast is very dense. There is a diffuse edema pattern with a marked increase in skin thickness (**arrow**) and prominence of the interstitium. The primary differentials in this patient are metastatic to the breast, inflammatory breast cancer, and edema secondary to axillary adenopathy.

IMPRESSION: Edema pattern, favoring metastases to the breast from endometrial cancer.

HISTOPATHOLOGY: Endometrial cancer metastatic to the breast.

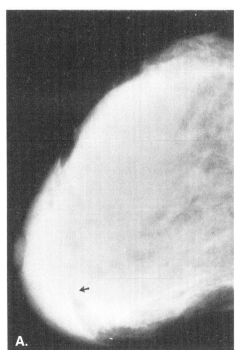
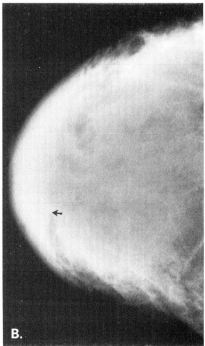

Figure 9.14

HISTORY: A 49-year-old woman with a history of melanoma, presenting with new heaviness and thickening of the left breast.

MAMMOGRAPHY: Left (**A**) and right MLO (**B**) views show marked asymmetry in the appearance of the breasts, with the left being diffusely more dense than the right. There is diffuse skin thickening over the left breast with prominence of the interstitial markings, also seen on the CC view (**C**). Melanoma is a tumor that metastasizes to the breast and should be considered when this mammographic pattern occurs.

IMPRESSION: Metastatic melanoma to the left breast.

HISTOPATHOLOGY: Metastatic melanoma involving breast, skin, and subcutaneous tissue.

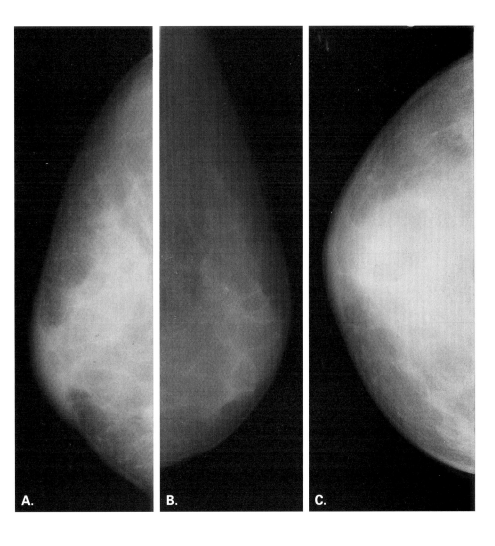

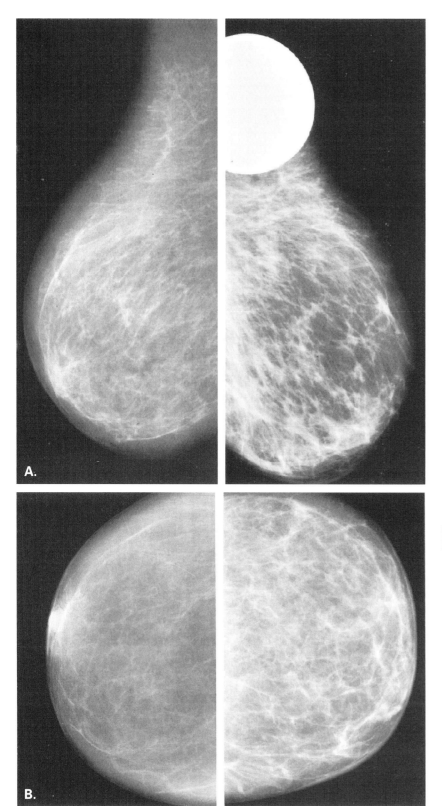

A.

B.

Figure 9.15

HISTORY: An 81-year-old woman with a right parotid gland mass and a right breast mass.

MAMMOGRAPHY: Bilateral MLO (**A**) and CC (**B**) views. There is generalized asymmetry between the breasts. The right breast is more dense, and there is a prominence of interstitial markings. There is slight skin thickening inferiorly. With the history of parotid gland tumor, one might consider metastatic disease to the breast or lymphoma or pseudolymphoma as high in the differential diagnosis.

HISTOPATHOLOGY: Lymphocytic infiltration of the breast (lymphoma found in the parotid gland). (Case courtesy of Dr. Melvin Vinik, Richmond, VA.)

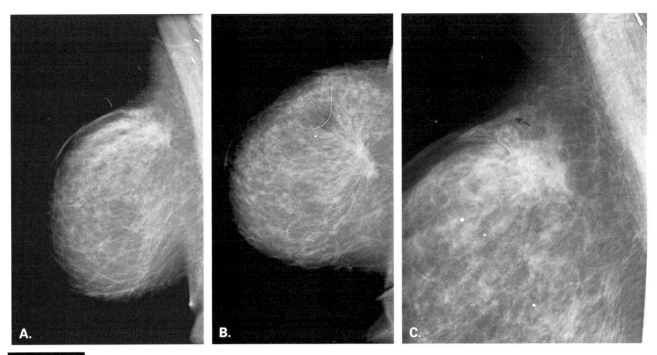

Figure 9.16

HISTORY: A 64-year-old woman who is 2 years status postlumpectomy and breast irradiation for invasive ductal carcinoma.

MAMMOGRAPHY: Left MLO **(A)** and CC **(B)** views show a postsurgical scar appearing as an area of architectural distortion in the 12 o'clock position. Diffuse skin thickening and trabecular thickening are present, as well as focal skin thickening and retraction **(arrow)** at the lumpectomy site, seen best on the magnification MLO view **(C)**. These changes were less prominent than on the prior posttreatment studies.

IMPRESSION: Edema pattern secondary to radiation therapy.

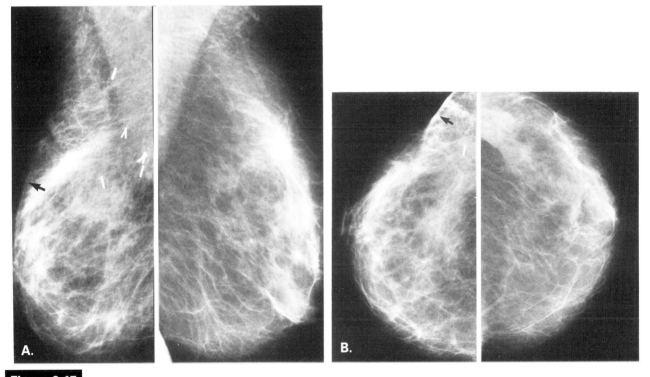

Figure 9.17

HISTORY: A 65-year-old woman 6 months after lumpectomy and radiotherapy for ductal carcinoma in situ in the left upper-outer quadrant.

MAMMOGRAPHY: Bilateral MLO views **(A)** and bilateral CC views **(B)**. There is diffuse increased density with interstitial edema involving the left breast. Surgical clips in the upper outer quadrant mark the lumpectomy site. Skin thickening is present **(arrow)** diffusely on the treated side. The diffuse changes are related to radiotherapy and are maximum on this study. The edema gradually decreases over time and approaches a normal skin thickness and breast density.

IMPRESSION: Skin thickening and interstitial thickening secondary to radiotherapy.

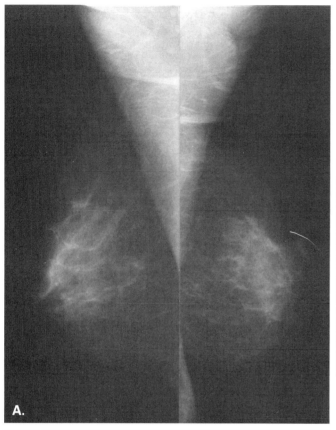

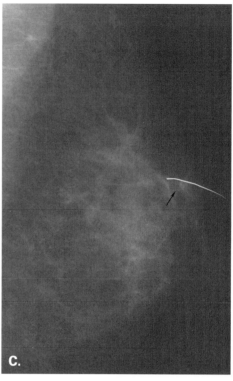

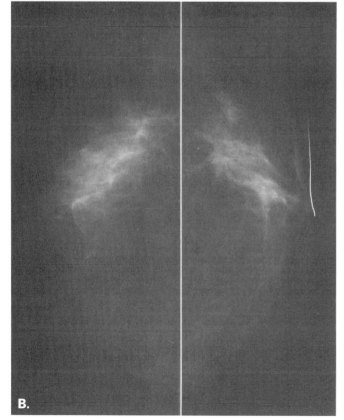

Figure 9.18

HISTORY: A 63-year-old woman status post-lumpectomy and radiation therapy for right breast cancer.

MAMMOGRAPHY: Bilateral MLO **(A)** and CC **(B)** views show a scar marker at the lumpectomy site. There is architectural distortion at the site, consistent with scar. Diffuse and focal skin thickening is present, related to the surgical scarring and the radiation effect. On the magnification view **(C)**, the architectural distortion is evident **(arrow)**.

IMPRESSION: Normal postlumpectomy and radiation changes.

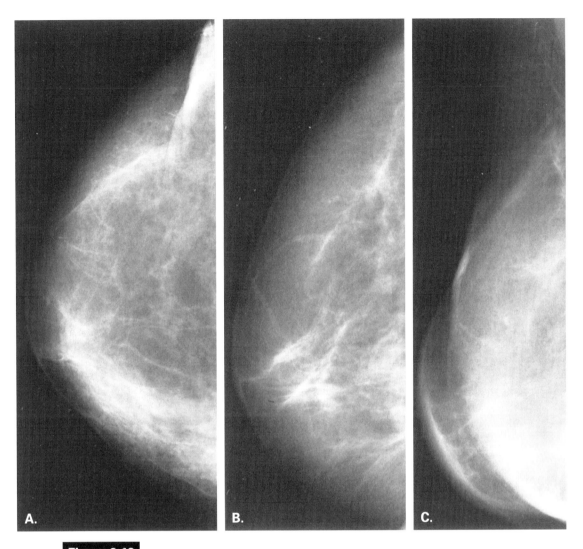

Figure 9.19

HISTORY: A 55-year-old woman who, in March 1982, had lumpectomy and radiation therapy for a carcinoma in the lower inner quadrant of the left breast. In 1985, she returned with an increase in thickness of the left breast.

MAMMOGRAPHY: Left ML (**A**) and CC (**B**) views in 1982 and left MLO view in 1985 (**C**). Three months after treatment, there is increased density of the trabeculae with mild skin thickening. There is focal increased density remaining at the lumpectomy site, presumed to be related to resolving hematoma. Three years later, on the left MLO view (**C**), there is marked skin thickening with greater density of the breast diffusely near the chest wall.

IMPRESSION: Recurrent carcinoma after lumpectomy and radiation therapy.

HISTOPATHOLOGY: Infiltrating ductal carcinoma.

NOTE: The skin thickening and edema of the breast that occur after radiation therapy are greater in the months immediately following treatment, and the changes gradually resolve over several years. The development of new skin thickening should alert the radiologist to the possible development of recurrent carcinoma. When the treated breast is being evaluated, it is very important to review the entire series of mammograms after treatment for subtle changes in skin thickness or parenchymal density.

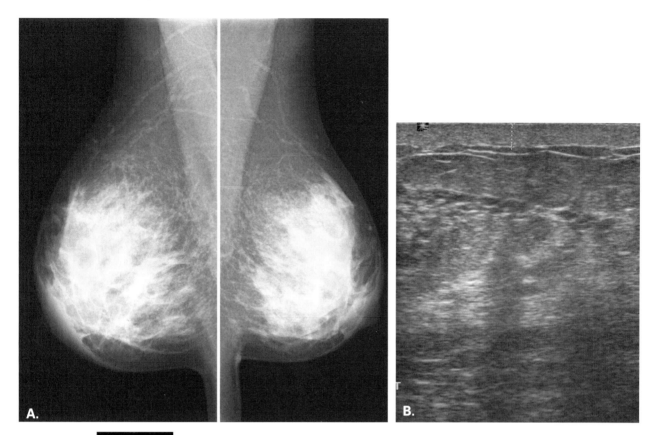

Figure 9.20

HISTORY: A 26-year-old woman who is 7 months pregnant and who presents with a painful, swollen, tender left breast. Clinical examination showed mild erythema in the periareolar area with mild skin thickening in this region.

MAMMOGRAPHY: Bilateral MLO **(A)** views show a mild degree of skin thickening, primarily in the left periareolar area. No underlying mass or calcifications were present. Sonography **(B)** showed thickening of the skin as well as edema in the subcutaneous tissue.

IMPRESSION: Mastitis.

MANAGEMENT: The patient was treated with oral antibiotics and improved symptomatically. Follow-up clinical examination and ultrasound showed resolution of the edematous changes. It is important to follow a possible mastitis to complete resolution, often also with follow-up imaging, to assure that malignancy is not present.

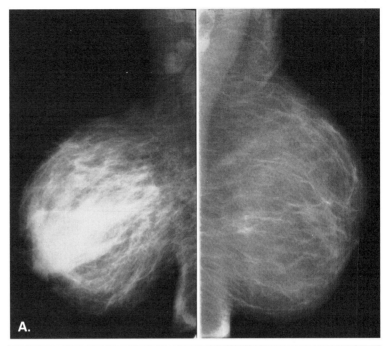

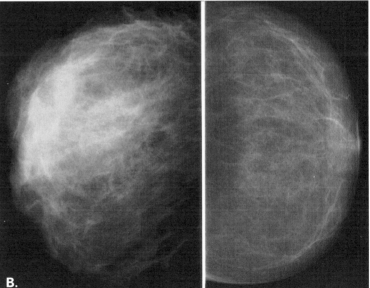

Figure 9.21

HISTORY: A 52-year-old gravida 4, para 4 woman presenting with fever, chills, and a large hard mass in the left breast.

MAMMOGRAPHY: Bilateral MLO (**A**) and CC (**B**) views. There is marked asymmetry in the appearance of the breasts. The left breast is diffusely dense with prominent interstitial markings. The left breast appears smaller than the right because of the thickening present and the lesser degree of compressibility of the tissue. Enlarged nodes are present in the left axilla. The differential diagnosis includes primarily acute mastitis versus inflammatory breast cancer. The extensive nature of the process is suspicious for neoplasm, but because of the patient's constitutional symptoms, mastitis is more likely.

HISTOPATHOLOGY: Fat necrosis, acute inflammation, abscess.

NOTE: The patient was treated with antibiotics, and the clinical examination returned to normal.

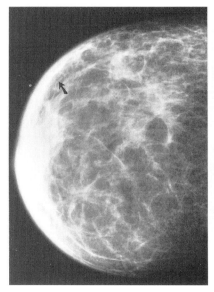

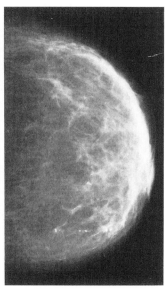

Figure 9.22

HISTORY: An 82-year-old gravida 1, para 1 woman with a history of melanoma. Clinical examination showed enlarged tender lymph nodes in the axilla and firmness diffusely throughout the left breast.

MAMMOGRAPHY: Bilateral CC views. Marked asymmetry in the appearance of the breasts is noted. There is diffuse increase in the density of the interstitium of the left breast with marked skin thickening **(arrow)**. Skin thickening in a patient with a history of melanoma could represent diffuse metastatic involvement of the breast with melanoma or edema secondary to lymphatic obstruction from axillary adenopathy. (Biopsy of the breast and axillary dissection were performed).

HISTOPATHOLOGY: Metastatic melanoma in 38 of 40 lymph nodes with no involvement of the breast.

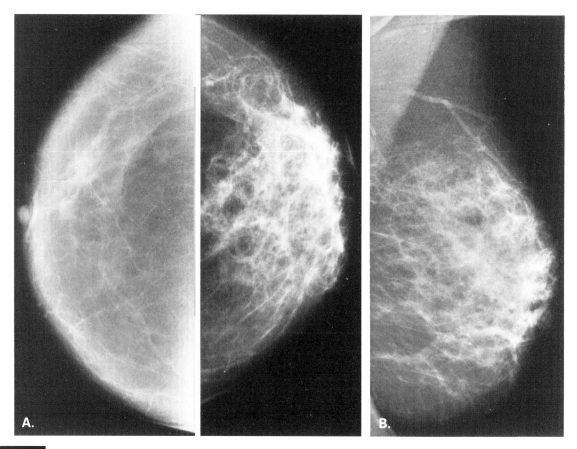

Figure 9.23

HISTORY: An 82-year-old gravida 5, para 5 woman with severe breast trauma to the right breast 6 months earlier, presenting with a right breast mass, which was unchanged in size since the trauma.

MAMMOGRAPHY: Bilateral CC **(A)** and right MLO **(B)** views. There is marked asymmetry in the appearance of the breasts **(A)**, with the right being diffusely more dense than the left. Prominence of the interstitium is present on the right **(A and B)**, but no significant skin thickening is noted. Given the clinical history, this finding is most consistent with a diffuse interstitial hematoma with fat necrosis. The time for resolution of a hematoma is variable, and late changes of fat necrosis may be palpated as a firm mass.

IMPRESSION: Interstitial hematoma with fat necrosis.

NOTE: The breast was biopsied because of clinical concern about the palpable finding, and the biopsy showed fat necrosis.

metastatic disease (i.e., melanoma) and skin thickening occurs, it is often impossible to determine on mammography if the finding represents metastatic involvement of the breast or impaired lymphatic drainage from surgery.

Sometimes lumpectomy or surgery that involves the upper outer quadrant or the axillary tail can also produce a mild degree of chronic breast edema. This condition is related to impaired lymph drainage caused by transection of lymphatic channels in the upper outer quadrant. The edematous changes may be evident clinically and mammographically.

Trauma

Fat necrosis and interstitial hematoma of the breast may produce focal or diffuse skin thickening. Generally, the edema is focal unless the trauma is severe or the hemorrhage is extensive (Fig. 9.23). Clinical history is key in suggesting the diagnosis, because posttraumatic changes with skin involvement may have an identical appearance with that of

locally advanced breast cancer. Patients who have been treated with Coumadin for thromboembolic disorders may develop acute breast necrosis, appearing mammographically as an edema pattern (29). Burns to the chest area with scarring can also produce prominent skin thickening of a chronic nature, and this is usually not associated with interstitial thickening (Figs. 9.24 and 9.25). There may be distortion of the normal breast contour because of contractures.

Fluid Overload

Systemic conditions that produce a fluid overload state are manifested in the breast as bilateral diffuse skin thickening (Figs. 9.26–9.30). Cardiac failure, renal failure, cirrhosis, and hypoalbuminemia are other benign causes of a thickened skin syndrome (5). In these patients, the breasts may feel heavy, and there is edema noted on clinical examination with a *peau d'orange*

(text continues on page 442)

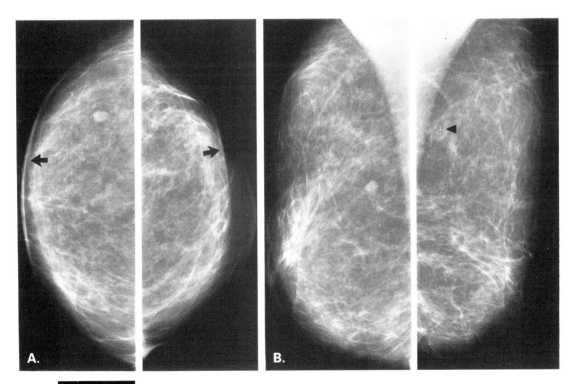

Figure 9.24

HISTORY: A 36-year-old gravida 4, para 4 woman who had suffered burns to the anterior chest area years ago, for screening mammography.

MAMMOGRAPHY: Bilateral CC **(A)** and MLO **(B)** views. There is distortion of the contour of the breasts bilaterally, with retraction centrally. Skin thickening **(arrows) (A)** is present bilaterally, consistent with scarring from the burns. Coarse dystrophic skin calcification, probably secondary to the scarring, is present on the right **(arrowhead) (B)**. Incidental note is made of a well-defined nodule in the left upper-outer quadrant, which was found to be cystic on ultrasound.

IMPRESSION: Skin thickening secondary to a burn injury.

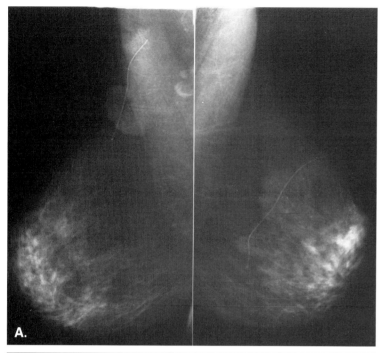

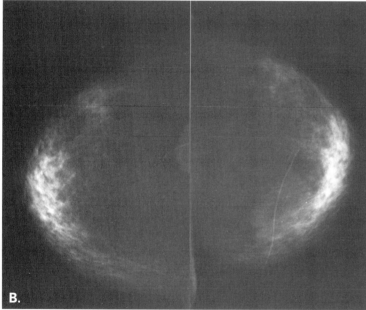

Figure 9.25

HISTORY: A 70-year-old woman with a history of benign breast biopsies for screening mammography.

MAMMOGRAPHY: Bilateral MLO (**A**) and CC (**B**) views show very-well-defined densities bilaterally, marked with wires indicating the biopsy sites. These densities have very defined edges, suggesting that the lesions are on the skin and are demarcated by an air halo. Clinical examination confirmed keloids.

IMPRESSION: Keloids at biopsy sites causing focal skin thickening.

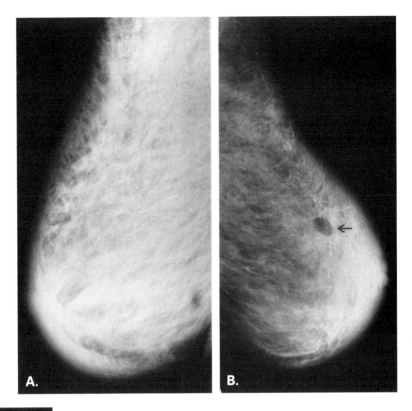

Figure 9.26

HISTORY: An 81-year-old woman with thickening of the left breast and no focal palpable mass.

MAMMOGRAPHY: Left MLO **(A)** and right MLO **(B)** views. There is bilateral skin thickening, worse on the left **(A)** than on the right **(B)**. A diffuse edema pattern is noted with thickening of the interstitial markings of the breasts. Incidental note is made of a small lipoma **(arrow)** in the right breast. The differential diagnosis for bilateral asymmetric skin thickening includes systemic causes, such as fluid overload states, congestive heart failure, renal failure, metastatic disease to the breast, and hemorrhage secondary to anticoagulant therapy.

IMPRESSION: Congestive heart failure producing an edema pattern in the breasts.

NOTE: The patient had been lying on the left side, presumably accounting for the asymmetric edema on the left.

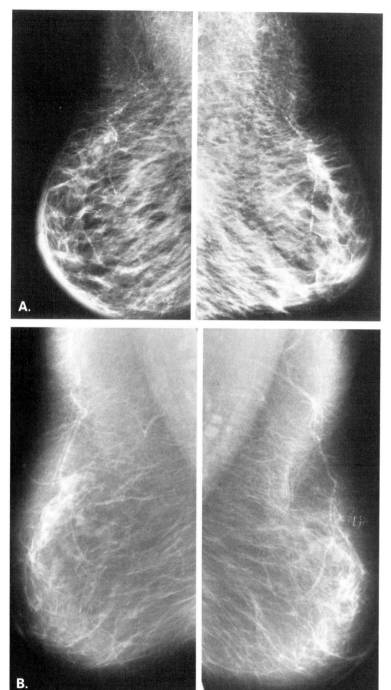

Figure 9.27

HISTORY: A 75-year-old woman for screening mammography. She has a history of chronic renal failure secondary to an allergic reaction to penicillin.

MAMMOGRAPHY: Bilateral MLO views **(A)** and bilateral MLO views before the onset of renal failure **(B)**. The breasts show a symmetrical edema pattern **(A)** characterized by increased interstitial markings and skin thickening. These findings were not present on the baseline mammogram **(B)**. Diffuse bilateral edema suggests a systemic origin and in this case is secondary to renal failure. There is a fluid overload state and an increase in thickness of the interstitium by this fluid filling.

IMPRESSION: Edema pattern secondary to renal failure. (Case courtesy of Dr. Cherie Scheer, Richmond, VA.)

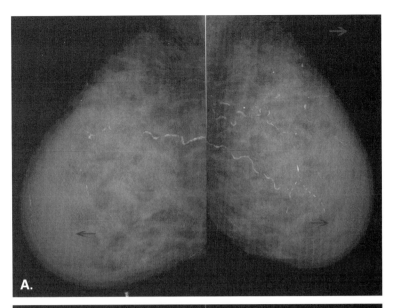

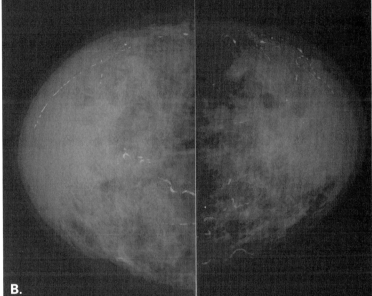

Figure 9.28

HISTORY: A 43-year-old woman with end-stage renal disease.

MAMMOGRAPHY: Bilateral MLO **(A)** and CC **(B)** views show marked increased density of both breasts. There is an edema pattern with marked skin thickening **(arrows)** and trabecular thickening. The thickness of the skin exceeds 10 mm bilaterally. Extensive arterial and punctuate calcifications are present bilaterally, associated with the renal failure and hypercalcemic state.

IMPRESSION: Edema pattern and arterial calcifications consistent with renal failure and fluid overload.

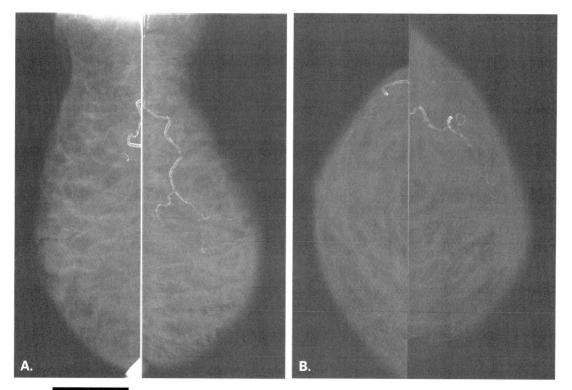

Figure 9.29

HISTORY: A 54-year-old woman with a history of renal disease, for screening mammography.

MAMMOGRAPHY: Bilateral MLO **(A)** and CC **(B)** views show extensive vascular calcifications in both breasts and a marked edema pattern. There is skin thickening and trabecular thickening diffusely and bilaterally, suggesting a systemic etiology.

IMPRESSION: Edema pattern and vascular calcifications consistent with renal disease and fluid overload.

appearance. However, the breasts are usually not8 erythematous or tender, and no mass is palpable. The thickening occurs mostly in the dependent aspect of the breast. If the patient has been lying on one side, the edema is unilateral in the dependent breast (30).

SUMMARY

The range of normal skin thickness varies from patient to patient, with the inferior and medial aspects of the breasts being thicker. When skin thickening is present, whether focally or diffusely, mammography and physical examination are important to the radiologist in suggesting the probable cause. Unilateral edema is caused by impairment of lymph drainage, as seen in mastitis, postradiation change, axillary lymphatic obstruction, and inflammatory carcinoma. A bilateral edema pattern

suggests a systemic etiology, such as congestive heart failure or renal failure.

Other image modalities, such as ultrasound and MRI, are particularly helpful in the patient with unilateral edema of unknown etiology. These may identify a suspicious mass in the patient with inflammatory carcinoma when the edema obscures the mass on mammography. If mastitis is suspected, treatment with antibiotics is performed, with immediate follow-up mammography and physical examination to assure complete resolution of the edema. The persistence of symptoms after 2 weeks should prompt biopsy of the skin to exclude inflammatory carcinoma.

In patients with bilateral edema, clinical examination and medical history are most helpful in identifying the etiology. In these patients with systemic causes of edema, mammography alone and no other imaging modalities are usually necessary to evaluate the breasts.

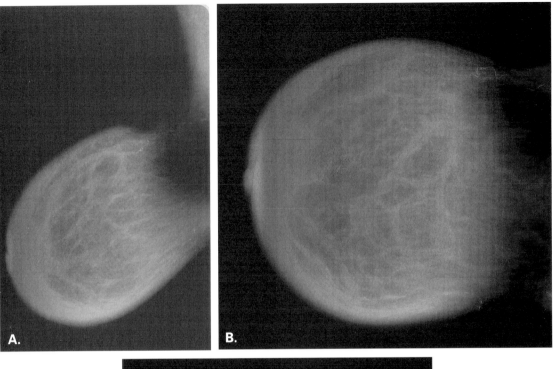

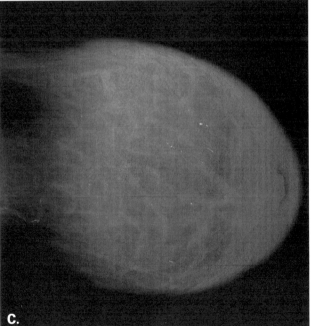

Figure 9.30

HISTORY: Elderly patient with a history of cardiac insufficiency, for screening mammography. Clinical examination showed mild pitting edema of the breasts with no erythema.

MAMMOGRAPHY: Left MLO (**A**) and left CC (**B**) and right CC (**C**) views show marked trabecular and skin thickening bilaterally, consistent with an edema pattern. There are also extensive vascular calcifications bilaterally.

IMPRESSION: Edema pattern secondary to congestive heart failure.

REFERENCES

1. Gold RH, Montgomery CK, Minagi H, et al. The significance of mammary skin thickening in disorders other than primary carcinoma: a roentgenologic-pathologic correlation. *AJR Am J Roentgenol* 1971;112:613–621.
2. Wilson SA, Adam EJ, Tucker AK. Patterns of breast skin thickness in normal mammograms. *Clin Radiol* 1982;33:691–693.
3. Pope TE Jr, Read ME, Medsker T, et al. Breast skin thickness: normal range and causes of thickening shown on film-screen mammography. *J Can Assoc Radiol* 1984;35:365–368.
4. Andersson I. Mammography in clinical practice. *Med Radiogr Photogr* 1986;62(2):1–41.
5. Dunkley B, Frankl G, Haile RWC, et al. The importance of skin thickening in breast cancer. *Breast Dis* 1988;1:205–210.
6. Bell C. *A System of Operative Surgery*, vol. 2. Hartford, CT: Hale & Hasmer, 1816:136.
7. Parker LM, Boyages J, Eberlein TJ. Inflammatory carcinoma of the breast. In: Harris JR, Hellman S, Henderson IC, et al., eds. *Breast Diseases*. 2nd ed. Philadelphia: Lippincott, 1991;775–782.
8. Swain SM, Lippman M. Locally advanced breast cancer. In: Bland KI, Copeland EM, eds. The Breast: *Comprehensive Management of Benign and Malignant Diseases*. Philadelphia: Saunders, 1991;843–862.
9. Kuerer AM, Wilson MW, Bowersox JC. Innominate vein stenosis mimicking locally advanced breast cancer in a dialysis patient. *Breast J* 2001;7(2):128.
10. Günhan-Bilgen I, Üstün EE, Memis A. Inflammatory breast carcinoma: mammographic ultrasonographic, clinical, and pathologic findings in 142 cases. *Radiology* 2002;223:829–838.
11. Kushwaha AC, Whitman GJ, Stelling CB, et al. Primary inflammatory carcinoma of the breast: retrospective review of mammographic findings. *AJR Am J Roentgenol* 2000;174:535–538.
12. Dershaw DD, Moore MP, Liberman L, et al. Inflammatory breast carcinoma: mammographic findings. *Radiology* 1994;190:831–834.
13. Whitman GJ, Kushwaha AC, Cristofanilli M, et al. Inflammatory breast cancer: current imaging perspectives. *Semin Breast Dis* 2001;4(3):122–131.
14. Droulias CA, Sewell CW, McSweeney MB, et al. Inflammatory carcinoma of the breast: a correlation of clinical, radiologic and pathologic findings. *Ann Surg* 1976;184:217–222.
15. Keller RJ, Herman G. Unilateral edema simulating inflammatory carcinoma of the breast. *Breast Dis* 1990;3:61–74.
16. Yasumura K, Ogawa K, Ishikawa H, et al. Inflammatory carcinoma of the breast: characteristic findings of MR imaging. *Breast Cancer* 1997;4(3):161–169.
17. Rieber A, Tomczak RJ, Mergo PJ, et al. MRI of the breast in the differential diagnosis of mastitis versus inflammatory carcinoma and follow-up. *J Comput Assist Tomogr* 1997;21:128–132.
18. Bohman LG, Bassett LW, Gold RH, et al. Breast metastases from extramammary malignancies. *Radiology* 1982;144:309.
19. Kwak JY, Kim EK, Chung SY, et al. Unilateral breast edema: spectrum of etiologies and imaging appearances. *Yonsei Med J* 2005;46(1):1–7.
20. Mambo NC, Burks JS, Butler JJ. Primary malignant lymphomas of the breast. *Cancer* 1977;39:2033–2040.
21. Meyer JE, Kopans DB, Long JC. Mammographic appearance of malignant lymphomas of the breast. *Radiology* 1980;135:623–626.
22. Sabaté JM, Gomez A, Torrubia S, et al. Lymphoma of the breast: clinical and radiologic features with pathologic correlation in 28 patients. *Breast J* 2002;8(5):294–304.
23. Liberman L, Giess CS, Dershaw DD, et al. Non-Hodgkin lymphoma of the breast: imaging characteristics and correlation with histopathologic findings. *Radiology* 1994;192:157–160.
24. Lin JJ, Farha GJ, Taylor RJ. Pseudolymphoma of the breast. I. In a study of 8,654 consecutive tylectomies and mastectomies. *Cancer* 1980;45:973–978.
25. Libshitz HI, Montague ED, Paulus DD. Skin thickness in the therapeutically irradiated breast. *AJR Am J Roentgenol* 1978;130:345–347.
26. Dershaw DD, Shank B, Reisinger S. Mammographic findings after breast cancer treatment with local excision and definitive irradiation. *Radiology* 1987;164:455–461.
27. Mendelson EB. Evaluation of the postoperative breast. *Radiol Clin North Am* 1992;30:107–138.
28. Crowe DJ, Helvie MA, Wilson TE. Breast infection: mammographic and sonographic findings with clinical correlation. *Invest Radiol* 1995;30(10):582–587.
29. Anderssen I, Adler DD, Ljungberg O. Breast necrosis associated with thromboembolic disorders. *Acta Radiol* 1987;28:517–521.
30. Oraedu CO, Pinnapureddy P, Alrawi S, et al. Congestive heart failure mimicking inflammatory breast carcinoma: a case report and review of the literature. *Breast J* 2001;7(2):117–119.

The Axilla

On routine mammography, the low axilla is visualized, and a variety of normal and abnormal findings in this region may be identified. Physical examination is extremely important in the evaluation of the axilla, particularly in the assessment of adenopathy and fixation of nodes associated with breast carcinoma. In addition to lymph nodes, a breast lesion occurring in the axillary tail may be identified as a mass on mammography.

AXILLARY LYMPH NODES

The axillary lymph nodes are divided into three levels based on their anatomic relationship to the pectoralis minor muscle: level I nodes are inferior to the pectoralis minor muscle, level II nodes are posterior to the muscle, and level III nodes are medial to the muscle.

On the routine mediolateral oblique (MLO) view, lymph nodes in the low to middle axillary region can normally be identified. An additional axillary view can yield more information about the upper aspect of the axilla, which may not be seen on the routine MLO projection. This is particularly important when a palpable mass is present and is not identified on mammography. However, three-dimensional imaging such as computed tomography (CT) or magnetic resonance imaging (MRI) are superior to mammography in visualizing the level I, II, and III nodal systems (1). Even so, CT has been found to have a sensitivity for tumor detection in axillary nodes of 50%, because in about one half of cases of metastases to the axilla, the tumor is a micrometastasis and occurs in normal-sized nodes (2).

Normal axillary nodes are very-well-defined, medium- to low-density nodules that are less than 1.5 cm in diameter (3) unless fatty replaced. Lymph nodes are round, ovoid, elliptical, or bean shaped. A lucent notch or center is often seen, representing fat in the hilum. This finding helps to confirm the diagnosis of a lymph node (Figs. 10.1–10.3). On ultrasound, normal nodes are well-defined, oval, hypoechoic masses with a central echogenic area representing the fatty hilum (Fig. 10.4). Malignant nodes may have eccentric cortical widening (4), an irregular border, and be enlarged, particularly in anteroposterior diameter (Fig. 10.5).

Lipomatosis or fatty infiltration occurs in axillary nodes and is commonly seen in older patients. The fat distends the capsule and enlarges the node, and the surrounding lymphoid tissue atrophies (5). On mammography, these nodes are crescentic and mainly fat containing, often demonstrating only a thin rim of cortex. The node may be 3.5 cm or more in length and be normal when fatty replaced (1,6,7).

In 1965, Leborgne et al. (5) described six patterns of fatty infiltration of nodes. The fatty replacement may occur centrally or eccentrically, producing densities of nodal tissue described as ring, sickle, or crescent in shape. As the fatty infiltration increases, the rim of the lymphoid tissue narrows, eventually leaving a distended capsule surrounding a fatty center (5). Large fatty-infiltrated nodes are more commonly seen in elderly obese women (3).

ADENOPATHY

When approaching adenopathy in the axillae, it is important to try to determine if the process is unilateral or bilateral (Table 10.1). Bilateral adenopathy suggests a systemic etiology that is benign or malignant. Unilateral adenopathy suggests a local or regional abnormality related to the breast or arm, such as breast cancer, mastitis, or an infection in the arm. Although systemic conditions may be associated with nodes that are asymmetrically enlarged, the approach to adenopathy based on unilateral versus bilateral involvement is most helpful in suggesting further management.

In a review of 94 patients with axillary abnormalities, Walsh et al. (7) found that in most cases, benign and malignant nodes could not be differentiated from each other by mammography. In this study, 76 of 94 patients had axillary lymphadenopathy, and the causes were as

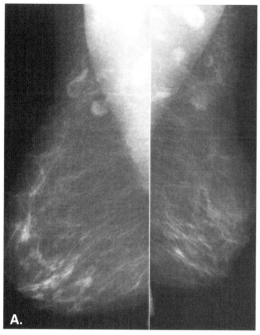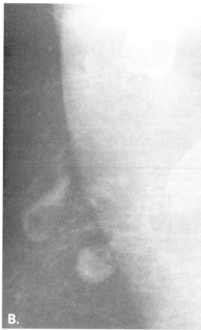

Figure 10.1

HISTORY: A 68-year-old woman for screening.

MAMMOGRAPHY: Bilateral MLO views **(A)** show prominent lymph nodes in both axillae. A coned-down image **(B)** shows the nodes to have a normal appearance. They are well defined, reniform, with central fatty hila, all features of benign nodes.

IMPRESSION: Normal axillary nodes.

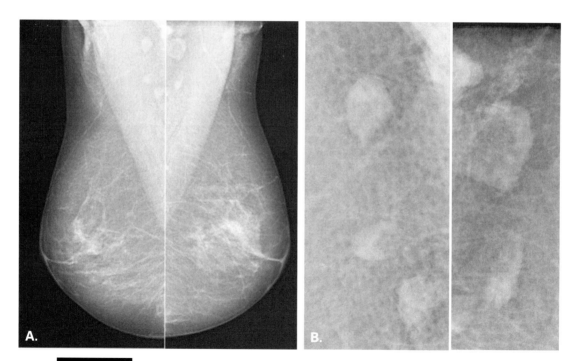

Figure 10.2

HISTORY: A 64-year-old woman for screening.

MAMMOGRAPHY: Bilateral MLO views **(A)** and enlarged images of the axillae **(B)** show normal-appearing nodes. These nodes are crescentic and well circumscribed with fatty hila.

IMPRESSION: Normal axillary nodes.

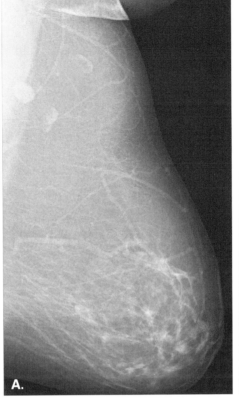

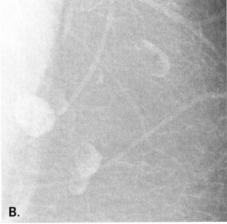

Figure 10.3

HISTORY: A 61-year-old woman for screening.

MAMMOGRAPHY: Right MLO view **(A)** shows multiple normal-sized lymph nodes in the axilla. On the enlarged image **(B)**, the very-well-defined reniform shapes are seen.

IMPRESSION: Normal fatty-replaced axillary nodes.

A.

B.

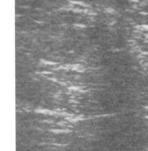

Figure 10.4

HISTORY: A 48-year-old woman for screening.

ULTRASOUND: Ultrasound of a low axillary mass shows it to be hypoechoic, elliptical, with a hyperechoic focus, consistent with the fatty hilum of a node.

IMPRESSION: Lymph node.

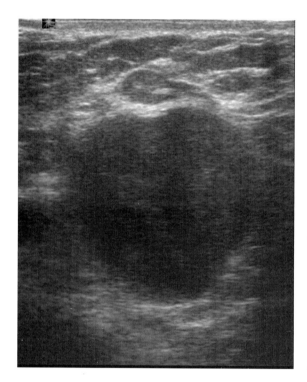

HISTORY: A 72-year-old woman with a large palpable mass in the left breast and a lump in the axilla.

ULTRASOUND: Sonography of the axillary mass shows a large hypoechoic lesion that is taller than wide. The margins are somewhat indistinct, and the lesion is markedly hypoechoic, all features suspicious for malignancy.

IMPRESSION: Metastatic disease in the axillary node.

HISTOPATHOLOGY: Metastatic ductal carcinoma involving a node.

follows: benign lymphadenopathy in 29%, metastatic breast cancer in 26%, chronic lymphocytic leukemia or well-differentiated lymphocytic lymphoma in 17%, and other causes (including collagen vascular disease, human immunodeficiency virus [HIV], sarcoidosis, nonbreast

metastases) in 28%. Lymph nodes that were not fatty replaced and larger than 33 mm, those that had spiculated margins, and those that contained intranodal microcalcifications were likely malignant.

When unilateral lymph nodes enlarge on otherwise normal mammograms, the etiology is most often benign. This is particularly so if there is no history of malignancy, the change in node size is small, and the node maintains a benign appearance (8). Lee et al. (8) in a study of 24 patients with unilateral enlarging nodes found that two had malignant biopsies. One of these patients had lymphoma and one had melanoma, and in both patients the size increase was greater than 100%.

Inflammatory nodes are usually dense, enlarged, and with defined margins (3). Coarse calcification may occur particularly with granulomatous infections. In sarcoidosis, enlarged axillary lymph nodes may occur as a manifestation of the generalized adenopathy that occurs in 23% to 50% of patients (9) (Figs. 10.6–10.8). Another inflammatory cause of axillary adenopathy is tuberculosis (10,11). The affected nodes in tuberculosis are usually unilateral and are large and dense on mammography. The margins are variable, and the nodes may be matted.

In patients with silicone implants, the rupture of the implant with extravasation of silicone may be associated with painful ipsilateral lymphadenopathy (Fig. 10.9). The nodes often contain the hyperdense deposits of free silicone that are associated with the leaking implant. Histologic evaluation of these nodes may reveal "silicone-induced granulomatous adenitis" (12). Other

▶ TABLE 10.1 Etiologies of Axillary Adenopathy

Unilateral Adenopathy
Metastatic breast cancer
Mastitis
Infection in the ipsilateral arm
Metastases from nonbreast primaries (melanoma)
Silicone induced adenitis

Bilateral Adenopathy
Lymphoma
Metastases
Sarcoidosis
Rheumatoid arthritis
Systemic lupus erythematosus
Scleroderma
Psoriasis
Sjögrens disease
Cat-scratch disease
Mononucleosis
Human immunodeficiency virus
Tuberculosis
Silicone-induced granulomatous adenitis
Lymphoid hyperplasia

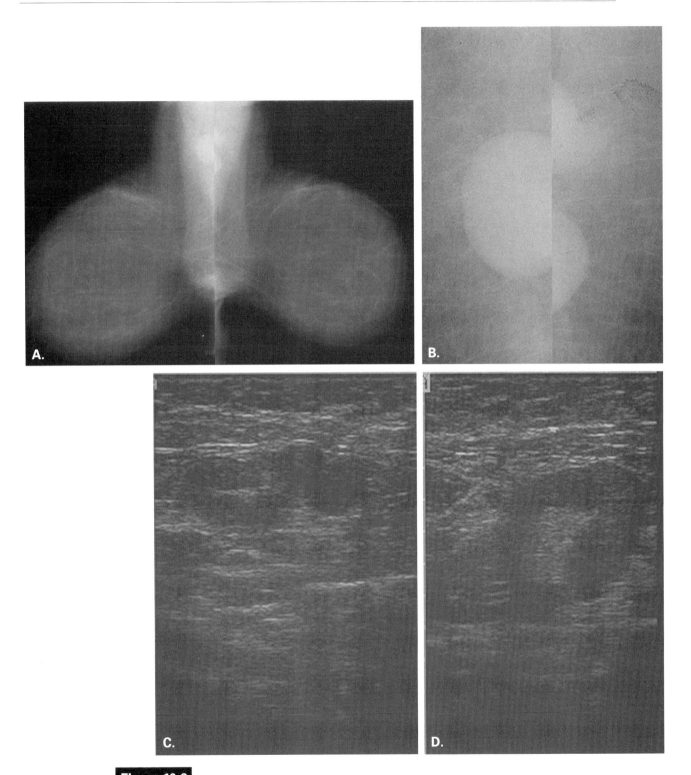

Figure 10.6

HISTORY: A 38-year-old woman with a history of sarcoidosis for screening mammography.

MAMMOGRAPHY: Bilateral MLO views **(A)** show mildly enlarged lymph nodes in both axillae. On the enlarged image **(B)**, the nodes are dense and very well defined. On ultrasound of the left **(C)** and right **(D)** axillae, the nodes are hypoechoic and lobulated, with fatty hila evident.

IMPRESSION: Mild adenopathy secondary to sarcoidosis.

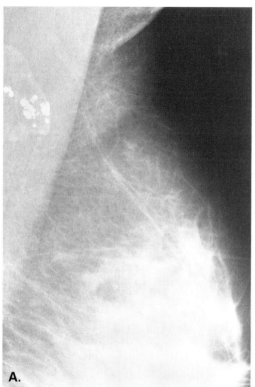

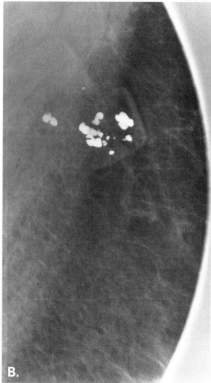

Figure 10.7

HISTORY: A 71-year-old gravida 2, para 2 woman with a lump in the left breast.

MAMMOGRAPHY: Right MLO (**A**) and enlarged (1.5×) axillary (**B**) views. There is an enlarged, fatty-replaced lymph node in the right axilla. Coarse calcification is present, consistent with previous granulomatous infection.

IMPRESSION: Granulomatous calcification in an axillary node.

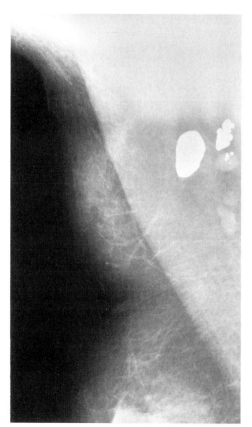

Figure 10.8

HISTORY: A 61-year-old gravida 0 woman for screening.

MAMMOGRAPHY: Left axillary view. There are three nodes in the left axilla that contain calcifications. Two of the nodes are completely calcified, and the third contains dense round calcifications. The finding is most consistent with old granulomatous infection.

IMPRESSION: Calcified axillary nodes secondary to old granulomatous changes.

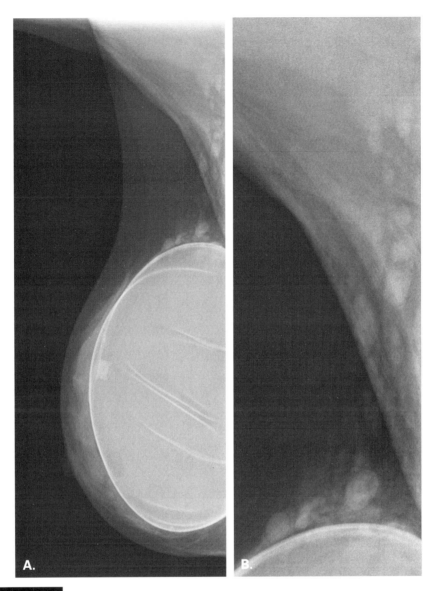

Figure 10.9

HISTORY: A 51-year-old woman with saline implants who previously had silicone implants that were removed.

MAMMOGRAPHY: Left MLO view **(A)** and enlarged image **(B)** show a prepectoral saline implant. There is residual free silicone present in the axillary tail, with silicone-laden lymph nodes being noted as well.

IMPRESSION: Silicone-laden lymph nodes from prior rupture.

inflammatory or infectious conditions associated with adenopathy include mastitis or infections in the arm, cat scratch disease, HIV (Figs. 10.10 and 10.11), and mononucleosis.

Axillary lymphadenopathy occurs in patients with rheumatoid arthritis (13–15), along with the generalized lymphadenopathy that occurs in about 50% to 80% of patients with the disease. Palpable enlarged nodes have

been found in a majority of patients with rheumatoid arthritis (Figs. 10.12 and 10.13) and are mostly located in the axillae (15). Abnormal axillary nodes in patients with rheumatoid arthritis are characterized by rounded shapes, higher density, little or no fatty replacement, and sizes of greater than 1 cm (14). Other arthritides and collagen vascular diseases associated with axillary adenopathy are psoriasis (Figs. 10.14 and 10.15), systemic lupus

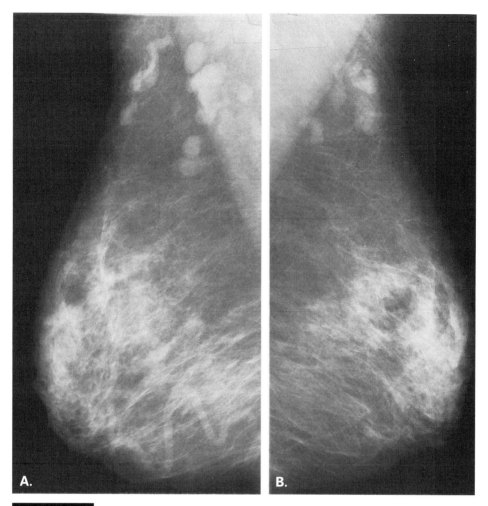

Figure 10.10

HISTORY: Baseline screening mammogram on a patient who is HIV positive.

MAMMOGRAPHY: Left **(A)** and right **(B)** MLO views show mildly enlarged axillary lymph nodes bilaterally. No breast abnormalities were found. The findings are consistent with the patient's history of acquired immunodeficiency syndrome (AIDS).

IMPRESSION: Adenopathy related to AIDS.

erythematosus (Figs. 10.16 and 10.17), scleroderma (14), and Sjögren's disease (Fig. 10.18). The frequency of palpable adenopathy in patients with lupus has been found to be 69%. In most cases of adenopathy related to collagen vascular disease, the nodes are slightly enlarged and more dense than normal nodes.

Malignant involvement of axillary nodes may occur as a result of primary lymphomatous tumors, metastatic disease from breast cancer, and metastatic disease from nonbreast primaries. An important first step in the evaluation of axillary adenopathy is to determine if the finding is unilateral or bilateral. Bilateral adenopathy is more typical of lymphoma, and unilateral adenopathy raises the concern for metastatic breast cancer that is involving the axilla.

In lymphoma, the involved axillary nodes are enlarged (greater than 2.5 cm) and dense (Figs. 10.19–10.23). The pericapsular fat line bordering the nodes is not obliterated (16). This finding is important in differentiating a primary lymph node tumor from metastatic involvement. The nodes are dense but retain their shape and are well marginated (3). Most often, the adenopathy is bilateral, and the nodes may be quite large and bulky, but they retain their smooth margination. In lymphoid hyperplasia, the adenopathy demonstrated on mammography cannot be distinguished from that found in lymphoma.

Metastatic nodes from breast carcinoma are generally enlarged (2–2.5 cm or more) (3), dense, and rounded (17)

(text continues on page 460)

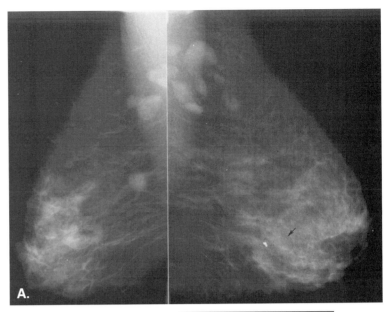

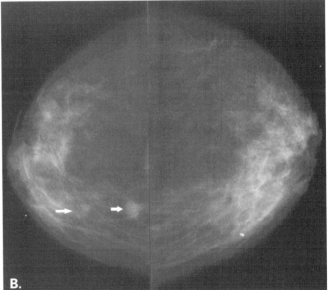

Figure 10.11

HISTORY: A 64-year-old for screening mammography. Patient had a history of being HIV positive.

MAMMOGRAPHY: Bilateral MLO **(A)** and CC **(B)** views show a high-density indistinct mass in the left breast at 11 o'clock. Two spiculated masses are seen in the left breast medially **(white arrows)** on the enlarged left CC **(C)** view. Bilateral adenopathy is seen, which may be related to the patient's history of AIDS or to metastatic breast cancer. On the right at 3 o'clock are multiple groups of amorphous microcalcifications **(arrow)**.

IMPRESSION: Left breast carcinoma, right breast calcifications, suspicious for malignancy. Bilateral adenopathy which may be related to AIDS or metastatic breast cancer.

HISTOPATHOLOGY: Invasive ductal carcinoma left breast; ductal carcinoma in situ and lobular carcinoma in situ right breast; negative left axillary nodes for metastatic disease.

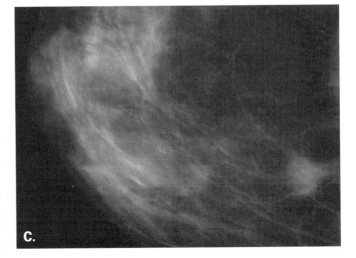

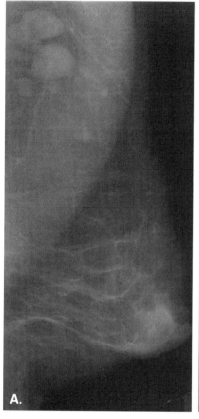

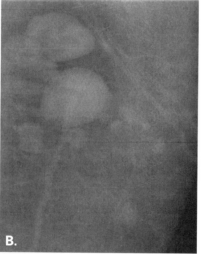

Figure 10.12

HISTORY: A 70-year-old woman with a history of rheumatoid arthritis, for screening mammography.

MAMMOGRAPHY: Right MLO view **(A)** shows multiple mildly enlarged lymph nodes in the axilla. On the enlarged image **(B)**, the nodes are very well defined, and in some the fatty hila are noted. The finding of enlarged lymph nodes was present bilaterally.

IMPRESSION: Mild adenopathy consistent with history of rheumatoid arthritis.

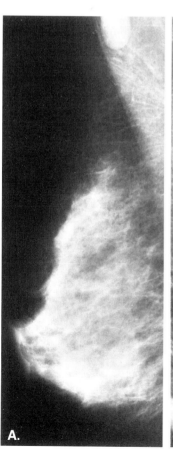

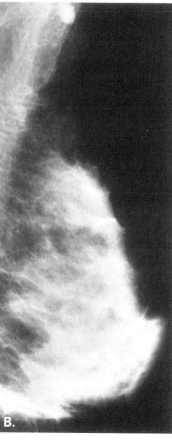

Figure 10.13

HISTORY: A 46-year-old woman with a history of rheumatoid arthritis, for screening mammography.

MAMMOGRAPHY: Left MLO **(A)** and right MLO **(B)** views. The breasts are dense for the age and parity of the patient. In the axillae bilaterally are non–fatty-replaced lymph nodes. The node on the right is not, by strict criteria, enlarged, but the node on the left is clearly greater than 1.5 cm. The adenopathy is consistent with the patient's known history of rheumatoid arthritis and is not suspicious.

IMPRESSION: Bilateral adenopathy secondary to rheumatoid arthritis.

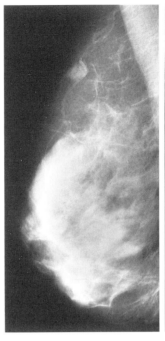
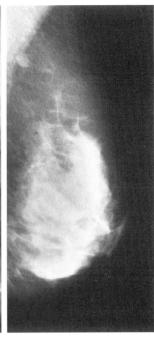

Figure 10.14

HISTORY: A 67-year-old gravida 4, para 4 woman with a history of psoriasis, for screening mammography.

MAMMOGRAPHY: Bilateral MLO views. Dense parenchyma is present bilaterally, with the right breast being smaller than the left. There are enlarged lymph nodes in both low axillary areas, consistent with benign adenopathy related to the patient's known psoriasis.

IMPRESSION: Benign adenopathy secondary to psoriasis.

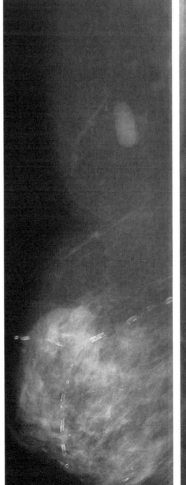
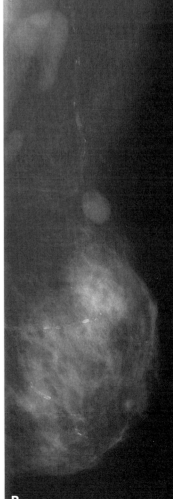

Figure 10.15

HISTORY: Screening mammogram on a patient with a history of psoriasis.

MAMMOGRAPHY: Left **(A)** and right **(B)** MLO views show mildly enlarged lymph nodes in both axillae. This appearance is consistent with the adenopathy related to psoriasis.

IMPRESSION: Adenopathy secondary to psoriasis.

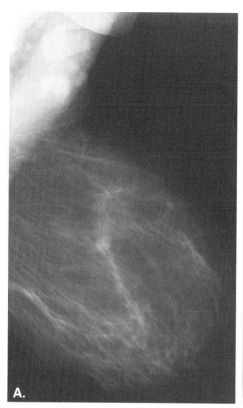

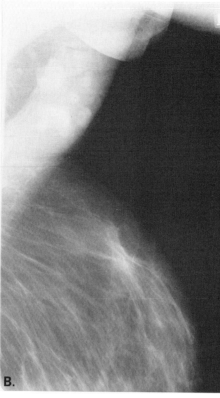

Figure 10.16

HISTORY: A 41-year-old woman with a history of lupus erythematosus for screening mammography.

MAMMOGRAPHY: Right MLO (A) and axillary (B) views show mildly enlarged lymph nodes in the axilla, consistent with the history of lupus.

IMPRESSION: Mild adenopathy secondary to lupus.

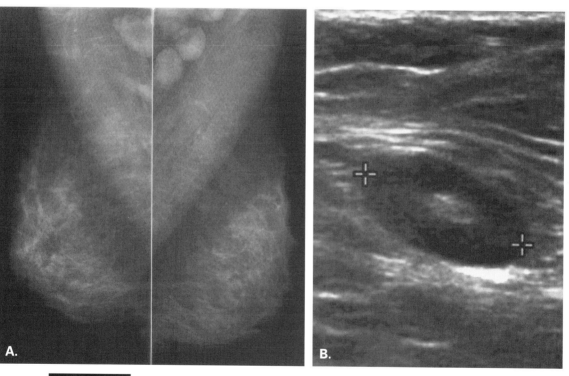

Figure 10.17

HISTORY: A 51-year-old woman with a history of systemic lupus erythematosus.

MAMMOGRAPHY: Bilateral MLO views (A) demonstrate mildly enlarged lymph nodes in both axillae. On ultrasound (B), the typical reniform shape and hyperechoic hilum of a node are noted.

IMPRESSION: Adenopathy secondary to lupus.

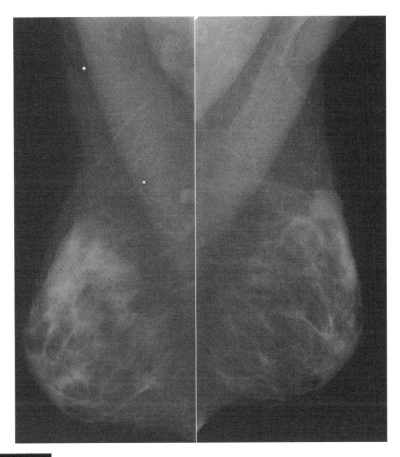

Figure 10.18

HISTORY: A 60-year-old woman for screening mammography. Her only medical problem was Sjögren's disease.

MAMMOGRAPHY: Bilateral MLO views show mild adenopathy in the low axillary regions. This degree of adenopathy suggests a benign etiology, such as is found in a connective tissue disorder.

IMPRESSION: Mild adenopathy related to Sjögren's disease.

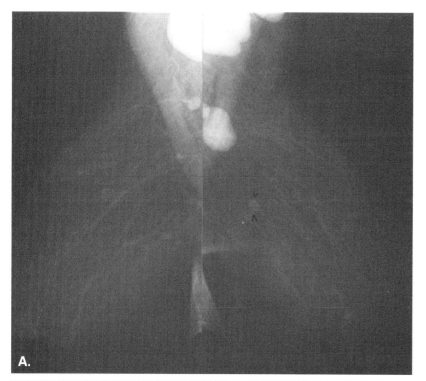

A.

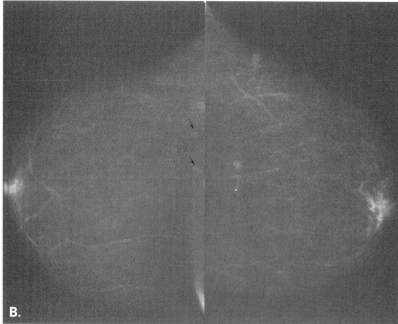

B.

Figure 10.19

HISTORY: A 65-year-old woman with a history of chronic lymphocytic leukemia for screening mammography.

MAMMOGRAPHY: Bilateral MLO **(A)** and CC **(B)** views show large dense nodes in both axillae. The size of these nodes suggests a neoplastic process. Multiple prominent intramammary nodes are also present bilaterally **(arrows)**. Core biopsy was performed for the central posterior mass on the right **(open arrow)**, and a clip was placed.

IMPRESSION: Recurrent leukemia.

HISTOPATHOLOGY: Chronic lymphocytic leukemia in axillary and intramammary nodes, including the right breast mass.

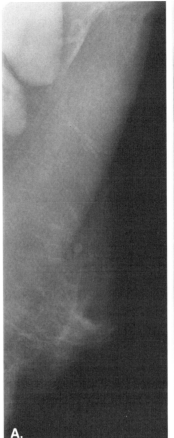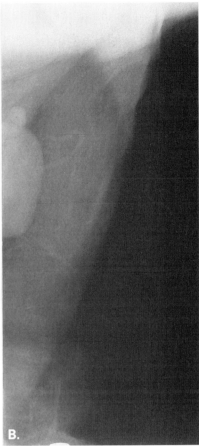

Figure 10.20

HISTORY: A 63-year-old woman with a history of lymphoma, for screening mammography.

MAMMOGRAPHY: Right MLO (**A**) and axillary (**B**) views. There are smoothly marginated, enlarged solid nodes in the axilla. An intramammary node is also present. The smoothly marginated, round enlarged nodes are more typical of lymphoma than of metastatic breast carcinoma. The findings are consistent with recurrence of lymphoma.

IMPRESSION: Recurrent lymphoma.

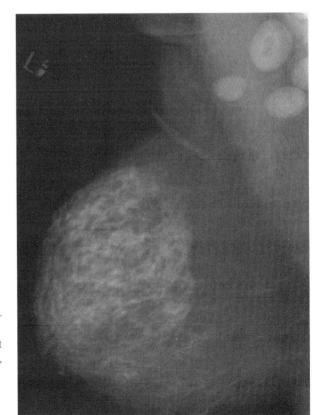

Figure 10.21

HISTORY: A 67-year-old woman with a history of lymphoma.

MAMMOGRAPHY: Left MLO view shows heterogeneously dense breast tissue and adenopathy in the axilla. The nodes are dense, enlarged, and very clearly marginated.

IMPRESSION: Adenopathy, suspicious for recurrence of lymphoma.

CYTOLOGY: Lymphoma.

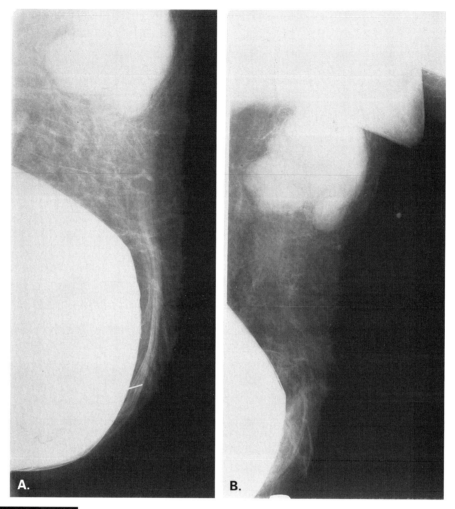

Figure 10.22

HISTORY: A 38-year-old woman presented with a mass in the right axilla and hoarseness.

MAMMOGRAPHY: Right MLO **(A)** and axillary **(B)** views show a normal-appearing subpectoral silicone implant. There are greatly enlarged, dense, circumscribed nodes in the axilla. There is no evidence for silicone rupture or free silicone adjacent to the implant or in the nodes. The constellation of findings and history are most suggestive of lymphoma involving the right axilla and mediastinum.

IMPRESSION: Lymphoma.

HISTOPATHOLOGY: Non-Hodgkins lymphoma.

(Figs. 10.24–10.26). The normal architecture is lost, and the pericapsular fat line is obliterated as the borders of the node are infiltrated by tumor (3). Metastatic nodes may be multiple and matted together, and nodes involved by metastatic breast cancer often have an indistinct or spiculated margin (18).

In a comparison of clinical examination and mammography with pathologic examination of axillary nodes, Kalisher et al. (19) found no significant difference in clinical examination and radiography in predicting metastatic involvement of nodes. When nodes were dense and greater than 2.0 cm in diameter, the true positive rate in predicting metas-

tases was 85%, and the false negative rate was 37%. When the criterion for abnormality was a nodal size of greater than 2.5 cm, the rates were 100% and 41%, respectively (19).

When metastatic carcinoma is found in axillary nodes, the primary breast cancer is usually seen, but occasionally it may not be identified (20–22) (Fig. 10.27). Occasionally, the patient presents with a palpable axillary mass that on biopsy is found to be a lymph node containing adenocarcinoma. The mammogram may reveal the clinically occult primary (23). Sometimes, however, the source of the metastasis is not evident, and screening ultrasound or MRI are used to search for the primary carcinoma.

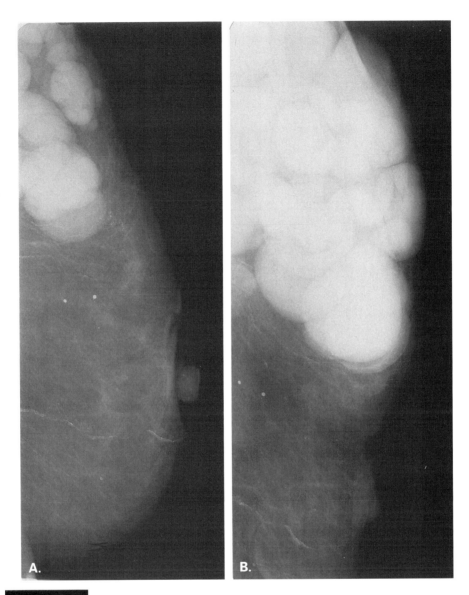

Figure 10.23

HISTORY: An 84-year-old woman with a history of left breast cancer and lymphoma, presenting with increasing adenopathy in the right axilla.

MAMMOGRAPHY: Right exaggerated CC lateral (**A**) and axillary views (**B**). There is massive solid adenopathy in the right axilla. Note the haloes that surround these large lobulated masses. Although one could not exclude involvement with metastatic breast cancer, this degree of adenopathy is more typical of lymphoma.

IMPRESSION: Lymphoma involving right axillary nodes.

HISTOPATHOLOGY: Malignant lymphoma.

Although microcalcifications are uncommon in an axillary node, this finding is most consistent with metastatic involvement (Fig. 10.28). Gold deposits can occur in axillary nodes of patients treated with chrysotherapy for rheumatoid arthritis and may simulate microcalcifications (24). The gold deposits appear stippled, fine, and dense compared with the calcifications that are associated with metastases (Fig. 10.29).

Lymphadenopathy in patients with rheumatoid arthritis treated with gold has also been found to be related to lymph node infarction (25). Rarely, metastases from non-breast primaries, such as mucin-producing tumors, may appear as adenopathy with fine psammomatous microcalcifications (Fig. 10.30).

(text continues on page 467)

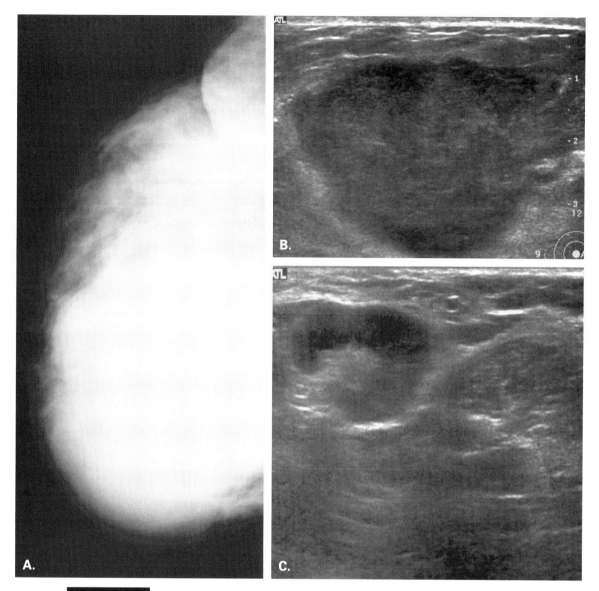

Figure 10.24

HISTORY: A 34-year-old woman who is 28 weeks pregnant and who presents with a large left breast mass.

MAMMOGRAPHY: Left CC view **(A)** shows a large, lobular, very-high-density mass with indistinct margins. On ultrasound **(B)**, the mass is solid, irregular, and inhomogeneous in echo pattern, all features of malignancy. Ultrasound of the axilla **(C)** showed multiple enlarged nodes with irregular margins and thickened cortices.

IMPRESSION: Carcinoma, metastatic to axillary nodes.

HISTOPATHOLOGY: Invasive ductal carcinoma, metastatic to the axilla.

Figure 10.25

HISTORY: A 45-year-old gravida 4, para 4 patient with a 3 × 3-cm mass in the right breast.

MAMMOGRAPHY: Right MLO **(A)** and CC **(B)** views. There is a large, high-density spiculated mass with linear extensions toward the nipple, having an appearance typical of carcinoma. Additionally, in the axillary tail there is a second smaller ill-defined mass **(arrow)** **(A** and **B)**. Although this could be a second primary lesion, because of its location and appearance, a metastatic node would be more likely diagnosis.

IMPRESSION: Carcinoma with metastatic adenopathy in the low axilla.

HISTOPATHOLOGY: Infiltrating ductal carcinoma, with 7 of 14 nodes with macroscopic foci of metastatic carcinoma.

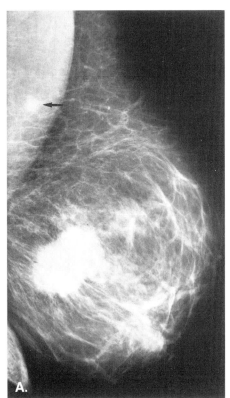
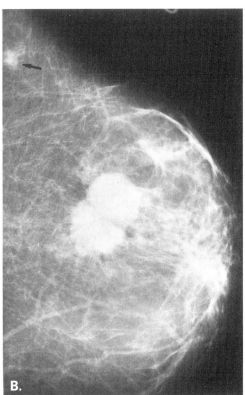

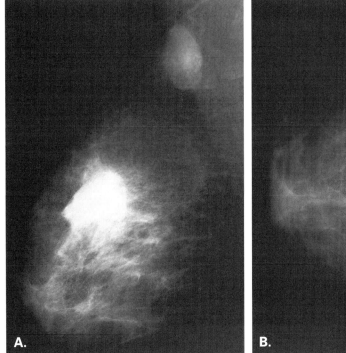
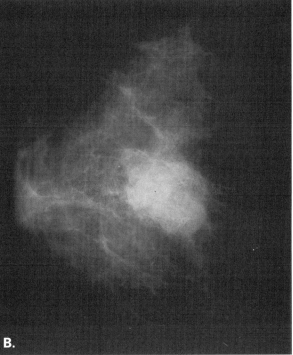

Figure 10.26

HISTORY: A 57-year-old woman with a large, firm palpable mass in the left breast.

MAMMOGRAPHY: Left MLO **(A)** and CC **(B)** views show a lobular high-density mass with indistinct margins in the 12 o'clock position of the left breast. There is also a large, dense, circumscribed node in the axilla.

IMPRESSION: Carcinoma, with nodal metastasis.

HISTOPATHOLOGY: Infiltrating ductal carcinoma with multiple positive axillary nodes.

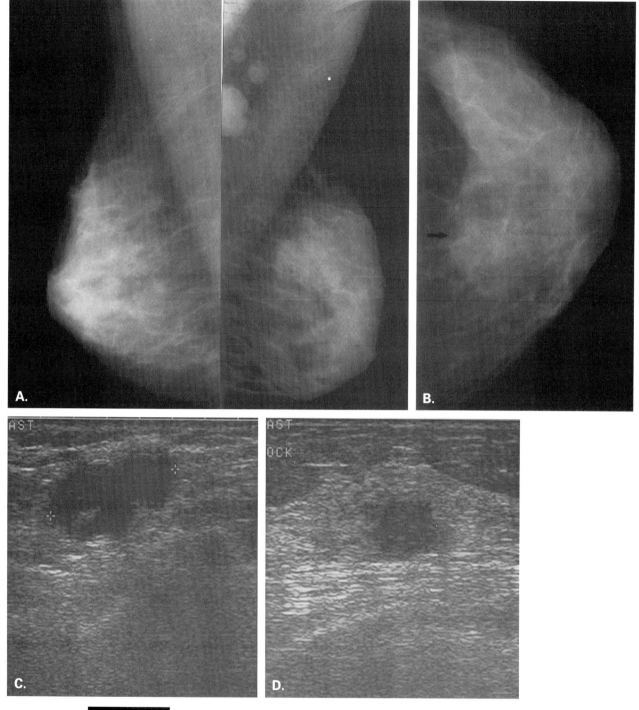

Figure 10.27

HISTORY: A 41-year-old woman who presents with a palpable mass in the right axilla and a normal breast examination otherwise.

MAMMOGRAPHY: Bilateral MLO views **(A)** show adenopathy in the right axilla corresponding to the palpable lump. On the right CC view **(B)**, a vague distortion is noted medially **(arrow)**. Sonography of the axilla **(C)** shows an enlarged, slightly irregular hypoechoic mass consistent with an abnormal node. Sonography of the area of distortion **(D)** shows an irregular hypoechoic mass, highly suspicious for malignancy.

IMPRESSION: Highly suspicious for carcinoma, metastatic to the axillary nodes.

HISTOPATHOLOGY: Invasive lobular carcinoma with positive axillary nodes.

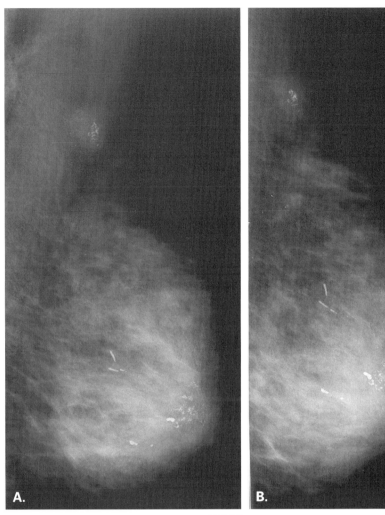

Figure 10.28

HISTORY: Patient recalled from a screening mammogram for microcalcifications.

MAMMOGRAPHY: Right MLO **(A)** and exaggerated CC lateral **(B)** views show highly pleomorphic microcalcifications in the subareolar area. There is also an oval mass with indistinct margins and associated pleomorphic microcalcifications in the low axilla. On the magnification view of the axilla **(C)**, the pleomorphic microcalcifications within the mass are noted, suggestive of metastatic carcinoma.

IMPRESSION: Ductal carcinoma with metastatic involvement of an axillary node.

HISTOPATHOLOGY: Invasive ductal carcinoma and ductal carcinoma in situ, positive axillary node.

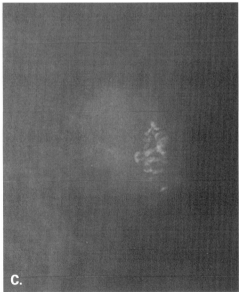

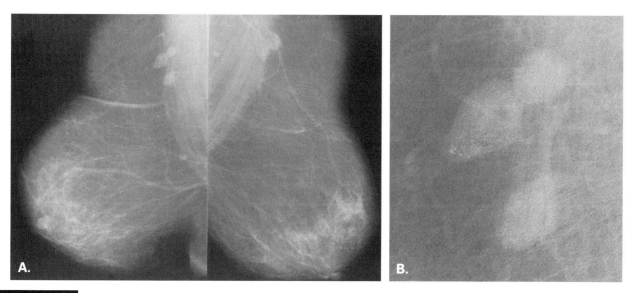

Figure 10.29

HISTORY: A 62-year-old woman treated with gold for rheumatoid arthritis.

MAMMOGRAPHY: Bilateral MLO views **(A)** show mildly prominent lymph nodes in the axillae. Within these are faint calcificlike densities, seen best on the magnified image **(B)**. These findings are typical of gold deposits in a patient treated with chrysotherapy for rheumatoid arthritis.

IMPRESSION: Gold deposits in axillary nodes.

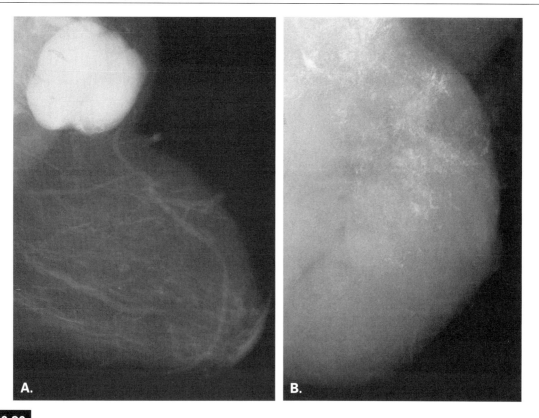

Figure 10.30

HISTORY: A 74-year-old woman with a history of carcinoma of the umbilicus, who presents with a palpable mass in the right axilla.

MAMMOGRAPHY: Right MLO view **(A)** shows a fatty-replaced breast with a large, lobulated, dense circumscribed mass in the axilla. On magnification **(B)**, the mass is noted to contain innumerable fine powdery microcalcifications.

IMPRESSION: Highly suspicious for malignancy, metastasis versus breast carcinoma.

HISTOPATHOLOGY: Mucin-producing carcinoma of the umbilicus, metastatic to an axillary node.

NOTE: Mucin-producing tumors may be associated with the formation of psammomatous calcifications.

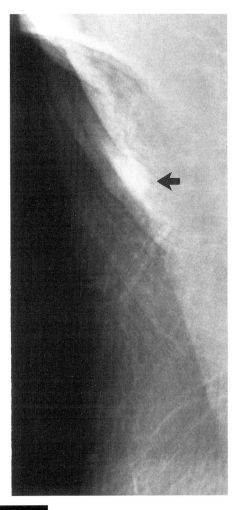

Figure 10.31

HISTORY: A 72-year-old gravida 0 woman for screening.

MAMMOGRAPHY: Left axillary view. There is a relatively well-circumscribed nodule **(arrow)** in the left axilla. Although a non–fatty-replaced node would be the most likely etiology of this mass, examination of the patient showed the nodule to correspond in location to a sebaceous cyst.

IMPRESSION: Sebaceous cyst.

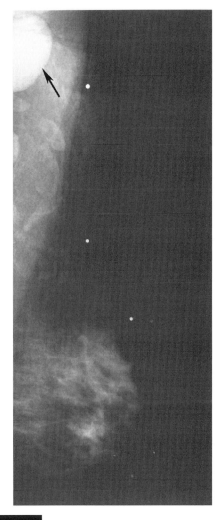

Figure 10.32

HISTORY: A 53-year-old woman with a history of neurofibromatosis.

MAMMOGRAPHY: Right MLO view shows a heterogeneously dense breast. Numerous skin lesions were marked with BBs. There is a large, dense circumscribed mass in the axilla **(arrow)**, which could represent an enlarged node, a cancer, or a skin lesion. Inspection of the skin showed a large pedunculated skin lesion.

IMPRESSION: Skin lesion, neurofibroma.

Other lesions that may occur in the axilla or axillary tail and that must be differentiated from lymph nodes are sebaceous cysts (Fig. 10.31), skin lesions (Fig. 10.32), hidradenitis suppurativa (Fig. 10.33), breast tumors (malignant and benign), cysts, lipomas, and ectopic breast tissue (Fig. 10.34). Ectopic breast tissue in the tail of Spence, or axillary tail, develops in the primitive milk streak. Ectopic breast tissue may be present with or without an overlying nipple or areola and is thought to occur in as many as 6% of women (26). It may be impossible to differentiate a primary tumor from an enlarged lymph node when a solitary, relatively well-defined mass in the axillary tail or axilla is present. Unless a patient has a reason to have generalized adenopathy, solid masses of greater than 1.5 cm in the axilla or smaller lesions without characteristic features of nodes should be regarded with suspicion.

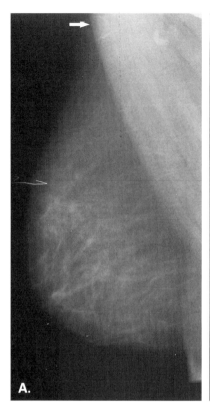

Figure 10.33

HISTORY: History of longstanding skin infections in the axillae bilaterally.

MAMMOGRAPHY: Left **(A)** MLO and right **(B)** axillary tail views show multiple nonenlarged lymph nodes in the axillae. There are also round, low-density, relatively circumscribed masses in the subcutaneous area bilaterally **(arrows)** consistent with the cystic inflammatory changes of hidradenitis suppurativa.

IMPRESSION: Hidradenitis suppurativa.

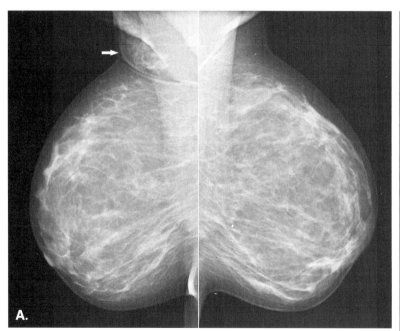

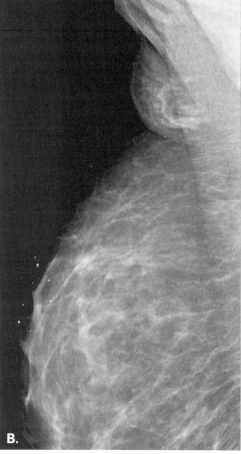

Figure 10.34

HISTORY: A 35-year-old asymptomatic woman for screening.

MAMMOGRAPHY: Bilateral MLO views **(A)** show a focal asymmetric area of glandular tissue in the left axilla. On the axillary tail view **(B)**, the glandularity is better seen.

IMPRESSION: Ectopic breast tissue in the tail of Spence.

REFERENCES

1. Venta LA. Evaluation of axillary node status with imaging modalities. *Semin Breast Dis* 1998;1(3):134–139.
2. March DE, Wechsler RJ, Kurtz AB, et al. CT-pathologic correlation of axillary lymph nodes in breast carcinoma. *J Comput Assist Tomogr* 1991;15:440–444.
3. Kalisher L. Xeroradiology of axillary lymph node disease. *Radiology* 1975;114:67–71.
4. Vassallo P, Wernecke K, Roos N, et al. Differentiation of benign from malignant superficial lymphadenopathy: the role of high-resolution US. *Radiology* 1992;183:215–220.
5. Leborgne R, Leborgne F, Leborgne JH. Soft-tissue radiography of axillary nodes with fatty infiltration. *Radiology* 1965;84:513–515.
6. Dershaw DD, Panicek DM, Osborne MP. Significance of lymph nodes visualized by the mammographic axillary view. *Breast Dis* 1991;4:271–280.
7. Walsh R, Kornguth PJ, Soo MS, et al. Axillary lymph nodes: mammographic, pathologic, and clinical correlation. *AJR Am J Roentgenol* 1997;68(1):33–38.
8. Lee CH, Giurescu ME, Philpotts LE, et al. Clinical importance of unilaterally enlarging lymph nodes on otherwise normal mammograms. *Radiology* 1997;203:329–334.
9. Lazarus AA. Sarcoidosis. *Otolaryngol Clin North Am* 1982;15(3):621–633.
10. Patel T, Given-Wilson RM, Thomas V. The clinical importance of axillary lymphadenopathy detected on screening mammography: revisited. *Clin Radiol* 2005;60(1):64–71.
11. Muttarak M, Pojchamarnwiputh S, Chaiwun B. Mammographic features of tuberculous axillary lymphadenitis. *Australas Radiol* 2002;46(3):260–263.
12. Vaamonde R, Cabrera JM, Vaamonde-Martin RJ, et al. Silicone granulomatous lymphadenopathy and siliconomas of the breast. *Histol Histopathol* 1997;12(4):1003–1011.
13. Weston WJ. Enlarged axillary glands in rheumatoid arthritis. *Australas Radiol* 1971;15(1):55–56.
14. Andersson I, Marsal L, Nilsson B, et al. Abnormal axillary lymph nodes in rheumatoid arthritis. *Acta Radiol (Diagn)* 1980;21:645–649.
15. Calgunneri M, Ozturk MA, Ozbalkan Z, et al. Frequency of lymphadenopathy in rheumatoid arthritis and systemic lupus erythematosus. *J Int Med Res* 2003;31(4):345–349.
16. Meyer JE, Kopans DB, Long JC. Mammographic appearance of malignant lymphoma of the breast. *Radiology* 1980;135:623–626.
17. Leborgne R, Leborgne F, Leborgne JH. Soft tissue radiography of the axilla in cancer of the breast. *Br J Radiol* 1963;36:494–496.
18. Dershaw DD, Selland DG, Tan LK, et al. Spiculated axillary adenopathy. *Radiology* 1996;201:439–442.
19. Kalisher L, Chu AM, Peyster RG. Clinicopathological correlation of xeroradiography in determining involvement of metastatic axillary nodes in female breast cancer. *Radiology* 1976;121:333–335.
20. Abrams RA, O'Connor T, May G, et al. Breast cancer presenting as an axillary mass: a case report and review of the literature. *Breast Dis* 1990;3:39–46.
21. Patel J, Nemoto T, Rosner D, et al. Axillary lymph node metastasis from an occult breast cancer. *Cancer* 1981;47:2923–2927.
22. Leibman AJ, Kossoff MB. Mammography in women with axillary lymphadenopathy and normal breasts on physical examination: value in detecting occult breast carcinoma. *AJR Am J Roentgenol* 1992;159:493–495.
23. Abrams RA, O'Connor T, May G, et al. Breast cancer presenting as an axillary mass: a case report and review of the literature. *Breast Dis* 1990;3:39–46.
24. Bruwer A, Nelson GW, Spark RP. Clinicopathological correlation of xeroradiography in determining involvement of metastatic axillary nodes in female breast cancer. *Radiology* 1976;121:333–335.
25. Roberts C, Batstone PJ, Goodlad JR. Lymphadenopathy and lymph node infarction as a result of gold injections. *J Clin Pathol* 2001;54(7):562–564.
26. De Cholnoky T. Accesory breast tissue in the axilla. *NY J Med* 1951;51:2245–2248.

Chapter 11

The Male Breast

Benign and malignant conditions affect the male breast to a much lesser degree than the female breast, and mammography is of help in the differentiation of some of these lesions. Although mammography, and particularly the craniocaudal (CC) view, may be difficult to perform unless the breast is enlarged, the mediolateral oblique (MLO) view can generally be quite satisfactorily obtained. Ultrasound may be a helpful modality in the evaluation of male breast enlargement (1), but it does not replace mammography, particularly in the evaluation of a unilateral breast mass (2).

A variety of diseases can occur in the male breast, but the most common diagnoses are gynecomastia and breast cancer. In a review of 236 male patients who underwent mammography, Günhan-Bilgen et al. (3) found that 206 had gynecomastia, 14 had primary breast cancer, 3 had metastases, and 13 had other benign lesions (including hematomas, fat necrosis, inclusion and sebaceous cysts, and lipomas). In another series of 263 men with breast abnormalities, Cooper et al. (4) found that the majority, 81%, had gynecomastia on mammography.

GYNECOMASTIA

Gynecomastia is the development of a male breast into the shape of a female breast and is clinically evident as a firm palpable breast mass in the subareolar area. Gynecomastia occurs most commonly in adolescent boys and in men older than 50 years, and the condition represents about 85% of breast masses in men (5). The etiologies of gynecomastia include (a) hormonal (related to an imbalance in estradiol-testosterone levels or to dysfunction of the adrenal, thyroid, or pituitary glands), (b) systemic (in cirrhosis, chronic renal failure with hemodialysis, chronic obstructive pulmonary disease, and tuberculosis), (c) drug induced (secondary to exogenous estrogens, digitalis, cimetidine, antihypertensives, ergotamine, tricyclic antidepressants, and marijuana), (d) tumors (particularly of testicular, pituitary, and adrenal origin or secondary to hepatomas or lung cancers), and (e) idiopathic.

The normal male breast contains subcutaneous adipose tissue and a few rudimentary ducts beneath the nipple. The appearance is similar to that of the prepubertal girl. Histologically, three forms of gynecomastia are noted: (a) florid, which usually occurs over a short duration and is seen to have an increase in the ducts with proliferation of the epithelium, edema, and an increase in the stroma and fat; (b) fibrotic, which is more chronic and seen in elderly men who have dilated ducts without an increase in stroma or edema; and (c) intermediate (5).

The most common mammographic appearance of gynecomastia (54%) in a series by Chandrakant and Pareck (5) was that of mild prominence of the subareolar ducts (Figs. 11.1 and 11.2). Dershaw (6) found the most common presentation of gynecomastia as a triangular or flame-shaped density symmetrically situated behind the nipple. The appearance, however, may range to diffuse ductal enlargement or even to a homogeneously dense breast having the appearance of that of a young woman (Figs. 11.3–11.9). The condition may be unilateral or bilateral. Günhan-Bilgen et al. (3) found that 55% of cases of gynecomastia were unilateral and 45% were bilateral. Cooper et al. (4) found that 72% of patients with gynecomastia had unilateral findings. Of importance in suggesting the diagnosis of gynecomastia on mammography is that the increased density or prominent ductal pattern be situated directly beneath the subareolar area and radiate out in a fan shape, as would be expected for the distribution of the ducts.

In most cases, mammography alone is sufficient as an imaging evaluation of the patient with gynecomastia. The findings of uniform subareolar parenchymal density in the patient with breast enlargement are typical of gynecomastia. Sonography may be helpful in questionable cases as it depicts normal-appearing ductal structures and no mass. Some authors have suggested sonography as the first-line imaging (7) in patients with suspected gynecomastia, although this is not a common practice.

Benign masses that have been described in the male breast include inclusion or sebaceous cysts (Fig. 11.10), abscesses, hematomas, fat necrosis (Fig. 11.11), enlarged

(text continues on page 476)

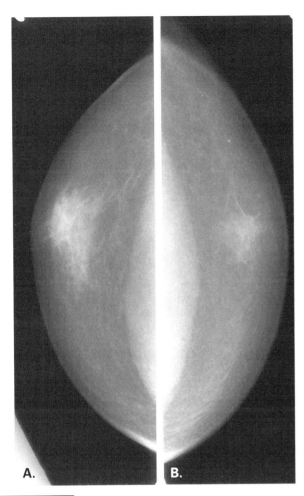

Figure 11.1

HISTORY: A 45-year-old man with a tender left breast mass.

MAMMOGRAPHY: Left **(A)** and right **(B)** CC views demonstrate flame-shaped densities in both subareolar areas. The findings are more prominent in the left breast than in the right.

IMPRESSION: Unilateral gynecomastia.

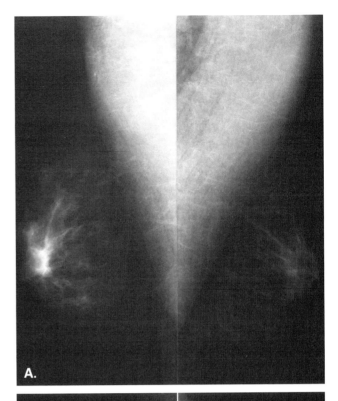

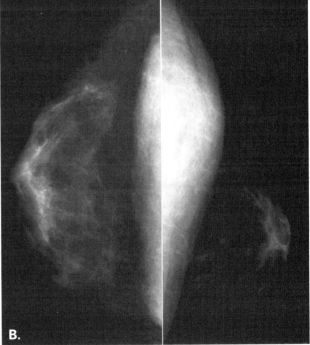

Figure 11.2

HISTORY: A 47-year-old man reporting left breast pain.

MAMMOGRAPHY: Bilateral MLO **(A)** and CC **(B)** views show breast enlargement with subareolar flame-shaped densities, on the left greater than the right, consistent with bilateral gynecomastia.

IMPRESSION: Bilateral gynecomastia.

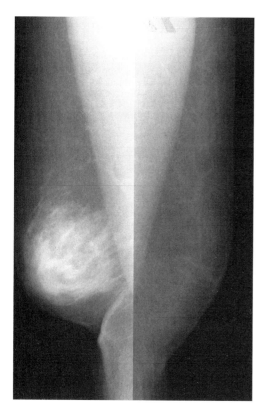

Figure 11.3

HISTORY: A 63-year-old man with soreness and a tender 3-cm lump in the left breast.

MAMMOGRAPHY: Bilateral views show marked asymmetry in the appearance of the breasts. The left breast is larger and markedly more dense than the right. On the right, only rudimentary ducts are present. The density in the left is radiating back from the nipple and is most consistent with gynecomastia.

IMPRESSION: Unilateral gynecomastia.

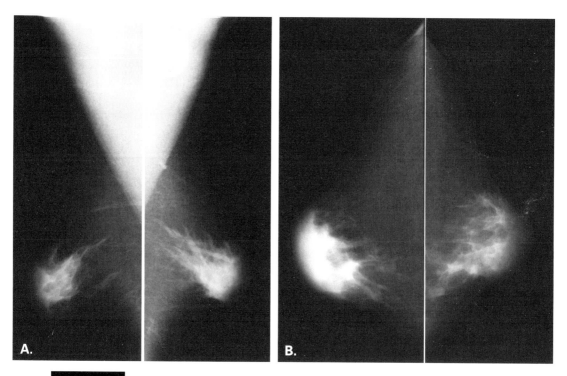

Figure 11.4

HISTORY: A 38-year-old man with breast enlargement.

MAMMOGRAPHY: Bilateral MLO **(A)** and CC **(B)** views show generalized enlargement bilaterally. There is diffuse increase in parenchymal density extending from the subareolar regions bilaterally.

IMPRESSION: Bilateral gynecomastia.

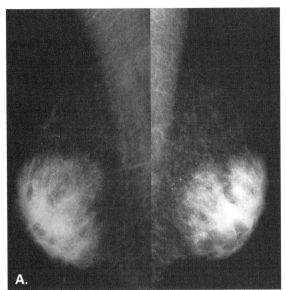
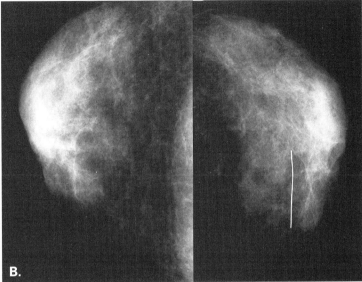

Figure 11.5

HISTORY: A 78-year-old man with history of bomb exposure in Hiroshima and a past medical history of multiple carcinomas. He had been treated recently with estrogen therapy for prostate cancer.

MAMMOGRAPHY: Bilateral MLO (**A**) and CC (**B**) views show enlargement of both breasts with increased parenchyma bilaterally. Also noted are extensive dermal calcifications.

IMPRESSION: Bilateral gynecomastia.

Figure 11.6

HISTORY: A 61-year-old man with right breast tenderness and induration.

MAMMOGRAPHY: Bilateral MLO (**A**) and CC (**B**) views show fatty enlargement of both breasts. In addition, on the right, there is diffuse parenchymal density extending from the nipple posterolaterally, typical of unilateral gynecomastia.

IMPRESSION: Unilateral gynecomastia.

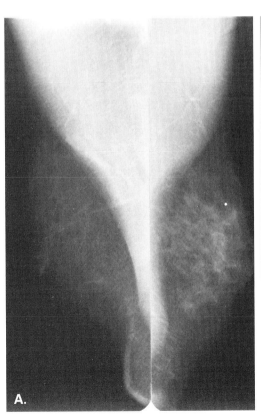
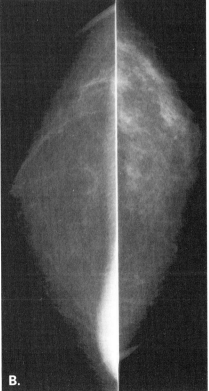

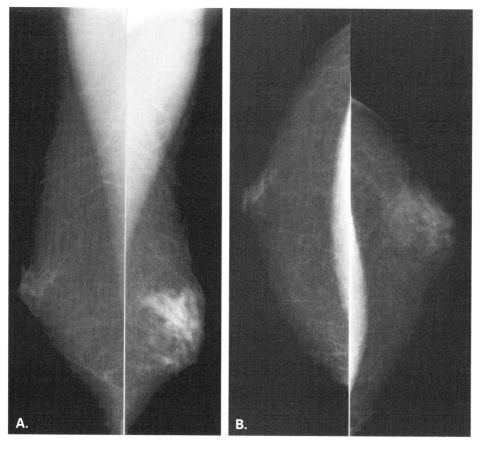

A.

B.

Figure 11.7

HISTORY: A 38-year-old man with liver failure and right breast enlargement.

MAMMOGRAPHY: On bilateral MLO (**A**) and CC (**B**) views, there is bilateral ductal prominence on the right greater than the left, consistent with gynecomastia. Findings of prominent pectoralis major muscle and relatively small breasts suggest a male patient.

IMPRESSION: Gynecomastia, right greater than the left.

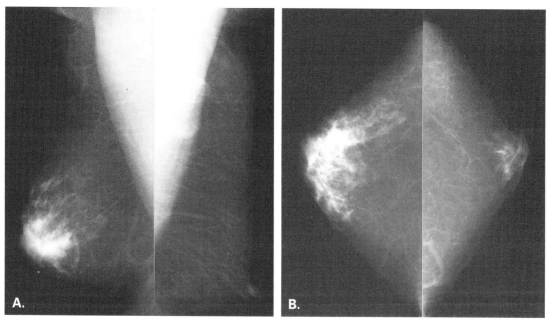

A.

B.

Figure 11.8

HISTORY: A 61-year-old man on steroids with left breast enlargement.

MAMMOGRAPHY: Bilateral MLO (**A**) and CC (**B**) views show generalized breast enlargement. There is parenchymal density in the subareolar areas bilaterally, seen on the left to a greater degree than on the right, consistent with gynecomastia.

IMPRESSION: Gynecomastia.

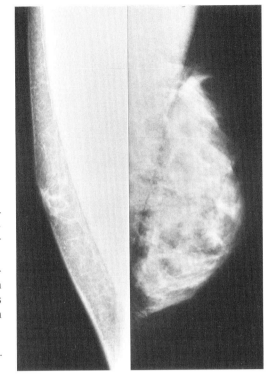

Figure 11.9

HISTORY: A 21-year-old man who presented with unilateral breast enlargement. He stated that he had sustained blunt trauma to the right chest 2 weeks earlier; no bruising, mass, or tenderness was found on physical examination.

MAMMOGRAPHY: Bilateral MLO views show striking asymmetry in the appearance of the breasts. The left breast has a normal appearance for a man, with minimal fat and rudimentary ductal structures noted. The right breast is striking enlarged and is dense and glandular, having the appearance of an adult female breast.

IMPRESSION: Unilateral gynecomastia.

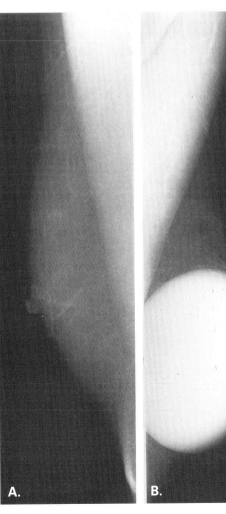

Figure 11.10

HISTORY: A 32-year-old man presenting with a large, tender palpable right breast mass.

MAMMOGRAPHY: Left **(A)** and right **(B)** MLO views show marked asymmetry in the appearance of the breasts. The left breast has a normal appearance for a male patient: prominent pectoralis major muscle and rudimentary ducts. There is a very large, circumscribed, high-density oval mass in the right breast. An occluded inflamed pore was noted on the skin overlying the mass.

IMPRESSION: Sebaceous cyst.

NOTE: The mass was drained and was a sebaceous cyst. This has the appearance of the "egg in the breast" in a male patient, which is typical for a large sebaceous cyst.

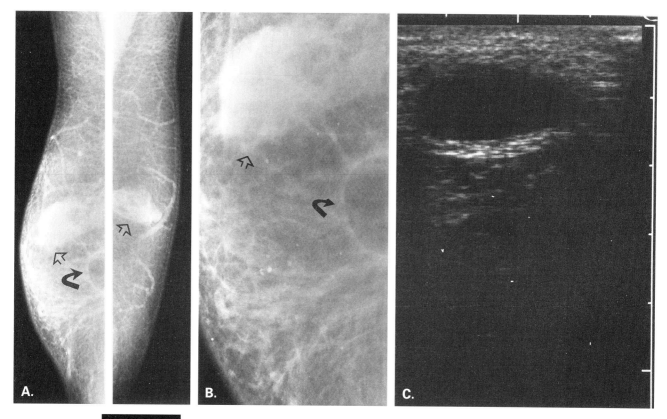

Figure 11.11

HISTORY: A 41-year-old man who had been bitten by a horse on the left breast 6 months earlier, presenting with a firm mass in the upper inner quadrant.

MAMMOGRAPHY: Bilateral MLO (**A**) and enlarged left CC (**B**) views and ultrasound (**C**). There is some prominent ductal tissue in both subareolar areas (**open arrows**) (**A** and **B**), consistent with a mild degree of gynecomastia. On the left, near the chest wall, there is a radiolucent, circumscribed encapsulated mass (**curved arrows**) (**A** and **B**) having the characteristic appearance of an oil cyst. Sonography (**C**) shows this mass to be relatively anechoic, with good through-transmission of sound and a well-defined back wall. These findings corresponded to the area of palpable abnormality. Incidentally noted also are extensive skin calcifications.

IMPRESSION: Large oil cyst secondary to previous trauma.

HISTOPATHOLOGY: Fibrous walled cyst, fat necrosis.

lymph nodes (5), intraductal papillomas, and fibroadenomas (2). The mammographic manifestations of these masses are similar to those found in the female breast. Because of the need for progesterone for lobular development, genetically normal men do not develop lobules and do not have the lesions that occur in the lobule. Therefore, fibrocystic changes and lobular carcinomas do not occur in genetically normal men. Instead, the parenchymal lesions that occur in the man are ductal in origin: gynecomastia and ductal carcinomas.

Carcinomas of the male breast accounts for about 0.9% of all breast cancers (8). The disease is more common in men older than 60 years, but breast cancer has been seen rarely in young men. Most patients present clinically with

a palpable breast lump (9). Factors that increase the risk of male breast cancer include advanced age, positive family history, Jewish origin, black race (10), altered estrogen metabolism, exogenous estrogens, infectious orchitis, Klinefelter syndrome, and radiation to the chest (11). The BRCA2 mutations are believed to account for the majority of inherited breast cancers in men (12,13).

In reviewing National Cancer Institute Surveillance, Epidemiology, and End Results (SEER) data from 1973 to 1998, Giordano et al. (14) found that the incidence for male breast cancer increased significantly from 0.86 to 1.08 per 100,000 population. In comparison with women, men had a higher median age at diagnosis, were more likely to have lymph node involvement, had a more advanced stage at

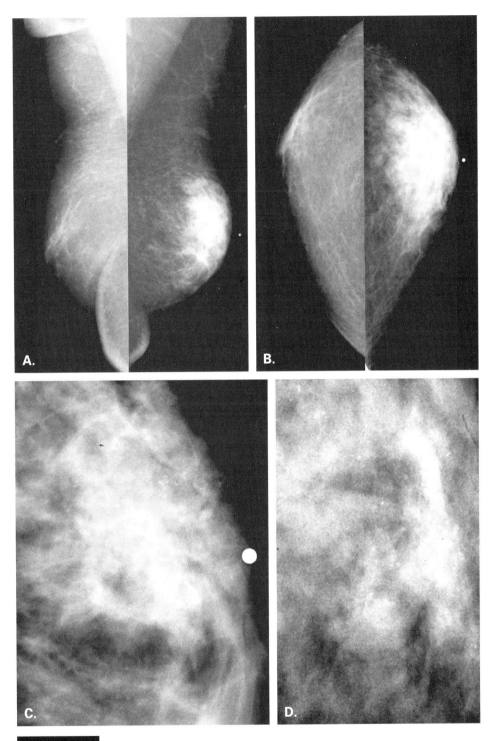

Figure 11.12

HISTORY: A 62-year-old man who presented with palpable thickening in the right breast.

MAMMOGRAPHY: Bilateral MLO (**A**) and CC (**B**) views show marked asymmetry in the appearance of the breasts. The right breast is noted to contain dense dilated ducts in the subareolar lesion. However, these ducts are associated with extensive pleomorphic microcalcifications, better seen on magnified CC (**C**) and ML (**D**) views. The presence of the microcalcifications is highly suspicious for malignancy.

IMPRESSION: BI-RADS® 5, highly suspicious for malignancy.

HISTOPATHOLOGY: DCIS.

diagnosis, and had tumors positive for estrogen and progesterone receptors. Relative survival rates for men and women were similar for similar stages and grade of tumors.

In comparison with breast cancers in women, when screening mammography is performed and detects in situ cancers, the rate of male ductal carcinoma in situ (DCIS) is small. DCIS accounts for about 5% of all male breast cancers (15), whereas in women, it often represents about one fourth of breast malignancies. DCIS in male patients presents with malignant microcalcifications associated with dilated ducts that are extensive (Fig. 11.12) and that present as palpable thickening or a nipple discharge. Although sex differences have been found with respect to tumor characteristics, sex has not been found to be a significant predictor of survival (16).

On mammography, male breast cancer usually presents as a spiculated mass, like scirrhous cancer of the female breast. A majority of male breast cancers are located in an eccentric position relative to the nipple, and they present as noncalcified masses (3). Calcifications may occur, but they are usually larger and fewer in number than those found in cancers of the female breast (5). Male breast carcinoma is distinguished from gynecomastia by its eccentric location, spiculation, microcalcifications, and secondary features (Figs. 11.13 and 11.14), such as skin or nipple retraction (17). Male breast cancers may also present as more circumscribed masses (Figs. 11.15 and 11.16) when the etiology is a specialized type of malignancy, such as the papillary, medullary, or mucinous types. If, however, gynecomastia presents in an eccentric location (6), it may not be readily distinguished from carcinoma, and biopsy is warranted.

(References begin on page 481)

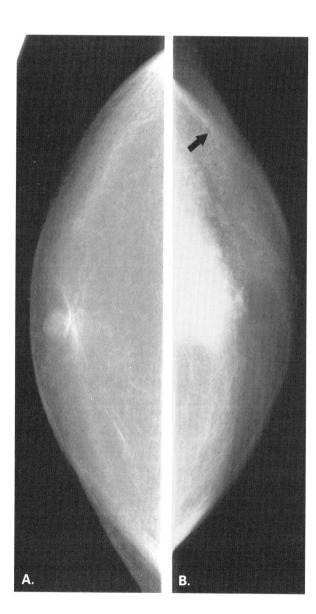

Figure 11.13

HISTORY: An 80-year-old man with fixed right breast mass.

MAMMOGRAPHY: Left **(A)** and right **(B)** CC views show a normal-appearing left breast and a large dense microlobulated mass in the posterolateral aspect of the right breast. This mass is not associated with the subareolar area and is eccentric relative to the nipple, all features that are suspicious for malignancy. There is also associated skin thickening laterally **(arrow)**.

IMPRESSION: Highly suspicious for carcinoma.

CYTOLOGY: Carcinoma.

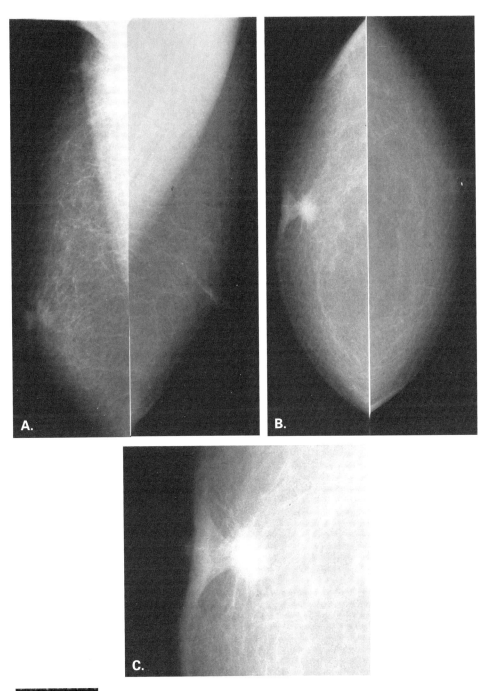

HISTORY: A 55-year-old male patient who presents with left nipple retraction and a firm palpable mass.

MAMMOGRAPHY: Bilateral MLO (**A**) and CC (**B**) views show a normal-appearing right breast and a mass in the subareolar area of the left breast. On the left CC spot-magnification view (**C**), the mass is spiculated and is associated with nipple retraction and mild skin thickening.

IMPRESSION: Highly suspicious for carcinoma.

HISTOPATHOLOGY: Invasive ductal carcinoma.

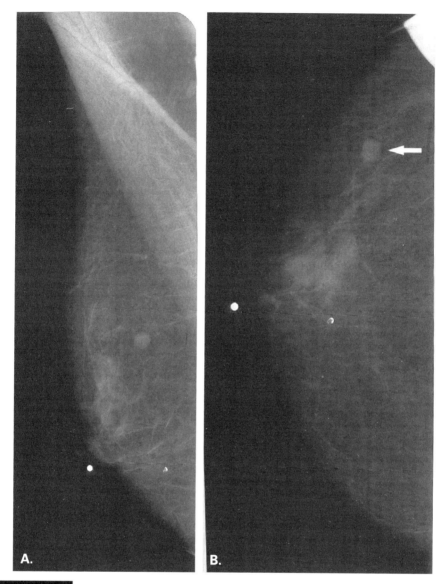

Figure 11.15

HISTORY: Male patient with an enlarged left breast and a palpable mass laterally.

MAMMOGRAPHY: Left MLO **(A)** and CC **(B)** views show a mild degree of gynecomastia, characterized by subareolar ductal prominence. There is also a round, dense, slightly indistinct mass in the upper outer quadrant **(arrow)**, suspicious for carcinoma.

IMPRESSION: Gynecomastia and probable carcinoma.

HISTOPATHOLOGY: Invasive ductal carcinoma.

REFERENCES

1. Cole-Beuglet C, Schwartz GF, Kurtz AB, et al. Ultrasound mammography for male breast enlargement. *J Ultrasound Med* 1982;1:301–305.
2. Jackson VP, Gilmor RL. Male breast carcinoma and gynecomastia: comparison of mammography with sonography. *Radiology* 1983;149:533–536.
3. Günhan-Bilgen I, Bozkaya H, Ustun EE, et al. Male breast disease: clinical, mammographic, and ultrasonographic features. *Eur J Radiol* 2002;43(3):246–255.
4. Cooper RA, Gunter BA, Ramamurthy L. Mammography in men. *Radiology* 1994;191(3):651–656.
5. Chandrakant CK, Pareck NJ. The male breast. *Radiol Clin North Am* 1983;21:137–148.
6. Dershaw DD. Male mammography. *AJR Am J Roentgenol* 1986; 146:127–131.
7. Daniels IR, Layer GT. Gynaecomastia. *Eur J Surg* 2001;167(12): 885–892.
8. Yap HY, Tashima CK, Blimensheim GR, et al. Male breast cancer: a natural history study. *Cancer* 1979;44:748–754.
9. Hultborn R, Friberg S. Hultborn KA. Male breast carcinoma. *Acta Oncol* 1987;26:241–256.
10. Meguerditchian AN, Falardeau M, Martin G. Male breast carcinoma. *Can J Surg* 2002;45(4):296–302.
11. Meyskins FL, Tormey DC, Neifeld JP. Male breast cancer: a review. *Cancer Treat Rev* 1976;3:83–93.
12. Weiss JR, Movsich KB, Swede H. Epidemiology of male breast cancer. *Cancer Epidemiol Biomarkers Prev* 2005;14(1):20–26.
13. Joseph A, Mokbel K. Male breast cancer. *Int J Fertil Womens Med* 2004;49(5):198–199.
14. Giordano SH, Cohen DS, Buzdar AU, et al. Breast carcinoma in men: a population-based study. *Cancer* 2005;103(2):432–433.
15. Pappo I, Wasserman I, Halevy A. Ductal carcinoma in situ of the breast in men: a review. *Clin Breast Cancer* 2005;6(4):310–314.
16. Hill TD, Khamis HJ, Tyczynski JE, et al. Comparison of male and female breast cancer: incidence trends, tumor characteristics, and survival. *Ann Epidemiol* 2005;15(10):773–780.
17. Michels LG, Gold RH, Arndt RD. Radiography of gynecomastia and other disorders of the male breast. *Radiology* 1977;122:117–122.

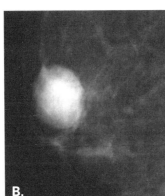

Figure 11.16

HISTORY: An 80-year-old man with a firm mass beneath the left nipple.

MAMMOGRAPHY: Left ML view (**A**) and magnified image (**B**). The breast is somewhat enlarged but fatty and not containing prominent ductal tissue, as would be found in gynecomastia. In the subareolar area, there is a well-defined high-density mass with slight microlobulation of the margins, suggesting a suspicious nature.

IMPRESSION: Mass in the left breast, highly suspicious for carcinoma.

HISTOPATHOLOGY: Medullary carcinoma.

NOTE: The scalloping of the edges of this lesion (**B**) and the high density are the features suggestive of malignancy. (Case courtesy of Dr. Luisa Marsteller, Norfolk, VA.)

Chapter 12

The Postsurgical Breast

A wide variety of mammographic findings are seen after surgical procedures on the breast. Surgical procedures—including core needle biopsy, excisional breast biopsy, wide excision or segmental mastectomy, subcutaneous or modified radical mastectomy with reconstruction, reduction mammoplasty, and lumpectomy with radiation therapy—produce a spectrum of classical and unusual findings. Critical to an accurate analysis of a mammogram and to determination that findings are of postsurgical origin is knowledge of the history and clinical examination of the patient.

It is of help to place a wire or BB marker on the skin to avoid repeating films because of uncertainty about positions of scars. If this is not done, then it is absolutely necessary that the technologist be responsible for clearly marking the location and orientation of any scars on a drawing of the breast. The surgical site is sometimes demarcated with surgical clips, particularly in cases of lumpectomy performed for carcinoma. Additionally, it is equally important to document the location and size of any palpable masses and particularly their relationship to the surgical scar.

In interpreting a mammogram of a postsurgical breast, it is important for the radiologist to compare present studies with previous studies. Temporal changes are reflective of the normal evolution of postsurgical findings. Also, knowledge of the appearance of the original lesion in patients who have undergone lumpectomy and correlation with the specimen film is helpful to identify residual disease.

POSTBIOPSY CHANGES

Immediately after a needle biopsy of a breast lesion, there may be a small amount of air at the biopsy site, especially when a vacuum-assisted biopsy is performed. Occasionally, there also may be irregular increased density at the site from edema and hematoma formation. Unless there is significant bleeding during the biopsy, the changes are subtle. If there is a puncture of a vessel during a needle biopsy, a hematoma may form. If the hematoma dissects through the tissue, an amorphous ill-defined density is seen on mammography. If a hematoma is more localized, then the appearance is that of a relatively circumscribed mass (Fig. 12.1). These findings are typically observed immediately after the biopsy on the postprocedure mammogram. In most cases, however, there is no long-term mammographic finding after a needle biopsy.

The mammographic findings associated with excisional biopsy are localized to the area of the biopsy site. It is, therefore, important to correlate the position of the scar to the mammographic findings and to be aware of the temporal changes that are expected postsurgically. In a study of 1,049 breast biopsies, Sickles and Herzog (1) found mammographic abnormalities attributed to postsurgical changes in 474 (45%). Normal postsurgical changes include localized skin thickening or retraction, an asymmetric glandular defect, architectural distortion, contour deformity of the breast, hematoma or seroma, fat necrosis formation, parenchymal scarring (Figs. 12.2–12.6), calcifications of fibrosis (Figs. 12.7 and 12.8), fat necrosis and sutures, and opaque foreign bodies (1,2) (Figs. 12.9–12.11).

Skin thickening is localized to the biopsy site unless there is superimposed infection, in which case a more generalized thickening is present. A contour deformity may be associated with the skin thickening. Skin thickening is maximum on mammography during the first 6 months after biopsy and gradually diminishes. In a majority of patients who have undergone a lumpectomy or excisional biopsy for benign disease, the focal skin thickening is nearly inapparent on mammography after several years.

A hematoma may be seen at the biopsy site on a mammogram performed soon after biopsy. Postoperative hematoma or seromas are seen more commonly if a drain has not been placed and may actually be related to an improved cosmetic result with a lesser degree of contour

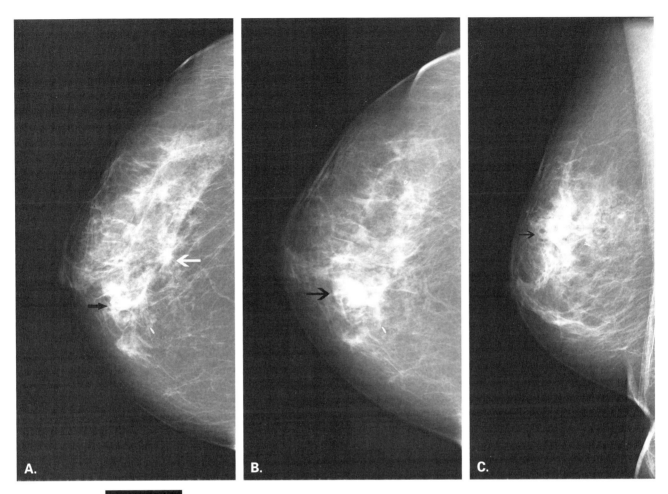

Figure 12.1

HISTORY: A 45-year-old woman for biopsy of multiple left breast lesions.

MAMMOGRAPHY: Left CC view **(A)** immediately after needle biopsy and left CC **(B)** and ML **(C)** views 2 hours later. A spiculated mass is present centrally **(white arrow)**, and an indistinct mass is located medially **(arrow)**, both of which were biopsied. There are also faint, pleomorphic microcalcifications laterally that were biopsied. Following vacuum-assisted core needle biopsies, the medial area was associated with the interval development of a lobulated circumscribed mass, consistent with a hematoma.

IMPRESSION: Hematoma following core needle biopsy of suspicious left breast lesion, multiple left breast lesions suspicious for carcinoma.

HISTOPATHOLOGY: Invasive ductal carcinoma, multicentric.

NOTE: The medial round mass represented a small hematoma secondary to core biopsy.

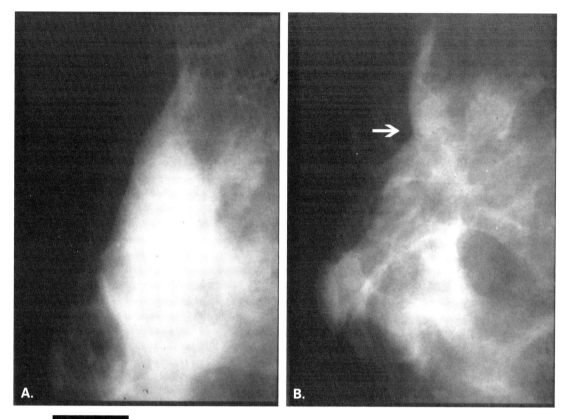

Figure 12.2

HISTORY: Routine mammography following surgical excision for left breast microcalcifications that were benign.

MAMMOGRAPHY: Left MLO **(A)** and left MLO **(B)** 1 year later, following surgical excision. There is dense parenchyma with some fine punctuate and amorphous microcalcifications in a regional distribution **(A)**. These were removed by surgical excision following needle localization.

IMPRESSION: Contour defect following surgical excision or lumpectomy.

deformity (3). On mammography, fluid collections are usually relatively circumscribed medium- to high-density masses and may range from 2 to 10 cm in diameter. In a series of postlumpectomy patients who were referred for radiotherapy, Mendelson (3) found postoperative fluid collections in 47%. On ultrasound, hematomas or seromas are relatively smooth and anechoic but may contain some internal echoes or debris, depending on the degree of organization (4). Because fluid collections may contain debris even if they are not infected, the clinical findings are of more help to suggest the presence of superimposed infection.

Areas of architectural disturbance are a common finding after surgery and include asymmetric decrease in glandular tissue from resection that does not change over time (1), architectural distortion, and focal increased density or parenchymal scar and fat necrosis. As a hematoma resolves, it is usual to see some residual, irregular increased density and/or distortion. Architectural distortion was the second most common postsurgical finding after skin thickening by Sickles and Herzog (1) in the evaluation of 474 postoperative breasts.

The changes of increased density and architectural distortion are maximum at 0 to 6 months after surgery and gradually diminish over time (1). The presence of entrapped fat within the distortion is also suggestive of scar. Scars also tend to have a different shape on two views, appearing as a spiculated area of architectural distortion on one view and as much less distorted on the orthogonal view. Often the extension of the distortion to the skin scar is also noted.

(text continues on page 490)

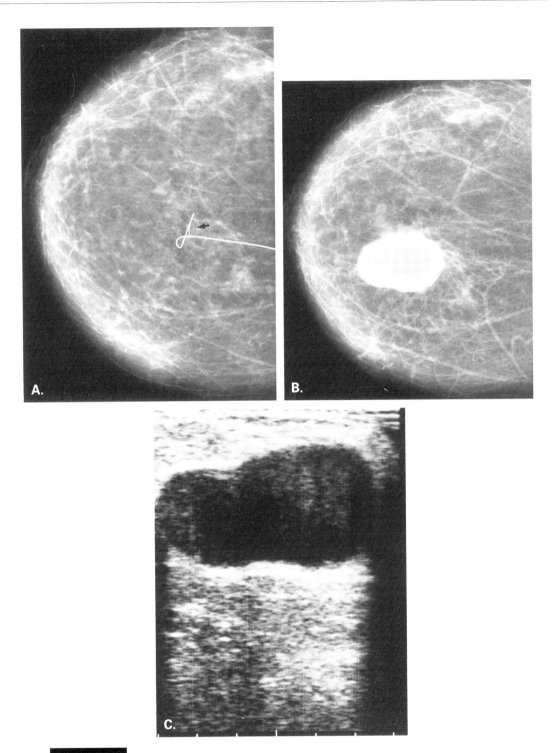

Figure 12.3

HISTORY: A 48-year-old gravida 2, para 2 woman 6 months after left breast biopsy, presenting with no new palpable findings.

MAMMOGRAPHY: Left CC view from a needle localization **(A)** and left CC view **(B)** and ultrasound **(C)** 6 months after biopsy. On the initial film **(A)**, a needle localization wire is marking a cluster of microcalcifications **(arrow)** for biopsy. The histopathology was benign. On the subsequent study **(B)**, there is a large, high-density, partially circumscribed mass at the biopsy site. On ultrasound **(C)**, the mass is complex, appearing circumscribed with some acoustic enhancement. The features are typical of a postoperative hematoma or seroma, and a fluid collection of this size may not be palpable. The patient was followed without aspiration of the seroma.

IMPRESSION: Large postoperative hematoma or seroma.

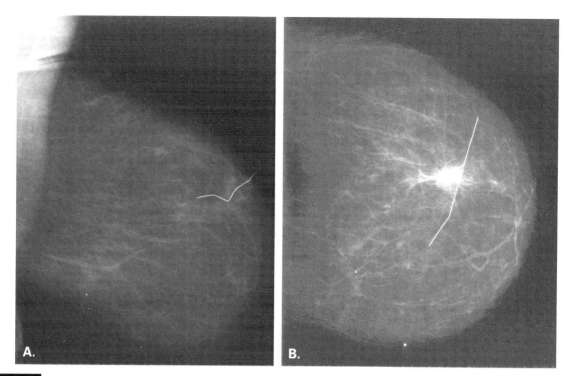

Figure 12.4

HISTORY: A 51-year-old woman status post–benign right breast biopsy.

MAMMOGRAPHY: Right MLO **(A)** and CC **(B)** views show an essentially fatty-replaced breast. The postsurgical site is indicated by a wire marker. This appears dense and spiculated on the CC view but is more amorphous and vertically oriented on the MLO view. The differing appearance on the two projections is typical of a scar.

IMPRESSION: Postsurgical scar.

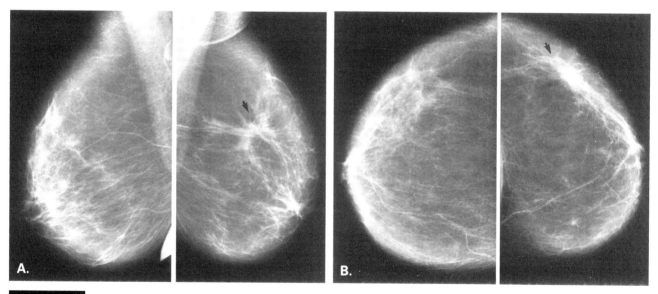

Figure 12.5

HISTORY: A 72-year-old gravida 2, para 2 woman for follow-up 1 year after a right breast biopsy that showed fibrocystic change.

MAMMOGRAPHY: Bilateral MLO **(A)** and CC **(B)** views. There is an irregular density in the right upper-outer quadrant **(arrows)**. On the MLO view **(A)**, the lesion appears somewhat less dense and spiculated than on the CC view **(B)**. The difference in shape of such a density suggests more likely a benign rather than a malignant etiology. This density was confirmed to be in the location of the scar from the previous biopsy.

IMPRESSION: Irregular density consistent with fat necrosis and scar after excisional biopsy.

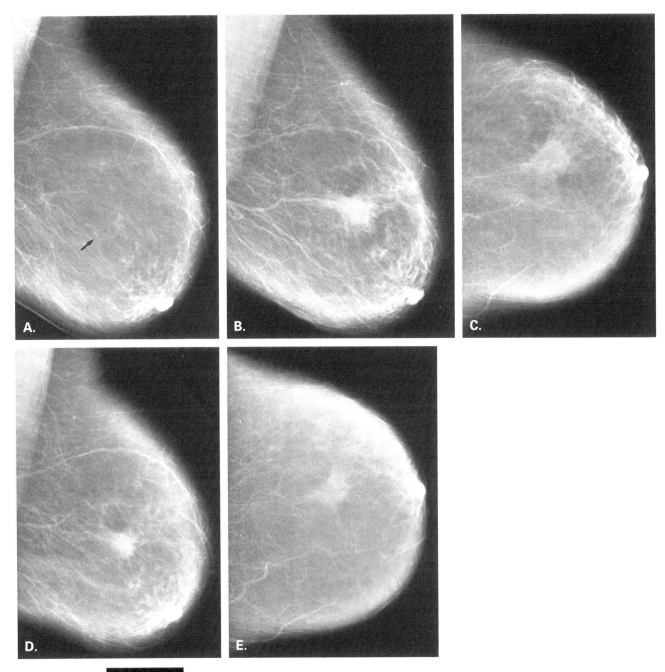

Figure 12.6

HISTORY: A 55-year-old gravida 0 woman for follow-up mammography after a benign biopsy in the right breast.

MAMMOGRAPHY: Right MLO film (preoperative) (**A**), right MLO (**B**) and CC (**C**) view 6 months after biopsy, and right MLO (**D**) and CC (**E**) views 12 months after biopsy. The preoperative film (**A**) demonstrates a small cluster (**arrow**) of microcalcifications that were biopsied and found to be benign. On the initial postoperative study (**B** and **C**), there is a 3-cm ill-defined area of increased density in the right middle-outer quadrant. On the CC view (**C**), the area is of lower density than would be expected for a neoplastic process. Because the location of the biopsy was in this area, the density is most consistent with scar and fat necrosis. Six months later (**D** and **E**), the area of that fat necrosis has decreased in size, as would be expected for normal postoperative changes.

IMPRESSION: Postoperative fat necrosis and scar, decreasing in size.

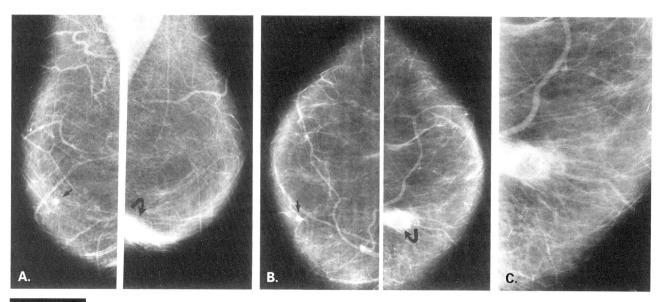

Figure 12.7

HISTORY: A 32-year-old gravida 0 woman who had had breast reduction 3 years ago, presenting with a firm irregular nodule in the right lower-inner quadrant.

MAMMOGRAPHY: Bilateral MLO **(A)**, CC **(B)**, and enlarged (2×) right CC **(C)** views. The breasts show fatty replacement. In the right lower-inner quadrant, there is an irregular area of increased density associated with a radiolucent mass containing eggshell calcification in the wall **(curved arrow)**. A radiolucent lesion is typical of an oil cyst and is most consistent with posttraumatic changes from reduction mammoplasty. The area was biopsied because of clinical concern about the palpable findings. Incidental note is also made of a small degenerating fibroadenoma in the left middle-inner quadrant **(arrow)**.

IMPRESSION: Fat necrosis, oil cyst.

HISTOPATHOLOGY: Fat necrosis.

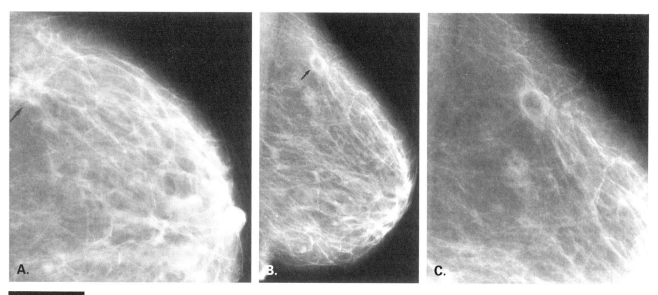

Figure 12.8

HISTORY: A 78-year-old gravida 2, para 2 woman after right breast biopsy for microcalcifications that were found to be epithelial hyperplasia, presenting for routine follow-up.

MAMMOGRAPHY: Right enlarged (2×) CC view **(A)** 6 months postoperatively and right MLO **(B)** and enlarged XCCL **(C)** views 12 months postoperatively. On the initial study **(A)**, there is an irregular area **(arrow)** of increased density in the outer aspect of the breast. This corresponded in location to the scar and was presumed to represent fat necrosis. Six months later **(B** and **C)**, the density has resolved and has been replaced by a lucent mass with a calcifying rim **(B, arrow)**, consistent with an oil cyst.

IMPRESSION: Postoperative fat necrosis evolving into an oil cyst.

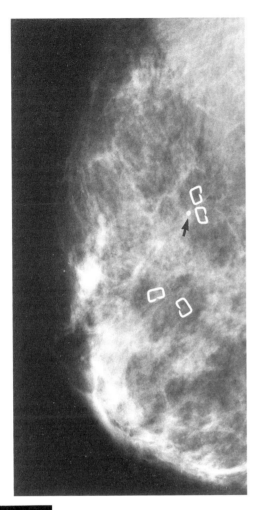

Figure 12.9

HISTORY: A 52-year-old woman 5 years after treatment for intra-ductal carcinoma of the left breast with lumpectomy and radiation therapy.

MAMMOGRAPHY: Left MLO view. The breast is moderately dense. Surgical clips have been placed at the lumpectomy site to outline the tumor bed for radiation therapy planning. A single calcification of fat necrosis **(arrow)** is noted at the tumor bed.

IMPRESSION: Foreign bodies: surgical clips marking tumor bed.

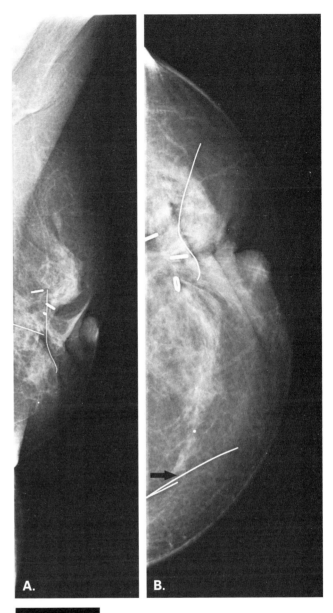

A.   B.

Figure 12.10

HISTORY: A 64-year-old woman status postlumpectomy and radiotherapy for right breast ductal carcinoma.

MAMMOGRAPHY: Right MLO **(A)** and CC **(B)** views show marked distortion and skin retraction related to postsurgical scar-ring. Surgical clips demonstrate the tumor bed, and wires have been placed on the skin to mark the surgical scars. In the medial aspect of the breast is a segment of the hook wire **(arrow)** used during a prior needle localization. The wire was present for three subsequent years and has not been associ-ated with any side effects.

IMPRESSION: Posttreatment changes, retained segment of local-ization hook wire.

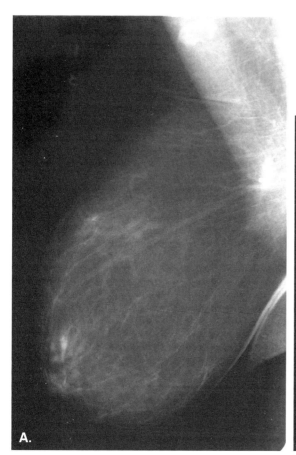

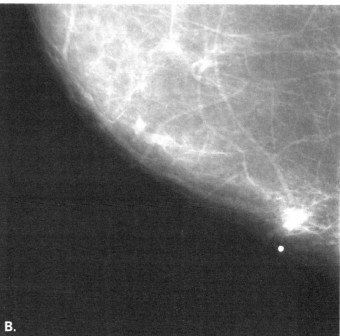

Figure 12.11

HISTORY: A 24-year-old woman with acute leukemia and neutropenia, presenting with a 2 × 2-cm tender mass in the left upper-inner quadrant. (A BB was placed over the palpable lesion for mammography).

MAMMOGRAPHY: Left MLO view **(A)** and left enlarged (2×) CC view **(B)**. There are scattered fibroglandular densities present. Far posteriorly in the upper inner quadrant in the area of palpable mass is a tubular intraparenchymal artifact. Some surrounding increased density is present **(A** and **B)**. This tubular structure is the tip of a catheter for chemotherapy, which had been removed several months earlier. The tip was severed and remained in the breast and had not been clinically evident until the surrounding inflammation occurred.

IMPRESSION: Catheter tip with surrounding inflammatory changes.

When one is interpreting a spiculated density as a postsurgical change, it is important to review the mammogram before biopsy to confirm that the lesion removed was in fact in the area of concern and, if nonpalpable, was present in the specimen. The most helpful factor that can aid one in making the diagnosis of "postsurgical change" on subsequent studies is a mammogram at 3 to 6 months after biopsy (1). This is particularly important when the biopsy demonstrated an atypical lesion.

Calcifications of fat necrosis form at variable times after biopsy but usually later than 6 months. These calcifications are typically ringlike, with lucent centers, and may be small (liponecrosis macrocystica calcificans) or larger oil cysts (radiolucent masses with eggshell calcifications). Occasionally, fat necrosis may be associated with clumps of irregular but rather coarse microcalcifications. Other forms of calcification that occur postoperatively include ringlike dermal calcifications in the scar, particularly in keloids. Calcified sutures, which are in linear or knot shapes, are observed postoperatively but more frequently in patients treated with radiotherapy (5).

Foreign bodies left in the breast include surgical clips (often used for marking a tumor bed for location of a boost dose of radiotherapy) and sutures that may calcify. Inadvertent transection of a needle localization wire and lack of its retrieval will result in the observation of a small segment of wire in the breast. Another cause of an iatrogenic foreign body in the breast is the inadvertent severing of the tip or cuff of a central venous catheter for chemotherapy, which may be embedded in the upper inner aspect of the breast (6).

REDUCTION MAMMOPLASTY

Breast reduction is performed for cosmetic reasons (to treat macromastia) or to achieve symmetry of the contralateral breast after the patient has undergone mastectomy with reconstruction. The surgical procedure involves elevation of the nipple, resection of glandular tissue, and skin removal (7). If there is a nipple transpo-

sition procedure, the nipple-areolar complex remains attached to the lactiferous ducts, and the whole complex is transposed upward. In a transplantation procedure, the nipple-areolar complex is severed from the ducts and is transplanted upward (7).

Mammographic findings vary with the type of procedure performed. In patients with a transposition, the subareolar ducts are in a normal relationship with the nipple-areolar complex, but there is a disruption of this orientation after transplantation procedures. Miller et al. (7) found parenchymal redistribution, with most of the fibroglandular tissue below the level of the nipple, as the most common finding in 24 patients who had undergone reduction mammoplasties. Elevation of the nipple was also a common finding, along with thickening of the skin of the lower aspect of the breast and the areola (7). There may be disorientation of the normal parenchymal pattern, with swirled patterns of tissue distribution (8). The scars on the skin may be evident on the mammogram as circumlinear densities traversing the inferior aspect of the breast (Figs. 12.12–12.19).

(text continues on page 495)

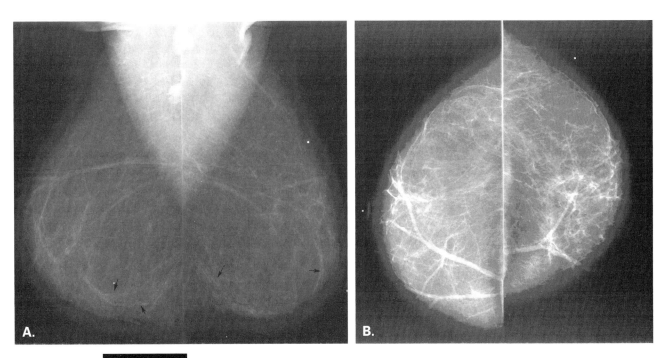

Figure 12.12

HISTORY: A 55-year-old woman who is status postreduction mammoplasty.

MAMMOGRAPHY: Bilateral MLO **(A)** and CC **(B)** views show fatty-replaced breasts. There is mild distortion of the tissue with linear swirling inferiorly **(arrows)**. The breasts have a flattened appearance on the MLO views, and the nipples are located more superiorly than in the normal state. This combination of findings is typical of postsurgical changes from reduction mammoplasty.

IMPRESSION: Postoperative changes secondary to reduction mammoplasty.

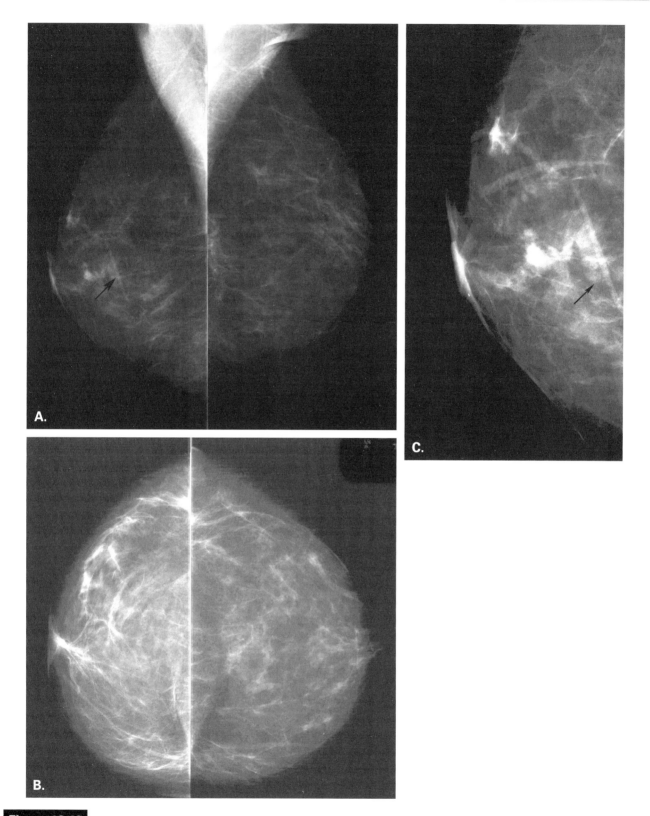

Figure 12.13

HISTORY: A 47-year-old woman is status postreduction mammoplasty, for routine screening.

MAMMOGRAPHY: Bilateral MLO **(A)** and CC **(B)** views show scattered fibroglandular densities. The breasts have a somewhat flattened appearance on the MLO views, and the nipples are situated higher than in the normal state. There are linear densities **(arrows)** inferiorly, best seen on a left MLO enlarged image **(C)**; these represent the scar lines related to the reduction procedure.

IMPRESSION: Postoperative changes from reduction mammoplasty.

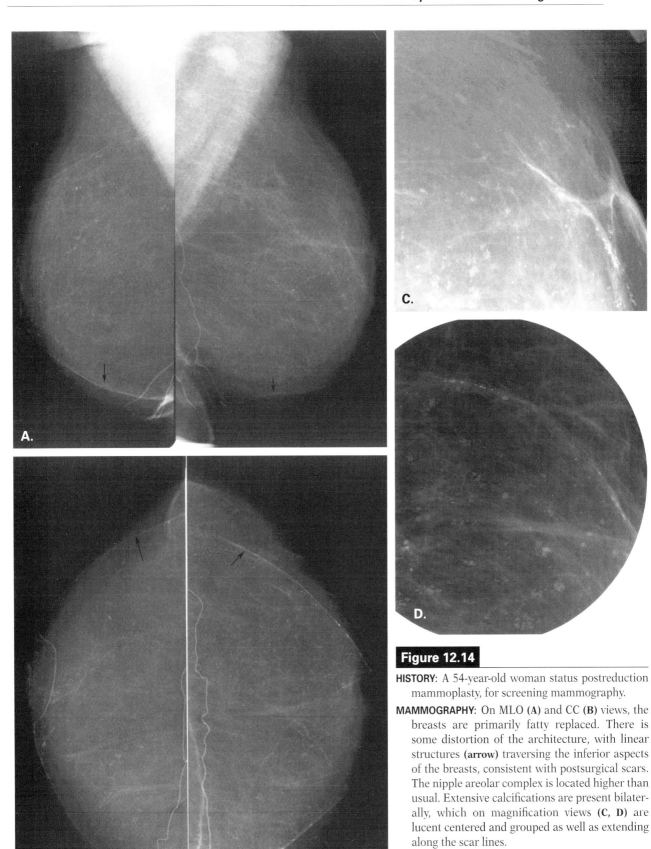

Figure 12.14

HISTORY: A 54-year-old woman status postreduction mammoplasty, for screening mammography.

MAMMOGRAPHY: On MLO **(A)** and CC **(B)** views, the breasts are primarily fatty replaced. There is some distortion of the architecture, with linear structures **(arrow)** traversing the inferior aspects of the breasts, consistent with postsurgical scars. The nipple areolar complex is located higher than usual. Extensive calcifications are present bilaterally, which on magnification views **(C, D)** are lucent centered and grouped as well as extending along the scar lines.

IMPRESSION: Postreduction mammoplasty changes with extensive dermal calcifications.

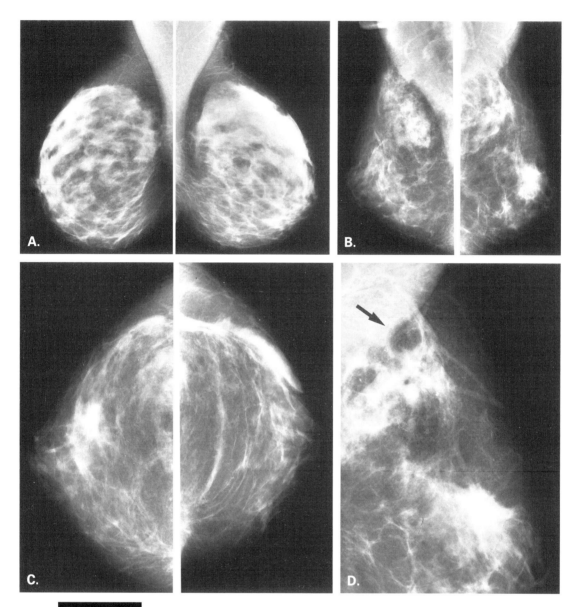

Figure 12.15

HISTORY: A 36-year-old woman who underwent reduction mammoplasties, for routine follow-up.

MAMMOGRAPHY: Baseline preoperative bilateral MLO views **(A)**, MLO **(B)** and CC **(C)** views 1 year postoperatively, and enlarged (2×) right MLO view **(D)** 2 years postoperatively. On the baseline mammogram **(A)**, the breasts are composed of dense, symmetrical fibroglandular tissue. After reduction **(B** and **C)**, a large amount of fibroglandular tissue has been removed, and there is disorientation of the remaining tissue and elevation of the nipple, consistent with normal changes after the procedure. This pattern should suggest to one the findings of a reduction procedure, even without knowledge of the clinical history. One year later **(D)**, there has been interval development of multiple oil cysts **(arrow)** and some smaller coarse calcifications of fat necrosis in the upper outer quadrant.

IMPRESSION: Postreduction changes, with development of fat necrosis. (Case courtesy of Dr. Cherie Scheer, Richmond, VA.)

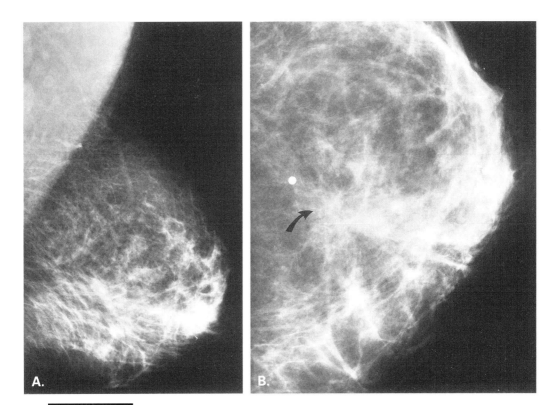

Figure 12.16

HISTORY: A 44-year-old gravida 3, para 3 woman after left mastectomy and reduction mammoplasty on the right.

MAMMOGRAPHY: Right MLO **(A)** and CC **(B)** views. There is distortion of normal architecture with disturbance of the normal orientation of the ducts toward the nipple. In the lower central aspect of the right breast, there is focal irregular increased density **(B, arrow)** along the direction of the reduction scar (marked by BBs). This finding is typical of the fat necrosis and scarring that is seen after reduction mammoplasty.

IMPRESSION: Postoperative changes after reduction mammoplasty.

Mandrekas et al. (9) described fat necrosis in 1.7% of patients following breast reduction. These patients all presented with a palpable mass that was located deep in the breast near the pectoralis major muscle. The lesion resembled a cancer on mammography and ultrasound.

Brown et al. (10) found that periareolar soft tissue changes and inferior pole alterations were present at 6 months in nearly all of 42 patients following breast reduction, and these findings regressed on subsequent studies. In 50% of patients, calcifications occurred after 2 years. In 10% of patients, there was evidence of fat necrosis on mammography.

Calcifications are a common finding in patients who have had breast reductions (3). Dermal calcifications, which are smooth and round, may occur in the areola (7) or in scars. Areas of fat necrosis are more common in patients who have undergone reduction than those who have had routine biopsies. Calcifications may be eggshell shaped in the walls of oil cysts or may be irregular (11) or even lacy in appearance (Fig. 12.20). The calcifications may be extensive and have a coarse pleomorphic appearance, sometimes raising a concern for cancer because of the pleomorphism. Importantly, these calcifications are oriented in the direction of the scars, and correlation with this distribution is helpful in confirming their etiology. Even sutural calcification may be identified after reduction procedures (8) (Fig. 12.21).

(text continues on page 498)

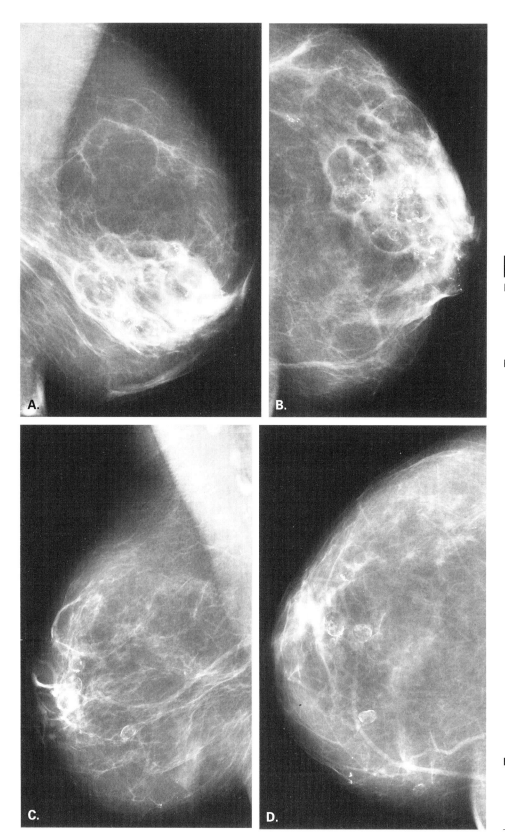

Figure 12.17

HISTORY: A 45-year-old woman after bilateral reduction mammoplasties, with firm nodularity in both subareolar areas.

MAMMOGRAPHY: Right MLO **(A)** and CC **(B)** views and left MLO **(C)** and CC **(D)** views. The breasts show primarily fatty replacement. There are extensive areas of calcification in both breasts, more prominent on the right than on the left. Many of the calcifications are thin eggshell or rimlike in areas of liponecrosis macrocystica (fat necrosis). On the right **(A** and **B)**, there is a mixture of the large oil cysts with coarse pleomorphic calcifications. The findings represent dystrophic changes of fat necrosis secondary to reduction mammoplasty. Generally, this extent of fat necrosis is not seen after biopsy or lumpectomy and instead represents a more significant trauma, such as a reduction procedure or severe nonsurgical breast trauma.

IMPRESSION: Extensive changes of fat necrosis, secondary to reduction mammoplasty. (Case courtesy of Dr. M. C. Wilhelm, Charlottesville, VA.)

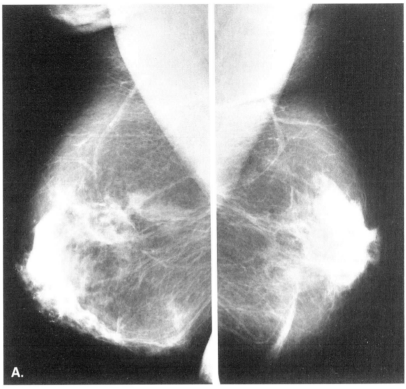

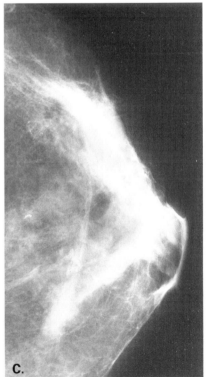

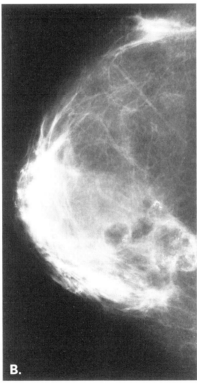

Figure 12.18

HISTORY: A 50-year-old woman after bilateral reduction mammoplasties, for routine mammogram.

MAMMOGRAPHY: Bilateral MLO (**A**), left CC (**B**), and right CC (**C**) views. There is disorientation of the parenchymal pattern, without the normal flow of ducts toward the nipples (**A**). This disorientation of parenchyma is a typical postreduction finding. On the CC views (**B** and **C**), there are circular, round, and lacy coarse calcifications associated with the dense areas of parenchymal scarring. These findings are seen after reduction mammoplasty and represent dystrophic changes of fat necrosis.

IMPRESSION: Fat necrosis secondary to reduction mammoplasty.

NOTE: The patient was followed for 18 months, and the calcifications were stable.

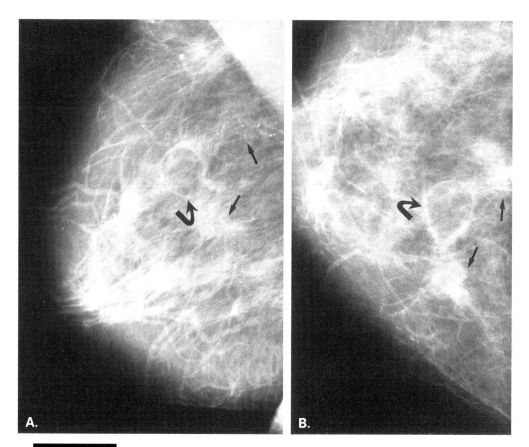

Figure 12.19

HISTORY: A 58-year-old gravida 6, para 6 woman with history of right breast cancer and of reduction mammoplasty on the left.

MAMMOGRAPHY: Left MLO **(A)** and enlarged (1.5×) CC **(B)** views. The breast is moderately dense. In the left upper-inner quadrant, there is a radiolucent well-circumscribed lesion **(curved arrow)** with early calcification in the rim, consistent with an oil cyst. Adjacent to the oil cyst are two clusters of coarse pleomorphic microcalcifications **(arrows)** that had developed since the prior mammogram. Because of their morphology and their association with the nearby oil cyst, these microcalcifications were thought to represent most likely fat necrosis and fibrosis. However, because of the risk status of the patient and the interval change, the area was biopsied.

IMPRESSION: Probable fat necrosis.

HISTOPATHOLOGY: Changes compatible with old biopsy, fat necrosis.

LUMPECTOMY AND RADIATION THERAPY

During the past two decades, there has been a striking increase in breast conservation procedures for treatment of carcinomas. Several studies (12,13) have shown that the long-term survival of women treated for grade I and II breast cancer with lumpectomy and radiation therapy is similar to that of those treated with mastectomy. Four large, randomized controlled trials evaluating lumpectomy with radiotherapy include the National Cancer Institute of Italy (13), the National Cancer Institute of the United States (14), the European Organization for Research and Treatment of Cancer (15), and the National Surgical

Adjuvant Breast Project (12). In these trials, the treatment included whole breast irradiation. Typical radiation therapy for breast cancer is a treatment course over 6 weeks using an external beam. More recently, partial breast accelerated radiotherapy or brachytherapy has been used for certain small invasive cancers. These treatments, which occur over a week, may be delivered through multiple catheters or a balloon inserted into the breast or by an accelerated dose by external beam (16).

Patients who have the option for breast conservation therapy are usually those who have tumor confined to the breast and ipsilateral nodes, a tumor size of <4 cm without fixation, and a size or location of tumor that, after

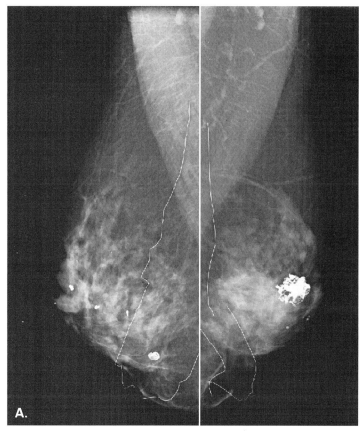

A.

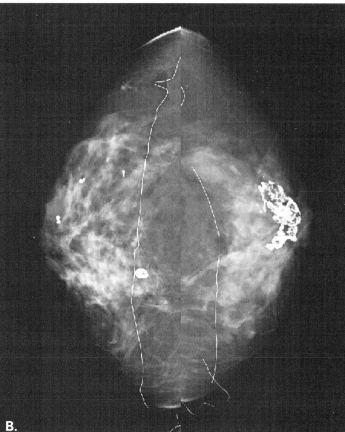

B.

Figure 12.20

HISTORY: A 62-year-old woman with a history of reduction mammoplasty.

MAMMOGRAPHY: Bilateral MLO (**A**) and CC (**B**) views show dense parenchyma and postsurgical scars delineated by wire markers in the skin. There is some parenchymal redistribution, with more tissue being located inferiorly and medially. The breasts appear somewhat flattened at the area of the nipple areolar complex, which is elevated in comparison with a nonreduced breast. In addition, there are coarse dystrophic calcifications bilaterally. Those on the right have a dense but eggshell appearance typical of fat necrosis and an oil cyst.

IMPRESSION: Postreduction changes.

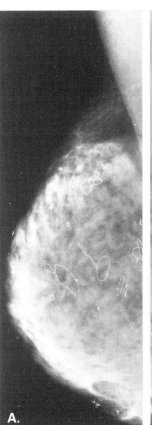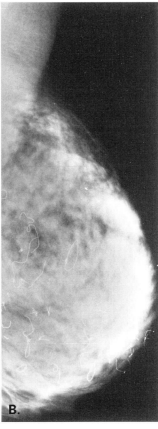

A. B.

Figure 12.21

HISTORY: A 35-year-old woman after reduction mammoplasty, for routine screening.

MAMMOGRAPHY: Left MLO (**A**) and right MLO (**B**) views. The breasts are very dense and glandular. Multiple calcified and radiopaque sutures are present bilaterally, corresponding to the scars involved with the reduction procedure.

IMPRESSION: Calcified sutures.

treatment, will yield satisfactory cosmetic results (3,12). Multicentric carcinoma (17) is also considered by many radiotherapists as a contraindication to breast conservation therapy.

In patients who are treated with lumpectomy and radiation therapy, the rate of local recurrence is in the range of 6% to 10% (18–20) and is at a rate of 2% per year (3). There is a significant salvage rate (58% at 5 years, 50% at 10 years) in patients who develop local recurrences after lumpectomy and radiation (21). In a study of treatment methods used for 124 cases of pure ductal carcinoma in situ (DCIS), Warneke et al. (22) found the local recurrence rates to be as follows: 1.3% following mastectomy, 3.2% following lumpectomy and radiation, and 11% following wide excision alone. All the local recurrences after lumpectomy were detected at mammography, and all lesions were salvaged by mastectomy. A majority of local recurrences occur in the same quadrant as the initial primary (20). Because of this, not only

whole breast irradiation but also a boost to the tumor bed may be given (23). Careful clinical and mammographic follow-up is necessary in order to detect these recurrences when they are early enough for the patient to be salvaged.

A thorough preoperative evaluation of the patient who is considering breast conservation is necessary to optimize the results. Importantly, the mammographic assessment of the size and extent of tumor is necessary. Ultrasound and magnetic resonance imaging (MRI) are important adjunctive examinations to answer this question. The presence of multiple lesions that are potentially malignant requires biopsy to determine the presence of multifocal (two or more foci in the same quadrant) or multicentric (two or more foci in different quadrants) disease.

An initial postlumpectomy/preradiotherapy mammogram is recommended to serve as a baseline for follow-up studies and to evaluate the breast for residual carcinoma (3,24–27) (Figs. 12.22 and 12.23). This study should be performed at least 10 days after surgery, allowing for time for the incision to heal. Comparison must be made with the preoperative mammogram to determine the exact location of the tumor and its appearance. Particularly if the tumor contained microcalcifications, the postoperative study can provide valuable information about the presence of residual calcifications (18,25). Pretreatment postoperative mammography is helpful as an indicator of the adequacy of tumor excision, particularly in cases in which the original tumor presented with microcalcifications. Gluck et al. (28) found the positive predictive value for residual tumor to be 0.69; when the tumor was DCIS and when more than five microcalcifications were present at the lumpectomy site, the positive predictive value was 0.90. However, the negative predictive value of the absence of residual microcalcifications was 0.64 for all tumor types and was 1.0 for the noncomedo subtype of DCIS.

In addition, the pretreatment mammogram can serve as a new baseline before radiotherapy. Teixidor et al. (29) found the preradiotherapy mammogram to be helpful for interpretation of the subsequent studies in 32% of patients. In 5% of patients, residual tumor was identified on the pretreatment study as well.

On this baseline, normal expected findings are skin thickening at the lumpectomy site, architectural distortion, and oftentimes a fluid collection. In a study of the imaging findings after breast conservation therapy, Mendelson (4) found that approximately one half of 110 patients had a fluid collection at the surgical site. Most often the size of the hematoma/seroma was 3 to 5 cm. Postoperative hematomas are of maximum size on this initial baseline study and gradually diminish in size, becoming more irregular in contour. When a patient is found to have irregular density on a 6-month posttreatment mammogram, it is extremely useful to have a baseline postoperative study that showed a larger hematoma at the site.

Normal mammographic and clinical changes that may be expected after breast conservation therapy include (a) local changes that the tumor bed related to surgery and (b) diffuse changes related to irradiation (Figs. 12.24–12.36). Mammography is necessary for accurate monitoring of the postirradiation changes as well as the possible development of recurrent carcinoma (24). DiPiro et al. (30) in a study of the role of routine magnification views in patients after breast conservation therapy for breast cancer, suggested that the magnification view was necessary to evaluate equivocal microcalcifications. In 4% of cases, the magnification view influenced the decision to perform a biopsy. However, the authors did not find the magnification views helpful when conventional views of the breast were not questionable.

At 6 to 12 months, the maximum changes of increased interstitial markings and skin thickening are seen. These diffuse findings are secondary to the edema from irradiation of the breast. These edematous changes will stabilize and then diminish, usually at 2 years or later (3). The skin thickness may increase to as much as 1 cm. Dershaw et al. (31) found that in 160 women treated with lumpectomy and radiation therapy, 96% had skin thickening, which stabilized by 1 year. At 3 years, 50% of women had persistent edema and skin thickening.

The latent normal changes after radiation are the development of calcifications of fat necrosis, developing usually after 1 year. Libshitz et al. (32) found that benign calcifications developed in treated breasts from 2 to 44 months after irradiation. These calcifications have the same mammographic appearance of liponecrosis microcystia secondary to trauma or biopsy, and they may occur at the lumpectomy site or elsewhere in the treated breast. Brenner and Pfaff (33) found that although all the normal postoperative changes other than calcifications resolved over time, architectural distortion showed the most significant change (p = 0.05).

In a study of 123 patients treated with breast conservation therapy, Cox et al. (34) found that 27% of patients never developed a scar on mammography; in the 73% of patients with a scar, the mean decrease in scar size was 16.7 mm over the study period of 4 years. Calcifications developed in 16% of patients between 6 and 48 months after treatment. Recurrent cancer was found in 2% of patients. Others (31,35) have described the development of calcifications that are coarse and round in one third to one half of irradiated breasts.

Serial mammography and clinical examination of the treated breast are complementary for the optimal detection of recurrence. Hassell et al. (36) found that in 24 patients with recurrent carcinoma, 7 had positive mammographic findings alone, 9 had positive clinical examination alone, and 8 had both positive mammography and clinical examination. Most common mammographic findings were new microcalcifications or a new mass. Orel et al. (37), in a series of 38 biopsy-proven recurrences, found that 34% were found by mammography alone, 45% with palpation alone, and 21% by both methods. A majority (55%) of recurrences were in the lumpectomy quadrant.

The findings of recurrent carcinoma include the development of new microcalcifications, increased skin thickening after stabilization, increased density (particularly at the tumor bed) after stabilization, and the development of a new mass (Figs. 12.37–12.41). Because of the difficulty in differentiating benign from malignant microcalcifications with certainty, biopsy is indicated unless the calcifications are those of fat necrosis.

New spiculated masses and irregular ductal-type malignant microcalcifications are highly suspicious for recurrence. Stomper et al. (38) found that 65% of recurrences in 23 women occurred at the primary site, 22%

(text continues on page 507)

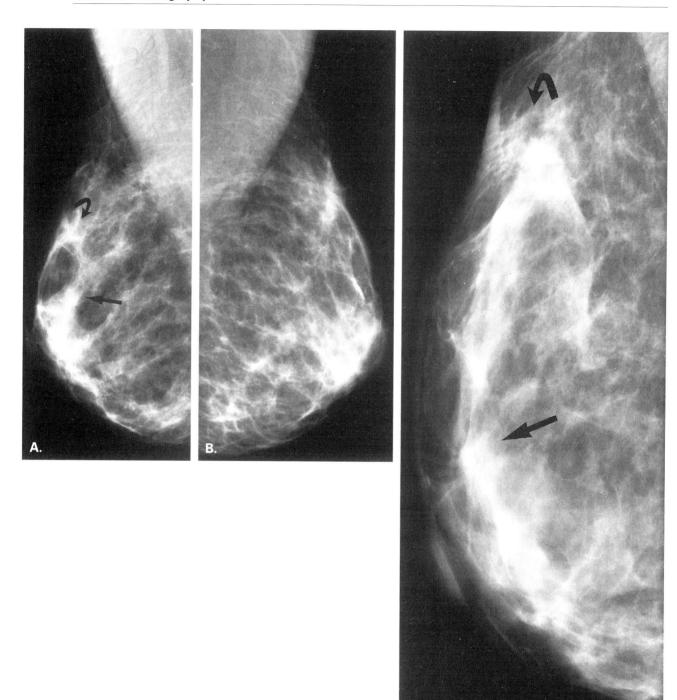

Figure 12.22

HISTORY: A 31-year-old woman who had a lumpectomy for a palpable carcinoma in the left axillary tail 3 weeks earlier. She was referred for radiation therapy, and a postoperative baseline mammogram was obtained.

MAMMOGRAPHY: Left MLO (**A**), right MLO (**B**), and left CC (**C**) views. The scar from the recent lumpectomy is evident as a flat irregular density in the upper outer quadrant (**curved arrow**) (**A** and **C**). There is asymmetry of the left supra-areolar area (**arrow**) in comparison with the right breast (**B**). A focal area of increased density is present, and on the CC views (**C**), it appears finely spiculated (**arrow**). This supra-areolar lesion is suspicious for residual multicentric nonpalpable carcinoma.

IMPRESSION: Highly suspicious for residual carcinoma, separate focus, left breast.

HISTOPATHOLOGY: Infiltrating ductal carcinoma.

NOTE: This case demonstrates the importance of obtaining a mammogram, even in a young patient, before definitive therapy to confirm the absence of residual carcinoma.

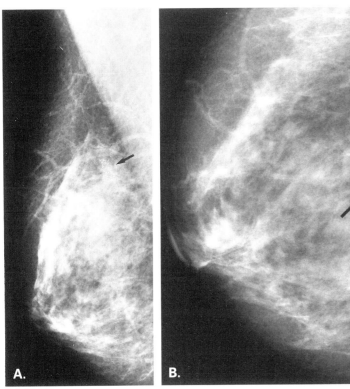

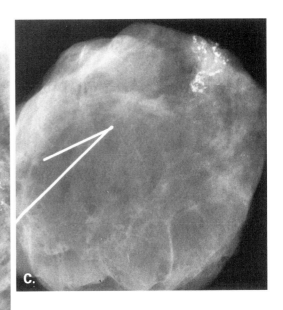

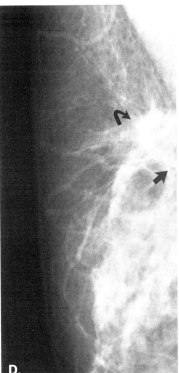

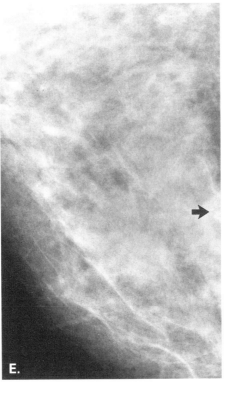

Figure 12.23

HISTORY: A 66-year-old gravida 2, para 2 woman with a family history of breast cancer, for screening.

MAMMOGRAPHY: Left MLO (**A**) and enlarged exaggerated CC lateral (**B**) views, specimen radiograph (**C**), and enlarged left ML (**D**) and CC (**E**) views after biopsy. On the initial mammogram, a cluster of innumerable, irregular malignant calcifications (**arrows**) is seen (**A** and **B**). The specimen radiograph (**C**) following needle localization and excision demonstrates the calcifications, which were noted to extend to the edge of the tissue. Histopathology demonstrated intraductal carcinoma of the comedo type, extending close to the surgical margin. The patient wished to have breast conservation therapy. The postbiopsy, preradiotherapy baseline mammogram (**D** and **E**) demonstrates residual malignant-appearing calcifications at the lumpectomy site (**arrows**). The spiculated soft-tissue density (**curved arrow**) represents postoperative hematoma.

IMPRESSION: Preradiotherapy baseline mammogram demonstrating residual carcinoma.

HISTOPATHOLOGY: Residual DCIS.

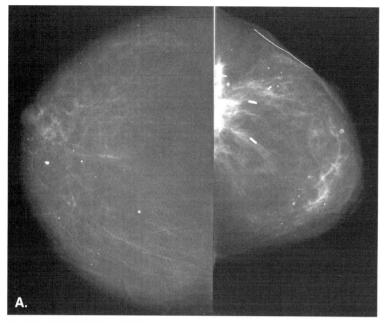

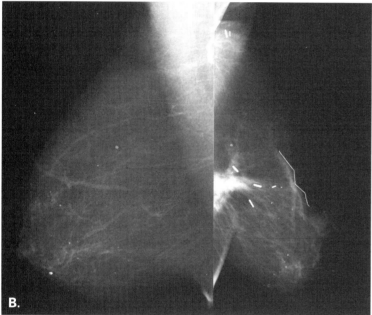

Figure 12.24

HISTORY: A 62-year-old woman who is status postlumpectomy and radiation for breast cancer.

MAMMOGRAPHY: Bilateral CC **(A)** and MLO **(B)** views show that the right breast is smaller and retracted in comparison with the left. There is an irregular spiculated mass at the lumpectomy site, consistent with postsurgical scar. There are dystrophic calcifications in the scar and scattered elsewhere throughout both breasts. Diffuse skin thickening is present on the right secondary to radiation therapy as well.

IMPRESSION: Postlumpectomy and radiation therapy changes, right breast.

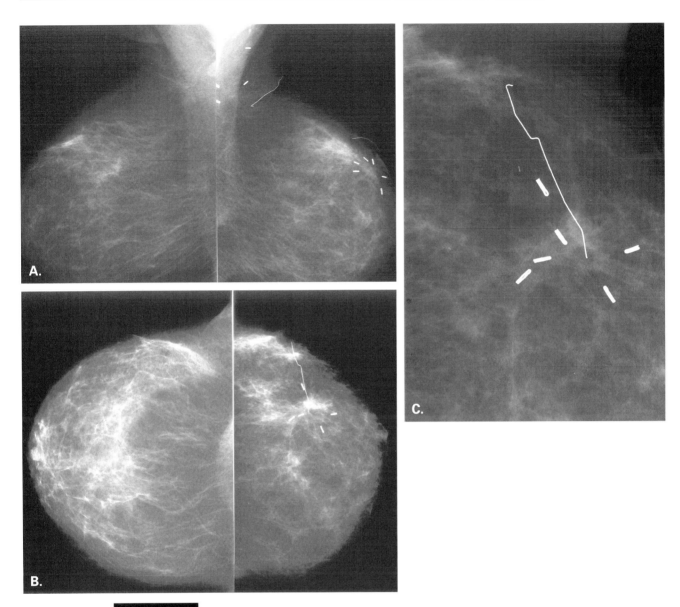

Figure 12.25

HISTORY: A 49-year-old woman who is status postlumpectomy and radiation therapy for right breast DCIS.

MAMMOGRAPHY: Bilateral MLO **(A)** and CC **(B)** views show marked asymmetry in the appearance of the breasts. The right is smaller and diffusely more dense than the left, related to the effects of radiation therapy. A postsurgical scar is demarcated by surgical clips in the 10 o'clock position. On the spot MLO magnification view **(C)**, the scar is better seen and is noted to contain radiolucencies consistent with evolving oil cysts.

IMPRESSION: Normal posttreatment changes.

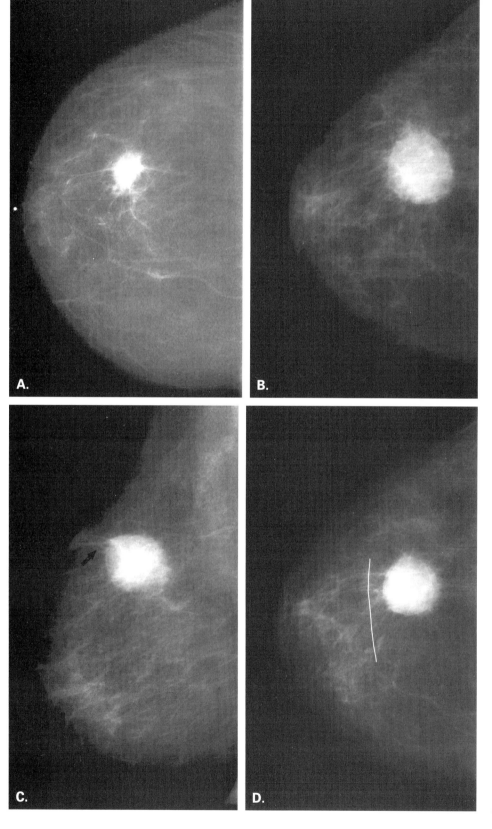

A.

B.

C.

D.

Figure 12.26

HISTORY: Patient with a history of left breast invasive ductal carcinoma, treated with lumpectomy and radiation therapy.

MAMMOGRAPHY: Left CC **(A)** view before surgery shows a high-density lobular mass with spiculated margins, consistent with carcinoma. Six months after treatment, the left CC **(B)** and MLO **(C)** views show a large round mass with somewhat indistinct margins extending toward the skin **(arrow)**. This is a normal postlumpectomy finding: hematoma or seroma. One year later, the left CC view **(D)** shows that the seroma is retracting and in doing so is more dense and spiculated.

IMPRESSION: Normal evaluation of seroma at lumpectomy site.

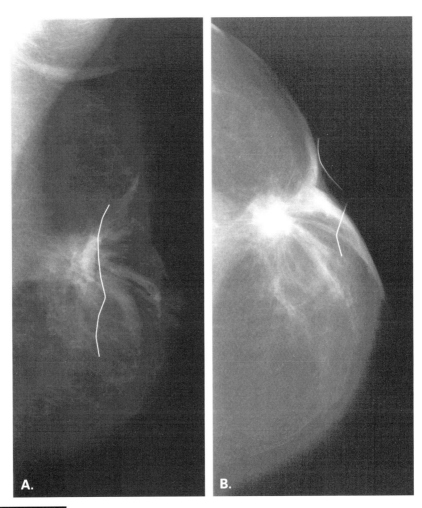

Figure 12.27

HISTORY: Postmenopausal patient who is status posttreatment of right breast cancer with lumpectomy and radiation therapy.

MAMMOGRAPHY: Right MLO **(A)** and CC **(B)** views show a spiculated mass at the surgical site, which is consistent with postsurgical scar. The area has a different appearance on the two views. On the MLO, it is contiguous with the skin and associated with the scar on the skin. Diffuse skin thickening related to radiation therapy is also noted.

IMPRESSION: Postsurgical and radiation changes.

recurred in different sites, and 13% were multifocal. Dershaw et al. (39) found that microcalcifications were the most common presentation of recurrence (19 of 29 cases), and a mass with or without calcifications was less frequent (10 of 29 cases). Two of the recurrences that were masses were evident as enlargement of the scar. The positives rates for recurrent tumor on biopsies for mammographic or clinical abnormalities in treated breasts range from 20% to 58% (26,40–42). A combination of clinical findings and mammographic findings is highly suspicious for recurrence; careful attention to and comparison with all previous studies, not just the most recent, are necessary.

The differentiation of posttreatment scar and recurrence can sometimes be difficult on mammography alone. The temporal changes from prior mammography determine the approach to patients. In cases in question, contrast-enhanced MRI is very helpful to differentiate scar from tumor. Heywang-Köbrunner et al. (43) found that in the early posttreatment period (up to 9 months), MRI was not helpful because of the strong enhancement present; however, after 18 months, MRI detected all recurrences correctly as diffuse or focal areas of enhancement.

(text continues on page 514)

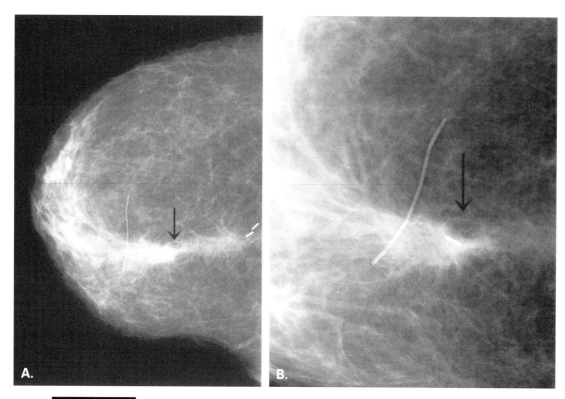

Figure 12.28

HISTORY: A 47-year-old woman with a history of DCIS treated with lumpectomy and radiation therapy.

MAMMOGRAPHY: Left CC views **(A)** show a wire marking the lumpectomy site. Postsurgical scarring is present, extending toward the chest wall. Within the scar, there is a small radiolucent mass **(arrow)** better seen on the magnification view **(B)**.

IMPRESSION: Oil cyst within the lumpectomy site, fat necrosis.

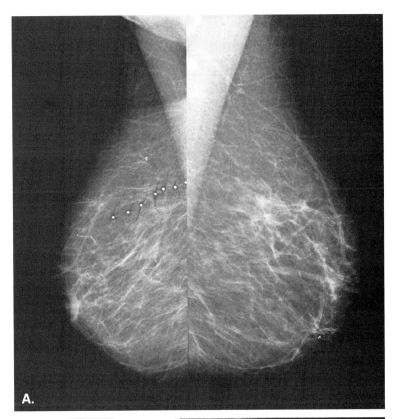

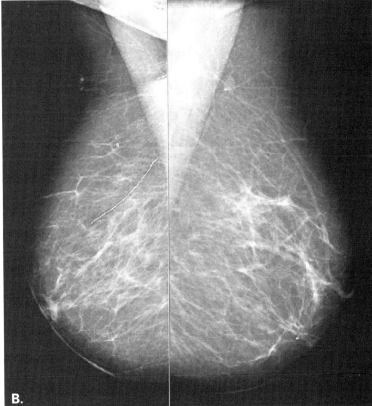

Figure 12.29

HISTORY: A 58-year-old woman who is 7 years status post–breast conservation therapy for left breast cancer.

MAMMOGRAPHY: Bilateral MLO views **(A)** 1 year ago demonstrate minimal distortion in the left breast superiorly, as demonstrated by a scar marker on the skin. Mild skin thickening is present as well, and the breast appears smaller and somewhat retracted compared with the right. On the current MLO views **(B)**, the scar is slightly less prominent, and the other changes are stable.

IMPRESSION: Normal changes following breast conservation with lumpectomy and radiation therapy.

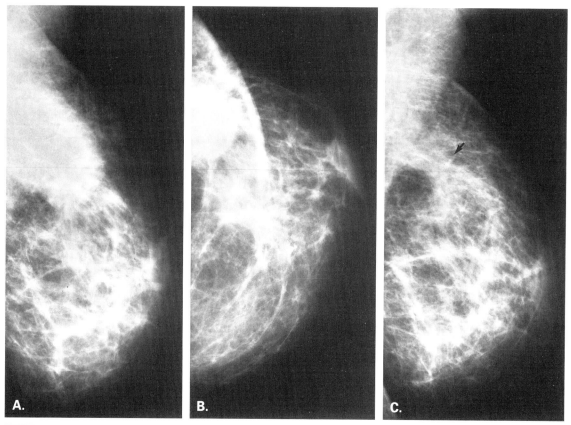

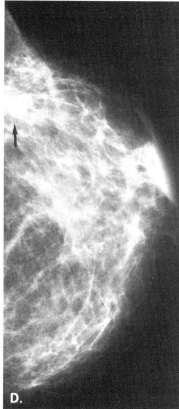

Figure 12.30

HISTORY: A 50-year-old gravida 4, para 4 woman after lumpectomy for a carcinoma in the right upper-outer quadrant and referred for radiation therapy. A preliminary mammogram, after lumpectomy and before radiotherapy, was obtained.

MAMMOGRAPHY: Right MLO **(A)** and CC **(B)** views 1 month after lumpectomy, and right MLO **(C)** and CC **(D)** views 6 months later. On the postlumpectomy films **(A** and **B)**, a large, medium-density, partially circumscribed mass is present at the surgical site and is consistent with a postoperative hematoma. Six months after therapy **(C** and **D)**, the hematoma has resolved, and there is a small residual area of increased density, consistent with scar and fat necrosis **(arrows)**. There is also a mild increase in the overall density of the interstitium and an increase in skin thickness that are normal postradiation changes.

IMPRESSION: Normal evolution of postlumpectomy and radiation changes in the acute-subacute phase.

NOTE: It is not unusual to see a hematoma on the baseline postlumpectomy study. The mammogram can usually be performed with adequate compression of the breast 10 days or more after lumpectomy.

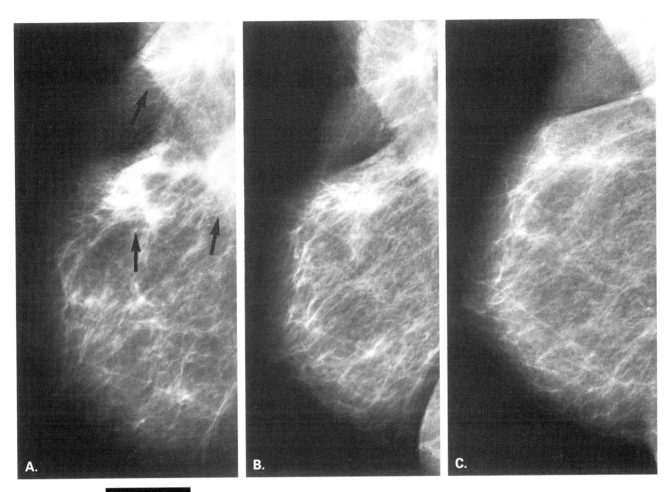

Figure 12.31

HISTORY: A 66-year-old gravida 3, para 3 woman who was referred for radiation therapy after a lumpectomy and axillary dissection in the left upper-outer quadrant.

MAMMOGRAPHY: Left MLO view 3 weeks after lumpectomy **(A)** and left MLO views 6 months **(B)** and 12 months **(C)** later. On the initial postoperative film **(A)**, there is architectural distortion associated with irregular areas of increased density in the left upper-outer quadrant and in the axilla **(arrows)**. The density represents hematoma and postsurgical change, and the examination will serve as a baseline for the follow-up after radiotherapy. Six months after treatment **(B)**, the distortion from the scar persists, but the hematoma and surrounding density have significantly decreased in size. Very minimal increase in interstitial markings is seen, an effect of radiotherapy. On the study 1 year after treatment **(C)**, further diminution in the density is seen as would be expected, and there are no new findings to suggest recurrence.

IMPRESSION: Postlumpectomy scarring showing resolution.

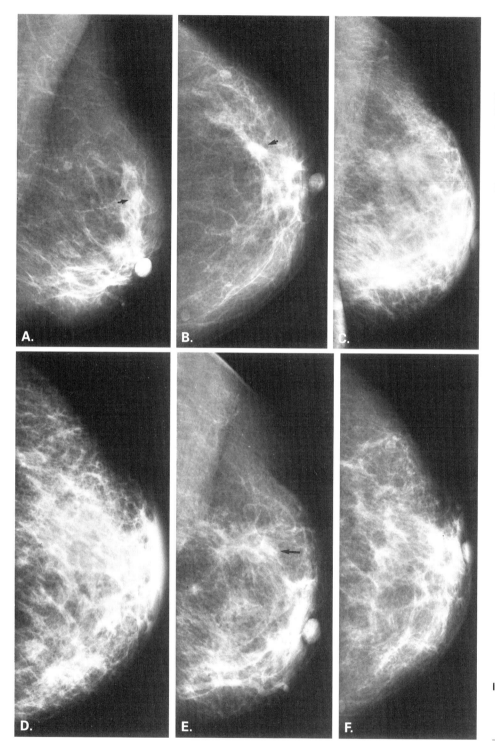

Figure 12.32

HISTORY: A 67-year-old gravida 6, para 5 woman with a positive family history of breast cancer, for routine screening.

MAMMOGRAPHY: Right oblique (**A**) and CC (**B**) views from April 1988, right MLO (**C**) and CC (**D**) views from April 1989, and right MLO (**E**) and CC (**F**) views from October 1989. On the initial screening examination (**A** and **B**), there is a high-density spiculated mass in the upper outer quadrant (**arrows**). The lesion was considered highly suspicious and was biopsied after needle localization. The histopathology demonstrated infiltrating ductal carcinoma, and the patient was treated with lumpectomy and radiation therapy. One year later (**C** and **D**), the breast is diffusely edematous, with prominent interstitial markings, increased density, and skin thickening. These are normal changes in the first year after radiation therapy. At 18 months after diagnosis (**E** and **F**), the edema pattern secondary to radiation is decreasing. There also has been a decrease in skin thickening. The scar in the upper outer quadrant is evident (**arrow**), but there are no changes to suggest recurrence.

IMPRESSION: Normal evolution of postradiation changes after treatment of primary breast carcinoma.

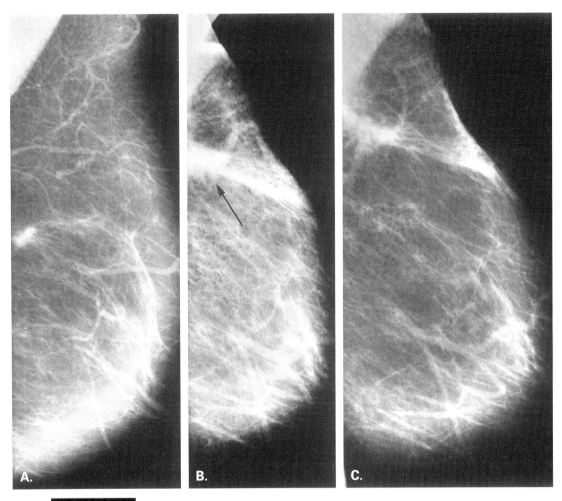

Figure 12.33

HISTORY: A 65-year-old woman treated with lumpectomy and radiation therapy for infiltrating ductal carcinoma of the right breast.

MAMMOGRAPHY: Prebiopsy right MLO view **(A)** and posttreatment right MLO views at 6 months **(B)** and at 12 months **(C)**. On the initial study **(A)**, there is a high-density spiculated mass deep in the right breast, consistent with carcinoma. This was biopsied after a needle localization, and histopathology revealed infiltrating ductal carcinoma. On the next examination **(B)**, 6 months after lumpectomy and radiation therapy, the breast is diffusely more dense and does not compress as well. There is a focal irregular density **(arrow)** at the lumpectomy site that is most consistent scar and fat necrosis. Subsequently, at 12 months posttreatment **(C)**, there has been a decrease in the edema of the breast as well as a decrease in the size and density of the scar and fat necrosis.

IMPRESSION: Normal evolution of postoperative and radiation changes.

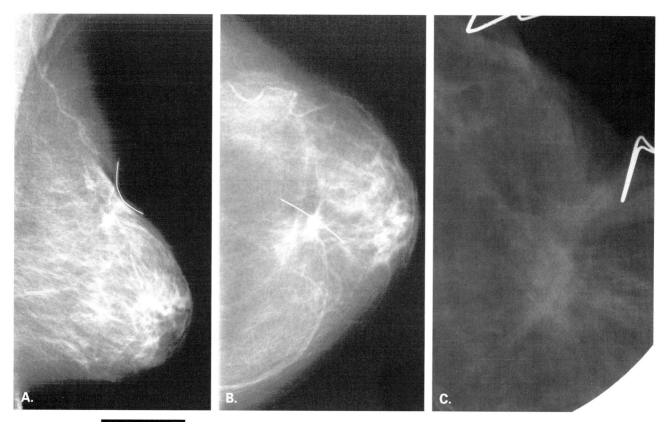

Figure 12.34

HISTORY: A 78-year-old woman with a history of right breast cancer, treated with lumpectomy and radiation therapy.

MAMMOGRAPHY: Right MLO **(A)** and CC **(B)** views show an area of architectural distortion beneath the wire marker, consistent with postsurgical scar. On the spot magnification **(C)**, the area is noted to be highly spiculated and contain small punctuate and amorphous microcalcifications.

IMPRESSION: Postsurgical scar containing indeterminate microcalcifications. Recommend needle biopsy.

HISTOPATHOLOGY: Fat necrosis, foreign body giant cell reaction, hemosiderin laden macrophages, microcalcifications.

A rare complication of breast irradiation is the development of radiation-induced sarcoma (RIS). The rate of RIS has been reported to be 0.18% (44), and the mean latency period after treatment is 5.5 to 9 years (45). Angiosarcoma typically presents as a painless mass that may be associated with overlying blue or purplish discoloration of the skin (45).

IMAGING OF THE MASTECTOMY SITE

Although a majority of physicians do not recommend routine imaging of the mastectomy site to search for cancer recurrence, there is some literature that sup-ports the value of mammography or sonography in these patients. Rissanen et al. (46) evaluated the roles of mammography and ultrasound in the diagnosis of local and regional recurrences in patients who had undergone mastectomy. The authors found the sensitivity of ultrasound to be the highest at 91%, with the sensitivities of clinical examination and mammography to be 79% and 45%, respectively. Most recurrent cancers were seen as circumscribed masses on mammography and hypoechoic lesions at ultrasound (Fig. 12.42). In addition, if the mastectomy site is imaged, benign lesions may be observed. Fat necrosis as evidenced by oil cysts or dystrophic calcifications may be seen on mammography (Fig. 12.43).

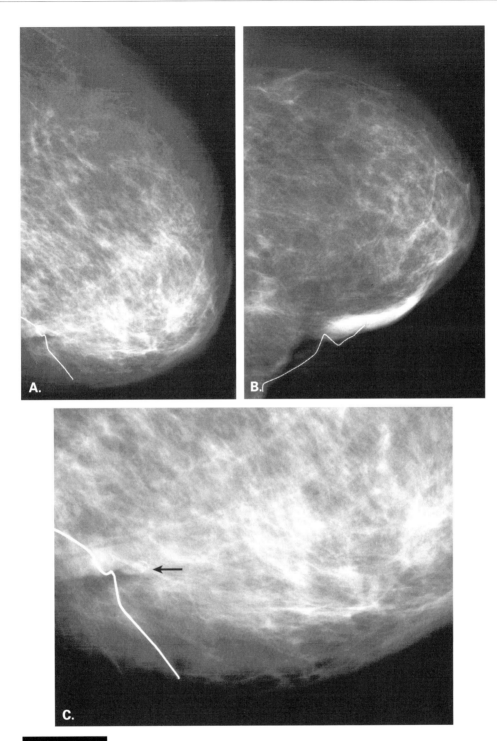

HISTORY: An 80-year-old woman who is 7 months status posttreatment of right breast cancer with lumpectomy and radiation therapy.

MAMMOGRAPHY: Right MLO **(A)** and CC **(B)** views show architectural distortion at the lumpectomy site, marked by a wire, consistent with postsurgical scar. On the magnification ML view **(C)**, there are fine linear microcalcifications **(arrow)** at the anterior edge of the biopsy site, suspicious for recurrence of carcinoma. Biopsy of these calcifications was performed.

IMPRESSION: Microcalcifications suspicious for recurrence of carcinoma.

HISTOPATHOLOGY: Benign breast tissue with fibrosis and microcalcifications.

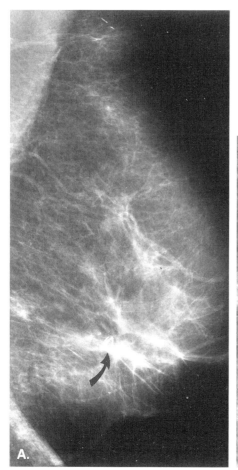

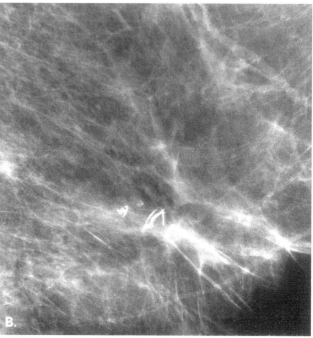

Figure 12.36

HISTORY: A 68-year-old gravida 6, para 4 woman for follow-up after lumpectomy and radiation therapy on the right for infiltrating lobular carcinoma. She had also undergone a re-excision at the tumor bed for new microcalcifications found to be atypical epithelial hyperplasia.

MAMMOGRAPHY: Right MLO **(A)** and magnification (2×) **(B)** views at the tumor bed 2 years after treatment. There is irregular increased density at the lumpectomy site, consistent with post-surgical scar. There are curvilinear coarse calcifications at the biopsy site **(A, curved arrow)** seen better on the magnification view **(B)**. Behind the curvilinear calcifications is a group of calcifications in a knotted shape **(A and B)**. The smooth curvilinear shape of the calcifications is typical of sutural calcification.

IMPRESSION: Sutural calcifications.

Certainly in patients in whom a prophylactic subcutaneous mastectomy has been performed, mammography is necessary. In these patients, the nipple areolar complex is not removed. Because the nipple remains, the ducts remain; therefore, carcinoma can still develop in the residual tissue.

In most cases, patients who have had a total or modified radical mastectomy and reconstruction are not imaged. The reconstruction may be performed by placement of an expandable implant or by plastic repair with a myocutaneous flap (Fig. 12.44). Several types of myocutaneous flaps have been used for breast

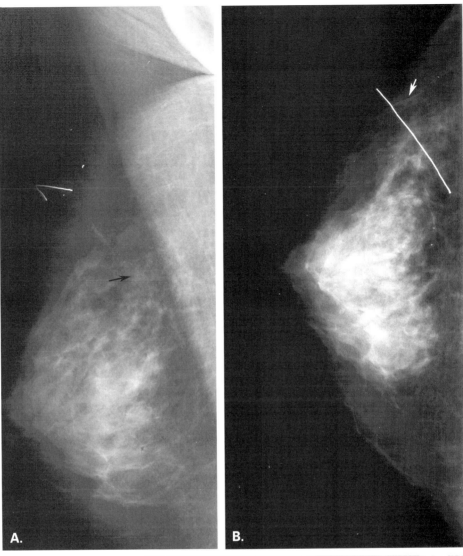

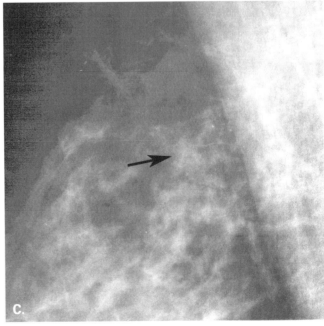

Figure 12.37

HISTORY: A 58-year-old woman who was status postlumpectomy and radiation therapy to the left breast, 20 years ago.

MAMMOGRAPHY: Left MLO **(A)** and CC **(B)** views show heterogeneously dense tissue and minimal scarring marked by a wire on the skin. In the 2 o'clock position, just posterior to the lumpectomy site, are clustered microcalcifications **(arrows)**. On the enlarged MLO image **(C)**, the pleomorphic and fine linear morphologies of the calcifications are noted.

IMPRESSION: Highly suspicious for recurrence of carcinoma.

HISTOPATHOLOGY: DCIS, intermediate grade, solid type.

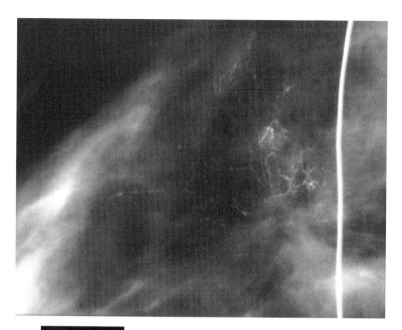

Figure 12.38

HISTORY: Routine follow-up for a 48-year-old patient who is status postlumpectomy and radiation therapy for left breast ductal carcinoma.

MAMMOGRAPHY: Left magnification CC view. There is architectural distortion at the site of the lumpectomy. Within this distortion are innumerable fine, pleomorphic, linear, and branching microcalcifications. This appearance is highly suggestive of carcinoma and is not a benign postsurgical change.

IMPRESSION: Highly suspicious for malignancy, BI-RADS® 5.

HISTOPATHOLOGY: High-grade DCIS with comedonecrosis.

reconstruction, including those from the transversus rectus abdominis muscle and the latissimus dorsi muscle. One complication of this procedure, which is related to maintaining an adequate blood supply, is fat necrosis of the flap (47) (Fig. 12.45). The patient presents with a firm mass (48,49), and the differential diagnosis includes recurrent carcinoma or fat necrosis. Mammography may be used in this circumstance and may demonstrate changes of fat necrosis ranging from an irregular increased density to radiolucent oil cysts to ringlike calcifications characteristic of a benign process. Recurrent carcinoma in the flap may be clinically suspected because of development of a palpable mass (Fig. 12.46). Mammography demonstrates a mass that is most often located peripherally, at the junction of the flap with the native tissue.

(References begin on page 526)

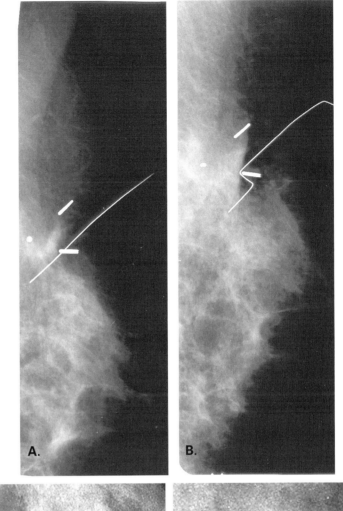

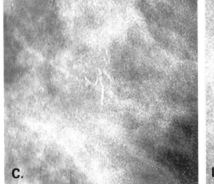

Figure 12.39

HISTORY: A 55-year-old woman 1 year status postlumpectomy and radiation therapy for right breast ductal carcinoma.

MAMMOGRAPHY: Right magnification ML (**A**) and MLO (**B**) and enlarged images (**C, D**) show the lumpectomy site delineated by surgical clips. There are a few very faint, fine linear microcalcifications just inferior to the tumor bed. Stereotactic core needle biopsy was performed.

IMPRESSION: Highly suspicious for recurrent carcinoma.

HISTOPATHOLOGY: High-grade DCIS.

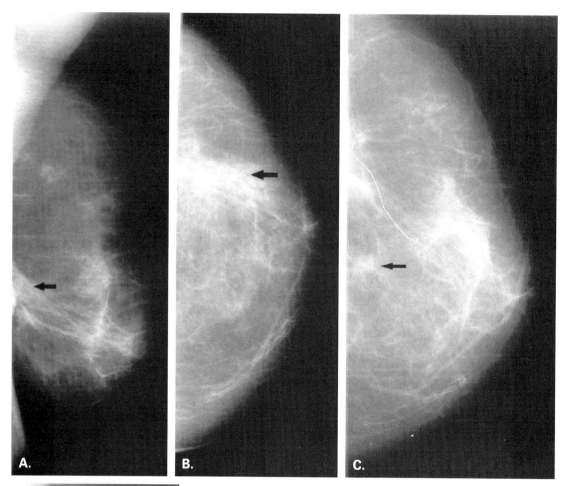

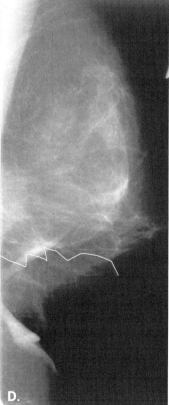

Figure 12.40

HISTORY: A 49-year-old woman who is status postlumpectomy and radiation therapy for right breast cancer.

MAMMOGRAPHY: Right MLO **(A)** and CC **(B)** views from 1993 show normal postoperative changes. There is a scar located posterolaterally **(arrow)** and skin thickening diffusely related to normal postradiation changes. On the subsequent mammogram **(C, D)** in 1994, there has been interval development of a new, small indistinct mass **(arrow)** medial to the tumor bed. Core needle biopsy was performed.

IMPRESSION: Findings suspicious for recurrent carcinoma.

HISTOPATHOLOGY: Recurrent invasive ductal carcinoma.

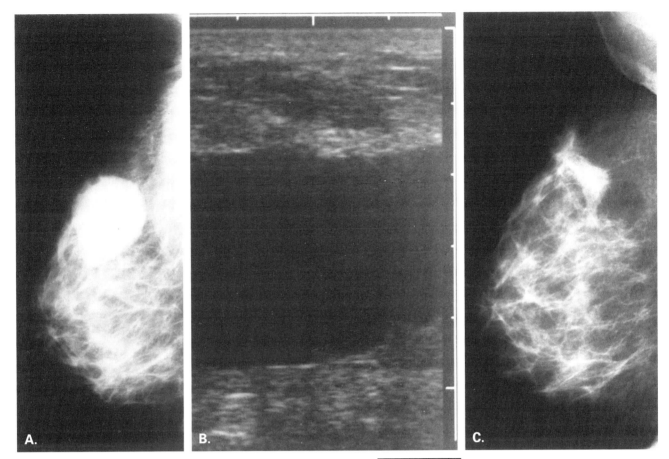

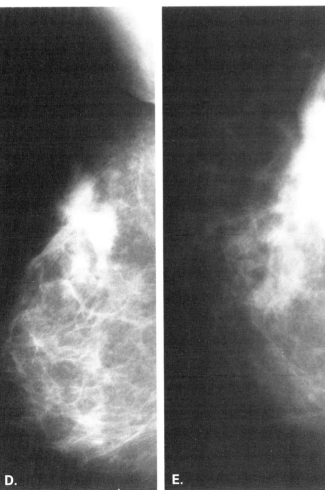

Figure 12.41

HISTORY: A 39-year-old gravida 1, para 1 woman 20 months after treatment for stage I breast carcinoma with lumpectomy and radiation therapy. She became pregnant and delivered a child approximately 12 months after radiation therapy was completed.

MAMMOGRAPHY: Left MLO view **(A)** and ultrasound **(B)** 4 weeks after lumpectomy, left MLO view **(C)** 14 months after lumpectomy and radiotherapy, and left MLO **(D)** and CC **(E)** views 18 months after lumpectomy. On the initial postlumpectomy mammogram **(A)**, there is a large, high-density, relatively circumscribed mass at the biopsy site. On ultrasound **(B)**, this mass is relatively anechoic, consistent with a postoperative hematoma or seroma. The mammogram 1 year later, when the patient was postpartum **(C)**, demonstrates an irregular medium-density mass at the lumpectomy site. This had decreased in size considerably from the postoperative mammogram and was thought to represent most likely postoperative scarring. However, because of the lack of sequential mammograms, a repeat study in 3 months was recommended. On the final films **(D** and **E)** 4 months later, there is a high-density spiculated lesion at the lumpectomy site. (Clinical examination revealed increased induration in this area.) The findings are highly consistent with recurrent carcinoma in the treated breast.

IMPRESSION: Sequence of changes demonstrating a recurrent carcinoma in the treated breast.

CYTOLOGY: Carcinoma.

NOTE: The lumpectomy site should never become larger. It may become more irregular and more dense as the hematoma retracts, but it should not increase in size.

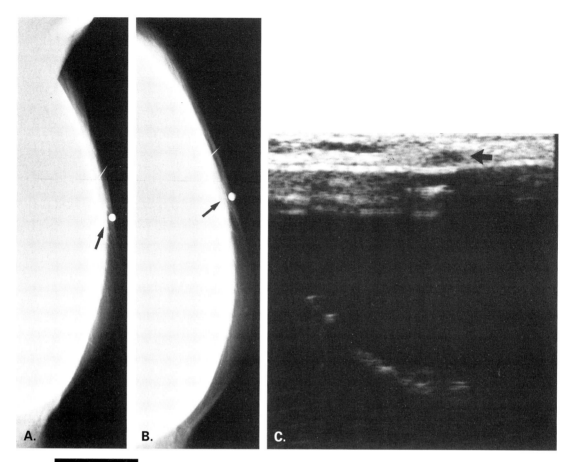

Figure 12.42

HISTORY: A 51-year-old woman 6 years after right mastectomy and reconstruction with an expandable implant. She presented with palpable thickening of questionable duration, inferior to the mastectomy scar.

MAMMOGRAPHY: Right MLO view **(A)**, right ML view **(B)**, and ultrasound **(C)**. A wire is present over the scar, and a BB overlies the palpable nodule. A small focal area of irregular tissue **(arrow)** is present beneath the BB **(A and B)**. The ultrasound **(C)** clearly demonstrates the hypoechoic nodule **(arrow)** in the subcutaneous area.

IMPRESSION: Recurrent carcinoma.

CYTOLOGY: Positive for malignancy.

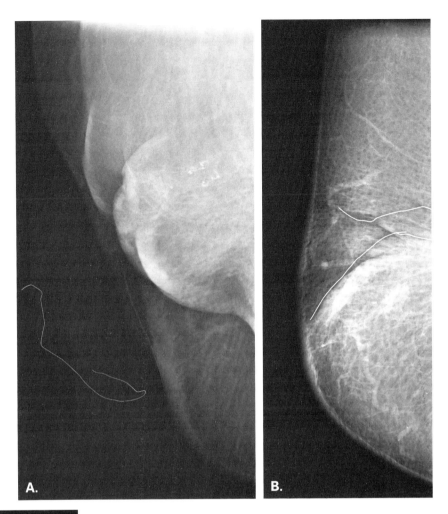

Figure 12.43

HISTORY: A 62-year-old woman who is status post–left mastectomy, who presents with an abnormal mammogram of the mastectomy site.

MAMMOGRAPHY: Left MLO (**A**) and exaggerated CC lateral (**B**) views show residual fatty tissue at the mastectomy site. In the upper outer aspect is a group of coarse calcifications that are forming a circle. The pattern of the dystrophic calcification is typical for fat necrosis.

IMPRESSION: Benign calcifications of fat necrosis in the mastectomy site.

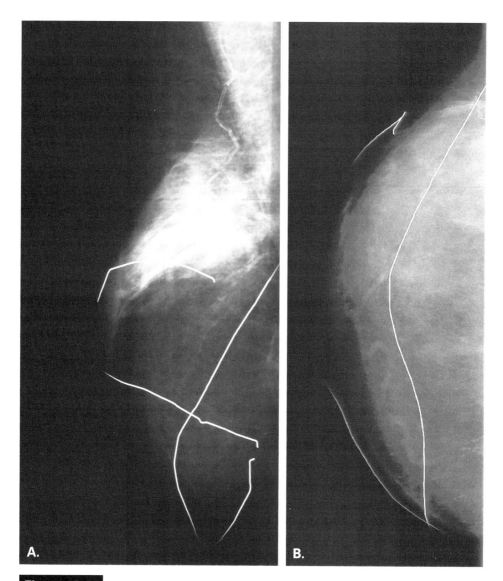

Figure 12.44

HISTORY: A 59-year-old patient who is status postmastectomy and reconstruction with a myocutaneous flap.

MAMMOGRAPHY: Left MLO **(A)** and CC **(B)** views show primarily fatty tissue with some density in the upper outer aspect of the flap. The shape of the breast is somewhat flattened and less pendulous than the normal breast, and the skin is slightly thickened. No ductal tissue is present.

IMPRESSION: Reconstructed breast with a transversus rectus abdominis myocutaneous (TRAM) flap.

Figure 12.45

HISTORY: A 51-year-old woman after left breast cancer treated with a modified radical mastectomy and reconstruction with a myocutaneous flap. She presents with a palpable mass in the upper aspect of the reconstruction breast.

MAMMOGRAPHY: Left MLO **(A)** and CC **(B)** views and ultrasound **(C** and **D)**. The wires mark the surgical scar, and the BB marks the palpable nodule. There is no ductal tissue present; instead, the reconstructed breast is composed of bandlike densities of muscle, fascia, and fatty tissue **(A** and **B)**. In the upper central aspect, there is an irregular mass **(arrow) (B)**. On ultrasound, the superior aspect of the density is complex, containing fluid and echogenic components **(C)**, most consistent with an organizing hematoma. Adjacent to the hematoma is a focal area of shadowing **(D, arrow)**, which could represent fat necrosis, fibrosis, or tumor. This shadowing corresponded to the palpable nodule and was biopsied.

IMPRESSION: Reconstructed left breast with a palpable hematoma and a solid shadowing area representing either fat necrosis or recurrent tumor.

HISTOPATHOLOGY: Fat necrosis, lipogranuloma, foreign body giant cell reaction.

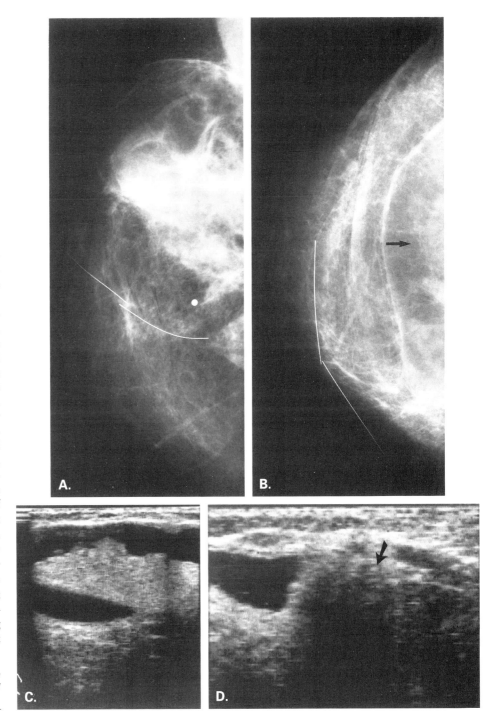

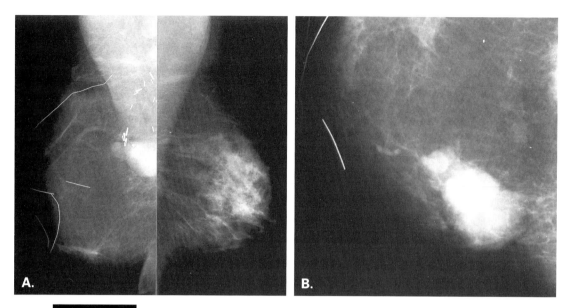

Figure 12.46

HISTORY: A 36-year-old woman who is status post–left mastectomy for invasive carcinoma and transverse rectus abdominis myocutaneous (TRAM) flap reconstruction. She presents with a palpable lump in the medial aspect of the reconstructed breast.

MAMMOGRAPHY: Bilateral MLO views (**A**) show a heterogeneously dense right breast. The TRAM flap on the left is completely fatty. There is a large, lobulated, relatively circumscribed mass in the left upper-inner quadrant. On the enlarged CC view (**B**), the multilobular dense mass is seen. The location in the upper inner quadrant and the appearance of the mass do not suggest fat necrosis.

IMPRESSION: Recurrence of carcinoma in the reconstructed breast.

HISTOPATHOLOGY: Poorly differentiated carcinoma.

REFERENCES

1. Sickles EA, Herzog KA. Mammography of the postsurgical breast. *AJR Am J Roentgenol* 1987;136:585–588.
2. Stigers KB, King JK, Davey DD, et al. Abnormalities of the breast caused by biopsy: spectrums of mammographic findings. *AJR Am J Roentgenol* 1991:156:287–291.
3. Mendelson EB. Imaging the postsurgical breast. *Semin Ultrasound CT MR* 1989;10(2):154–170.
4. Mendelson EB. Evaluation of the postoperative breast. *Radiol Clin North Am* 1992;30(1):107–138.
5. Davis SP, Stomper PC, Weidner N, et al. Suture calcification mimicking recurrence in the irradiated breast: a potential pitfall in mammographic evaluation. *Radiology* 1989;172:247–248.
6. Beyer GA, Thorsen MK, Shaffer KA, et al. Mammographic appearance of the retained Dacron cuff of a Hickman catheter. *AJR Am J Roentgenol* 1990;155:1203–1204.
7. Miller CL, Feig SA, Fox JW. Mammography changes after reduction mammoplasty. *AJR Am J Roentgenol* 1987;149:35–38.
8. Swann CA, Kopans DB, White G, et al. Observations on the postreduction mammoplasty mammogram. *Breast Dis* 1989;1:261–267.
9. Mandrekas AD, Assimakopoulos GI, Mastorakos DP, et al. Fat necrosis following breast reduction. *Br J Plast Surg* 1994;47:560–562.
10. Brown FE, Sargent SK, Cohen SR, et al. Mammographic changes following reduction mammoplasty. *Plast Reconst Surg* 1987;80:691–698.
11. Baber CE, Linshitz HI. Bilateral fat necrosis of the breast following reduction mammoplasties. *AJR Am J Roentgenol* 1977;128:508–509.
12. Fisher B, Redmond C, Poisson R, et al. Eight-year results of a randomized clinical trial of comparing total mastectomy and lumpectomy with or without irradiation in the treatment of breast cancer. *N Engl J Med* 1989;320:822–828.
13. Veronesi U, Zucali R, Luini A. Local control and survival in early breast cancer: the Milan trial. *Int J Radiat Oncol Biol Phys* 1986;12:717–720.
14. Bader J, Lippman ME, Swain SM, et al. Preliminary report of the NCI early breast cancer (BC) study: a prospective randomized comparison of lumpectomy (L) and radiation (XRT) to mastectomy (M) for stage I and II BC [abstract]. *Int J Radiat Oncol Biol Phys* 1987;13[Suppl 1]:160(abst).
15. Bartelink H, van Dongen JA, Aaronson N, et al. Randomized clinical trial to assess the value of breast conserving therapy (BCT) in stage II breast cancer: EORTC trial 10801 [abstract]. In: Proceedings of the 7th Annual Meeting of the European Society for Therapeutic Radiology and Oncology (ESTRO). Den Haag, the Netherlands: ESTRO, 1988;211.
16. Trivedi AM, Saady M, Cuttino LW, et al. Imaging findings in patients following brachytherapy for the treatment of breast cancer. Presented at the Radiologic Society of North America meeting, 2005.
17. Peters ME, Fagerholm MI, Scanlan KA, et al. Mammographic evaluation of the postsurgical and irradiated breast. *RadioGraphics* 1988;8(5):873–899.

18. Romsdahl MM, Montague ED, Ames FC, et al. Conservative surgery and irradiation as treatment for early breast cancer. *Arch Surg* 1983;118:521–528.
19. Stehlin JS, de Ipolyi PD, Greeff PJ, et al. A ten year study of partial mastectomy for carcinoma of the breast. *Surg Gynecol Obstet* 1987;165:191–198.
20. Fisher ER, Sass R, Fisher B, et al. Pathologic findings for the National Surgical Adjuvant Breast Project: relation of local breast recurrence to multicentricity. *Cancer* 186;57:1717–1724.
21. Harris JR, Recht A, Amalric R, et al. Time course and prognosis of local recurrence following primary radiation therapy for early breast cancer. *J Clin Oncol* 1984;2(1):37–41.
22. Warneke J, Grossklaus D, Davis J, et al. Influence of local treatment on the recurrence rate of ductal carcinoma in situ. *J Am Coll Surg* 1995;180:683–688.
23. Krishnan I, Krishnan EC, Mansfield C, et al. Treatment options in early breast cancer. *RadioGraphics* 1989;9(6):1067–1079.
24. Paulus DD. Conservative treatment of breast cancer: mammography in patient selection and follow-up. *AJR Am J Roentgenol* 1984;143:483–487.
25. Homer MJ, Schmidt-Ullrich R, Safaii H, et al. Residual breast carcinoma after biopsy: role of mammography in evaluation. *Radiology* 1989;170:75–77.
26. Spaulding C, Shaw de Paredes E, Anne P, et al. Detection of recurrence after breast conservation treatment with radiotherapy. *Breast Dis* 1992;5:75–90.
27. Gefter WB, Friedman AK, Goodman RL. The role of mammography in evaluating patients with early carcinoma of the breast for tylectomy and radiation therapy. *Radiology* 1982;142:77–80.
28. Gluck BS, Dershaw DD, Liberman L, et al. Microcalcification on postoperative mammograms as an indicator of adequacy of tumor excision. *Radiology* 1993;188:469–472.
29. Teixidor HS, Chu FC, Kim YS, et al. The value of mammography after limited breast surgery and before definitive radiation therapy. *Cancer* 1992;69:1418–1423.
30. DiPiro PJ, Meyer JE, Shaffer K, et al. Usefulness of the routine magnification view after breast conservation therapy for carcinoma. *Radiology* 1996;198:341–343.
31. Dershaw DD, Shank B, Reisinger S. Mammographic findings after breast cancer treatment with local excision and definitive irradiation. *Radiology* 1987;164:455–461.
32. Libshitz HI, Montaque ED, Paulus DD. Calcifications and the therapeutically irradiated breast. *AJR Am J Roentgenol* 1977;128:1021–1025.
33. Brenner RJ, Pfaff JM. Mammographic features after conservation therapy for malignant breast disease: serial findings standardized regression analysis. *AJR Am J Roentgenol* 1996;167:171–177.
34. Cox CE, Greenberg H, Fleisher D, et al. Natural history and clinical evaluation of the lumpectomy scar. *Am Surg* 1993;59:55–59.
35. Dershaw DD. Mammography in patients with breast cancer treated by breast conservation (lumpectomy with or without radiation). *AJR Am J Roentgenol* 1995;164:309–316.
36. Hassell PR, Olivotto IA, Mueller HA, et al. Early breast cancer: detection of recurrence after conservative surgery and radiation therapy. *Radiology* 1990;176:731–735.
37. Orel SG, Troupin RH, Patterson EA, et al. Breast cancer recurrence after lumpectomy and irradiation: role of mammography in detection. *Radiology* 1992;183:201–206.
38. Stomper PC, Recht A, Berenberg AL, et al. Mammographic detection of recurrent cancer in the irradiated breast. *AJR Am J Roentgenol* 1987;148:39–43.
39. Dershaw DD, McCormick B, Osborne MP. Detection of local recurrence after conservative therapy for breast carcinoma. *Cancer* 1992;70:493–496.
40. Dershaw DD, McCormick B, Cox L, et al. Differentiation of benign and malignant local tumor recurrence after lumpectomy. *AJR Am J Roentgenol* 1990;155:35–38.
41. Rebner M, Pennes DR, Adler DD, et al. Breast microcalcifications after lumpectomy and radiation therapy. *Radiology* 1989;170:691–693.
42. Solin LJ, Fowble BL, Troupin RH. Biopsy results of new calcifications in the post irradiated breast. *Cancer* 1989;63:1956–1961.
43. Heywang-Köbrunner SH, Schlegel A, Beck R, et al. Contrast-enhanced MRI of the breast after limited surgery and radiation therapy. *J Comput Assist Tomogr* 1993;17:891–900.
44. Pierce SM, Recht A, Lingos T, et al. Long-term radiation complications following conservation surgery and radiation therapy in patients in early stage breast cancer. *Int J Radiat Oncol Biol Phys* 1992;23:915–923.
45. Chahin F, Paramesh A, Dwivedi A, et al. Angiosarcoma of the breast following breast preservation therapy and local radiation therapy for breast cancer. *Breast J* 2001;7(2):120–123.
46. Rissanen TJ, Makarainen HP, Mattila SJ, et al. Breast cancer recurrence after mastectomy: diagnosis with mammography and US. *Radiology* 1993;188:463–467.
47. Shermis RB, Adler DD, Smith DJ, et al. Intraductal silicone secondary to breast implant rupture: an unusual mammographic presentation. *Breast Dis* 1990;3:17–20.
48. Rebner M, Stevenson TR. Fat necrosis of bilateral musculocutaneous flap breast reconstruction. *Breast Dis* 1988;1:199–203.
49. Holmes FA, Singletary ES, Kroll S, et al. Fat necrosis in an autogenously reconstructed breast mimicking recurrent carcinoma at mammography. *Breast Dis* 1988;1:121–218.

Chapter 13

The Augmented Breast

More than 250,000 women in the United States undergo an augmentation mammoplasty annually. Two studies (1,2) have reported the incidence of implants in American women to range from 3.3 to 8.1 per 1,000. The augmented breast presents a challenge to the radiologist to image the residual parenchyma adequately and to detect any abnormalities. The presence of implants may interfere with routine mammography and therefore has the potential to delay the diagnosis of breast cancer (3,4).

Fortunately, most women in the United States who have had augmentation mammoplasty have undergone placement of implants rather than direct silicone or paraffin injection. Augmentation may be performed for cosmetic reasons: to increase the size of both breasts unilaterally for an asymmetric hypoplastic breast, or after mastectomy for reconstruction. Augmentation procedures have included direct injection of silicone or paraffin into the breast, placement of a variety of types of implants in either a subpectoral or retroglandular location, and the use of several types of autologous myocutaneous flaps for reconstruction. In this chapter, the mammographic findings associated with the augmented breast will be discussed.

DIRECT INJECTION FOR AUGMENTATION

Silicone injection for breast augmentation was never approved in the United Stated by the Food and Drug Administration (FDA) (5). Many patients seen in the United States with augmentation by direct injection have had the procedure performed in Asia or Mexico (6). Because of the intense response to the foreign material, management of the patient is quite difficult. Clinically, the breasts are quite hard or lumpy, and the exclusion of a tumor by palpation is impossible (6). Parsons and Thering (6) found that mastodynia was the most common presenting symptom in 28 patients with silicone-injected breasts. Another problem that these patients face is the tendency for the silicone to migrate far outside the breasts (7). Histologically, the silicone incites areas of fat

necrosis, infiltration with fibrocytes, and cystlike spaces lined by fibrous tissues (7). There may be hyaline degeneration with calcifications of the inner surface of the fibrous capsule of the siliconoma (8). The calcification may represent deposition of calcium and phosphates near necrotic tissue (8).

Mammography is markedly limited in patients who have undergone augmentation by injection, because the breasts are thick and hard and therefore difficult to compress well (Figs. 13.1 and 13.2). The injected substances and the fibrous response create a very dense appearance requiring a long exposure. Technically, by increasing the kVp to 30 or 32 or by using a tungsten target, one is sometimes able to penetrate the breasts adequately. Ultrasound shows numerous areas of dense shadowing related to the reaction to the injected substances. Because of this, sonography is usually not helpful to evaluate for malignancy.

Magnetic resonance imaging (MRI) can be very helpful to assess for tumors in a patient who has a compromised mammogram because of the density related to augmentation by injection. In a study of 16 patients who had undergone silicone injection breast augmentation and who underwent breast MRI, Cheung et al. (9) found that four of four cancers were accurately identified by using contrast enhancement techniques. In this series, the silicone granulomas were nonenhancing on MRI or were associated with a benign rimlike enhancement.

Koide and Katayama (8) found differences in the mammographic findings in breasts augmented by injection, depending on the substances used for injection. In patients who had paraffin injections, radiolucent masses were seen; 75% of these patients developed extensive small annular calcifications, and lymphadenopathy was common. In patients who received silicone injections, the mammographic nodules were of high density, and 29% of these women were found to have large, localized, eggshell calcifications in the breasts. Others (10,11) have found calcifications in patterns varying from irregular to small ringlike to eggshell shaped in patients with silicone injections.

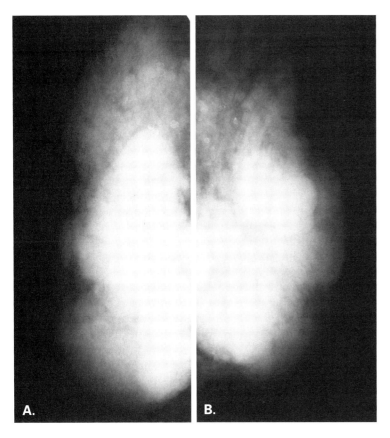

Figure 13.1

HISTORY: A 41-year-old woman after augmentation mammoplasty with silicone injections, presenting with numerous hard masses and distortion of the contour of the breasts bilaterally.

MAMMOGRAPHY: Left MLO **(A)** and right MLO **(B)** views. Technically, the examination is limited by the extreme density of the breasts and the inability to compress them adequately. The study was performed at 32 kVp with a tungsten target and rhodium filtration to attempt to penetrate the tissue. The breasts are extremely dense, with multiple soft tissue masses bilaterally. There are also innumerable circular calcifications bilaterally that represent dystrophic and granulomatous reaction to the silicone injections. Ultrasound was not of help because of diffuse shadowing from this process.

IMPRESSION: Extensive reactive changes secondary to silicone injection for augmentation mammoplasty.

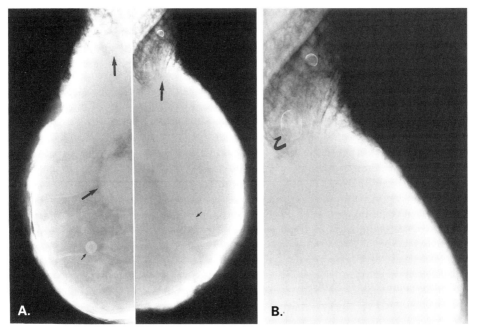

Figure 13.2

HISTORY: A 40-year-old woman after augmentation mammoplasty with silicone injections and saline implants. On clinical examination the breasts were filled with hard nodules, particularly in the upper outer quadrants.

MAMMOGRAPHY: Bilateral MLO **(A)** and right enlarged (2X) MLO **(B)** views. The breasts are very difficult to image because of the postsurgical changes. Saline implants are present bilaterally, and the valves of these prosthesis are seen **(A, small arrows)**. There are also extremely dense nodules bilaterally **(A, large arrows)** that are related to the silicone injections. On the enlarged view **(B)**, these very dense masses are seen, and some areas of fat necrosis (rimlike calcifications, secondary to the injections) are also identified **(B, curved arrow)**.

IMPRESSION: Postoperative changes of augmentation mammoplasty with both implants and direct silicone injections. (Case courtesy of Dr. Cherie Scheer, Richmond, VA.)

AUGMENTATION WITH IMPLANTS

Implants are most often placed for augmentation for cosmetic reasons, but also are frequently used for breast reconstruction after mastectomy. In patients with asymmetric breast size, a hypoplastic breast, or a chest wall deformity, an implant may be placed to achieve symmetry. Some of the types of implants used for augmentation have included saline filled, silicone gel, inflatable double lumen, and polyurethane coated (12,13). Commonly encountered silicone implants are those composed of a silicone gel contained within a silicone elastomer shell. The single lumen gel-filled implant can have a smooth or a textured shell; the textured shell was designed to reduce the incidence of capsular contraction (14). Another type of single-lumen implant that was designed to reduce capsular contraction is polyurethane covered. In this type of prosthesis, a thin layer of polyurethane foam is adherent to the gel-filled implant.

Saline implants are composed of a silicone elastomer shell that is filled with saline. These implants usually have a fill valve that is used for inflation of the implant. Double-lumen implants typically are composed of an inner lumen of silicone gel that is encased within an outer lumen of saline. Other double-lumen implants are reversed, with saline internally and silicone in the outer lumen.

When an implant is placed into the breast, the body reacts to the prosthesis by forming a fibrous capsule around it. This fibrous capsule surrounds the implant and can thicken and contract. The capsule can also calcify, which is visible on mammography and is often associated with capsular contraction (15). The use of implants with a textured surface or polyurethane coating has been found to decrease the severity of encapsulation (14).

Goodman et al. (16) in a meta-analysis of literature evaluating implant rupture found that the estimated median life span of a silicone gel implant was 16.4 years. In the event of a rupture of a silicone implant, the intact fibrous capsule may contain the extruded silicone, so the contour of the implant both clinically and on mammography is unchanged. If the fibrous capsule also tears, the silicone can extend outside the capsule and into the surrounding breast tissue. This finding is termed an *extracapsular rupture*. The relationship of the implant wall to the capsule in the normal implant, in intracapsular rupture and extracapsular rupture is shown in Figure 13.3.

In the patient with a saline prosthesis, the implant is identified as saline filled because it is not of homogeneous density. The wall of the implant is more dense than the contents because the shell is a silicone elastomer that is more dense than the contained saline. Often folds and a fill valve are visible, and these are normal findings (Fig. 13.4). The density of a silicone implant is homogeneous because the wall and the contents are both silicone, and overall, the silicone implant is more dense than a saline implant (Figs. 13.5 and 13.6).

POSITIONING THE AUGMENTED BREAST

Implants may be placed beneath the pectoralis major muscle or may be located anteriorly, in the retroglandular or prepectoral area. The imaging of a patient with implants is limited in that on routine mammography the prosthesis may obscure large areas of glandular tissue. The use of manual techniques (17) rather than phototiming is usually of help in imaging these patients.

Eklund et al. (18) have described a modified positioning technique in which the implant is displaced posteriorly and the breast tissue is pulled anteriorly as compression is applied. This technique allows for improved compression and visualization of the parenchyma (Fig. 13.7). The implant-displacement views have become a standard part of the mammographic examination for patients with implants. This technique is more easily performed on patients with a moderate amount of native tissue over the implant or in patients with subpectoral implants. The description of Eklund et al. (18) for imaging the augmented breast includes (a) standard mediolateral oblique (MLO) and craniocaudal (CC) views using normal positioning techniques and (b) modified MLO and CC views with phototiming and implant displacement. In those patients who have encapsulated implants or in whom implant displacement is not successful, a third view, the lateromedial oblique (LMO), can prove useful in imaging the upper inner and the inner lower quadrants that are obscured on the routine views. Some authors also routinely perform a 90-degree lateral (mediolateral [ML]) view with the implant displaced (19). This may include tissue that may not be visualized otherwise on the MLO or CC implant-displaced view.

IMPLANT COMPLICATIONS

Complications associated with implants include infection, hematoma formation, encapsulation, leakage or rupture, and collapse. In the immediate postoperative period following augmentation mammoplasty, infections or hematomas may occur. These are usually clinically evident, and ultrasound may be used for confirmation of a fluid collection. Treatment includes drainage and antibiotics if needed.

In the 2 to 3 weeks after an implant has been inserted, a fibrous capsule is deposited around it (12). This capsule may become fibrotic and contract, which is the most commonly associated complication with

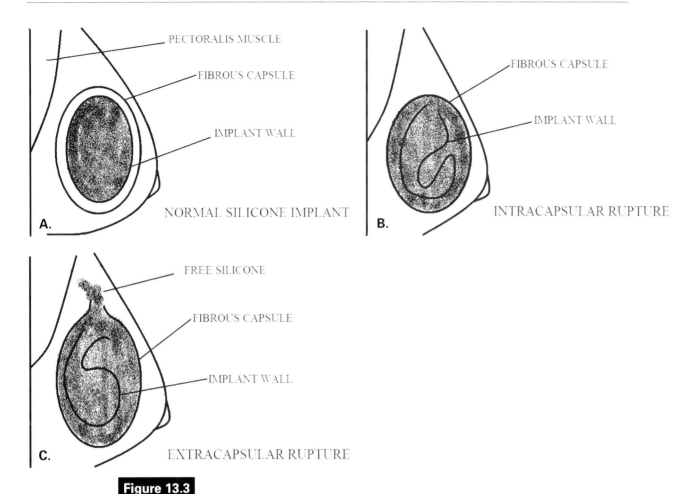

Figure 13.3

A: Schematic of the normal anatomy related to a single-lumen silicone implant. The implant is contained by a fibrous capsule. **B**: Intracapsular implant rupture shows the broken wall of the implant floating in the silicone and contained by the intact fibrous capsule. **C**: Extracapsular rupture showing the disruption of the fibrous capsule and the extrusion of the silicone into the breast.

implants (20); encapsulation may occur in as many as 10% to 40% of patients (20,21). Retromuscular implants are much less likely to develop contractures (12). On mammography, the findings of a crenulated or irregular contour of the implant may suggest capsular contraction (13) (Fig. 13.8). A very rounded contour of the implant is also seen in patients with encapsulation. Irregularity of the implant contour may be palpated as a mass (11,13,22), but the irregular contour, as opposed to a parenchymal mass, can be differentiated with mammography and ultrasound if needed.

The capsule around the implant may become calcified. This is thought to be related to inflammation of the capsule and encapsulation. This is evident on mammography as curvilinear plaquelike calcifications (Figs. 13.9–13.11). Calcifications that are coarse and ringlike may also develop in the capsule of the implant and are indicative of an inflammatory reaction to the prosthesis (13) but not

leakage of silicone. Irregularity of the contour of the implant may be caused by distortion or herniation of the prosthesis without a rupture (Figs. 13.12 and 13.13). Herniation has the appearance of a smooth bulge in the implant contour.

Rupture of an implant may be manifested clinically in a variety of ways. A saline implant that ruptures typically suddenly collapses, and there is an obvious decrease in the size of the breast. On mammography, the collapsed saline implant infolds on itself like a crumpled bag and the saline is absorbed (Figs. 13.14 and 13.15). The presentation is dramatic both clinically and on mammography. The rupture of a silicone implant may be associated clinically with pain, a change in contour of the implant, or a palpable mass.

The rupture of a silicone implant in the intracapsular space may cause a subtle change in contour of the implant but no obvious change in size or shape of the breast.

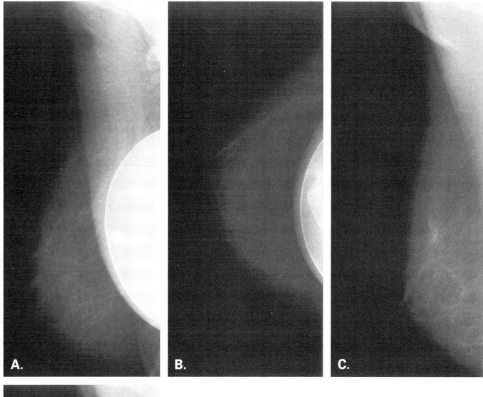

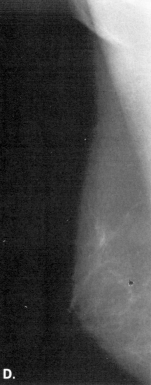

Figure 13.4

HISTORY: A 49-year-old woman who is status post–right mastectomy and reconstruction with augmentation on the left.

MAMMOGRAPHY: Left MLO **(A)** and CC **(B)** views show a subpectoral saline implant. This can be identified as saline filled, because the valve is evident and the inner aspect of the wall is seen. Implant-displaced MLO **(C)** and CC **(D)** views show normal parenchyma.

IMPRESSION: Normal saline subpectoral implant.

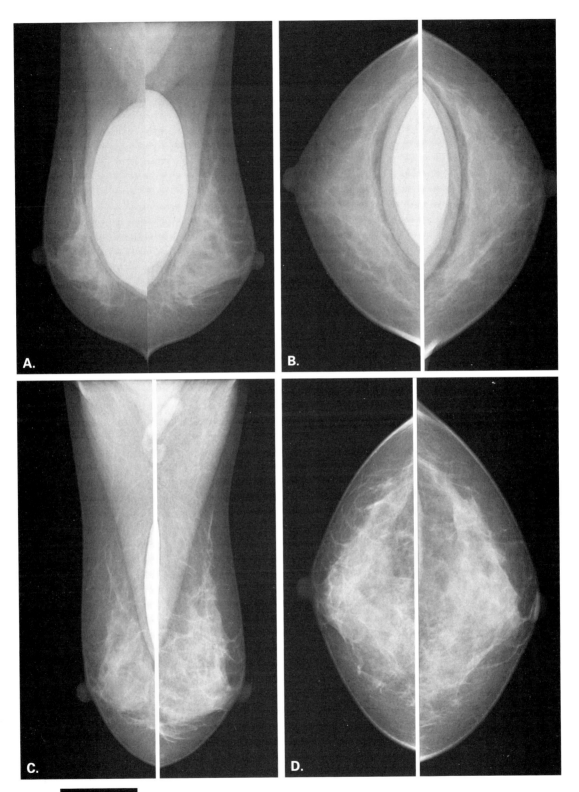

Figure 13.5

HISTORY: Routine mammogram on a patient with a history of breast augmentation.

MAMMOGRAPHY: Bilateral MLO **(A)** and CC **(B)** views show normal-appearing subpectoral silicone implants. On the implant-displaced MLO **(C)** and CC **(D)** views, the implants have been moved posteriorly out of the field of view, and the anterior breast tissue and anterior edge of the pectoralis major muscle are well compressed and in the field of view.

IMPRESSION: Images demonstrating proper positioning of normal subpectoral silicone implants.

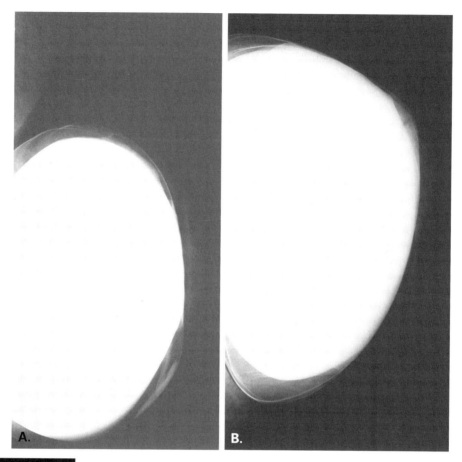

Figure 13.6

HISTORY: A 45-year-old patient with a history of implants, for routine mammography.

MAMMOGRAPHY: Right MLO **(A)** and CC **(B)** views show a normal double-lumen implant. In this case, the inner lumen is silicone and is very dense, and the outer lumen is saline and is less dense.

IMPRESSION: Normal double-lumen implant.

Mammography is typically normal, and the rupture is identified only on three-dimensional imaging, such as ultrasound or MRI. With an extracapsular rupture, the silicone extends beyond the edge of the capsule into the surrounding parenchyma, and this complication may be diagnosed on mammography as well as on ultrasound or MRI.

Palpable irregularity may also be associated with rupture of the implant with silicone extravasation. Mammography can identify the dense globules of silicone that may be calcified outside the contour of the implant, indicating rupture (12) (Figs. 13.16–13.20). The leaking silicone not only can form calcified nodules but also can present as intraductal casts of silicone (23) (Fig. 13.21). Silicone that is free in the breast is sometimes cleared by lymphatics and drains into the intramammary or axillary nodal chain. Nodes containing dense silicone may be seen on mammography and sometimes on ultrasound (Fig. 13.22). In patients with saline implants that were placed after a prior rupture of a silicone implant, residual free silicone that was not removed at surgery may be manifested clinically, mammographically, and on ultrasound (Figs. 13.23–13.26).

ROLE OF ULTRASOUND

Sonography is most helpful for the evaluation of possible implant rupture, and ultrasound is best performed by using a linear array transducer. Scanning both superficially and deep is necessary to evaluate the entire implant and the

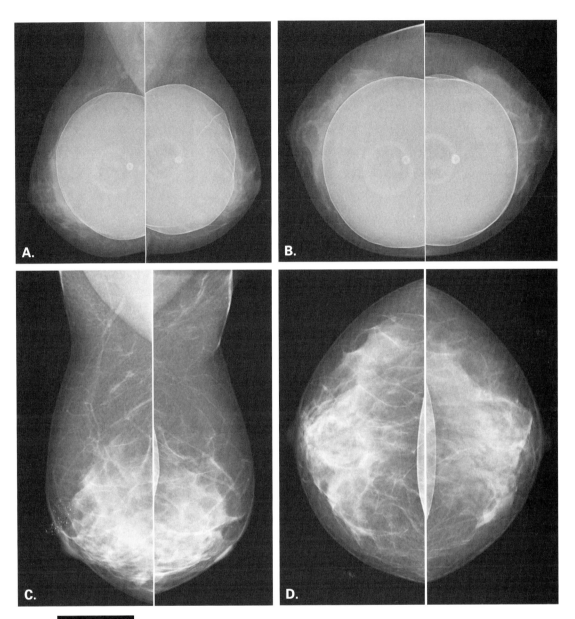

Figure 13.7

HISTORY: Routine mammogram on a woman with a history of breast implants.

MAMMOGRAPHY: Bilateral MLO **(A)** and CC **(B)** views show normal prepectoral saline implants. The valves and some folds are evident bilaterally. On the implant-displaced MLO **(C)** and CC **(D)** views, only a sliver of the anterior edge of the implants is seen, and the anterior breast tissue is well compressed and well visualized.

IMPRESSION: Normal prepectoral saline implants; normal mammogram demonstrated on routine and implant-displaced views.

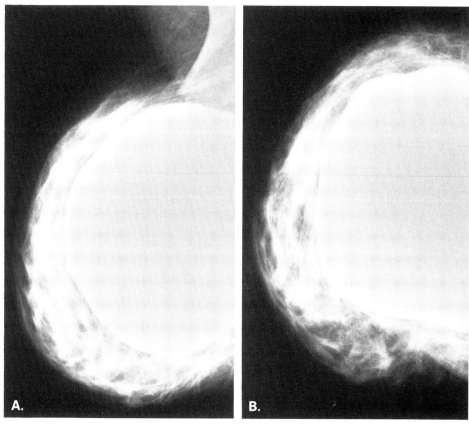

Figure 13.8

HISTORY: A 45-year-old gravida 2, para 2, abortus 1 woman after bilateral augmentation mammoplasty, with a smooth nodule in the left breast.

MAMMOGRAPHY: Left MLO **(A)**, exaggerated CC medial **(B)**, and CC **(C)** views. There is a prepectoral silicone implant in a breast that is heterogeneously dense. There is irregularity of the contour of the implant, particularly medially **(C, arrow)**, and this irregularity corresponds to the palpable finding for which the patient was referred. Such irregularity may indicate encapsulation of the implant.

IMPRESSION: Irregularity of the left implant; possible encapsulation.

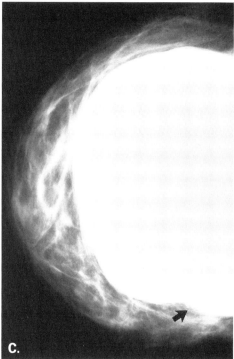

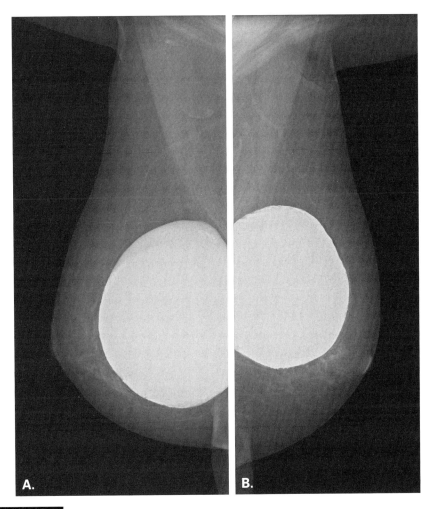

Figure 13.9

HISTORY: Patient with a history of augmentation, for routine mammography.

MAMMOGRAPHY: Left **(A)** and right **(B)** MLO views show that the patient has prepectoral saline implants. The capsule surrounding the implant in each breast is heavily calcified.

IMPRESSION: Calcified implants.

peri-implant space; this may require a lower power for the deeper area of the implant and a 5- to 7-MHz transducer (24). Scanning of the soft tissues and the axilla is also important to assess for signs of extracapsular rupture and free silicone.

The normal appearance of implants depends on the type of prosthesis. Saline and silicone single-lumen implants have a similar appearance: an anechoic oval structure that has a prominent anterior reverberation artifact. Anterior to this component is an echogenic line that represents the wall of the implant and the fibrous capsule. The port of the saline implant is often visible on ultrasound as an echogenic focus. Double-lumen implants and particularly expander implants are more complicated on

ultrasound. In particular, the inner lumen may appear as echogenic line within the lumen and may simulate an intracapsular rupture.

With an intracapsular rupture, the wall of the implant is broken and is floating in the lake of silicone contained by the fibrous capsule that formed around the prosthesis. Because of this, the mammogram is normal. On ultrasound, the broken segments of implant wall are identified as a stairstep pattern within the silicone. Diffuse internal factors are also sometimes identified on sonography (Figs. 13.27 and 13.28). Mammography is limited in its ability to detect intracapsular ruptures (25,26). Ultrasound has a

(text continues on page 547)

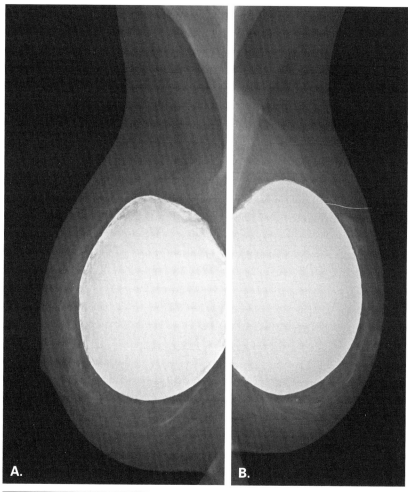

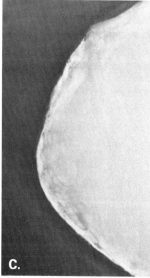

Figure 13.10

HISTORY: A 67-year-old woman with a history of breast implants.

MAMMOGRAPHY: Left MLO (**A**) and right MLO (**B**) views show rounded, calcified saline implants bilaterally. On the enlarged left MLO view (**C**), the dense calcification in the fibrous capsule around the implant is noted.

IMPRESSION: Calcified implant capsules.

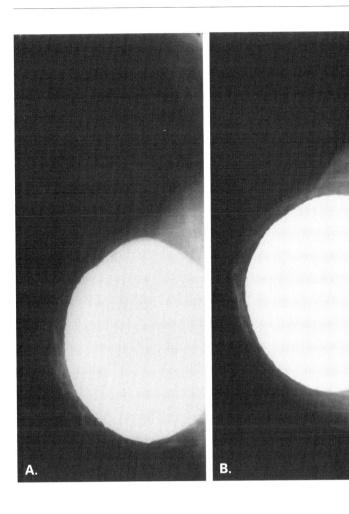

Figure 13.11

HISTORY: A 56-year-old woman with a history of implants, for screening mammography.

MAMMOGRAPHY: Left MLO (**A**) and CC (**B**) views show a silicone prepectoral implant. Slight irregularity of the contour is noted. The periphery of the implant is calcified, consistent with capsular calcification.

IMPRESSION: Capsular calcification of a silicone implant.

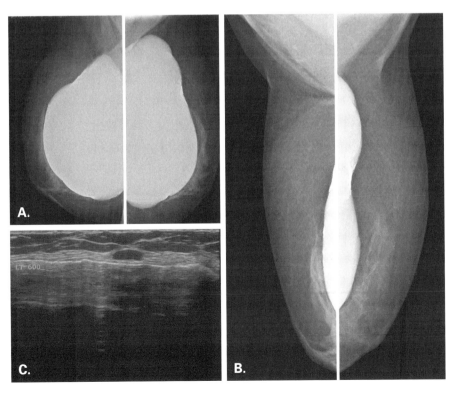

Figure 13.12

HISTORY: A 58-year-old woman with a history of implants with a palpable mass in the left breast at 4 o'clock.

MAMMOGRAPHY: Bilateral MLO views (**A**) show distorted calcified silicone prostheses in both breasts. On the implant displaced MLO views (**B**), the capsular calcification is evident, and the herniation and distortion of the right implant is present superiorly. The palpable mass is not seen on mammography. Ultrasound of the palpable region (**C**) shows a small simple cyst. Ultrasound of the implants shows dense shadowing related to extracapsular leakage of silicone in both axillary tail regions.

IMPRESSION: Simple cyst left breast, bilateral herniated, calcified implants with extracapsular free silicone.

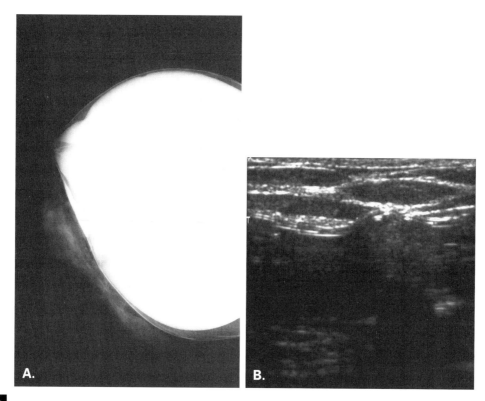

Figure 13.13

HISTORY: Patient who presents with a change in the shape of the left implant and a palpable mass.

MAMMOGRAPHY: Left CC views **(A)** show a distorted double-lumen implant. The palpable mass corresponded to the focal bulging in the subareolar region of the implant. On ultrasound **(B)**, irregularity of the contour of the implant is noted that suggests rupture. The implants were removed and replaced with saline prostheses.

IMPRESSION: Possible rupture of the double-lumen implant.

SURGICAL FINDINGS: Volvulus of the implant with the posterior margin and fill valve rotated anteriorly. No rupture was found.

NOTE: Ultrasound of a double-lumen implant is difficult to interpret because of the presence of the bands within the outer lumen that are caused by the inner lumen.

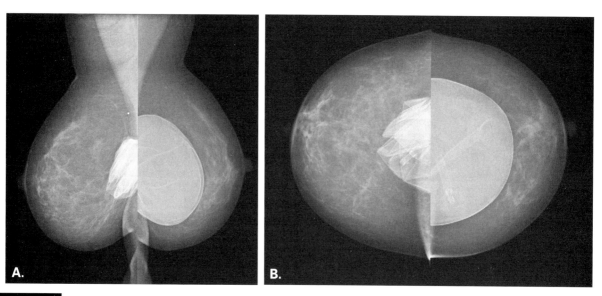

Figure 13.14

HISTORY: A 60-year-old woman who reports pain in the left axilla and who has a history of breast implants.

MAMMOGRAPHY: Bilateral MLO **(A)** and CC **(B)** views with the implants in place show a normal right saline implant with several folds. On the left, the implant has collapsed, with a typical appearance of a saline implant rupture.

IMPRESSION: Ruptured left saline implant.

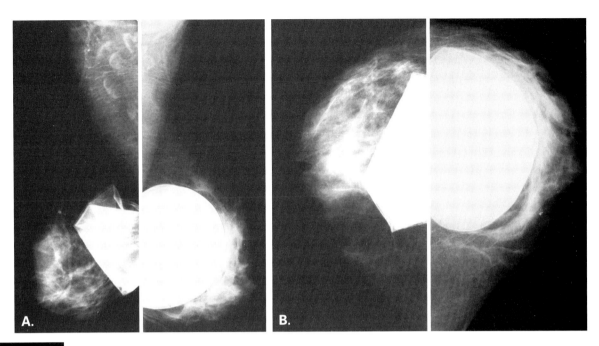

Figure 13.15

HISTORY: Patient with implants who reports decrease in size of the left breast.

MAMMOGRAPHY: Bilateral MLO **(A)** and CC **(B)** views show a normal prepectoral saline implant in the right breast. The left saline implant has collapsed in a typical form.

IMPRESSION: Collapsed left prepectoral saline implant.

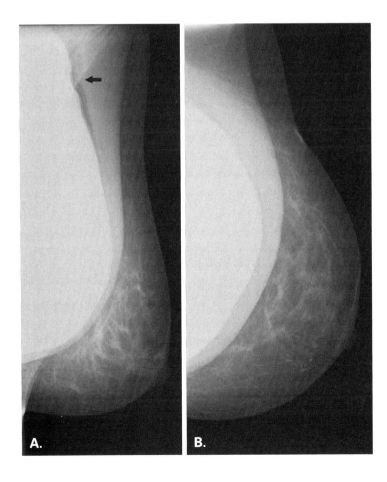

Figure 13.16

HISTORY: A 43-year-old woman who reports firmness in the right breast.

MAMMOGRAPHY: Right MLO **(A)** and CC **(B)** views show a subpectoral silicone implant. On the MLO view **(A)**, there is deformity of the shape of the implant, with apparent extension of silicone into the axillary region **(arrow)**. This finding is very suspicious for rupture of the implant. Extracapsular rupture was confirmed on ultrasound.

IMPRESSION: Extracapsular leak of silicone implant.

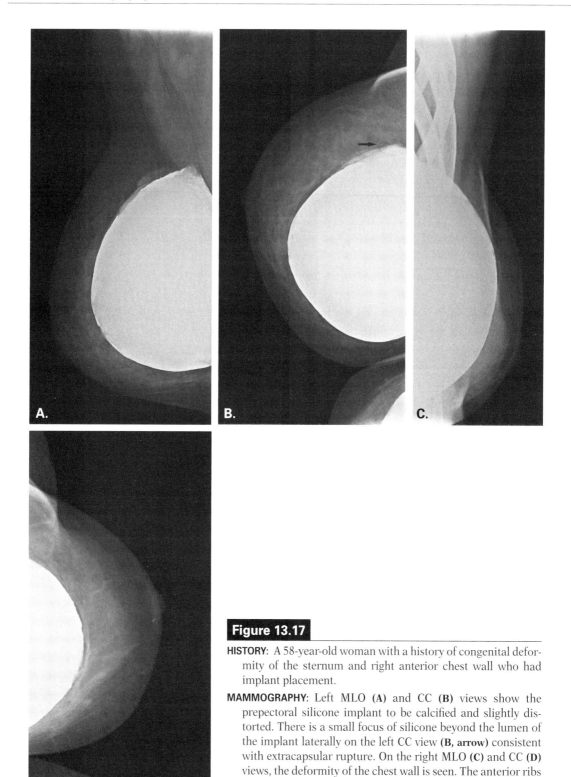

Figure 13.17

HISTORY: A 58-year-old woman with a history of congenital deformity of the sternum and right anterior chest wall who had implant placement.

MAMMOGRAPHY: Left MLO **(A)** and CC **(B)** views show the prepectoral silicone implant to be calcified and slightly distorted. There is a small focus of silicone beyond the lumen of the implant laterally on the left CC view **(B, arrow)** consistent with extracapsular rupture. On the right MLO **(C)** and CC **(D)** views, the deformity of the chest wall is seen. The anterior ribs are visible, yet no pectoralis major muscle is seen.

IMPRESSION: Implant placement for congenital deformity of the chest wall with an extracapsular rupture on the left.

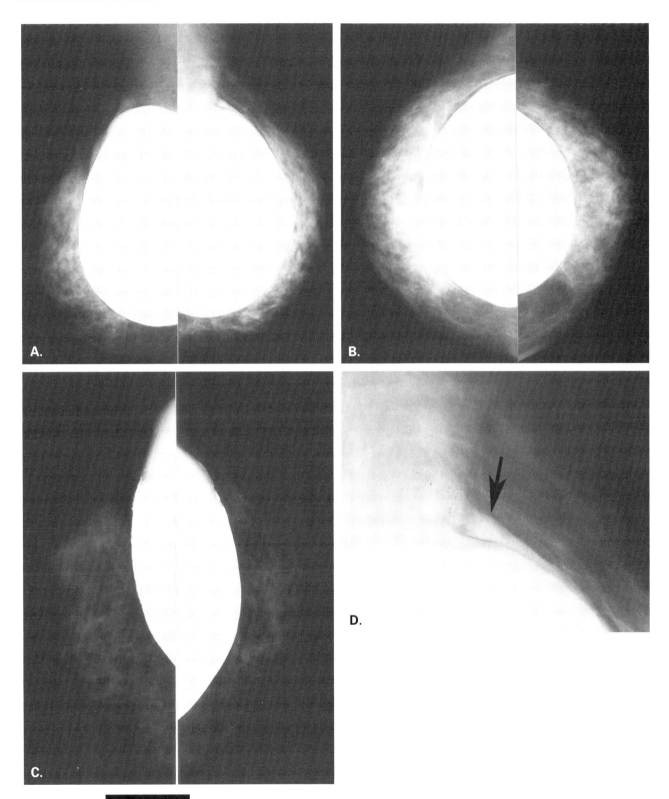

Figure 13.18

HISTORY: A 48-year-old woman with history of breast implants.

MAMMOGRAPHY: Bilateral MLO **(A)** and CC **(B)** views show prepectoral silicone implants. Calcification of the capsules is seen best on implant displaced MLO views **(C)**. A coned image **(D)** of the superior margin of the right implant shows a contour irregularity with high-density streaks **(arrows)** outside the implant, consistent with rupture.

IMPRESSION: Right extracapsular implant rupture.

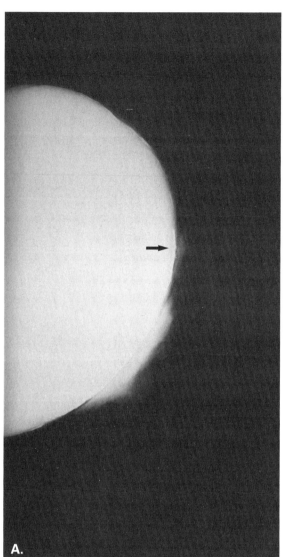

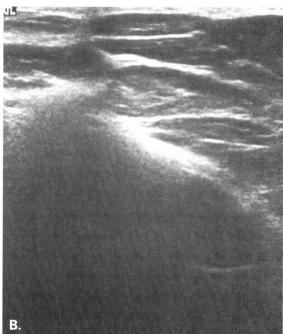

Figure 13.19

HISTORY: A 63-year-old patient with a history of implants.

MAMMOGRAPHY: Right CC view (**A**) shows that the patient has a prepectoral silicone implant. Capsular calcification (**arrow**) is present around the implant. There is a very-high-density irregular band surrounding the anterior margin of the implant, suggestive of extracapsular rupture. On ultrasound (**B**), a snowstorm appearance of dense shadowing related to this free silicone is seen, consistent with extracapsular rupture.

IMPRESSION: Left capsular calcifications surrounding implant with extracapsular rupture.

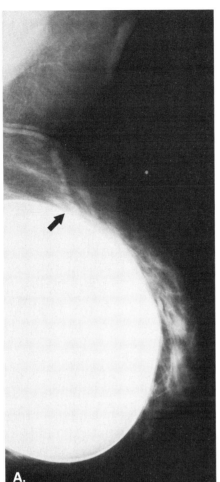

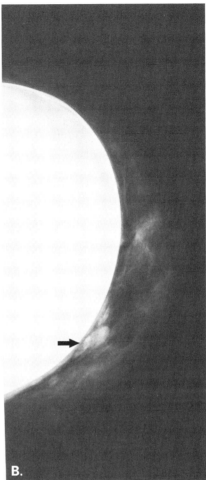

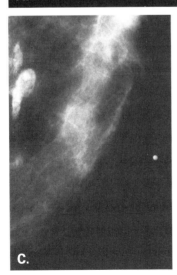

Figure 13.20

HISTORY: A 49-year-old woman with a history of ruptured implants that were replaced, now presenting with a palpable right breast mass.

MAMMOGRAPHY: Right MLO **(A)** and CC **(B)** views show the saline implant to be intact. There is hyperdense nodularity **(arrows)** surrounding the implant, including in the region of palpable concern. On the spot implant-displaced magnification CC view **(C)**, the palpable mass is noted to correspond to the droplets of residual silicone from the prior rupture.

IMPRESSION: Free silicone from prior rupture corresponding to palpable mass.

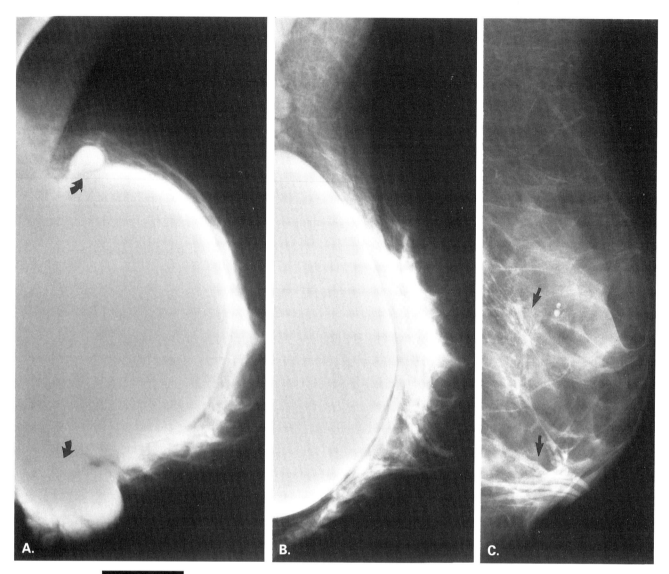

Figure 13.21

HISTORY: A 44-year-old woman after bilateral augmentation mammoplasties who presents with a firm nodule in the inferior aspect of the right breast.

MAMMOGRAPHY: Right MLO view **(A)** and right MLO **(B)** and implant-displaced MLO **(C)** views 1 year later. On the initial study, a prepectoral silicone implant is present. There are globules of free silicone beneath and above the implant in the surrounding parenchyma **(A, arrows)**. This silicone was leaking from a rupture in the implant and was removed at the same time as a replacement of the implant. On the subsequent mammogram **(B and C)**, the silicone globules have been removed. There is, however, a dense cast of the ductal system **(C, arrows)** consistent with silicone in the lactiferous ducts.

IMPRESSION: Rupture of implant treated surgically, with the development of silicone casts of lactiferous ducts. (Case courtesy of Dr. Cherie Scheer, Richmond, VA.)

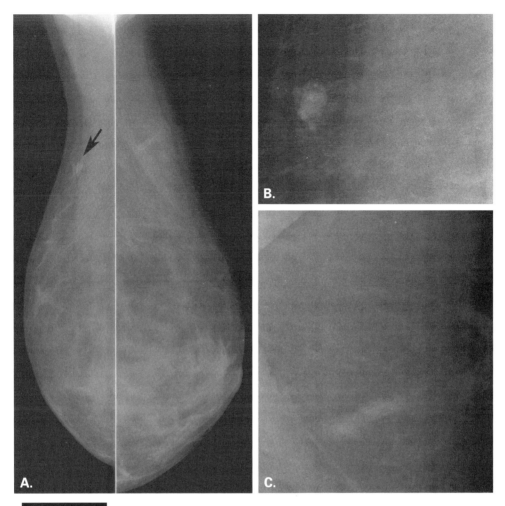

Figure 13.22

HISTORY: A 79-year-old woman with saline implants and a history of prior silicone implants that were removed.

MAMMOGRAPHY: Bilateral MLO implant-displaced views (**A**) show a small high-density mass (**arrow**) in the axillary tail of the left breast. On spot magnification (**B**), the mass is very high density and is consistent with a focus of free silicone from prior rupture. A spot-magnification view of the right axilla (**C**) at a palpable lump shows a silicone-laden lymph node as well.

IMPRESSION: Bilateral free silicone from prior implant rupture.

reported sensitivity for implant rupture of 70% and a specificity of 92% (27).

Sonographic features of extracapsular rupture include disruption of the echogenic line surrounding the implant, "silicone cysts," echogenic foci around the implant, and the snowstorm appearance of shadowing (Figs. 13.29 and 13.30). This noisy shadow is created by the tissue reaction to the free silicone. Ultrasound misdiagnoses of rupture have been caused by intrinsic changes in polyurethane implants, the structure of double-lumen implants, and extracapsular silicone from a prior rupture (28).

ROLE OF MAGNETIC RESONANCE IMAGING

MRI is an excellent method to evaluate silicone implants for rupture, particularly if mammography and ultrasound

(text continues on page 553)

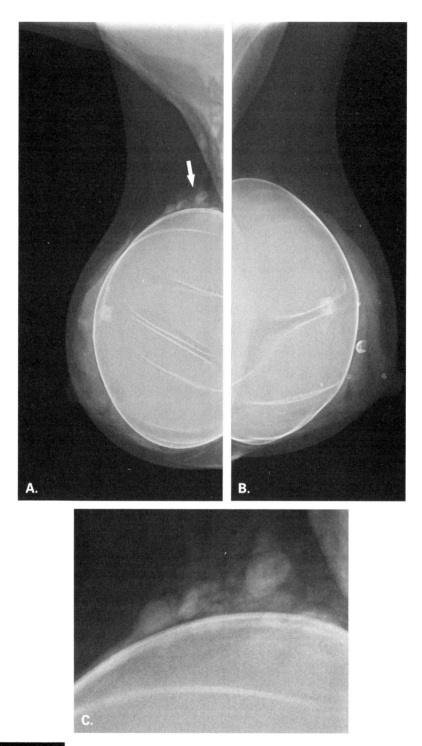

Figure 13.23

HISTORY: A 52-year-old woman with a history of prior silicone implants, replaced with saline implants.

MAMMOGRAPHY: Left (**A**) and right (**B**) MLO views show normal-appearing prepectoral saline implants. Benign eggshell calcifications are present in the right breast. On the left, multiple droplets of free silicone are seen (**arrows**) in the axillary tail. On the enlarged MLO image (**C**), the free silicone in the tissue is seen, as well as some silicone-laden lymph nodes in the axilla.

IMPRESSION: Normal saline implants, free silicone in the left breast and axillary nodes from prior rupture.

Figure 13.24

HISTORY: A 58-year-old woman for routine mammography. She has a history of silicone implant removal and replacement with saline implants.

MAMMOGRAPHY: Left MLO (**A**) and CC (**B**) views show a normal-appearing saline implant. A valve is present, as well as some normal folds. In the medial aspect of the breast, overlapping the implant in part, are two lobular high-density masses (**arrows**). These extend beyond the implant on the CC view (**B**) and are typical of residual silicone from the prior rupture.

IMPRESSION: Normal saline implant, residual silicone from prior rupture.

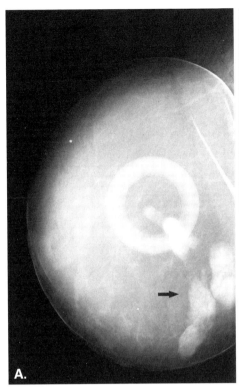

A.

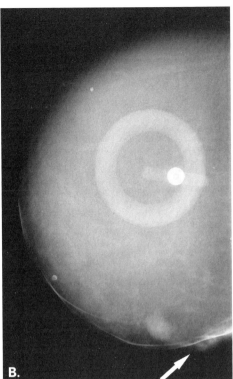

B.

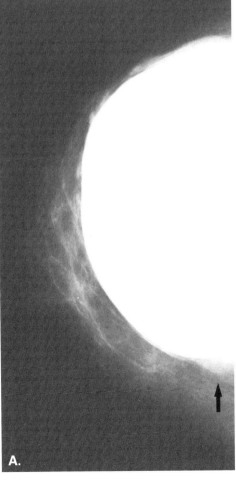

A.

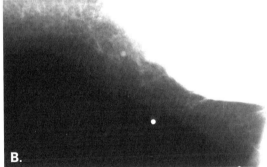

B.

Figure 13.25

HISTORY: A 45-year-old woman with implants who reports a new palpable mass in the left breast medially. She had prior silicone implants that were replaced.

MAMMOGRAPHY: Left CC view (**A**) and left ML spot view (**B**) over the palpable mass show a very-high-density region around the edge of the implant. This finding is typical of free silicone from the prior implant rupture that was not removed completely. Often, there is a foreign body reaction and granuloma formation around the silicone that may be clinically evident as a palpable mass.

IMPRESSION: Free silicone from prior rupture creating a palpable mass.

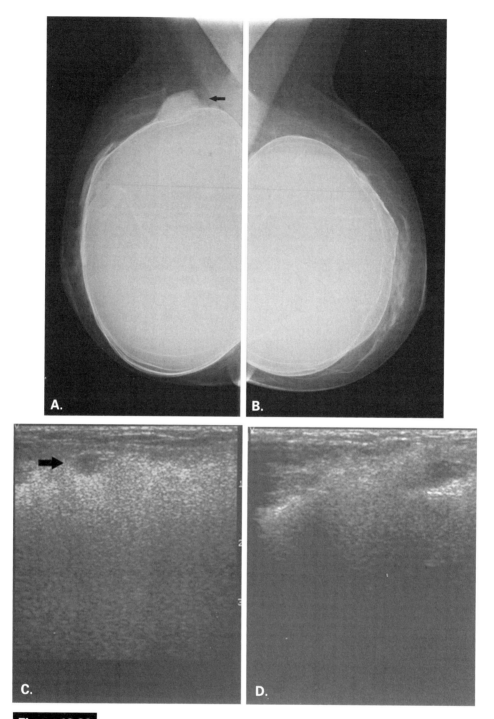

Figure 13.26

HISTORY: A 62-year-old woman with a history of silicone implant rupture and replacement with saline implants.

MAMMOGRAPHY: Left (**A**) and right (**B**) MLO views show bilateral, normal-appearing, prepectoral saline implants. There is residual free silicone present in the left axillary tail (**arrow**), as evidenced by a very-high-density region adjacent to the implant capsule. Normal folds are noted in the implants. Ultrasound (**C, D**) of the left implant shows echogenic shadowing diffusely consistent with free silicone. There is also a small hypoechoic mass that represents a "silicone cyst."

IMPRESSION: Normal saline implants, residual free silicone from extracapsular rupture of prior left implant.

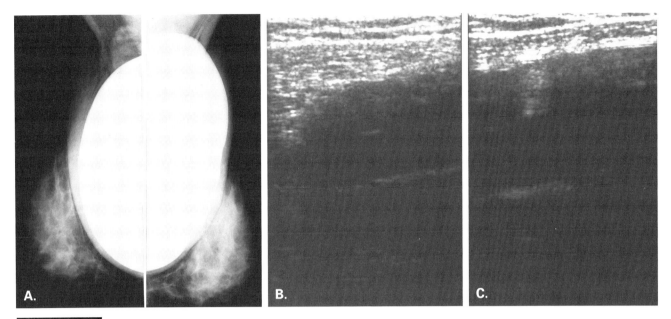

Figure 13.27

HISTORY: A 48-year-old woman who reported some change in contour of her right breast implant.

MAMMOGRAPHY: Bilateral MLO views (**A**) show subpectoral silicone implants. The right implant is situated slightly higher than the left, and it has some bulging of its superior border. Ultrasound of the right (**B**) and left (**C**) implants showed similar findings. The normal anechoic implant is not present. Instead, multiple bands traverse the implant lumen in a stairstep pattern. These findings are consistent with intracapsular rupture of the implant, and the bands represent the broken segments of the implant wall contained within the collection of silicone. The fibrous capsule contains the silicone, so it maintains a relatively normal shape.

IMPRESSION: Intracapsular silicone implant ruptures bilaterally.

NOTE: The implants were removed, and bilateral intracapsular rupture was confirmed at surgery.

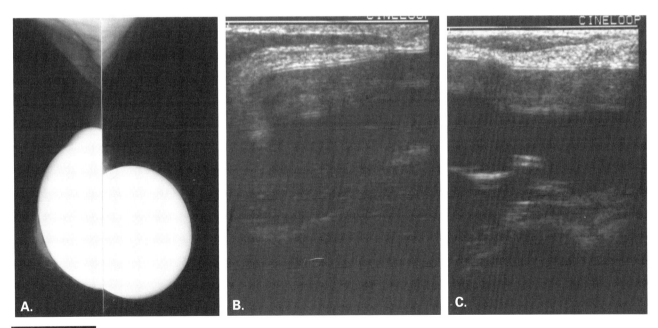

Figure 13.28

HISTORY: A 43-year-old patient with a history of silicone implants.

MAMMOGRAPHY: Bilateral MLO views (**A**) show prepectoral silicone implants to be present. There is distortion in the shape of the left implant. Ultrasound of the right (**B**) and left (**C**) implants shows internal echoes within the silicone with a stairstep pattern, consistent with intracapsular rupture.

IMPRESSION: Bilateral intracapsular rupture.

NOTE: The stairstep structures represent broken implant wall, floating in the silicone, which is contained within the fibrous capsule that formed around the implant.

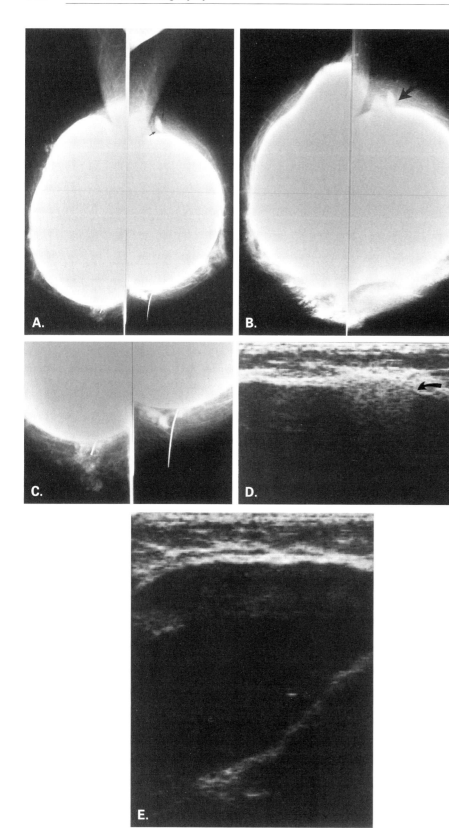

Figure 13.29

HISTORY: A 42-year-old woman after bilateral augmentation mammoplasty, presenting with bilateral palpable nodularity at the inferior aspects of the implants.

MAMMOGRAPHY: Bilateral MLO views (**A**), CC views (**B**), coned-down MLO view (**C**), and ultrasound (**D** and **E**). Bilateral, retroglandular silicone-filled implants are present. There is some deformity of the contour of both implants, which may be associated with encapsulation. There are multiple areas (**arrows**) of high-density nodularity near the border of the implants, both inferiorly and superiorly. On the enlargement (**C**), these nodules contain densities that appear to be calcific. Ultrasound (**D**) in the region of the palpable nodularity showed disruption of the border of the implant and a hyperechoic region (**arrow**) with vague irregularity in the capsule at the point of disruption. This contrasts with other areas (**E**) where the capsule is intact and the overlying parenchyma is normal.

IMPRESSION: Bilateral leakage of silicone implants.

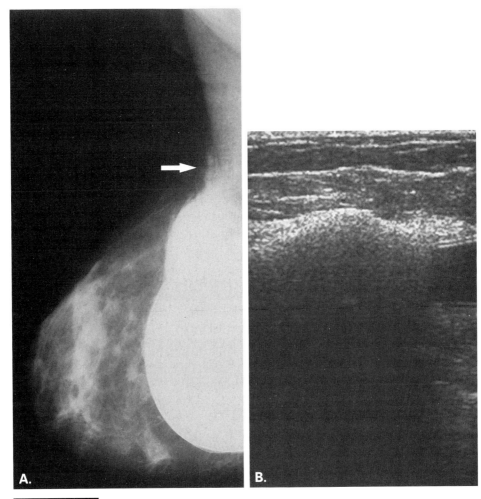

Figure 13.30

HISTORY: A 61-year-old woman with a history of implants, who presents for routine follow-up.

MAMMOGRAPHY: Left MLO view (**A**) shows a prepectoral silicone implant with a deformity along the superior aspect. Extending into the axilla are multiple high-density nodules and strands consistent with free silicone (**arrows**). On ultrasound (**B**) of the axillary region, the typical features of free silicone are seen: disruption of the wall of the implant, hyperechogenicity superficial to the implant with very prominent shadowing, and the snowstorm appearance related to the free silicone.

IMPRESSION: Ruptured silicone implant with extracapsular free silicone.

are negative or equivocal, and there is concern about leakage. Typical sequences are fast-spin echo (FSE) with T_2 weighting in axial and sagittal planes, T_1-weighted images with silicone suppression, and FSE T_2-weighted images with water suppression (24). Radial folds are a common finding and represent infolding of the elastomer shell; radial folds connect to at least one surface of the implant.

A rupture of the silicone implant into the intracapsular space is identified on MRI as the so-called linguine sign (29,30). This is the fragmented elastomer shell that is floating in the silicone and contained within the fibrous capsule (Figs. 13.31 and 13.32). Extrusion of the silicone beyond the capsule is depicted on MRI in the case of extracapsular rupture. In patients with a double-lumen implant that has failed internally, there may be admixing of the saline and silicone components without rupture of the outer lumen.

In a meta-analysis of articles that examined the diagnostic accuracy of various imaging techniques for implant rupture, Goodman et al. (16) found that the sensitivities and specificities for rupture were as follows: mammography, 28.4% and 92.9%; ultrasound, 59.0% and 76.8%; MRI,

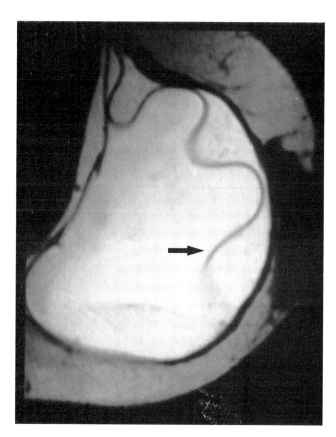

Figure 13.31

Sagittal T2 weighted MRI image of a patient with silicone implants. Within the fibrous capsule that surrounds the implant and within the pool of silicone is a circumlinear structure **(arrow)** that is the broken implant wall. There is no evidence for extracapsular extension of silicone.

IMPRESSION: Intracapsular rupture (the "linguine sign") (Case courtesy of Dr. Patricia Abbitt, Gainesville, Fl).

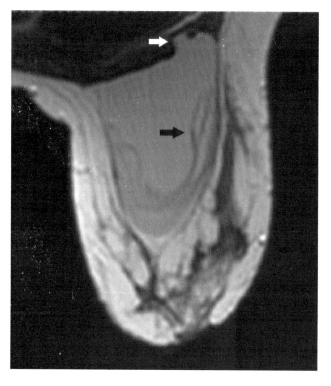

Figure 13.32

Axial T2 weighted image (TR 5500, TE 81.7) in a patient with silicone implants shows signs of intracapsular rupture and focal extracapsular rupture.

Within the silicone is a linear structure that is coiled in the anterior aspect, consistent with the broken implant wall (the "linguine sign") **(black arrow)**. Posteriorly, is a small focus of silicone **(white arrow)** behind the fibrous capsule. This represents an extracapsular rupture as well.

IMPRESSION: Ruptured silicone implant (Case courtesy of Dr. Neeti Goel, Harrisburg, Pa).

78.1% and 80.0%. In a study of 81 patients with 160 implants that were removed and who had preoperative MRI and ultrasound, Weizer et al. (28) found an additive benefit by using the two modalities. Twenty percent of the implants were ruptured. The sensitivity and specificity of ultrasound were found to be 47% and 83%, respectively. For MRI, the sensitivity and specificity were 46% and 88%, respectively. Other authors have found that the sensitivity of MRI for implant rupture was 76% and the specificity was 97% (29).

OTHER IMPLANT COMPLICATIONS

Gel bleed is a term that is used to describe the microscopic diffusion of silicone gel through the elastomer shell that is an intact semipermeable structure. This may be evident on ultrasound as echogenic lines separate from the fibrous capsule. On MRI, the elastomer shell appears folded with silicone gel on both sides of the fold (24) when gel bleed has occurred.

Peri-implant fluid collections may occur as a result of several causes, including infections, ruptured saline components, malignancy, and inflammation. In patients with polyurethane-covered silicone gel implants, peri-implant fluid collections are very common and have been described in 48% of patients (31). The fragmentation of the polyurethane in vivo creates a foreign-body reaction with chronic inflammation (24). Very large fluid collections surrounding an intact implant that has been in place for years should raise the concern for malignancy. Lymphoma may present in this manner and is diagnosed on cytologic examination of the aspirate of the effusion.

Various authors have described a group of symptoms and disorders that are known as silicone-related disease. These include various connective tissue disorders, such as rheumatoid arthritis, Sjögren syndrome, scleroderma, systemic lupus erythematosus, and fibromyalgia (32–35). Others have not proven any significant relationship of implants with these disorders (29,36–39). As a result of these concerns, in 1992 the FDA decided to limit the use of breast implants to clinical trials only (40). Subsequently, the use of silicone implants for breast reconstruction was once again approved.

PARENCHYMAL ABNORMALITIES

Parenchymal abnormalities can be demonstrated with imaging, but it is important to maximize information obtained by tailoring the examination to the patient. Both benign and malignant lesions may be demonstrated in the augmented breast (Figs. 13.33–13.38). Masses may be less readily detected than microcalcifications (13) on mammography, but ultrasound may be of help in the

evaluation of dense parenchyma over the prostheses and of palpable masses (41).

The diagnosis of breast cancer may be delayed in women who have undergone breast augmentation (3,4,42,43). The use of implant-displacement views is important to optimize visualization of the parenchyma, yet in most patients, areas of breast parenchyma may still be obscured by the implants. Brinton et al. (44) found that women with breast augmentation and breast cancer had later stage disease than women without augmentation. Skinner et al. (3) found that mammography was less sensitive in women with augmentation than in women without implants (66.3% versus 94.6%). In a prospective study of women identified through seven mammography registries, Miglioretti et al. (42) found that breast augmentation decreased the sensitivity of screening mammography among asymptomatic women, but the prognostic characteristics of tumors were not affected by augmentation. The location of the implant may affect visibility of breast tissue and also potentially the cancer detection rate. Silverstein et al. (45) found that 39% to 49% of breast tissue is obscured by prepectoral implants, but only 9% to 28% of the tissue is concealed by subpectoral prostheses.

THE EXPLANT SITE

After a breast implant is removed, the fibrous capsule may remain in the breast. Particularly, if the capsule's wall is thick or calcified, it will not collapse as a thin-walled capsule often does. Instead, a seroma may form within the fibrous capsule and may be evident on mammography as a mass.

The findings after explanation have been described previously (46–48). The capsule is visible in the position and orientation in which the implant was located. An oval mass parallel to the pectoralis muscle and located in the posterior third of the breast is commonly seen. The margins may be circumscribed or indistinct, and the mass may simulate cancer (Figs. 13.39–13.44). Residual silicone droplets may be evident within or adjacent to the seroma. The seroma may be so large and dense that it has the appearance of a saline implant on mammography. Calcification of the residual fibrous capsule may be present.

BREAST RECONSTRUCTION

After mastectomy, an immediate or a delayed breast reconstruction may be performed. This is accomplished either by placement of an implant or by recreating a breast mound by moving an autologous myocutaneous flap. A skin-sparing mastectomy is often performed if

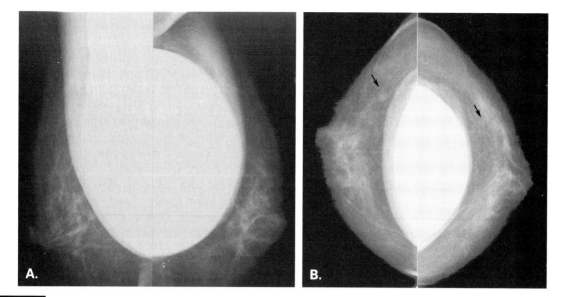

Figure 13.33

HISTORY: A 50-year-old woman with a history of breast implants.

MAMMOGRAPHY: Bilateral MLO (**A**) and CC (**B**) views show subpectoral silicone implants bilaterally. On the left MLO view, there is extension of the silicone density into the axilla, consistent with implant rupture. Also noted are small bilateral circumscribed masses (**arrows**) that were found to be cystic on ultrasound.

IMPRESSION: Left extracapsular implant rupture.

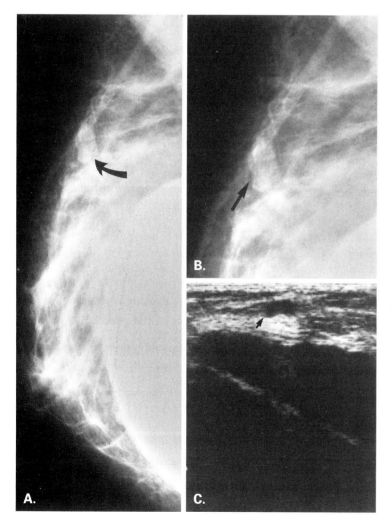

Figure 13.34

HISTORY: A 38-year-old woman with bilateral breast implants and a palpable nodule in the left axillary tail.

MAMMOGRAPHY: Left MLO view (**A**), coned-down MLO view (**B**), and ultrasound (**C**). A retroglandular implant and a moderate amount of overlying glandular tissue are present. There is a well-circumscribed lobulated nodule (**arrow**) in the upper outer quadrant of the left breast (**A** and **B**). Ultrasound (**C**) demonstrates the nodule to be a cyst (**arrow**), and this corresponded to the palpable nodule.

IMPRESSION: Simple cyst anterior to the retroglandular implant.

Figure 13.35

HISTORY: A 46-year-old woman with a history of implants who now presents with two new left palpable masses.

MAMMOGRAPHY: Bilateral CC views (**A**) show normal-appearing saline implants. The palpable masses were not evident on mammography. On ultrasound, the left 12 o'clock mass (**B**) is hypoechoic, oval, and smoothly marginated, suggestive of a fibroadenoma. The left 5 o'clock mass (**C**) is more vertically oriented and is hypoechoic and lobulated. A small simple cyst was seen at 6 o'clock (**D**).

IMPRESSION: Normal implants; two solid masses corresponding to palpable lesions, possible fibroadenomas; recommend biopsy.

HISTOPATHOLOGY: Fibrosis at 12 o'clock, fibroadenoma at 5 o'clock.

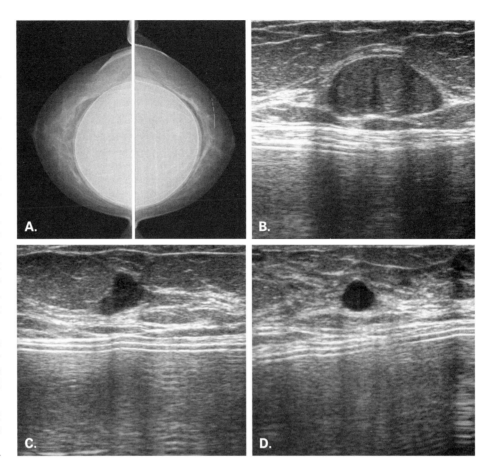

Figure 13.36

HISTORY: Routine mammogram on a postmenopausal patient with prepectoral implants.

MAMMOGRAPHY: Left MLO (**A**) and CC (**B**) implant-displaced views show heterogeneously dense tissue. A small, isodense indistinct mass (**arrows**) is present in the upper outer quadrant. On the spot-identification CC magnification view (**C**), the indistinct borders of the mass are evident.

IMPRESSION: Suspicious mass anterior to the implant.

HISTOPATHOLOGY: Invasive ductal carcinoma, negative axillary nodes.

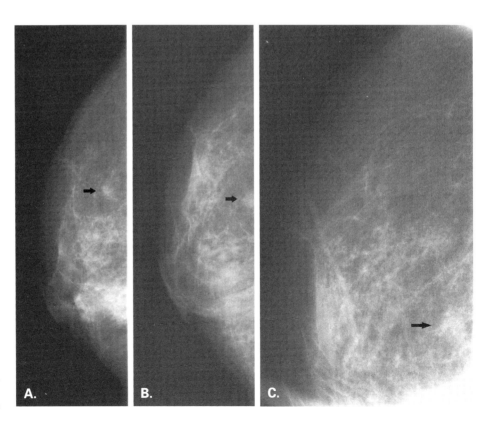

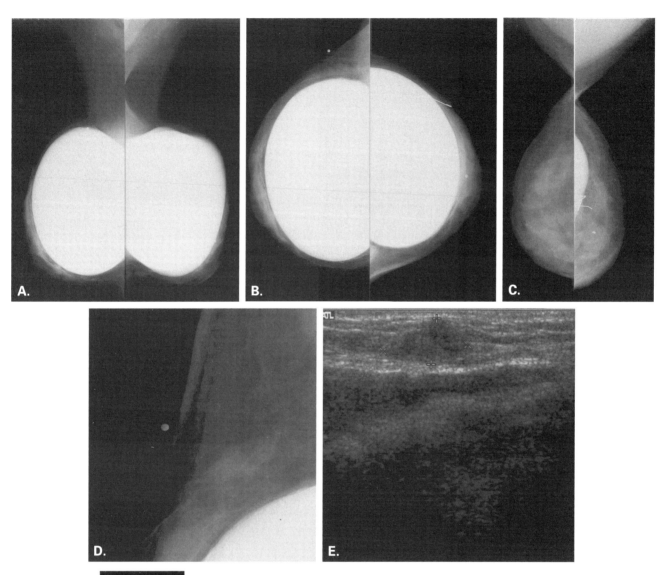

Figure 13.37

HISTORY: A 50-year-old woman with a history of implants and a new small palpable mass in the left breast at 2 o'clock.

MAMMOGRAPHY: Bilateral MLO **(A)** and CC **(B)** views show prepectoral silicone implants. A BB marks the palpable area in the left breast. The area is not visible on the implant-displaced MLO view **(C)**. On the spot CC, implant-displaced views **(D)**, a focal asymmetry is present at the BB. Ultrasound **(E)** of the palpable lump shows a hypoechoic irregular mass, suspicious for malignancy.

IMPRESSION: Solid mass, suspicious for carcinoma.

HISTOPATHOLOGY: Infiltrating ductal carcinoma, low nuclear grade.

possible when reconstruction is planned to facilitate the cosmetic procedure. Most often the mastectomy site or the reconstructed breast is not imaged. However, occasionally, especially if there is a clinical question about a recurrence that is not on the skin, mammography may be performed.

With implant placement for reconstruction, an expander is first positioned following the mastectomy. The expander is then gradually inflated to allow the skin to adapt and stretch. Ultimately, the expander is replaced with a permanent implant, and the nipple-areolar complex is reformed.

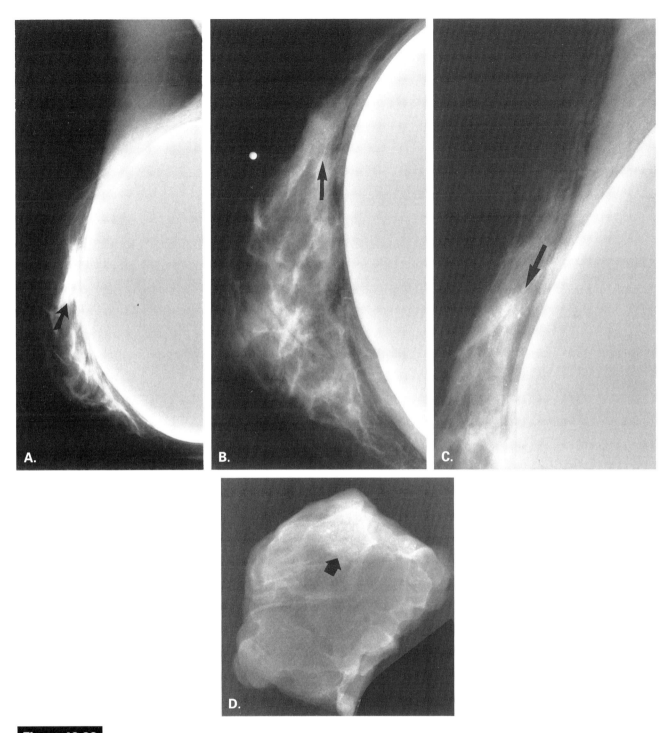

Figure 13.38

HISTORY: A 40-year-old gravida 6, para 2 woman with bilateral breast implants, for screening.

MAMMOGRAPHY: Left MLO (**A**), CC (**B**), enlarged (2X) CC (**C**), and specimen (**D**) views. A subpectoral implant is present, and heterogeneously dense glandular tissue overlies the prosthesis. In the left upper-outer quadrant (**A–C**), there is a focal area of increased density associated with fine, granular microcalcifications **(arrows)**. The area was considered suspicious for malignancy and was localized under mammographic guidance by placement of a skin marker rather than a needle over the lesion. The specimen film (**D**) confirms the removal of the suspicious area.

IMPRESSION: Irregular density with microcalcifications anterior to the implant, moderately suspicious for carcinoma.

HISTOPATHOLOGY: Infiltrating ductal carcinoma.

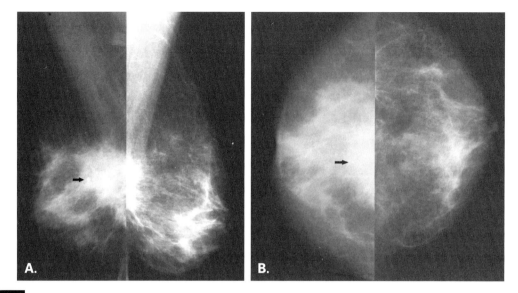

Figure 13.39

HISTORY: Postmenopausal patient with a history of silicone implant removal who also presents with left breast pain.

MAMMOGRAPHY: Bilateral MLO (**A**) and CC (**B**) views show the breasts to be heterogeneously dense. There are oval indistinct masses in both breasts having a relatively symmetrical appearance. The left mass (**arrow**) is slightly larger than the right. The densities are oriented along the plane of the chest wall and are most consistent with explant sites. Because of the symptoms on the left, the density was excised.

IMPRESSION: Fibrous capsules from explant sites.

HISTOPATHOLOGY: Left breast: Fibrous capsule, scar.

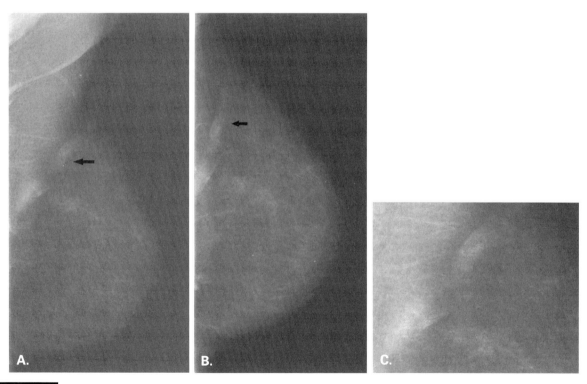

Figure 13.40

HISTORY: A 66-year-old woman with a history of silicone implants that were removed, who now presents for screening mammography.

MAMMOGRAPHY: Right MLO (**A**) and exaggerated CC lateral (**B**) views show the breast to be fatty replaced. Located posteriorly and parallel to the pectoralis major muscle is an ovoid low-density structure (**arrows**). This is better visualized on the enlarged MLO image (**C**).

IMPRESSION: Explant site from prior silicone implant removal.

NOTE: These findings are typical of the explant site, which typically is oriented along the plane of the pectoralis major muscle in the position in which the implant was located.

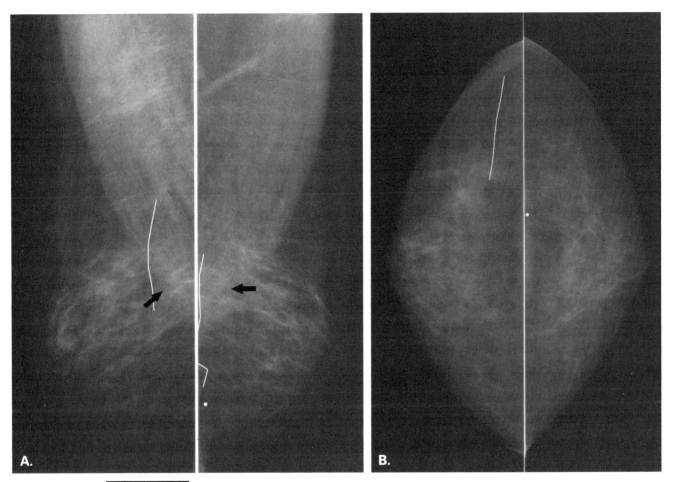

Figure 13.41

HISTORY: A 59-year-old woman with history of implant removal.

MAMMOGRAPHY: Bilateral MLO (**A**) and CC (**B**) views show scattered densities bilaterally. Deep in both breasts at the chest wall, marked by wires at the explant sites, are vague indistinct densities (**arrows**) oriented along the pectoralis major muscles. This finding represents the residual fibrous capsule at the explant site.

IMPRESSION: Explant sites bilaterally.

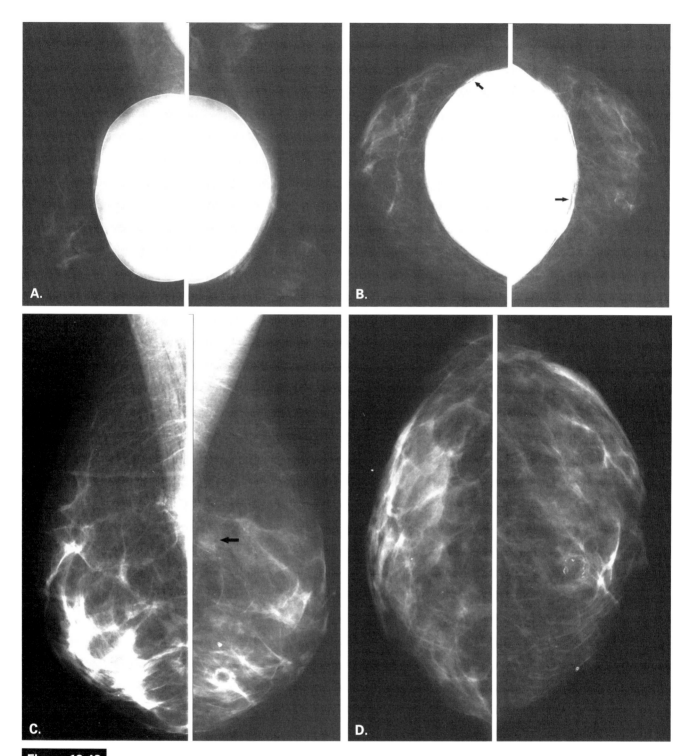

Figure 13.42

HISTORY: A 48-year-old woman with a history of implant rupture and replacement with saline implants.

MAMMOGRAPHY: Bilateral MLO **(A)** and CC **(B)** views show that the saline implants have a normal appearance. On the CC views **(B)**, a thin bandlike density surrounds the anterior edge of each of the implants **(arrows)**. This finding is consistent with the explant site from the prior implants. Three years later, after the saline implants also were removed, typical changes after implant removal are noted. On the bilateral MLO **(C)** and CC **(D)** views, postsurgical changes are seen. There is an oval density parallel to the pectoralis muscle seen on the right **(arrow)** more prominently than on the left, consistent with the residual fibrous capsule after explantation. Coarse eggshell calcifications are also noted.

IMPRESSION: Postexplantation findings.

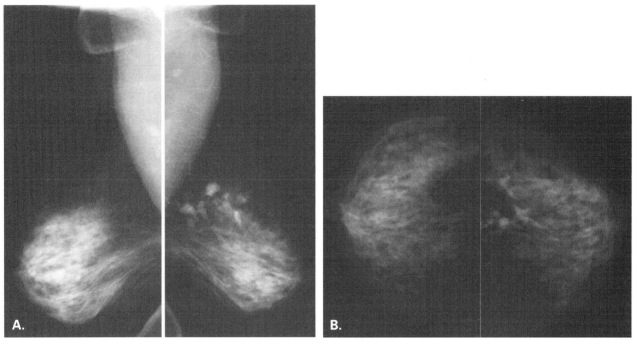

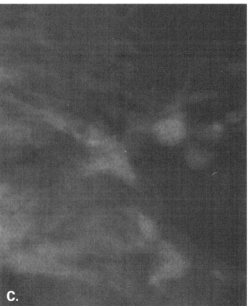

Figure 13.43

HISTORY: A 43-year-old woman for screening, with a history of removal of silicone implants.

MAMMOGRAPHY: Bilateral MLO **(A)** and CC **(B)** views show very dense parenchyma. On the right, there are multiple high-density round and lobular circumscribed masses at the 12 o'clock position. On enlarged CC image **(C)**, these are oriented in part around a somewhat circumscribed lucency where the implant had resided. The findings represent residual silicone at the explant site.

IMPRESSION: Explant site with free silicone.

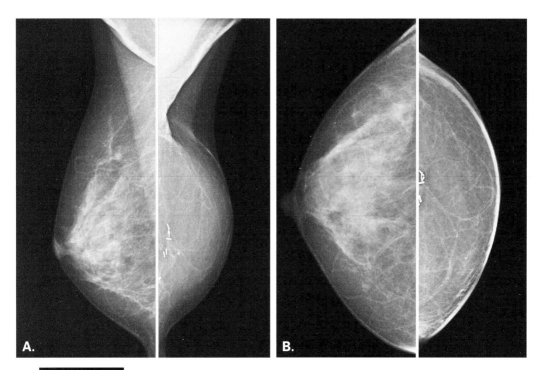

Figure 13.44

HISTORY: 53 year-old patient with history of right breast cancer treated with mastectomy and TRAM flap reconstruction.

MAMMOGRAPHY: Bilateral MLO **(A)**, and CC **(B)** views show marked asymmetry in the appearance of the breasts. The left breast has a normal appearance, and it is composed of scattered fibroglandular elements. The right breast is fatty, without any ductal tissue and has mild skin thickening. The shape of the right breast is slightly flatter and wider than the left, all of which are typical features of a myocutaneous flap reconstruction.

IMPRESSION: Normal TRAM flap breast reconstruction.

When a reconstruction is performed using a myocutaneous flap, the graft is derived from the transverse rectus abdominis muscle (TRAM), the gluteus maximus, or the latissimus dorsi. The flap is turned to create the breast mound, and the blood supply is maintained through a pedicle. In the case of reconstruction from the gluteus maximus, a free flap is raised and moved, with microsurgical technique used to maintain perfusion. One complication of a myocutaneous flap is fat necrosis, which may occur if the blood supply is compromised. Fat necrosis presents as a palpable mass that is firm or hard.

Like the patient who has had a breast reconstruction with an implant, the reconstructed breast is not usually imaged. If mammography is performed, the striking finding is the marked asymmetry in the appearance of the breasts and the complete lack of any density that appears to be ductal or glandular on the reconstructed side. Autologous flaps are primarily fatty on mammography, with minimal density related to the muscle component that is visualized on the MLO view, anterior to the pectoralis major muscle (49). Fat necrosis may occur

and has a similar appearance to fat necrosis in the breast itself. Fat necrosis has been reported to occur in 10% to 26% of TRAM flaps (50,51). The flap often compresses somewhat differently from the native breast, and the shape is slightly wider and thicker superiorly than the native breast. The skin over the flap is often slightly thicker than the normal breast as well. Occasionally, the patient may have a combined reconstruction that includes both a myocutaneous flap and an implant (Fig. 13.45).

The findings related to recurrent carcinoma at the mastectomy site are discussed in Chapter 12. Of concern for recurrence of cancer are the presence of findings that are suspicious otherwise: irregular or spiculated masses or suspicious microcalcifications. Imaging of the mastectomy site or the reconstructed breast is not routinely performed to search for recurrence. Often recurrence is manifested as a nodule in the skin or as erythema. If there is a palpable mass, mammography may be performed before biopsy to assess for fat necrosis versus a suspicious mass indicative of recurrent carcinoma.

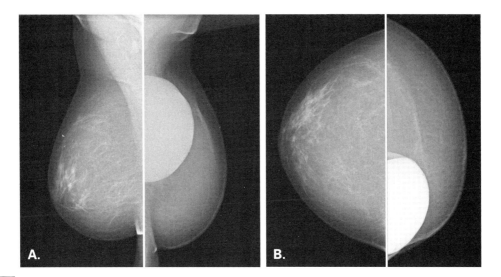

Figure 13.45

HISTORY: 49 year-old woman with a history of right breast cancer treated with mastectomy and subsequent reconstruction with both a TRAM flap and a small silicone implant.

MAMMOGRAPHY: Bilateral MLO **(A)**, and CC **(B)** views show a marked difference in the appearance of the breasts. The left breast is composed of scattered fibroglandular tissue. The reconstructed right breast is completely fatty, with no ductal tissue, consistent with a mastectomy site and reconstruction with a myocutaneous flap. The contour of the right breast is somewhat flatter and wider than the left. A small silicone implant also was placed medially as part of the reconstruction procedure to improve the overall symmetry.

IMPRESSION: Normal reconstructed right breast with a TRAM flap and a silicone implant.

REFERENCES

1. Bright RA, Jeng LL, Moore RM. National survey of self-reported breast implants: 1988 estimates. *J Long Term Eff Med Implants* 1993;3:81–89.
2. Cook RR, Delongchamp RR, Woodbury M, et al. The prevalence of women with breast implants in the United States—1989. *J Clin Epidemiol* 1995;48:519–525.
3. Skinner KA, Silberman H, Dougherty W, et al. Breast cancer after augmentation mammoplasty. *Ann Surg Oncol* 2001;8: 138–144.
4. Handel N, Silverstein MJ, Gamagami P, et al. Factors affecting mammographic visualization of the breast after augmentation mammoplasty. *JAMA* 1992;268:1913–1917.
5. Steinbach BG, Hardt NS, Abbitt PL, et al. Breast implants, common complications and concurrent breast disease. *RadioGraphics* 1993;13:95–118.
6. Parsons RW, Thering HR. Management of the silicone-injected breast. *Plast Reconstr Surg* 1977;60(4):534–538.
7. Delage C, Shane JJ, Johnson FB. Mammary silicone granuloma. *Arch Dermatol* 1973;108:104–107.
8. Koide T, Katayama H. Calcification in augmentation mammoplasty. *Radiology* 1979;130:337–340.
9. Cheung YC, Su MY, Ng SH, et al. Lumpy silicone-injected breasts enhanced MRI and microscopic correlation. *Journal of Clinical Imaging* 2002;26:397–404.
10. Jenson SR, Mackey JK. Xeromammography after augmentation mammoplasty. *AJR Am J Roentgenol* 1985;144:629–633.
11. Segel MC, Schnitt EL, Binns JH. Carcinoma of the breast associated with silicone paraffin injections. *Breast Dis* 1988;1: 225–229.
12. McGrath MH, Burkhardt BR. The safety and efficacy of breast implants for augmentation mammoplasty. *Plast Reconstr Surg* 1984;74(4):550–560.
13. Dershaw DD, Chaglassion TA. Mammography after prosthesis placement for augmentation or reconstructive mammoplasty. *Radiology* 1989;170:69–74.
14. Smahel J. Tissue reactions to breast implants coated with polyurethane. *Plast Reconstr Surg* 1978;61:80–85.
15. Peters W, Smith D. Calcification of breast implant capsules: incidence, diagnosis, and contributing factors. *Ann Plast Surg* 1995;34:8–11.
16. Goodman CM, Cohen V, Thornby J, et al. The life span of silicone gel breast implants and a comparison of mammography, ultrasonography, and magnetic resonance imaging and detecting implant rupture: a meta-analysis. *Ann Plast Surg* 1998;41(6):577–585.
17. Mitnick JS, Harris MN, Roses DF. Mammographic detection of carcinoma of the breast in patients with augmentation prostheses. *Surg Gynecol Obstet* 1989;168:30–32.
18. Eklund GW, Busby RC, Miller SH, et al. Improved imaging of the augmented breast. *AJR Am J Roentgenol* 1988;151:469–473.
19. Piccoli CW. Imaging of the patient with silicone gel breast implants. *MRI Clinics of North America* 2001;9(2):393–406.
20. Biggs TM, Cukier J, Worthing LF. Augmentation mammoplasty; a review of 18 years. *Plast Reconstr Surg* 1982;69(3):445–449.
21. McKinney P, Tresley G. Long-term comparison of patients with gel and saline mammary implants. *Plast Reconstr Surg* 1983; 72:27–29.
22. Grant EG, Cigtay OS, Mascatello VJ. Irregularity of Silastic breast implants mimicking a soft tissue mass. *AJR Am J Roentgenol* 1978;130:461–462.
23. Shermis RB, Adler DD, Smith DJ, et al. Intraductal silicone secondary to breast implant rupture: an unusual mammographic presentation. *Breast Dis* 1990;3:17–20.
24. O'Toole M, Caskey CI. Imaging spectrum of breast implant complications: mammography, ultrasound, and magnetic resonance imaging. *Semin Ultrasound CT MR* 2000;21(5):351–361.
25. Destouet JM, Monsees BS, Oser RF, et al. Screening mammography in 350 women with breast implants: prevalence and findings of implant complications. *AJR Am J Roentgenol* 1992;159:973–978.
26. Gorczyca DP, Debruhl MD, Ohn CY, et al. Silicone breast implant ruptures in an animal model: comparison of

mammography, MR imaging, US imaging and CT. *Radiology* 1994;190:227–232.

27. Debruhl MD, Gorczyca DP, Ohn CY, et al. Silicone breast implants: US evaluation. *Radiology* 1993;189:95–98.

28. Weizer G, Malone RS, Netscher DT, et al. Utility of magnetic resonance imaging and ultrasonography in diagnosing breast implant rupture. *Ann Plast Surg* 1995;34(4):352–361.

29. Gorczyca P, Sinha S, Ohn N, et al. Silicone breast implants in vivo: MR imaging. *Radiology* 1992;185:407–410.

30. Safvi A. Linguine sign. *Radiology* 2000;216:838–839.

31. Caskey CI, Berg WA, Hamper UM, et al. Imaging spectrum of extracapsular silicone: correlation of US, MR imaging, mammographic and histopathologic findings. *Radiographics* 1999;19:S39–S51.

32. Borenstein D. Siliconosis: a spectrum of illness. *Semin Arthritis Rheum* 1994;42:1–7.

33. Freundlich B, Altmann C, Sandorfi N, et al. A profile of symptomatic patients with silicone breast implants: a Sjörgens-like syndrome. *Semin Arthritis Rheum* 1994;24:44–53.

34. Solomon G. A clinical and laboratory profile of symptomatic women with silicone breast implants. *Semin Arthritis Rheum* 1994;24:29–37.

35. Cuellar ML, Gluck O, Molina JF, et al. Silicone breast implant-associated musculoskeletal manifestations. *Clin Rheumatol* 1995;14:667–672.

36. Blackburn WD, Grotting JC, Everson MP. Lack of systemic inflammatory rheumatoid disorders in symptomatic women with breast implants. *Plast Reconstr Surg* 1997;99:1054–1060.

37. Gabriel SE, O'Fallon WM, Kurland TL, et al. Risk of connective tissue disease and other disorders after breast implantation. *N Engl J Med* 1994;1697–1702.

38. Sanchez-Guerrero J, Colditz GA, Karlson EW, et al. Silicone breast implants and the risk of connective tissue diseases and symptoms. *N Engl J Med* 1995;332:1666–1670.

39. Berner I, Gaubitz M, Jackisch C, et al. Comparative examination of complaints of patients with breast cancer with and without silicone implants. *Eur J Obstet Gynecol Reprod Biol* 2002;102:61–66.

40. Kessler DA, Merkatz RB, Schapiro R. A call for higher standards for breast implants. *JAMA* 1993;270:2607–2608.

41. Cole-Reuglet C, Schwartz G, Kurtz AB, et al. Ultrasound mammography for the augmented breast. *Radiology* 1983;146:737–742.

42. Miglioretti DL, Rutter CM, Geller BM, et al. Effect of breast augmentation on the accuracy of mammography and cancer characteristics. *JAMA* 2004;291:442–450.

43. Fajardo LL, Harvey JA, McAleese KA, et al. Breast cancer diagnosis in women with subglandular silicone gel-filled augmentation implants. *Radiology* 1995;194:859–862.

44. Brinton LA, Lubin JH, Burich MC, et al. Breast cancer following augmentation mammoplasty (United States). *Cancer Causes Control* 2000;11:819–827.

45. Silverstein MJ, Handel N, Gamagami P, et al. Mammographic measurements before and after augmentation mammoplasty. *Plast Reconstr Surg* 1990;86:1126–1130.

46. Soo MS, Kornguth PJ, Georgiade GS, et al. Seromas in residual fibrous capsules after explantation: mammographic and sonographic appearances. *Radiology* 1995;194:863–866.

47. Hayes MK, Gold RH, Bassett LW. Mammographic findings after the removal of breast implants. *AJR Am J Roentgenol* 1993;160:487–490.

48. Stewart NR, Monsees BS, Destouet JM, et al. Mammographic appearance following implant removal. *Radiology* 1992;185:83–85.

49. Hogge JP, Zuurbier RA, Shaw de Paredes E. Mammography of autologous myocutaneous flaps. *Radiographics* 1999;19:S63–S72.

50. Helvie MA, Wilson TE, Roubidoux MA, et al. Mammographic appearance of recurrent breast carcinoma in six patients with TRAM flap breast reconstructions. *Radiology* 1998;209:711–715.

51. Mund DF, Wolfson P, Gorczyca DP, et al. Mammographically detected recurrent nonpalpable carcinoma developing in a transverse rectus abdominis myocutaneous flap. *Cancer* 1994;74:2804–2807.

Chapter 14

Galactography

The lactiferous ducts develop from epithelial buds and are affected by the hormonal milieu. The ducts drain the parenchyma and are the conduits of milk in the lactating woman. The duct system is the site of development of most benign and malignant epithelial lesions, and some of these may be associated with nipple discharge.

The evaluation of patients who present with an abnormal nipple discharge includes clinical examination and a variety of tests, such as cytologic analysis, mammography, ultrasound, magnetic resonance imaging (MRI), galactography, and ductoscopy. This chapter will focus on the role, technique, and interpretation of galactography.

Nipple discharge in a nonlactating breast can be produced by a variety of conditions, including duct ectasia, fibrocystic change, inflammation, intraductal papilloma, and intraductal carcinoma. The most common cause of a bloody or discharge at all ages is an intraductal papilloma (1). Galactography or ductography can be useful in the evaluation of a spontaneous nipple discharge, particularly when there are no mammographic or physical findings to account specifically for the etiology of the leakage.

EVALUATION OF NIPPLE DISCHARGE

Clinical assessment of the patient who presents with nipple discharge is the first step in determining the potential significance of the symptom and the next step in management. Important clinical history includes the duration of symptoms, the color of the discharge, history of trauma, the laterality (unilateral vs. bilateral) and spontaneity of the discharge, and the history of medications, including hormones or hormonal imbalances (2). Clinical examination should include a general examination of the breast with expression of the discharge. A trigger point that when compressed produces the discharge may be identified. This point may indicate the orientation of the abnormal duct. Observation of the color of the discharge and the location of the orifice are important in planning the management and identifying the potential etiology of this symptom. The determination of whether the discharge is uniorificial is an important step in determining whether galactography is necessary.

Nipple discharge from the nonlactating breast may be white, creamy, yellowish, clear, green, serosanguineous, or bloody. Guaiac testing may be useful to analyze for blood in nipple discharge. The most suspicious discharges are those that are uniorificial and serous, serosanguinous, or bloody. The exceptions are bloody discharge related to pregnancy or to trauma. The absence of blood in nipple discharge, however, does not exclude carcinoma (3,4). Ciatto et al. (5) found that a bloody discharge was more frequently associated with cancer than other patterns of discharge. However, serous discharge that is heme negative may be found with carcinoma.

In most cases, yellow, white, or green discharge is related to a systemic etiology and occurs bilaterally and from multiple ducts. This type of discharge is usually not spontaneous and is associated with duct ectasia, fibrocystic change, or hormonal or medicinal causes (6). Discharges that are not spontaneous and are expressible only are usually of benign origin and related to fibrocystic change (7).

The frequency of malignancy in a patient with bloody nipple discharge has been found to be 5% to 28% (1); however, the frequency of carcinoma is 1.6% to 13% in patients with serous discharge (1,8). In a study of 174 women with uniorificial discharge (31% serous and 69% bloody), Tabar et al. (1) found carcinoma in 18 of 174 (10%) patients. Serous discharge was present in 3 of 18 (17%) patients with cancer; 15 of 18 (83%) patients with cancer had bloody discharge. In this study, cytologic analysis of the discharge was not sensitive, with only 2 of 18 of the cancers having suspicious cytology.

Occasionally pregnant women may develop nipple discharge that is bloody. LaFreniere (9) found that both mammography and cytology were negative in five pregnant women with unilateral bloody multiorificial discharge. In all cases, the discharge resolved within 2 months of onset. Table 14.1 describes the etiologies of nipple discharge based on color.

In the presence of a suspicious nipple discharge, further evaluation beyond mammography is indicated. This

▶ **TABLE 14.1** **Etiologies of Nipple Discharge**

Color of Discharge	Etiologies
White	Galactorrhea, lactation, hormonal imbalances, medications, duct ectasia
Yellow	Hormonal, duct ectasia, infection, fibrocystic changes
Green	Fibrocystic changes
Clear	Papilloma, carcinoma, hyperplasia
Serosanguinous	Papilloma, carcinoma, hyperplasia, trauma
Bloody	Papilloma, carcinoma, hyperplasia, trauma, pregnancy

may include cytology of the discharge, galactography, MRI, ductoscopy, or duct excision. Cytology has shown variable results with a sensitivity ranging from 11% to 31% (10,11). Therefore, the presence of negative cytology does not confirm that an intraductal malignancy is not present. Galactography is the only method to determine preoperatively the nature, location, and extent of the lesion producing the discharge, and it allows for more precise and limited surgical excision of the area of abnormality. Galactography was first described in the 1930s (12,13) but was not commonly used until mammography became established. If a duct excision without a prior contrast study is performed, the surgery may be unnecessary or more extensive than needed. Also, a blind duct excision has the potential to miss an intraductal lesion in a small peripheral duct. As many as 40% of ductal tumors have been found to lie in a nonsubareolar location, which may cause a lesion to be missed at surgery if a duct excision without preoperative galactography is performed (14).

The sensitivity of galactography has been studied by several authors (11,15,16). In a comparison of galactography and exfoliative cytology, Dinkel et al. (11) found the sensitivities for malignancy for each procedure to be 83% and 31.2% and the specificities to be 41% and 99%, respectively. The authors (11) found that one half of the cancers in the study demonstrated no palpable, mammographic, or cytologic abnormality and were identified only by galactography.

Van Zee et al. (17) found that localizing the lesion causing nipple discharge by preoperative galactography increased the likelihood that a specific pathology was found at surgery. In this study, 67% of patients who did not undergo galactography preoperatively did not have a specific pathology on excision. Cardenosa (18) found that galactography was positive in 32 of 35 (91%) of patients with spontaneous nipple discharge. In another study, however, King et al. (19) suggested that patients with nipple discharge should have breast imaging, and if this is negative, should be offered duct excision. The authors found no role for ductography, cytology, or laboratory studies. Dawes et al. (20) found that in 91 women with nipple discharge,

only 5% were due to cancers and that galactography did not confirm or refute the presence of an intraductal lesion.

GALACTOGRAPHY

Galactography is a contrast study that outlines the intraductal lumina. The purpose of galactography is to identify the presence and location of an intraductal lesion. The indication for galactography is the presence of a suspicious type of nipple discharge—that is, a spontaneous, uniorificial, serous, serosanguinous, or bloody discharge. Galactography depicts the course of the ducts and the location and extent of intraductal lesions. Preoperative galactography facilitates a more directed surgery and can avert unnecessary surgery when findings are benign (21).

Galactography is performed only when discharge is present. The breast interventionist must visualize the orifice from which the discharge is occurring in order to cannulate the correct duct. The discharge is expressed, and the orifice is visualized. Identifying a trigger point is helpful to determine the orientation of the duct (7) before attempting duct cannulation. The supplies for the procedure include a 27- to 30-g cannula with tubing, a 5-cc syringe, water-soluble contrast, sterile gauze, antiseptic solution, and Steristrips (Fig. 14.1).

The nipple areolar complex is cleansed with an antiseptic solution, and the breast is draped. Small amounts of discharge are expressed from the breast until the orifice of the duct is identified. A blunt cannula—such as a 27-gauge pediatric sialography cannula with a straight end, a right angle, or an olive tip—is filled with water-soluble radiographic contrast. It is important to remove any air bubbles from the catheter, because when injected, they

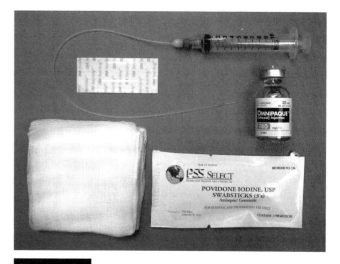

Figure 14.1

Supplies for galactography: cannula, syringe, water-soluble contrast, antiseptic solution, Steristrips, and sterile gauze.

may simulate intraductal masses. The duct is cannulated, and a small amount of contrast is injected. The most difficult step is cannulation of the duct, particularly if it is not dilated. Very gentle placement of the cannula is necessary to avoid penetration of the duct wall and extravasation of contrast. The cannula is taped in place with Steristrips. The amount of contrast needed ranges from 0.1 to 3.0 cc and varies with the number of secondary ducts draining into the main lactiferous duct and the degree of dilatation.

As the contrast is injected, the patient is asked to state when she feels tightness or pressure in the breast. At this point, the injection is terminated, the cannula is left in place, and images are obtained with mild compression. Should the patient experience pain, indicating possible extravasation of contrast, injection should be terminated immediately. The patient is positioned at the mammographic unit, and the craniocaudal (CC) view is obtained. If duct filling is incomplete, more contrast may be injected, and the CC view is repeated. With an obstruction of the distal duct, rapid backflow of contrast occurs.

Routine images include CC and mediolateral (ML) views. Magnification views are often helpful in the observation of small filling defects (21), and digital imaging is helpful to expedite the study. At the completion of imaging, the catheter is withdrawn with the breast still in compression, and a final image of the distal aspect of the duct is made. After the procedure, the patient is asked to express the residual contrast from the breast.

Complications of galactography include duct rupture with extravasation of contrast, lymphatic intravasation (Fig. 14.2), contrast reaction, and infection. In the patient with purulent discharge or signs of infection, galactography should not be performed, because the infection can be spread via retrograde injection.

The normal ducts converge toward the nipple into dilated ampullae, the lactiferous sinuses, which are then drained by thin 2- to 3-mm-diameter (1) collecting ducts (Fig. 14.3). As the ducts arborize back into the breast, the caliber gradually decreases. The walls of the lumina are smooth, and no beading, angulation, or abrupt narrowing should be present (Fig. 14.4).

In duct ectasia or secretory disease, the ducts are dilated, may be tortuous, and may contain filling defects from inspissated secretions (16). Cystic areas of dilatation may be present, particularly in the subareolar area, and a contrast-fluid level may be seen on the ML view (Figs. 14.5 and 14.6). The ducts may be up to 8 mm in diameter, and there may be some beading present (1). In fibrocystic

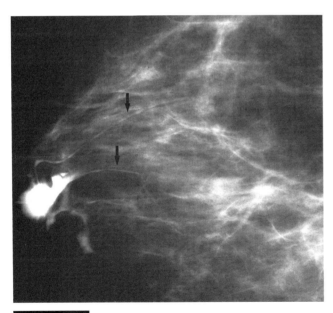

Figure 14.2

HISTORY: Patient who presents with serous nipple discharge.

MAMMOGRAPHY: Left ML view from a galactogram shows dense contrast in the subareolar area consistent with extravasation of contrast. There is filling of two tubular serosanguineous structures that are nonbranching and that extend from the areolar area toward the axilla.

IMPRESSION: Extravasation of contrast with lymphatic intravasation.

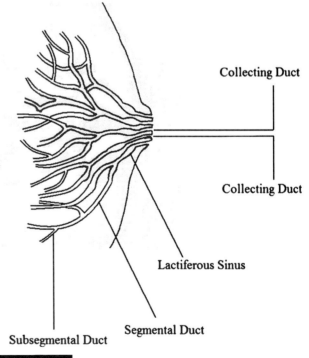

Figure 14.3

Anatomy of the major lactiferous duct system.

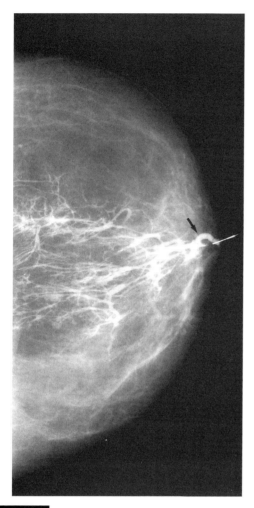

Figure 14.4

HISTORY: A 39-year-old woman with yellowish nipple discharge.

MAMMOGRAPHY: Right CC view from galactography shows the cannula in place and contrast filling the duct system drained by the collecting duct. Minimal dilatation in the collecting duct is seen **(arrow)**. The ducts arborize normally, and no filling defects are present.

IMPRESSION: Normal galactogram.

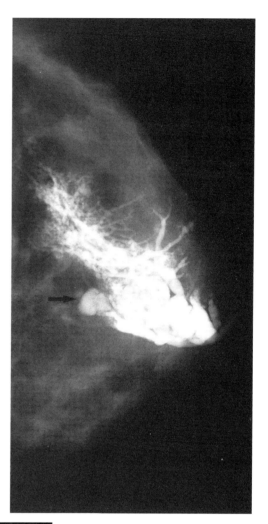

Figure 14.5

HISTORY: A 40-year-old woman who presents with serous right nipple discharge.

MAMMOGRAPHY: Right CC view from galactography shows marked distension of the subareolar collecting and segmental ducts. There is cystic dilatation noted as well **(arrow)**. Posterior to the subareolar region, the ducts appear pruned. No intraluminal filling defects were seen.

IMPRESSION: Marked duct ectasia.

change, the ducts may be slightly irregular in diameter, and there may be filling of multiple tiny or even large cysts (16) (Fig. 14.7). In intraductal hyperplasia, multiple small filling defects may be seen within the ductal lumen (Fig. 14.8).

Intraductal filling defects may be solitary or multiple. Filling defects identified on galactography may be iatrogenic (air bubbles), pseudolesions (clot, debris), or true epithelial lesions, including papilloma, papillomatosis, duct adenoma, intraductal hyperplasia, and ductal carcinoma. The etiologies of filling defects on galactography are listed in Table 14.2.

▶ **TABLE 14.2 Etiologies of Filling Defects on Galactography**

Solitary	Multiple
Papilloma	Ductal carcinoma in situ
Air bubble	Papillomatosis/hyperplasia
Clot	Multiple papillomas
Debris	Air bubbles
Duct adenoma	Duct adenoma
Intraductal hyperplasia	
Ductal carcinoma in situ	

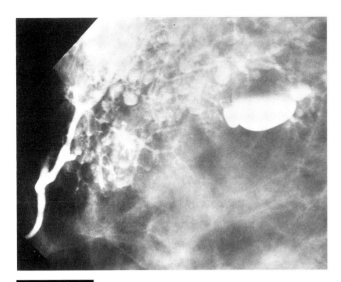

Figure 14.6

HISTORY: Spontaneous serous left nipple discharge.

MAMMOGRAPHY: Left ML view from a galactogram shows marked distention of the collecting and segmental ducts in the subareolar area. There is filling of a small cyst, with a contrast fluid level being noted. No filling defects to suggest intraductal pathology were noted.

IMPRESSION: Cystic duct ectasia.

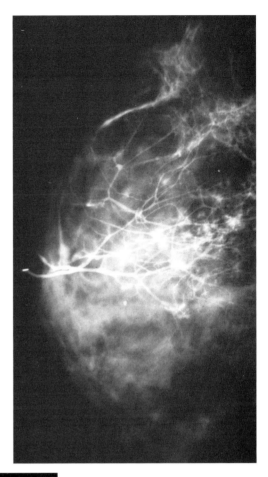

Figure 14.7

HISTORY: Premenopausal patient who presents with uniorificial yellowish clear discharge.

MAMMOGRAPHY: Left CC view from the galactogram shows the cannulated duct system filled with contrast. The duct system is not dilated, and the ducts arborize normally. There is filling of small distal cystic structures consistent with mild fibrocystic change.

IMPRESSION: Mild fibrocystic changes.

The etiology of a solitary defect is most often an intraductal papilloma, and these more commonly occur near the nipple-areolar complex (1). Hou et al. (8) found that 88 of 113 (77.9%) of benign intraductal lesions on galactography were located in main lactiferous ducts. It is important that the most terminal portion of the duct be filled during galactography to avoid bypassing a small papilloma in the nipple or subareolar area with the cannula. The borders of the papilloma are usually rounded or lobulated, and if the lesion is large, it may completely obstruct the duct (Figs. 14.9–14.16). Papillomatosis, which is a form of intraductal hyperplasia, produces multiple small defects and may appear as an irregularity of the luminal wall of the affected duct (16) (Fig. 14.17).

The appearance of intraductal carcinoma on galactography may be a solitary irregular mass, multiple intraluminal filling defects, encasement and abrupt areas of narrowing and dilatation of the duct, distortion of the arborization, and obstruction of the duct lumen (7) or multiple filling defects (Figs. 14.17–14.20). Multiple filling defects are suspicious for ductal carcinoma in situ, papillomatosis, or multiple papillomas. Encasement of the ducts, areas of abrupt termination, or multiple small filling defects are findings suspicious for intraductal

malignancy. If these findings are present, it is important that multiple biopsies or needle localization with bracketing wires be performed to identify the extent of the disease. Rongione et al. (15) found that galactographic findings associated with carcinoma included multiple irregular filling defects, ductal irregularity, ductal obstruction, and contrast extravasation. Hou et al. (8), in a review of 37 patients with cancers identified on galactography, found that 70.3% of these lesions were located in the smaller peripheral ducts.

Ciatto et al. (16) found that galactographic findings associated with malignancy in 200 patients with bloody

(text continues on page 576)

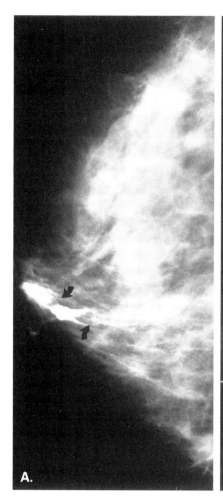
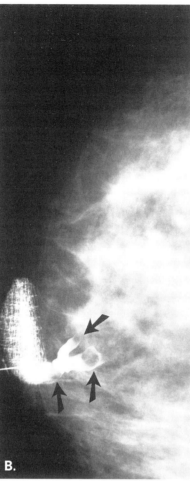

Figure 14.8

HISTORY: A 72-year-old gravida 3, para 3 woman with a bloody left nipple discharge.

MAMMOGRAPHY: Left galactogram ML **(A)** and magnification (2X) **(B)** views. The left breast is very dense for the patient's age. No abnormalities were noted on routine mammography. Galactography was performed because of the nipple discharge, but only a small amount of contrast could be injected without retrograde flow. On galactography, there are at least three intraductal filling defects **(arrows)**. There is incomplete filling of the duct system drained by this major duct. The filling defects are rather smooth, and there is no encasement present, suggesting more likely a benign etiology. However, the termination of the duct lumen is of some concern. The differential diagnosis includes papillomas, papillomatosis, duct hyperplasia, and intraductal carcinoma.

IMPRESSION: Intraluminal filling defects of uncertain nature, favoring a benign process.

HISTOPATHOLOGY: Atypical ductal hyperplasia.

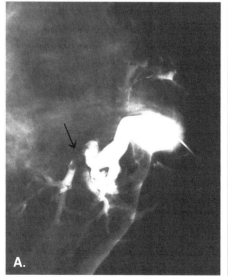
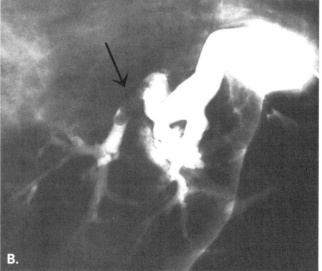

Figure 14.9

HISTORY: A 52-year-old woman with unilateral brownish nipple discharge.

MAMMOGRAPHY: Right CC **(A)** and enlarged CC **(B)** images from a galactogram show a dilated duct with minimal ramifications. There is a solitary intraluminal filling defect present **(arrows)** that, based on the imaging, most likely represents a papilloma.

IMPRESSION: Intraductal papilloma.

HISTOPATHOLOGY: Sclerotic ductal papilloma.

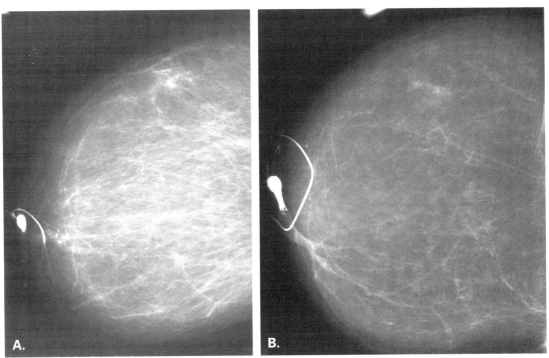

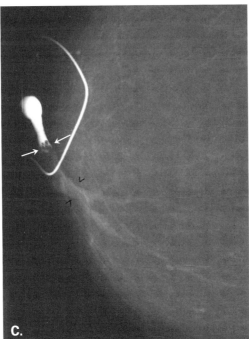

Figure 14.10

HISTORY: A 48-year-old woman with left spontaneous serous nipple discharge.

MAMMOGRAPHY: Left ML **(A)** and CC **(B)** views from a galactogram demonstrate an obstructed duct in the subareolar area. The enlarged image **(C)** shows an irregular intraluminal filling defect **(arrow)**. Posterior to this obstruction is a bifurcating distended duct **(arrowheads)**. Needle localization and excision were performed.

IMPRESSION: Filling defect, likely papilloma.

HISTOPATHOLOGY: Intraductal papilloma.

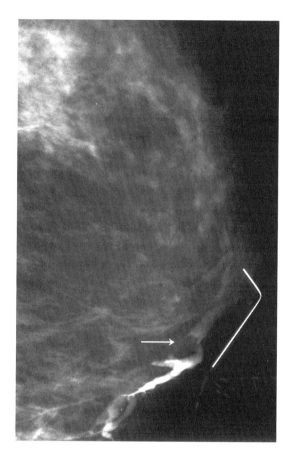

Figure 14.11

HISTORY: A 64-year-old woman with uniorificial heme-positive right nipple discharge.

MAMMOGRAPHY: Right ML galactographic view shows a distended duct delineated by contrast. There is a large polypoid filling duct **(arrow)** nearly completely obstructing the duct.

IMPRESSION: Filling defect, likely a papilloma.

HISTOPATHOLOGY: Sclerotic intraductal papilloma.

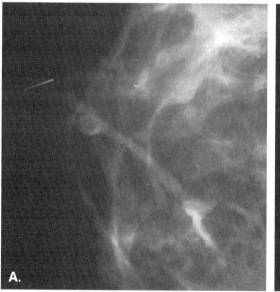 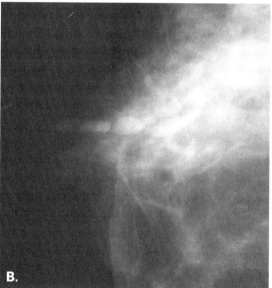

Figure 14.12

HISTORY: A 57-year-old woman with spontaneous serous nipple discharge.

MAMMOGRAPHY: Left ML **(A)** and CC **(B)** views show a solitary duct that has been cannulated. In the immediate subareolar area is a round intraluminal filling defect, and just posterior to this are two other small filling defects.

IMPRESSION: Intraluminal filling defects, likely papillomas.

HISTOPATHOLOGY: Papilloma.

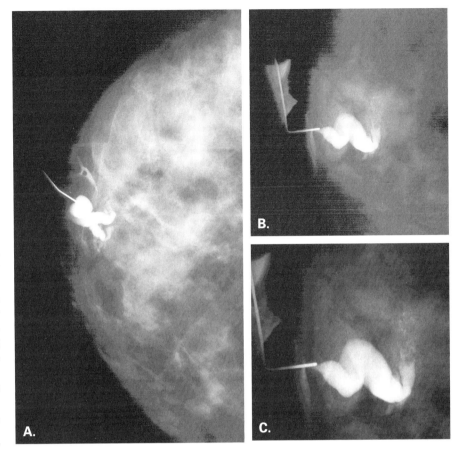

Figure 14.13

HISTORY: A 49-year-old woman reporting bloody left nipple discharge.

MAMMOGRAPHY: Left CC **(A)** and ML **(B)** views from a galactogram show the cannulated duct to be dilated. There is an intraluminal filling defect causing duct obstruction, seen best on the enlarged image **(C)**.

IMPRESSION: Filling defect, possible papilloma.

HISTOPATHOLOGY: Papilloma, partially sclerotic.

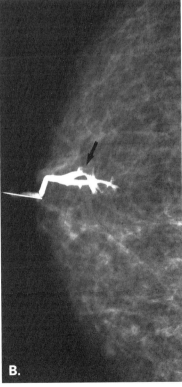

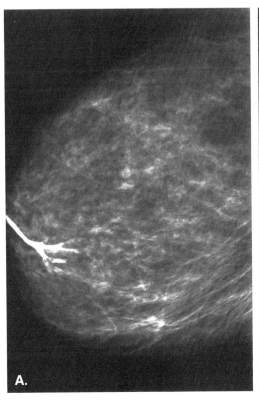

Figure 14.14

HISTORY: A 39-year-old woman with bloody spontaneous left nipple discharge.

MAMMOGRAPHY: Left ML view **(A)** from a galactogram and enlarged CC image **(B)** show the cannulated duct containing contrast. There is nearly complete obstruction of the duct by an intraluminal filling defect **(arrow)**. On the enlarged image, the polypoid filling defect with a multilobulated edge is noted.

IMPRESSION: Solitary defect, likely papilloma. Recommend biopsy.

HISTOPATHOLOGY: Intraductal papilloma with epithelial hyperplasia.

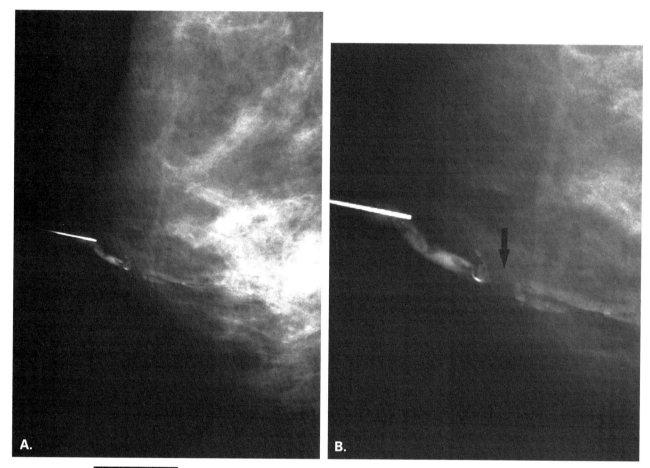

Figure 14.15

HISTORY: A 45-year-old woman with left bloody nipple discharge.

MAMMOGRAPHY: Left ML view **(A)** and enlarged image **(B)** from a galactogram show the cannulated duct containing contrast. There is nearly complete obstruction of the duct in the immediate subareolar area. An irregular filling defect is present within the duct **(arrow)**.

IMPRESSION: Solitary defect, likely papilloma. Recommend biopsy.

HISTOPATHOLOGY: Sclerotic intraductal papilloma.

nipple discharge were multiple filling defects; no solitary intraluminal-filling defect was malignant on excision. Funovics et al. (22) reported the following
sensitivities/specificities in detecting cancer in 134
galactography cases: filling defect (55.6%/62.1%), duct
ectasia (22.2%/94%), and obstructed duct (5.6%/77.6%).
Normal galactograms had a sensitivity of 78% and a
specificity of 93% in predicting the absence of disease
(22). Dinkel et al. (23), however, found no statistically
significant relationship between the galactographic filling defect and the presence of malignancy.

When an intraluminal filling defect is identified,
biopsy or surgical excision is needed to diagnose its etiology. Stereotactic breast biopsy of the filling defect identified on galactography can be performed (24,25) (Figs.

14.21 and 14.22). With the catheter in place and contrast
filling the duct, the lesion can be targeted stereotactically
and biopsied. Guenin (25) found that nipple discharge
ceased after vacuum-assisted biopsy of papillomas in five
patients, suggesting a potential therapeutic value of needle biopsy.

Alternatively, needle localization with excision of the
ductal abnormality duct is performed. The duct may be
visible in retrospect on mammography, and if so, can be
localized for excision based on mammographic findings.
If the location of the lesion is uncertain, repeat galactography at the time of needle localization is performed to
guide the procedure. Tabar et al. (1) described the use of

(text continues on page 582)

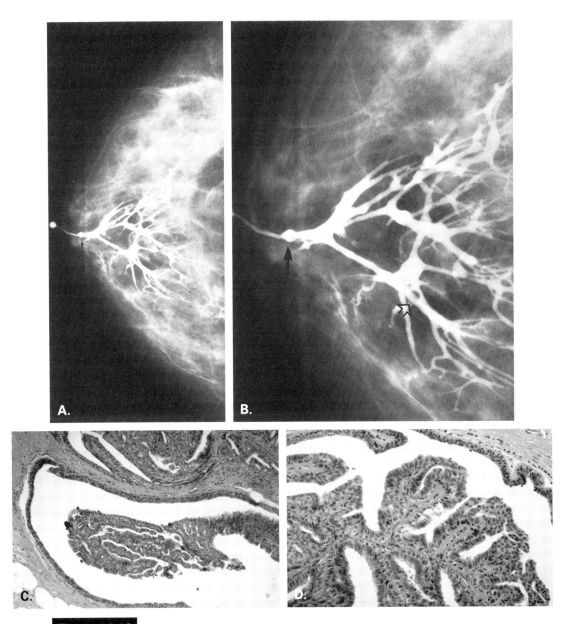

Figure 14.16

HISTORY: A 38-year-old woman with a bloody left nipple discharge.

MAMMOGRAPHY: Left CC view from galactography **(A)** and enlarged (2X) CC view **(B)**. The cannulated duct arborizes into mildly dilated lactiferous ducts. There is a solitary filling defect approximately 1 cm deep to the nipple **(closed arrow)**. This defect expands the duct and is well circumscribed and persistent, consistent with an intraductal lesion. A second well-circumscribed defect is seen more peripherally in the medial aspect of the breast **(open arrow) (B)**, and this was found to represent an air bubble. The differential diagnosis of the subareolar defect includes an intraductal papilloma, hyperplasia, or carcinoma (less likely).

HISTOPATHOLOGY: Intraductal papilloma. The histologic sections at low **(C)** and high **(D)** power shows the papilloma filling the duct lumen. The frondlike epithelium covers the papillary fibrovascular stalks.

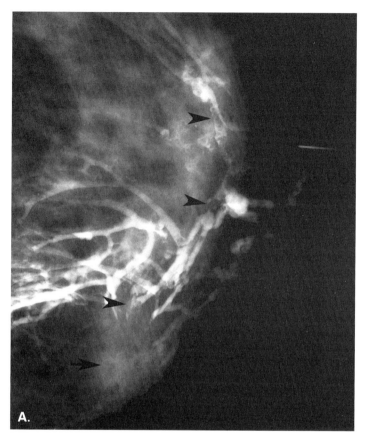

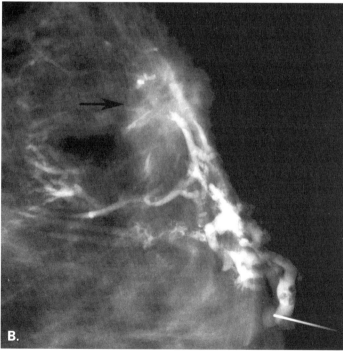

Figure 14.17

HISTORY: A 50-year-old woman with bloody nipple discharge from the right breast.

MAMMOGRAPHY: Right CC **(A)** and ML **(B)** views from a galactogram show contrast filling multiple ducts drained by the cannulated collecting duct. There are multiple small filling defects in the cannulated duct system **(arrowheads)**. There is also a spiculated mass **(arrow)** located medially that is associated with narrowing encasement and abrupt termination of the ducts.

IMPRESSION: Multiple filling defects most consistent with ductal carcinoma in situ and invasive carcinoma.

HISTOPATHOLOGY: Ductal carcinoma in situ, intermediate nuclear grade, solid type. Invasive ductal carcinoma.

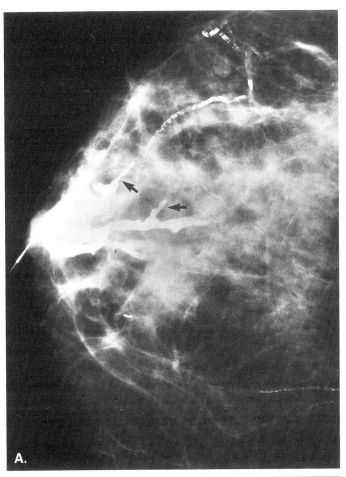

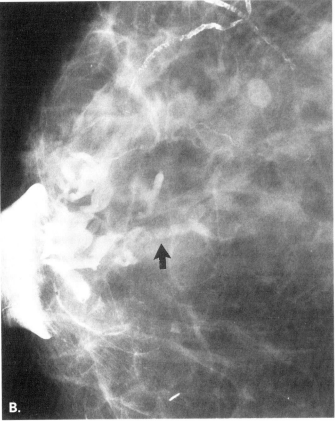

Figure 14.18

HISTORY: A 78-year-old gravida 4, para 4 woman with a bloody discharge from the left nipple.

MAMMOGRAPHY: Left CC **(A)** and magnification (2X) CC **(B)** views from a galactogram. The cannulated duct and its branches are dilated in the subareolar area. There are multiple areas of encasement **(arrows)** with narrowing and changes in caliber **(A)**, as well as irregular filling defects **(arrow) (B)** and areas of abrupt termination of the lactiferous ducts. These findings are highly suggestive of intraductal carcinoma.

IMPRESSION: Extensive intraductal carcinoma.

HISTOPATHOLOGY: Intraductal carcinoma, solid and cribriform varieties.

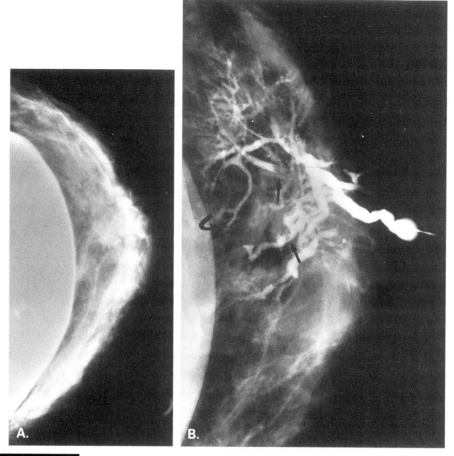

Figure 14.19

HISTORY: A 39-year-old gravida 3, para 4 woman with a bloody right nipple discharge.

MAMMOGRAPHY: Right CC **(A)** and magnification (1.5×) CC **(B)** views from a galactogram. On the initial film **(A)**, a breast implant is noted, and the breast tissue is heterogeneously dense. On the galactogram **(B)**, the injected ducts are mildly dilated. There are multiple irregular filling defects **(straight arrows)** and some areas of abrupt termination **(curved arrow)** of the ductal lumen. The filling defects could represent papillomatosis, hyperplasia, or carcinomas, but the finding of the abrupt terminations is more suspicious for intraductal carcinoma.

IMPRESSION: Multiple filling defects suspicious for intraductal carcinoma.

HISTOPATHOLOGY: Intraductal carcinoma.

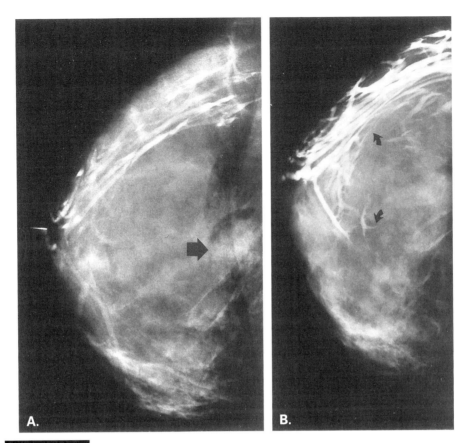

Figure 14.20

HISTORY: A 33-year-old woman with a 2-cm palpable mass at the 6 o'clock position in the left breast and bloody left nipple discharge.

MAMMOGRAPHY: Left CC views with early filling **(A)** and with late filling **(B)** during galactography. On the initial film **(A)**, the breast is very dense, consistent with the patient's age. There is multinodular mass **(arrow)** deep in the breast, corresponding to the palpable lesion and suspicious for carcinoma. It is important to evaluate the patient via galactography, because the lesion lies very deep in the breast, and the nipple discharge suggests the possibility of intraductal extension. On the galactogram **(B)**, there is a straightening of the ducts, with multiple areas of narrowing and abrupt termination **(arrows)** suspicious for intraductal extension of tumor.

IMPRESSION: Probable carcinoma with extensive intraductal extension.

HISTOPATHOLOGY: Infiltrating ductal carcinoma, extensive intraductal carcinoma, and comedocarcinoma.

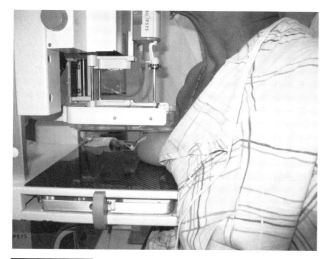

Figure 14.21

Patient in position for stereotactic biopsy of a galactographic finding. The galactography cannula is in place, taped to the nipple. The lesion has been targeted stereotactically on an upright unit. The vacuum-assisted probe has been inserted into the breast for lesion sampling.

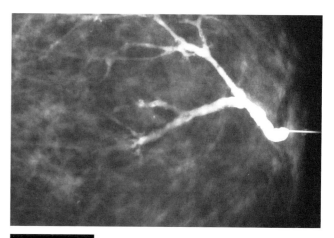

Figure 14.22

HISTORY: A 36-year-old woman with bloody nipple discharge.

MAMMOGRAPHY: Enlarged right CC view from a galactogram shows the filled duct to be irregular in contour. There are numerous small irregular filling defects causing a cobblestone appearance of the duct wall. Areas of narrowing and obstruction are noted medially as well. These filling defects were biopsied stereotactically using vacuum assistance.

IMPRESSION: Highly suspicious for malignancy.

HISTOPATHOLOGY: Ductal carcinoma in situ.

retrograde injection of methylene blue into the duct to guide surgical excision. With imaging guidance to identify and localize the lesion(s) preoperatively, surgical excision of the abnormalities is optimized.

In summary, galactography is performed to evaluate the patient with a suspicious type of nipple discharge. Galactography is not used to differentiate with certainty benign papillomas or papillomatosis from intraductal malignancy. Instead, galactography is important in identifying an intraluminal defect and its exact location for biopsy or surgical removal.

REFERENCES

1. Tabar L, Dean PB, Pentek Z. Galactography: the diagnostic procedure of choice for nipple discharge. *Radiology* 1983;149: 31–38.
2. Shaw de Paredes E, Hijaz TA, Trivedi AM. Assessment of the abnormal lactiferous duct. *Semin Breast Dis* 2004;7:21–48.
3. Leis HP. Management of nipple discharge. *World J Surg* 1989;13: 736–742.
4. Jardines L. Management of nipple discharge. *Am Surg* 1996;62: 119–122.
5. Ciatto S, Bravetti P, Cariaggi P. Significance of nipple discharge clinical patterns in the selection of cases for cytologic examination. *Acta Cytol* 1986;30(1):17–20.
6. Sakorafas GH. Nipple discharge: current diagnostic and therapeutic approaches. *Cancer Treat Rev* 2001;27:275–282.
7. Slawson SH, Johnson BA. Ductography: how to and what if? *RadioGraphics* 2001;21:133–150.
8. Hou MF, Huang TJ, Liu GC. The diagnostic value of galactography in patients with nipple discharge. *Clin Imaging* 2001;25(2):75–81.
9. Lafreniere R. Bloody nipple discharge during pregnancy: a rationale for conservative treatment. *J Surg Oncol* 1990;43:228–230.
10. Sardanelli F, Imperiale A, Zandrino F, et al. Breast intraductal masses: US-guided fine-needle aspiration after galactography. *Radiology* 1997;204:143–148.
11. Dinkel HP, Gassel AM, Muller T, et al. Galactography and exfoliative ectology in women with abnormal nipple discharge. *Obstet Gynecol* 2001;97(4):625–629.
12. Ries E. Diagnostic lipoidal injection into milk ducts followed by abscess formation. *Am J Obstet Gynecol* 1930;20: 414–416.
13. Hickman NF. Mammography: the roentgenographic diagnosis of breast tumors by means of contrast media. *Surg Gynecol Obstet* 1937;64:593–603.
14. Logan-Young W, Hoffman NY. *Breast Cancer: A Practical Guide to Diagnosis.* Rochester, NY: Mt Hope, 1994;193–209.
15. Rongione AJ, Evans BD, Kling KM, et al. Ductography is a useful technique in evaluation of abnormal nipple discharge. *Am Surg* 1996;62:785–787.
16. Ciatto S, Bravetti P, Berni D, et al. The role of galactography in the detection of breast cancer. *Tumori* 1988;74:177–181.
17. Van Zee KJ, Perez GO, Minnard E, et al. Preoperative galactography increases the diagnostic yield of major duct excision for nipple discharge. *Cancer* 1998;82(10): 1874–1880.
18. Cardenosa G, Doudna C, Eklund GW. Ductography of the breast: technique and findings. *AJR Am J Roentgenol* 1994; 621:1061–1087.
19. King TA, Carter KM, Bolton JS, et al. A simple approach to nipple discharge. *Am Surg* 2000;66:960–966.
20. Dawes LG, Bowen C, Venta LA, et al. Ductography for nipple discharge: no replacement for ductal excision. *Surgery* 1998;124:685–691.
21. Diner WC. Galactography: mammary duct contrast examination. *AJR Am J Roentgenol* 1981;137:853–856.

22. Funovics MA, Philipp MO, Lackner B, et al. Galactography: method of choice in pathologic nipple discharge? *Eur Radiol* 2003;13(1):94–99.
23. Dinkel H-P, Trusen A, Gassel AM, et al. Predictive value of galactographic patterns for benign and malignant neoplasms of the breast in patients with nipple discharge. *Br J Radiol* 2000;73:706–714.
24. Hijaz TA, Shaw de Paredes E, Sydnor MK, et al. Combined galactography and stereotactic core needle breast biopsy for diagnosis of intraductal lesions. *Contemp Diagn Radiol* 2004;27(18):1–8.
25. Guenin MA. Benign intraductal papilloma: diagnosis and removal at stereotactic vacuum-assisted directional biopsy guided by galactography. *Radiology* 2001;218:576–579.

Needle Localization

The preoperative localization of a nonpalpable breast abnormality is necessary for the accurate identification of the lesion and its removal. The procedure involves an integration of breast imaging, surgery, and pathology, with close interaction by all members of this team to assure optimization of the procedure. Careful communication of the information regarding the case is needed among the radiologist, surgeon, and pathologist to confirm that the correct area is removed and that the lesion is identified within the specimen.

The preoperative localization of a nonpalpable mammographic abnormality offers multiple advantages. Using preoperative localization, a smaller amount of tissue can be excised than without radiographic guidance. This is important not only from the patient's standpoint, because of a lesser degree of postoperative deformity, but also from the pathologist's standpoint, because the ease and accuracy of identifying a tiny focus of carcinoma in situ are improved when the amount of tissue to be sectioned is less.

PRIOR TO THE PROCEDURE

Prior to the procedure, the radiologist must carefully review the mammogram, other imaging studies, and pathology records if the lesion already has been biopsied. As percutaneous breast biopsy has evolved, the vast majority of suspicious lesion on mammography are biopsied by core biopsy methods instead of surgical excision. Prior to this era, clinically occult, mammographically detected lesions were excised following needle localization. Now, few lesions are excised for diagnosis. Instead, the vast majority of needle-localized lesions are cancers, high-risk lesions, or lesions that were insufficiently sampled or unable to be sampled percutaneously.

Prior to the procedure, it also is important that the complete imaging evaluation be performed of the patient who has not already undergone a percutaneous biopsy. A complete diagnostic mammogram is needed to confirm that the lesion is actually suspicious and warrants biopsy. For example, magnification views and a mediolateral

(ML) view are necessary in the case of microcalcifications, to evaluate them and to confirm that they do not represent milk of calcium. The ML view also is necessary to plan the approach to the lesion, because it is the orthogonal view to the craniocaudal (CC) view.

If the lesion has been already biopsied, the post-biopsy mammogram should be reviewed for several reasons. First, one must determine if the mammographic finding is still present. Second, if a clip was placed following biopsy, one should verify whether the clip is at the biopsy site or if it is deep or shallow to it. If one is planning to target the clip, it is critical to know that the clip is deployed at the biopsy site. Once the image review and plan for the procedure are complete, the procedure is explained to the patient, and informed consent is obtained.

MAMMOGRAPHICALLY GUIDED NEEDLE LOCALIZATION

The techniques for localization are varied, and have included triangulation and needle placement (1), needle localization with dye injection (2,3), and needle localization with wire placement (4–6). A number of wires are available, most of which have a type of hook (4) (Fig. 15.1) or J configuration (5) when released from the needle. The spring hookwire breast lesion localizer designed by Kopans (4,7), combined with a rigid compression plate, allows for accurate and safe localization of breast lesions. The compression plate has a fenestrated window, which maintains the breast in position and allows for insertion of the needle containing the hookwire in a direction parallel to the chest wall. Once deployed, the wire is in position and cannot be repositioned or withdrawn. In the situation in which a hookwire is placed in a position suboptimal for surgical excision, a second wire should be placed rather than trying to reposition the first wire.

A J-wire was designed by Homer (8,9) to allow retraction and repositioning of the wire if needed. The curved-end wire has a memory that allows it to be retracted into the needle and readvanced into the breast tissue in the

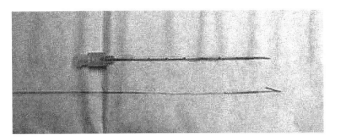

Figure 15.1

A typical needle and hookwire used for needle localization. The
wire has a stiffener near the distal end that aids the surgeon
in identifying it on palpation.

same shape. This type of wire is also thicker and not transected during surgical dissection.

Many mammographic units are equipped with a localization device. Two basic designs are available: a rectangu-
lar aperture or multiple 1-cm round perforations (6) in a
plastic compression plate (Fig. 15.2). The technical performance of needle localization is improved with the use of
digital mammography. Dershaw et al. (10) found that the
time to complete a needle localization was reduced by 50%
when digital mammography was used, and the mean glandular dose was reduced by a similar amount.

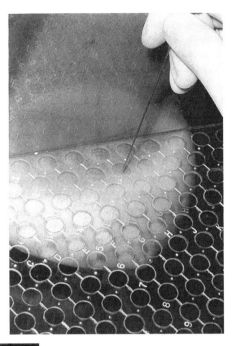

Figure 15.2

A localization plate with 1-cm round perforations is in place
with the breast compressed for needle localization.

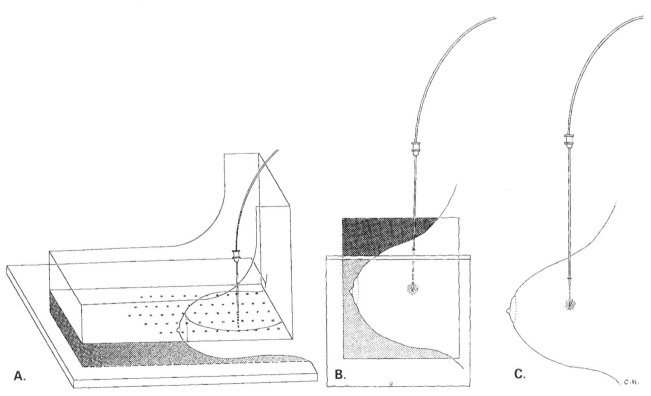

Figure 15.3

Procedure for mammographically guided needle localization. The needle is placed into the breast
through the appropriate aperture **(A)**, the opposite view is made to determine the depth of the
needle, the needle position is adjusted if necessary **(B)**, and the wire is ejected **(C)**.

Prior to the localization, a 90-degree lateral (ML) view is obtained if only CC and mediolateral oblique (MLO) projections are available. From these images, the closest skin surface to the abnormality is determined—superior, medial, lateral, or inferior. The localization plate is placed over the surface determined, and an image is obtained (Fig. 15.3). While the patient remains in position with her breast compressed, the coordinates of the aperture overlying the lesion are determined. A localization needle is placed into the breast, parallel to the chest wall at the indicated location; the depth of placement is estimated only, because the breast is compressed by the localization device. An image is obtained with the needle in place, to determine if the placement is accurate.

The localization plate is then carefully removed, leaving the needle in place, and the orthogonal view is made. If the needle is too deep, it is withdrawn until the tip is within the lesion, and then the wire is deployed. Most wires have a mark that, when positioned at the hub of the needle, indicates that the tip of the wire is at the tip of the needle. The wire is deployed by advancing this mark into the needle hub by about 1 cm. The needle is removed, the wire is taped to the skin, and two final images—CC and ML views—are made to show the position of the hook relative to the lesion (Fig. 15.4). Information regarding the procedure is communicated to the surgeon. This should include the location of the lesion targeted, the approach to the lesion used, the length of wire within the breast, the position of the hook relative to the lesion, and the need for a specimen radiograph.

For a dye localization, the needle is placed in a similar manner but, instead of placing a hookwire through the needle, dye is injected. Because the dye dissipates rather quickly, the scheduling of the localization and the operating room must be coordinated carefully to avoid a prolonged lapse between the two procedures. Because of the

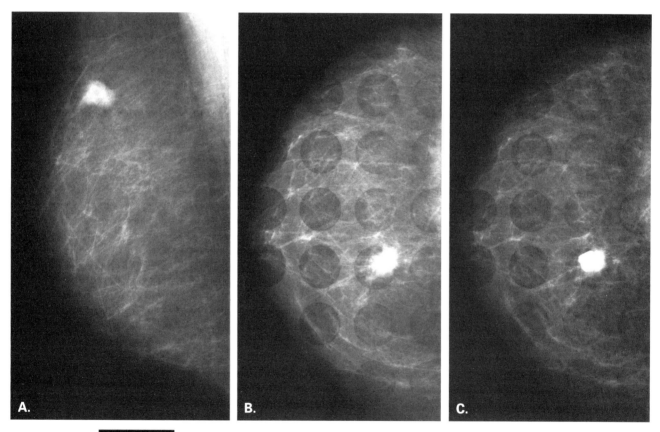

Figure 15.4

Needle localization series performed for a mass in the left breast that was found to be malignant. Left ML (**A**) and CC (**B**) views show the dense, lobular, indistinct mass in the 12 o'clock position. On the CC image, the localization plate is in place over the superior surface of the breast. Because the lesion is closest to the superior aspect of the breast (12 o'clock position), the localizer plate was placed in this position to provide the shortest distance for needle insertion. The needle has been placed into the aperture directly over the lesion on the CC view (**C**). *(continued)*

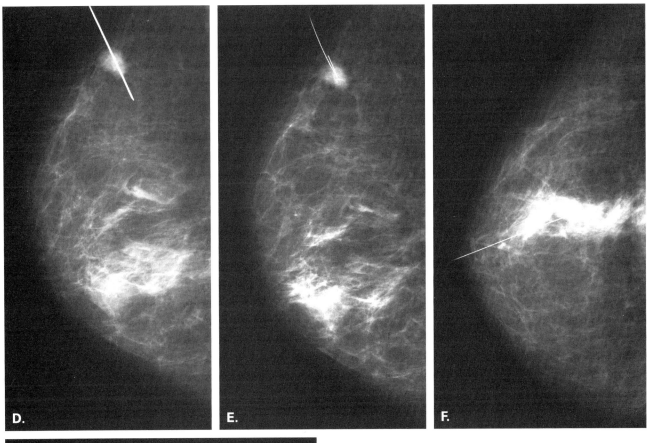

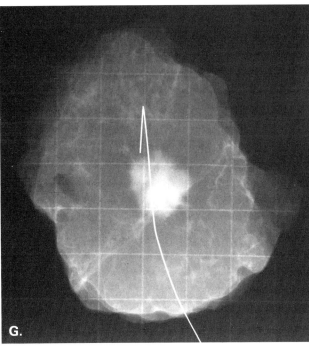

Figure 15.4 *(CONTINUED)*

The localizer plate has been removed, and the ML view **(D)** obtained, showing that the needle is directly through the lesion. Focal asymmetry is present inferior to the mass, which developed during the procedure, representing a small hematoma. The needle was withdrawn slightly and the wire was deployed.

Postprocedure ML **(E)** and CC **(F)** views show that the hookwire position is accurate. The specimen film **(G)** shows that the lesion is contained within the specimen and that a margin of normal tissue appears to be present around it.

dissipation of the dye, a prolonged time lapse leads to the excision of an unnecessarily large specimen. Dye alone is uncommonly used today, but some surgeons prefer a combined localization using both dye and a wire in case the wire is inadvertently displaced.

The types of dye that have been used include methylene blue, isosulfan blue, and toluidine blue. Methylene blue may interfere with estrogen-receptor assays (11). Isosulfan blue has been developed as an alternative to methylene blue (12), because it does not interfere with receptors, and it is commonly used for sentinel node mapping as well. Toluidine blue has also been suggested as an alternative to methylene blue because it diffuses less quickly (13).

STEREOTACTICALLY-GUIDED NEEDLE LOCALIZATION

Stereotaxis affords a rapid and precise way to visualize and localize a lesion for surgical excision. Early experience with stereotactic guidance was negative (14,15), because the hookwires were deployed either too shallowly or too deeply, relative to the lesion. The challenge with stereotaxis is understanding how to handle the wire with the breast compressed along the plane of insertion, as it is in stereotactic procedures. Once this is understood, the procedure is a very accurate and fast way of localizing the lesion.

For stereotactic localization (16), the breast is compressed with the aperture placed over the skin surface at a point that represents the shortest distance to the lesion. If

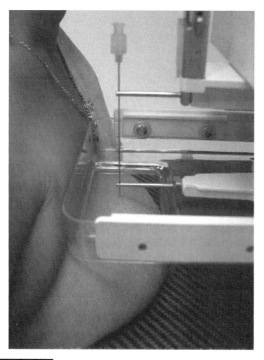

Figure 15.5

Patient in position for needle localization with stereotactic guidance using an upright unit. She is seated because a superior approach to the lesion is being utilized for this case. She would be lying on her side if an inferior, medial, or lateral needle placement were being performed. If the localization were performed on a stereotactic prone table, the patient would be lying prone for any needle placement.

the lesion has already been biopsied percutaneously, the same trajectory used for the biopsy is used for the localization procedure (Fig. 15.5). The technologist positions the patient with the aperture of the compression plate over the area of the lesion. A 0-degree scout image for confirmation may be obtained, followed by a stereotactic pair of images at a fixed angle of obliquity specific to the type of unit (usually 10 or 15 degrees) (Figs. 15.6 and 15.7). The reference point on the stereotactic images is confirmed, and the target point is identified. The length of the localization needle (not the wire) is programmed into the unit, and the coordinates are transferred to the table or are entered. The needle guides are positioned over the lesion on the X and Y axes by dialing the guides to a $\Delta X = 0$ and $\Delta Y = 0$ position. At this position, no difference is present in the position of the target point in the lesion and the needle guide on the X or Y axes. For needle localizations, the ΔZ-position of the needle is ideally placed at 10 mm deep to the lesion. This is a vital step for a successful procedure. Depending on the type of stereotactic unit, this may be a plus or minus ΔZ-position.

After the needle has been placed at $\Delta X = 0$, $\Delta Y = 0$, $\Delta Z = (\pm)$ 10.0, a stereotactic pair of images is obtained. On this set of images, the needle tip should appear to be just through the lesion on both views, because the ΔZ is set past or deep to the lesion. Once the needle position has been confirmed, the wire is deployed. Errors can occur in this second vital step. The wire is inserted until its tip is at the needle tip. On most wires, an indicator mark on the wire is present that, when placed at the level of the needle hub, indicates that the wire tip is at the needle tip. The wire is not inserted further. Instead, the wire is grasped firmly, and the needle is withdrawn over it. Compression is released, the patient is moved from the stereotactic unit, and the final postprocedure CC and mediolateral (ML) views are obtained. Because the breast is compressed along the plane of needle insertion, any advancement of the wire can cause it to be very deep to the lesion, once the compression is released. Similarly, allowing the wire to slip back as the needle is withdrawn causes the hook to deploy very superficially to the lesion.

ULTRASOUND-GUIDED NEEDLE LOCALIZATION

Ultrasound guidance is an excellent method for needle localization (17,18). For lesions visible on sonography, guidance using ultrasound affords a fast and accurate method for localization that is associated with no radiation exposure. Sonography is particularly useful for localization of a mass that is awkward to approach using a fenestrated plate, or for patients who have difficulty sitting up.

Several companies have developed clips embedded in materials (collagen, Gelfoam) that are visible on ultrasound.

If a patient has a percutaneous breast biopsy, and one of these clips is placed, the area may be evident on ultrasound several weeks later. If surgical excision is needed, the clip may be evident on ultrasound and is used as the target point for the localization procedure using sonographic guidance.

When ultrasound guidance is used for needle localization, a vertical needle insertion (Fig. 15.8) is preferred (18). The technique, as described by Fornage (18), allows for the shortest distance to the lesion from the skin. The lesion is visualized in the middle of the scan field, and the needle is inserted at the transducer's midpoint. The degree of obliquity of the needle insertion depends on the depth of the lesion. A more vertical angle is used for deeper lesions. Using this method, the needle tip is not seen until it crosses the scan plane at the depth of the lesion. Care must be taken to not penetrate the chest wall;

therefore, this technique is not for inexperienced interventionalists.

A safer angle of insertion is an oblique (Fig. 15.9) or horizontal placement of the needle. The lesion is visualized at the edge of the scan field, and the needle is placed at the end of the transducer. The needle is visualized in its entirety when it is within the scan plane. This technique is best for lesions located near the chest wall, in patients with very thick breasts, and in patients with implants. This technique also should be used by those with less interventional experience. The disadvantage is that the length of wire within the breast is greater than it is for the vertical procedure and, therefore, the surgery may be more difficult. With either a vertical or horizontal approach, however, ultrasound guidance is a fast and accurate method of needle localization that has a high level of patient comfort and acceptance (Fig. 15.10).

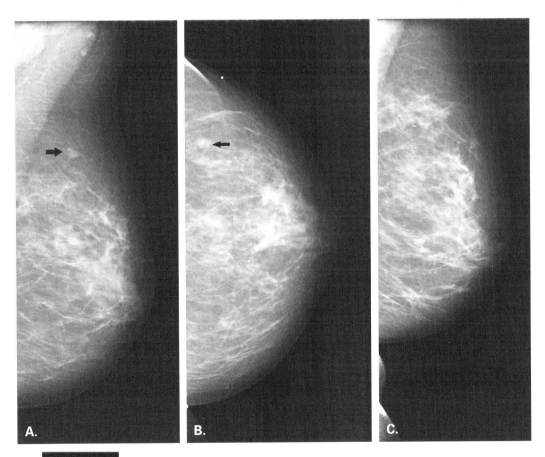

Figure 15.6

HISTORY: 31-year-old with a palpable thickening in the right upper outer quadrant.

MAMMOGRAPHY: Right MLO **(A)** and CC **(B)** views show a small indistinct mass located at 11 o'clock **(arrow)**. This was biopsied using ultrasound guidance, and a clip was placed. Pathology showed invasive ductal carcinoma.

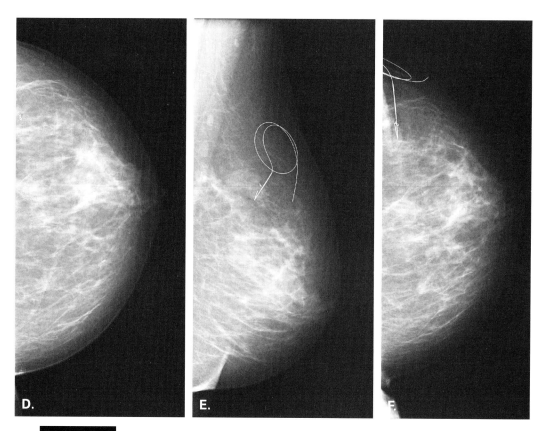

Figure 15.6 *(CONTINUED)*

Post biopsy images **(C)** and **(D)** show the clip at the site of the abnormality, which is no longer evident after core biopsy. Stereotactic needle localization was performed, and post–wire placement ML **(E)** and CC **(F)** views show accurate hookwire placement at the site.

IMPRESSION: Successful localization of invasive ductal carcinoma. Surgical pathology from the lumpectomy showed residual invasive ductal carcinoma.

PROBLEMATIC LOCALIZATIONS

Problems in localizing lesions are sometimes caused by lack of clear visibility of the lesion while the localization device is in place, a very posterior lesion that is difficult to keep in position for the localization procedure, and lesions that are evident on only one mammographic view. Prior to the procedure, it is important to completely work up the lesion with imaging to establish a clear understanding of where the lesion is expected to be, so that the localization plate is positioned correctly. The mediolateral view is used for a variety of reasons including determining the position of a lesion seen only on the MLO view. Rolled CC views help to identify whether a lesion seen only on the CC view is in the upper or lower half of the breast.

At times, the localization plate can obscure faint abnormalities. The comparison with the preprocedure films is important to focus on the area in which the lesion is expected to be located. Repositioning the breast slightly is sometimes helpful to move the lesion under an aperture and to visualize it.

For a very posterior lesion, the patient must be encouraged to stay in position, leaning forward, to avoid the breast slipping back during the procedure. Marking the skin near the aperture of the compression plate is also important to observe if any patient motion has occurred.

For lesions seen on only one view, a parallax approach, with the placement of several needles using mammographic guidance, has been described (19). A far simpler method is the use of stereotactic guidance (16). Using stereotaxis, the patient is positioned with the aperture over the breast on the view on which the lesion is seen. Stereotactic images are obtained to determine the depth for needle placement.

LOCALIZATION OF KNOWN CANCERS

The localization of lesions that represent known cancers must take into consideration the goal of the procedure. In this situation, the goal is to remove the entire tumor with a clear margin. This objective differs from the case in which localization of an indeterminate lesion is being performed for biopsy, when margins are much less important and removing the lesion with the least amount of normal tissue is performed. In the cancer patient, the role of the radiologist is to map out the extent of the mammographic lesion for the surgeon, to optimize exci-sion of all the tumor, thus reducing the likelihood of the need for re-excision.

Depending on the type of lesion, one or more wires may be used. For the solitary mass, the placement of a single hookwire through the lesion is ideal. However, for a mass with associated surrounding calcifications or for a

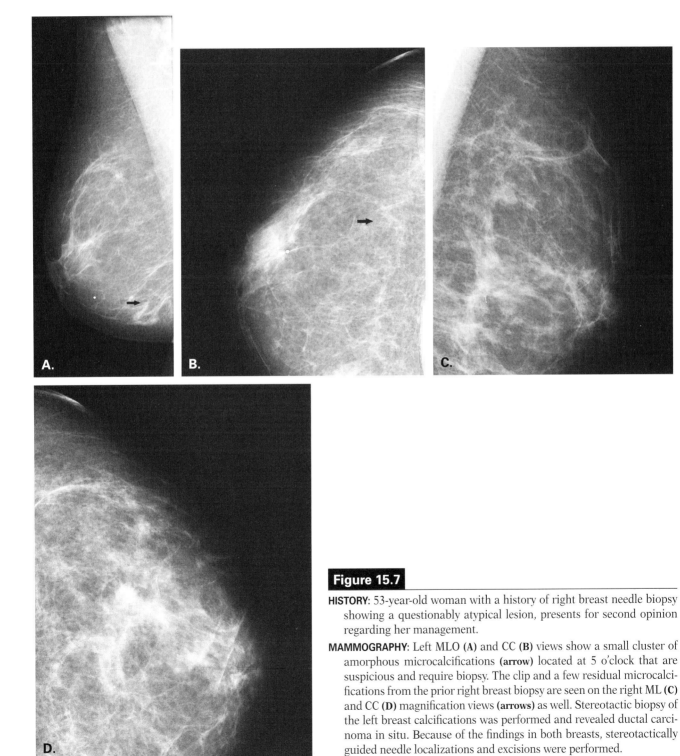

Figure 15.7

HISTORY: 53-year-old woman with a history of right breast needle biopsy showing a questionably atypical lesion, presents for second opinion regarding her management.

MAMMOGRAPHY: Left MLO **(A)** and CC **(B)** views show a small cluster of amorphous microcalcifications **(arrow)** located at 5 o'clock that are suspicious and require biopsy. The clip and a few residual microcalcifications from the prior right breast biopsy are seen on the right ML **(C)** and CC **(D)** magnification views **(arrows)** as well. Stereotactic biopsy of the left breast calcifications was performed and revealed ductal carcinoma in situ. Because of the findings in both breasts, stereotactically guided needle localizations and excisions were performed.

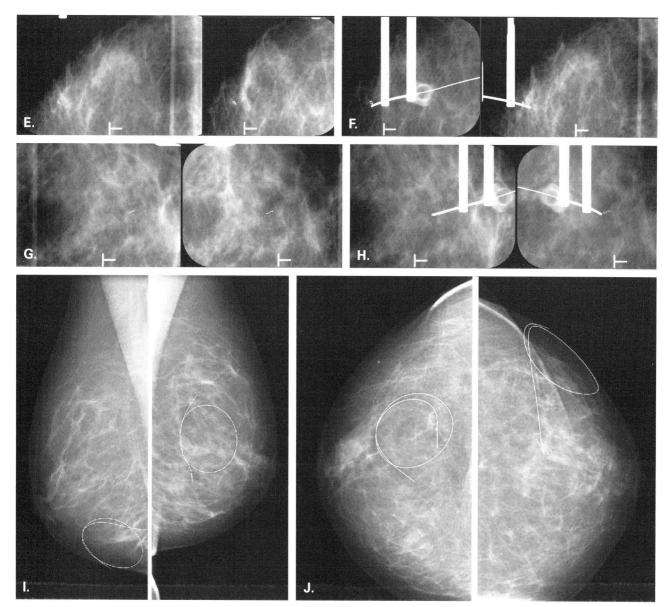

Figure 15.7 *(CONTINUED)*

Left stereotactic pair **(E)** shows the clip marking the biopsy site. The T at the bottom of the field is the reference point used for calculation of the Z position of the lesion. The clip was targeted, and the needle is in accurate position on the subsequent stereotactic pair **(F).**

Right stereotactic pair **(G)** shows the clip to be targeted. Post–needle placement stereotactic pair shows the needle in correct position **(H).**

Final wire placement ML **(I)** and CC **(J)** images show accurate hookwire position in the lesions.

IMPRESSION: Successful localization of left DCIS and right atypia. Histopathology from the excisions showed ductal carcinoma in situ bilaterally.

segment or region of calcifications that are ductal carcinoma in situ (DCIS), one wire is not the best choice. Instead, the placement of several wires to bracket the margins of the region of mammographic abnormality will guide the surgeon better in understanding the orientation and scope of the lesion (Fig. 15.11). Marking the anterior and posterior borders and/or the medial and lateral or superior and inferior margins can be performed. The choice of which borders to bracket depends on the orientation of the lesion. For example, if the lesion is a large linear area of calcifications extending from the subareolar area posteriorly, two wires marking the anterior and posterior margins are sufficient. However, for a lesion that extends transversely as well, medial and lateral wires may

(text continues on page 596)

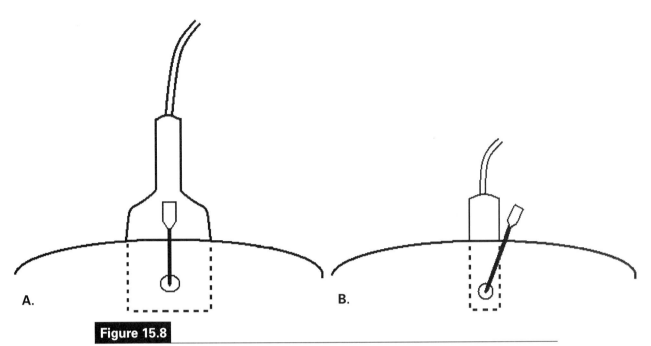

Figure 15.8

Vertical needle localization with ultrasound guidance. The needle is placed vertically into the breast in the center of the long axis of the transducer **(A).** When viewed from the opposite direction, at the short end of the transducer, the needle tip is seen at the lesion as it bisects the scan plane **(B).** The angle of the needle insertion depends on the depth of the lesion.

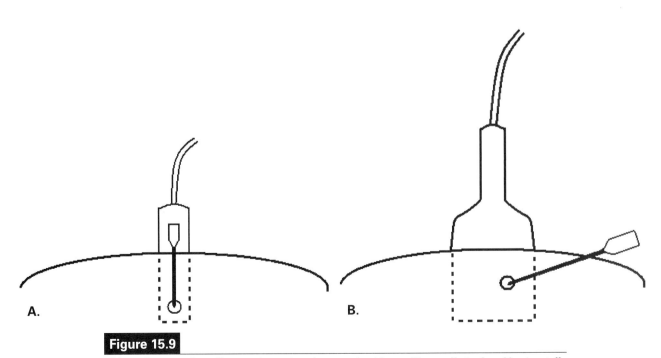

Figure 15.9

Oblique/horizontal needle insertion using ultrasound guidance. The needle is placed horizontally into the breast along the short end of the transducer and is visualized in its entirety as it is inserted **(A)** toward the lesion. When viewed enface **(B),** it is seen to be parallel to the scan plane. This technique is required for core biopsies, but it is optional for cyst aspiration or for needle localization.

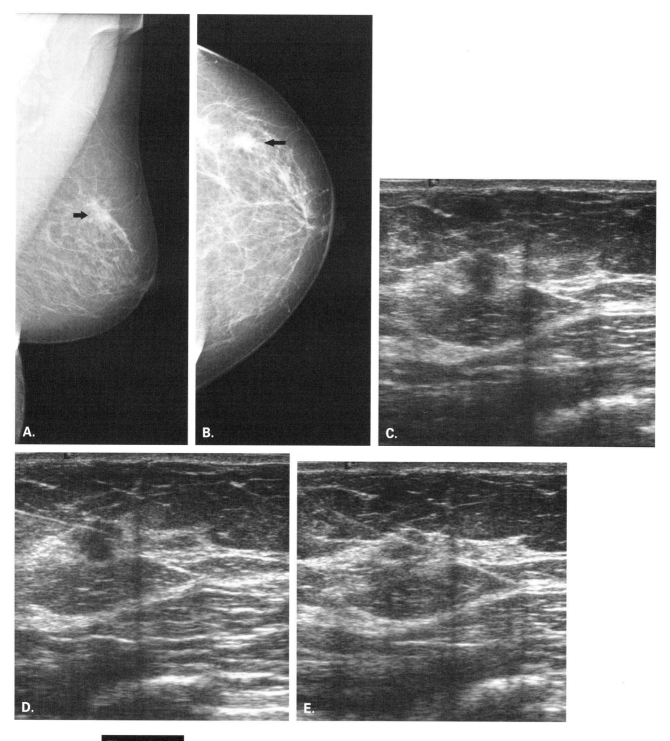

Figure 15.10

Right MLO **(A)** and CC **(B)** views show a small, dense, indistinct mass located laterally **(arrow)**. This was biopsied using ultrasound guidance and found to be an infiltrating ductal carcinoma. Subsequently, the area was needle localized using ultrasound guidance prior to lumpectomy. Preprocedure sonography **(C)** shows the microlobulated mass. Using an oblique insertion, the needle has been placed through the lesion in **D,** and it is visualized along the path leading to the lesion. The needle tip is just through the lesion. In **E,** the needle has been removed, and the wire has been deployed in the mass. *(continued)*

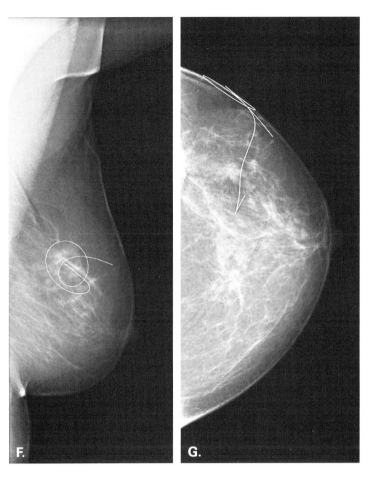

Figure 15.10 *(CONTINUED)*

Postprocedure ML **(F)** and CC **(G)** views show the hook-wire in position with the hook just through the mass.

IMPRESSION: Successful needle localization of right breast cancer using ultrasound guidance.

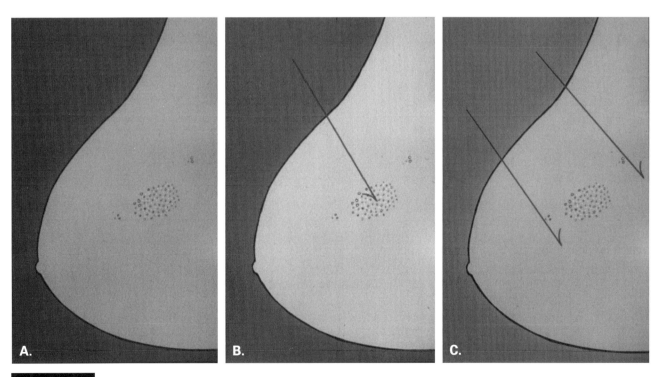

Figure 15.11

Schematic showing the procedure for localization of a region of microcalcifications. **A:** If one wire is placed in the center of the region **(B)**, the majority of calcifications may be excised, but the others that represent extension of carcinoma in the periphery may be missed. By placing two wires to bracket the anterior and posterior margins **(C)** the entire lesion is more accurately excised.

be used instead of or in addition to the anterior/posterior markers (Fig. 15.12).

MAGNETIC RESONANCE IMAGING-GUIDED LOCALIZATION

As magnetic resonance imaging (MRI) has evolved and is utilized for the evaluation of the extent of disease, so has the need for MRI-guided interventions. If the lesion identified on MRI is visible in retrospect on mammography or ultrasound, biopsy or needle localization is performed using the simpler methods. However, if the lesion is visible only on MRI, the biopsy or needle localization using MRI guidance is necessary.

MRI breast coils and biopsy devices that compress the breast and help to localize the lesion are used. A high-resolution study is performed and, if the lesion is visible

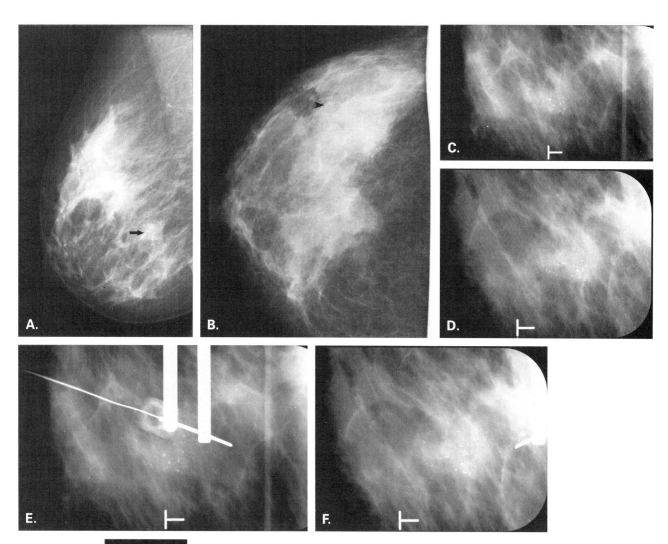

Figure 15.12

HISTORY: A 38-year-old referred for an abnormal baseline mammography.

MAMMOGRAPHY: Left MLO **(A)** and CC magnification **(B)** views show heterogeneously dense tissue. Segmentally oriented pleomorphic microcalcifications are located at 4 o'clock **(arrows)**. These were biopsied stereotactically, showing ductal carcinoma in situ (DCIS), high nuclear grade. A second small focus of amorphous microcalcifications **(arrowhead)** laterally was also biopsied and was benign. A clip was deployed at this second site.

A bracketing procedure using stereotactic guidance was performed for the needle localization of the region of DCIS prior to lumpectomy. Preliminary stereotactic images **(C, D)** show the region of calcifications in the field of view. Needles were placed to mark the superior and inferior margins of the abnormality, and needle placement is shown on the stereotactic pairs **(E, F and G, H)**. *(continued)*

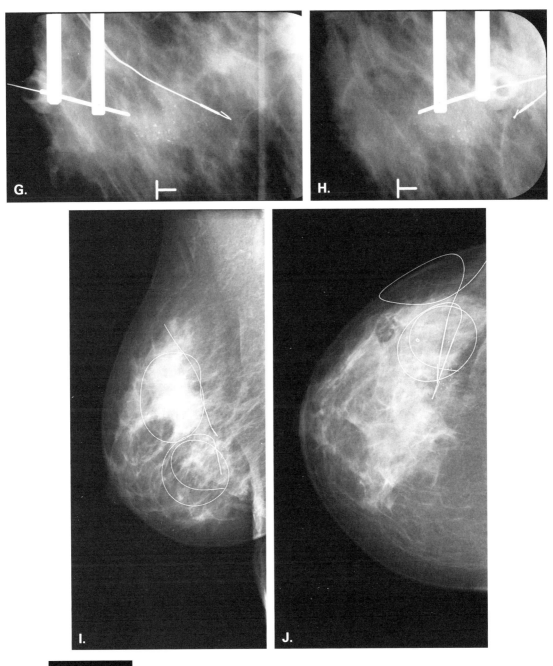

Figure 15.12 *(CONTINUED)*

Final wire placement ML **(I)** and CC **(J)** images show the hookwires marking the superior and inferior margins of the mammographic finding.

IMPRESSION: Successful bracketing of area of DCIS using stereotactic guidance. Clear margins were obtained at surgery.

without contrast, the needle may be placed through the localizer grid at the proper coordinates. An MRI-visible marker, such as vitamin E, is used as a fiducial and placed on the skin to help to orient the location of the lesion. Contrast is injected to confirm the needle position at the lesion, and the wire is deployed. MRI-compatible needles and hookwires are available for the procedure (20–22).

COMPLICATIONS AND RISKS

The potential complications of needle localization include bleeding and hematoma formation, infection, wire migration, vasovagal reaction, pneumothorax, and allergic reaction to dye that may be used. The most common problem by far is vasovagal reactions, which may occur in up to 7% of patients (23). Because of this, the team should be prepared by having a stretcher available and by having ammonia capsules and ice on hand. The interventional team should be experienced and able to keep the patient comfortable during the procedure, to distract her from the procedure with conversation, to perform the procedure as quickly and efficiently as possible, and to be ready to manage a vasovagal reaction if it occurs.

Prolonged bleeding is an uncommon problem during needle localization. Helvie et al. (24), in a review of 370 procedures, reported a 1% rate of bleeding for more than 5 minutes. Hematomas are infrequent and, if significant, are usually related to a vascular puncture (25). If care is used in needle placement, the risks of the procedure are minimal. Although a pneumothorax could occur, attention to placement of a localization wire parallel to the chest wall should avoid this problem. To avoid migration or a lost wire, it is important that a wire to be used of sufficient length to allow at least 10 cm to protrude from the breast at the end of the procedure (26).

The wire may be transected during the procedure, and the surgeon may lose perspective as to the location of the lesion and the hook, accounting for unsuccessful excision of the lesion. Some surgeons make an incision somewhere near the wire entry point in the direction of the lesion, intentionally clip the wire at the skin and excise the tissue en bloc, pulling the remainder of wire in. Others, who follow the wire down to the lesion, prefer a stiffener on the wire near the hook to help to locate it by palpation in case the distal wire is inadvertently transected.

In patients treated for breast cancer diagnosed by a needle-localization biopsy procedure, no documented increase has been noted in local recurrence rate to suggest seeding of tumor cells along the wire tract (27). In patients with implants, a potential exists for rupture during localization. Care must be taken during the localization of a lesion in a breast augmented with a prosthesis to avoid puncturing the prosthesis, particularly if it contains silicone. Robertson et al. (28) described wire localization in eight patients with implants, with placement of the needle using the implant displacement technique (29). Another option in these patients is to place the localization grid over the breast and mark the lesion with skin markers only, giving instructions as to the depth of the lesion from the skin surfaces.

Failure to surgically excise a localized lesion has been reported to occur in 0% to 17.9% of cases (30–33). Jackman et al. (34) reported a biopsy failure rate of 2.5% in 280 lesions. Unsuccessful localizations (34) were associated with smaller lesions, small specimens, more than one lesion in the breast, and microcalcifications. Removal of a second specimen converted the failed procedure to a successful one in 67% of cases (34). Causes

of lesion missed at surgery are a poorly positioned wire, transection of the wire at surgery, wire migration in a fatty breast, movement of the wire in preparing the patient for surgery or in performing the surgery, and poor communication between the radiologist and the surgeon about the position of the hook relative to the lesion. The miss rates reported with dye localization have been 2.2% (34) and 1.3% (32). A successful localization has been described as having the wire tip within 5 mm of the lesion (35).

SPECIMEN RADIOGRAPHY

Specimen radiography is an integral part of the needle localization and excisional biopsy procedure and should be performed in all cases (36–39). The specimen is radiographed for several reasons including: (a) to verify that the lesion is included, (b) to verify that the hookwire has been removed, and (c) to describe the relationship of the lesion to the margins of the specimen radiographically.

The technique for specimen radiography of a mammographically visible lesion involves an analog or digital radiograph. A mammographic unit or a dedicated specimen radiographic unit may be utilized. Magnification and compression (40) are used with low kVp techniques (22–23 kVp) and low mAs (39). Specimen containers are available that are ideal for transportation of the tissue; these contain a fenestrated compression plate that compresses the tissue (Fig. 15.13). Care must be taken to not overcompress the tissue, which could potentially lead to distortion of the margins (41). In addition, the fenestrated grid allows the radiologist to identify the location of the abnormality within the tissue for the pathologist (Fig. 15.14). Additional levels or cuts through the area of greatest interest may be performed. At times, radiography of the sliced specimen block is performed to localize the microcalcifications for pathologic analysis. When calcifications on the localized lesion are not evident to the pathologist on the initial slides, polarized light should be used to look for calcium oxalate crystals, which are not evident on routine hematoxylin and eosin staining. If calcium oxalate is not seen, the tissue block is radiographed and recut, with new slides made to search for the lesion (39).

For noncalcified lesions, Stomper et al. (37) found that film screen specimen radiography was a highly effective procedure for correctly identifying the presence of the mammographic abnormality. In a study of 104 specimen radiographs after excision of a clinically occult noncalcified lesion, the authors found that 93% of the lesions were visible on the specimen films. On comparison with the original mammograms, the specimen films showed better anatomic detail of the lesion in 35% of cases (37).

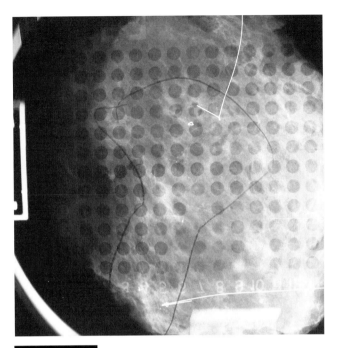

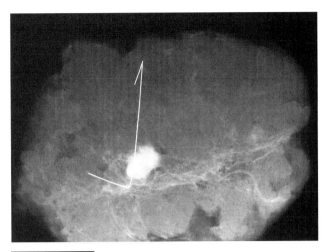

Figure 15.14

Specimen radiography shows a small cancer contained within the specimen. It does not appear to extend to the margins. The hookwire is included.

Figure 15.13

The patient had undergone core biopsy of a region of microcalcifications showing DCIS at two foci. Clips were placed after the biopsy. Needle localization using two hookwires was performed prior to lumpectomy. The specimen has been placed in a container with a fenestrated plate over it, compressing the tissue. The tissue is radiographed in this manner so that the region of interest can be indicated to the pathologist. The extent of the calcifications indicating the area of DCIS have been marked for the pathologist to focus on in sectioning and analyzing the tissue. The tissue is sent to the lab in the container and with the radiograph as marked.

Two orthogonal views of the specimen may be performed routinely and are particularly helpful in specific circumstances. When the lesion is not clearly seen on one view, the orthogonal view may demonstrate the abnormality. For cancers, in which the relationship of the abnormality to the surgical margins should be described to the surgeon while the patient is still in the operating room, the analysis of two views of the specimen is more complete (Fig. 15.15).

The specimen radiograph is certainly not sufficient to determine the presence or absence of tumor at the surgical margin, but it is helpful to the surgeon in deciding whether to excise more tissue at the initial lumpectomy. The false-negative rate of specimen radiography for tumor was found to be 44% and the false-positive rate was 21% (42).

For lesions localized using ultrasound and seen only on ultrasound, specimen radiography may demonstrate the lesion. However, sonography of the specimen using a high-resolution transducer and a stand-off pad may be

necessary (43–45). Following MRI localization, specimen radiography remains a challenge (46). The deployment of a clip, if MRI biopsy is performed first, may aid in specimen radiography; however, for lesions excised for diagnosis, this is not feasible.

Most series report a true-positive rate of 10% to 35% in needle localization series (47–60). Much of this data precedes the advent of stereotactic biopsy and reflects more the positive predictive value of a suspicious mammographic lesion. The vast majority of benign lesions biopsied represent some form of fibrocystic disease, although proliferative lesions, which increase the risk of the patient to develop breast cancer by 1.9 (without atypia) to 5.3 (with atypia) times, account for a significant number of nonpalpable lesions biopsied (57). Without meticulous techniques and attention to subtle signs of malignancy, early breast cancers will be missed. Rosenberg et al. (56) found that, in a series of 927 needle-guided breast biopsies, 29% were malignant, and 30% of the patients with invasive lesions had axillary nodal metastases. Hermann et al. (60) retrospectively reviewed the mammograms of 220 women who underwent needle localization biopsy procedures and classified the lesions as "probably benign" or "probably malignant." The radiologic diagnosis was correct in 68% of cases; 27 of the cancers were retrospectively interpreted as "probably benign" and would have been missed had there not been an aggressive approach to indeterminate lesions. A high-quality screening program coupled with percutaneous biopsy and needle localization biopsy procedures for suspicious or indeterminate lesions will yield increasing numbers of early breast cancers at biopsy.

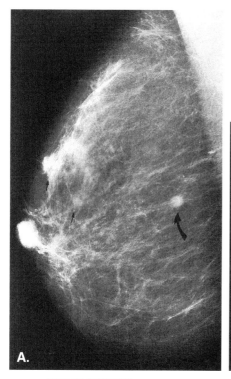
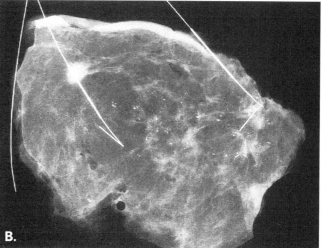

Figure 15.15

HISTORY: A 56-year-old woman who had presented for screening mammography.

MAMMOGRAPHY: Left ML view **(A)** and specimen film **(B).** A high-density spiculated lesion is present deep in the breast **(curved arrow)**, and two other areas of nodularity are located more superficially **(straight arrows) (A).** Between these nodules are extensive ductal-type microcalcifications. These findings are highly suspicious for extensive malignancy, and it is important that the extent of disease be demonstrated. In approaching the interventional procedure for this patient, it is best to place two wires for needle localization, with one marking the anterior extent of the abnormality, and the other the more posterior extent. The specimen radiograph shows the region of interest included, as demonstrated by the two hookwires that were placed for the needle localization procedure.

IMPRESSION: Two needle localization wires placed to mark extensive area of microcalcifications and nodularity, consistent with breast carcinoma.

HISTOPATHOLOGY: Infiltrating ductal and extensive intraductal carcinoma.

REFERENCES

1. Kalisher L. An improved needle for localization of nonpalpable breast lesions. *Radiology* 1978;128:815–817.
2. Edeiken S, Suer WD, Vitale SF, et al. Needle localization of nonpalpable breast lesions using methylene blue. *Breast Dis* 1990;3:75–80.
3. Raininko R, Linna MI, Rasanen O. Preoperative localization of nonpalpable breast tumours. *Acta Chir Scand* 1976;142:575–578.
4. Kopans DB, DeLuca S. A modified needle-hookwire technique to simplify preoperative localization of occult breast lesions. *Radiology* 1980;134:781.
5. Homer MJ. Nonpalpable breast lesions localization using a curved-end retractable wire. *Radiology* 1985;157:259–260.
6. Goldberg RP, Hall FM, Simon M. Preoperative localization of nonpalpable breast lesions using a wire marker and perforated mammographic grid. *Radiology* 1983;146:833–835.
7. Kopans DB, Lindfors K, McCarthy KA, Meyer JE. Spring hookwire breast lesion localizer: Use with rigid-compression mammographic systems. *Radiology* 1985;157:537–538.
8. Homer MJ, Pile-Spellman RE. Needle localization of occult breast lesions with a curved-end retractable wire: technique and pitfalls. *Radiology* 1986;161:547–548.
9. Homer MJ. Nonpalpable breast lesion localization using a curved-end retractable wire. *Radiology* 1985;157:259–260.
10. Dershaw DD, Fleischman RC, Liberman L, et al. Use of digital mammography in needle localization procedures. *Am J Roentgenol* 1993;161:559–562.
11. Hirsch JI, Banks WL, Sullivan JS, Horsley JS. Effect of methylene blue on estrogen-receptor activity. *Radiology* 1989;171:105–107.
12. Hirsch JI, Banks WL, Sullivan JS, Horsley JS. Noninterference of isosulfan blue on estrogen-receptor activity. *Radiology* 1989;171:109–110.
13. Czarnecki DJ, Feider HK, Splittgerber GF. Toluidine blue dye as a breast localization marker. *Am J Roentgenol* 1989;153:261–263.

14. Jackson VP. Needle localization to guide excisional biopsy. *RSNA Categorical Course in Breast Imaging*. RSNA Publications, Radiological Society of North America, Oak Brook, IL. 1995; 161–166.

15. Jackson VP, Bassett LW. Stereotactic fine-needle aspiration biopsy for nonpalpable breast lesions. *Am J Roentgenol* 1990; 154:1196–1197.

16. Shaw de Paredes E, Langer TG, Cousins J. Interventional breast procedures. *Curr Probl Diagn Radiol* 1998;27:133–184.

17. D'Orsi CJ, Mendelson EB. Interventional breast ultrasonography. *Semin Ultrasound CT MRI* 1989;10:132–138.

18. Fornage BD, Coan JD, David CL. Ultrasound-guided needle biopsy of the breast and other interventional procedures. *Radiol Clin N Am* 1992;30:167–185.

19. Kopans DB, Waitzkin ED, Linesky L, et al. Localization of breast lesions identified on only one mammographic view. *Am J Roentgenol* 1987;149:39–41.

20. Fischer U, Vosshenrich R, Keating D, et al. MR-guided biopsy of suspect breast lesions with a simple stereotaxic add-on device for surface coils. *Radiology* 1994;192:272–273.

21. Schnall MD, Orel SG, Connick TJ. MR guided biopsy of the breast. *MRI Clin North Am* 1994;2:585–589.

22. Gorczyca DP. Interventional breast imaging resonance imaging. In: *Interventional Breast Procedures*, 1996. New York: Churchill Livingstone; 1996:147–153.

23. Dershaw DD. Needle localization for breast biopsy. In: Dershaw DD, ed. *Interventional Breast Procedures*. New York: Churchill Livingstone; 1996:25–35.

24. Helvie MA, Ikeda DM, Adler DD. Localization and needle aspiration of breast lesions: complications in 370 cases. *Am J Roentgenol* 1983;41:929–930.

25. Sistrom C, Abbitt PL, Shaw de Paredes E. Hematoma of the breast: a complication of needle localization. *Va Med* 1988; 115:78–79.

26. Davis PS, Wechsler RJ, Feig SA, March DE. Migration of breast biopsy localization wire. *Am J Roentgenol* 1988;150: 787–788.

27. Kopans DB, Gallagher WJ, Swann CA, et al. Does preoperative needle localization lead to an increase in local breast cancer recurrence? *Radiology* 1988;167:677–668.

28. Robertson CL, Kopans DB, McCarthy KA, Hart NE. Nonpalpable lesions in the augmented breast: preoperative localization. *Radiology* 1989;173:873–874.

29. Eklund GW, Busby RC, Miller SH, Job JS. Improved imaging of the augmented breast. *Am J Roentgenol* 1988;151:469–473.

30. Landercasper J, Gundersen SB Jr., Gundersen AL, et al. Needle localization and biopsy of nonpalpable lesions of the breast. *Surg Gynecol Obstet* 1987;164:399–403.

31. Parker SH, Lovin JD, Jobe WE, et al. Stereotactic breast biopsy with a biopsy gun. *Radiology* 1990;176:741–747.

32. Alexander HR, Candela FC, Dershaw DD, Kinne DW. Needle-localized mammographic lesions: results and evolving treatment strategy. *Arch Surg* 1990;125:1441–1444.

33. Winchester DP. Limitations of mammography in the identification of noninfiltrating carcinoma of the breast. *Surg Gynecol Obstet* 1988;167:135–140.

34. Jackman R, Marzoni FA. Needle-localization breast biopsy: why do we fail? *Radiology* 1997;204:677–687.

35. Abrahamson PE, Dunlap LA, Amamoo A, et al. Factors predicting successful needle-localized breast biopsy. *Acad Radiol* 2003;10:610–606.

36. Snyder RE. Specimen radiography and preoperative localization of nonpalpable breast cancer. *Cancer* 1980;46:950–956.

37. Stomper PC, Davis SP, Sonnenfeld MR, et al. Efficacy of specimen radiography of clinically occult noncalcified breast lesions. *Am J Roentgenol* 1988;151:43–47.

38. Rebner M, Pennes DR, Baker DE, et al. Two view specimen radiography in surgical biopsy of nonpalpable breast masses. *Am J Roentgenol* 1987;149:283–285.

39. D'Orsi CJ. Management of the breast specimen. *Radiology* 1995;194:297–302.

40. Chilcote WA, Davis GA, Suchy P, Paushter DM. Breast specimen radiography: evaluation of a compression device. *Radiology* 1988;168:425–427.

41. Clingan R, Griffin M, Phillips J, et al. Potential margin distortion in breast tissue by specimen mammography. *Arch Surg* 2003;138:1371–1374.

42. Lee CH, Carter D. Detecting residual tumor after excisional biopsy of impalpable breast carcinoma: efficacy of comparing preoperative mammograms with radiographs of the biopsy specimen. *Am J Roentgenol* 1995;164:81–86.

43. Frenna TH, Meyer JE, Sonnenfeld MR. US of breast biopsy specimens. *Radiology* 1994;190:573.

44. Laing FC, Jeffrey RB, Minagi H. Ultrasound localization of occult breast lesions. *Radiology* 1984;151:795–796.

45. Mesurolle B. El-Khoury M, Hori D, et al. Sonography of post-excision specimens of nonpalpable breast lesions: value, limitations, and description of a method. *Am J Roentgenol* 2006;186:1014–1024.

46. Morris EA, Liberman L, Dershaw DD, et al. Preoperative MR-imaging-guided needle localization of breast lesions. *Am J Roentgenol* 2002;178:1211–1220.

47. Libshitz HI, Feig SA, Fetouh S. Needle localization of nonpalpable breast lesions. *Radiology* 1976;121:557–560.

48. Hall FM, Frank HA. Preoperative localization of nonpalpable breast lesions. *Am J Roentgenol* 1979;132:101–105.

49. Gisvold JJ, Martin JK Jr. Prebiopsy localization of nonpalpable breast lesions. *Am J Roentgenol* 1984;143:477–481.

50. Oppedal BR, Drevvatne T. Radiographic diagnosis of nonpalpable breast lesions: correlation to pathology. *Acta Radiol (Diagn)* 1983;24:259–265.

51. Meyer JE, Kopans DB, Stomper PC, Lindfors KK. Occult breast abnormalities: percutaneous preoperative needle localization. *Radiology* 1984;150:335–337.

52. Hoehn JL, Hardacre JM, Swanson MK, Williams GH. Localization of occult breast lesions. *Cancer* 1982;49:1142–1144.

53. Yankaskas BC, Knelson MH, Abernathy ML, et al. Needle localization biopsy of occult lesions of the breast: experience in 199 cases. *Invest Radiol* 1988;23:729–733.

54. Hall FM, Storella JM, Silverstone DZ, Wyshak G. Nonpalpable breast lesions: recommendations for biopsy based on suspicion of carcinoma at mammography. *Radiology* 1988;167:353–358.

55. Ciatto S, Cataliotti L, Distanne V. Nonpalpable breast lesions detected with mammography: review of 512 consecutive cases. *Radiology* 1987;165:99–102.

56. Rosenberg AL, Schwartz GF, Feig SA, Patchefsky AS. Clinical occult breast lesions: localization and significance. *Radiology* 1987;162:167–170.

57. Rubin E, Visscher DW, Alexander RW, et al. Proliferative disease and atypia in biopsies performed for nonpalpable lesions detected mammographically. *Cancer* 1988;161:2077–2082.

58. Hallgrimsson P, Karesen R, Artun K, Skjennald A. Nonpalpable breast lesions: diagnostic criteria and preoperative localization. *Acta Radiol* 1988;29:285–288.

59. Meyer JE, Sonnenfeld MR, Greene RA, Stomper PC. Preoperative localization of clinically occult breast lesions: experience at a referral hospital. *Radiology* 1988;169: 627–628.

60. Hermann G, Janus C, Schwartz IS, et al. Nonpalpable breast lesions: accuracy of prebiopsy mammographic diagnosis. *Radiology* 1987;165:323–326.

Chapter 16

Percutaneous Breast Biopsy

The capability of diagnosing a breast lesion percutaneously has dramatically improved the management of breast abnormalities over the last two decades. Prior to the development of these techniques, surgical excision was the procedure performed to identify the etiology of a nonpalpable mammographically detected lesion. The majority of these lesions, now classified as BIRADS 4—suspicious for malignancy—actually are benign. Until percutaneous breast biopsy was developed, many women underwent surgery for benign abnormalities to diagnose them.

Initially, fine needle aspiration biopsy (FNAB) was performed with mammographic (1) or sonographic guidance. The limitation of FNAB is the limited sampling and the need for an experienced cytopathologist for interpretation. Bolmgren (1) described the use of a stereotactic table that allowed for precise placement of a needle into a small lesion in the breast. Using this technology, percutaneous breast biopsy began its evolution. Core-needle biopsy techniques evolved as biopsy guns with Tru-cut-type automated needles of varying caliber were designed. Initially, 18-gauge core needles were used, followed by 16-gauge and subsequently 14-gauge automated core needles. The automated 14-gauge core needle is still used for the biopsy of masses, particularly with ultrasound guidance. Early results of core biopsy using a 14-gauge automated needle showed a sensitivity for malignancy of 85% (2) and a concordance between the pathologic results of core biopsy and surgery ranging from 87% to 96% (2–5). Parker et al. (3), in 1990, described biopsy utilizing stereotactic guidance in 103 patients, using a biopsy gun and automated cutting needles ranging from 18- to 14-gauge. The use of the 14-gauge needle improved the sample size and the results at pathology and, with this improvement, the management of breast abnormalities changed considerably.

Prior to the advent of the larger needles, a limited number of lesions were biopsied percutaneously—particularly cancers, complicated cysts, and fibroadenomas. However, many lesions, particularly fibrocystic lesions that were manifested as microcalcifications, yielded very nonspecific results on cytology and therefore were better diagnosed by surgical excision. With the development of percutaneous tissue sampling techniques, many more lesions could be biopsied by core biopsy instead of surgery.

The biopsy of microcalcifications has been challenging using core needles, because the volume of tissue removed is important to the accuracy of diagnosis for proliferative lesions. Vacuum-assisted breast biopsy probes have evolved to answer this problem, and larger samples can be obtained quickly and accurately using these devices. With the advent of vacuum-assisted biopsy, the speed of tissue acquisition, the volume of tissue acquired, and the accuracy for certain types of lesions have improved. Liberman et al. (6) showed that for calcifications that are highly suggestive of malignancy, the use of stereotactic 11-gauge vacuum-assisted biopsy was significantly more likely than the 14-gauge core needle or 14-gauge vacuum-assisted probe to spare a surgical procedure and was associated with the highest cost savings.

The advantages of percutaneous needle biopsy are many and include:

- Improved cosmesis
- Elimination of unnecessary surgery
- Reduced cost
- Improved efficiency in diagnosing a breast abnormality
- Reduced patient morbidity
- Less discomfort

Using percutaneous breast biopsy, benign lesions can be diagnosed accurately and do not require surgical excision in most cases.

Lesions that are suspicious for carcinoma can be proven to be cancer preoperatively. This is important in planning the proper surgery for the patient. Instead of performing a surgical excision for diagnosis, a lumpectomy with sentinel node biopsy can be performed with knowledge of the diagnosis. In particular, the diagnosis of invasive breast cancer on core biopsy allows for definitive therapy and increases the possibility of a single surgery. King et al. (7) reported that 90% of patients with invasive carcinoma on core biopsy could have a single surgery for definitive therapy. Liberman et al. (8) found that a single surgery was performed in 84% of women for whom the diagnosis of cancer was made on core biopsy, in comparison with 29% of women in whom the diagnosis was made by surgical biopsy. Jackman et al. (9) found that a single surgery was performed in 90% of patients whose cancers were found on percutaneous biopsy, versus 24% of patients whose cancers were diagnosed surgically.

For multiple suspicious lesions, percutaneous biopsy is a very important tool to define the extent of disease. The presence of multiple cancers in one breast that involve more than one quadrant indicates multicentric disease

(Fig. 16.1). This condition usually requires mastectomy for treatment. Therefore, the patient may be assessed by imaging and percutaneous biopsy, and be managed with definitive therapy—all without the need for unnecessary preliminary excisions. Rosenblatt et al. (10) found that multisite stereotactic biopsy had a positive effect on patient care in 80% of patients by helping to confirm the need for mastectomy or by documenting benign disease at multiple sites and avoiding unnecessary surgery.

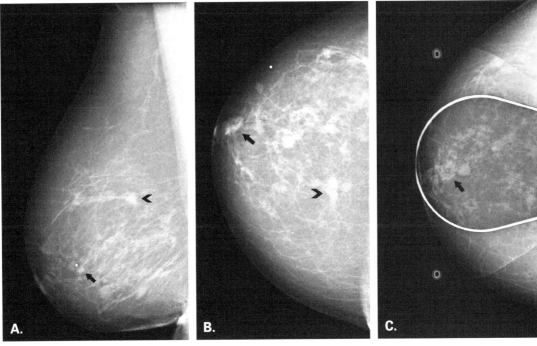

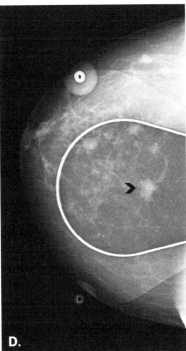

Figure 16.1

HISTORY: 74-year-old woman with a palpable thickening in the left periareolar area, for second opinion after being told that she had multiple "cysts."

MAMMOGRAPHY: Left MLO **(A)** and CC **(B)** views show multiple small masses in the left breast. The palpable thickening corresponded to a small indistinct mass at 4 o'clock, seen also on spot compression **(C)** **(arrows)**. An indistinct mass is also noted in the upper inner quadrant **(arrowheads)**, appearing spiculated on spot compression **(D)**. Multiple other small round masses are present, primarily in the lower outer quadrant. Ultrasound demonstrated 10 small solid masses, including those seen on spot compression. Biopsy of five of these lesions was performed. Sonographic images of the palpable mass **(E)** and three other biopsied masses **(F, G, H)** are shown.

HISTOPATHOLOGY: Invasive ductal carcinoma, all sites. The patient underwent mastectomy for multicentric disease.

NOTE: Percutaneous biopsy is an ideal method to assess extent of disease in a patient with multicentric carcinoma. (*continued*)

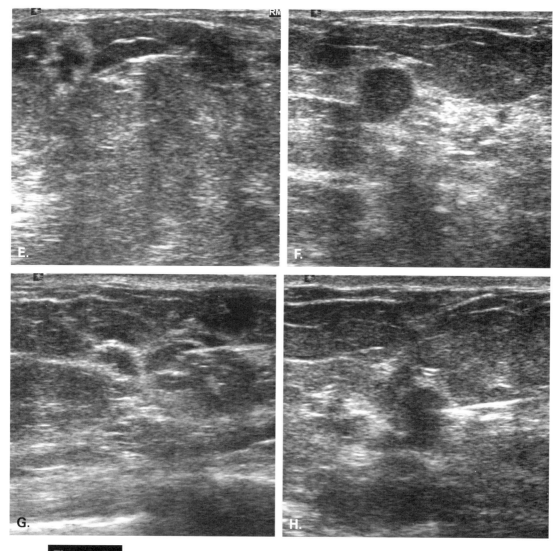

Figure 16.1 *(CONTINUED)*

Percutaneous biopsy is a less costly way of diagnosing a breast lesion than is surgery. Lee et al. (11) found an average cost savings of stereotactic biopsy versus open biopsy of $741 per case. The greatest savings occurred with indeterminate masses. Lindfors (12), in a study of the cost-effectiveness of core biopsy found that the marginal cost per year of life saved by screening mammography was reduced a maximum of 23% (from $20,770 to $15,934) with the use of core biopsy instead of surgical biopsy. Liberman et al. (13) found that stereotactic biopsy decreased the cost of a breast lesion diagnosis by over 50%. Lind et al. (14) found that stereotactic core biopsy shortened the time from detection at mammography to diagnosis and breast-conserving therapy, permitted discussion with the patient of treatment options, reduced the positive margin rate and re-excision rate, and represented a cost savings in the management of nonpalpable breast cancer.

ULTRASOUND-GUIDED BIOPSY

Ultrasound guidance is excellent for needle biopsy procedures in the breast. Cyst aspiration, fine-needle aspiration biopsy, and core biopsy can be performed readily for lesions that are visible sonographically. The benefits of ultrasound guidance include the ease of patient positioning, speed of the procedure, real-time visualization of the needle trajectory, low cost, lack of use of ionizing radiation, and the use of nondedicated equipment (15). Gordon et al. (16) found a sensitivity of 95% in 213 malignant lesions biopsied using ultrasound guidance and fine needle aspiration with a 20-gauge needle. Parker et al. (17) found that ultrasound-guided core biopsy using a free-hand technique with a long-throw 14-gauge core needle was a highly accurate alternative to open biopsy for the diagnosis of breast masses. Vacuum-assisted biopsy is

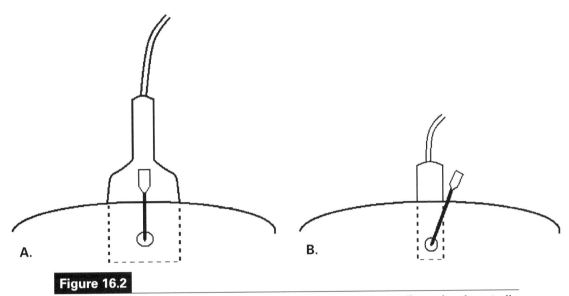

Figure 16.2

Schematic for ultrasound-guided cyst aspiration shows that the needle is placed vertically, directly toward the mass. The needle tip is visible when it bisects the scan plane at the level of the lesion.

also performed with ultrasound guidance (18) and offers a rapid and accurate method to biopsy lesions.

For cyst aspiration or fine-needle aspiration biopsy, a small-gauge hypodermic needle is used. The needle may be connected with thin, short tubing to a 20 cc syringe, allowing the interventionalist to handle the needle with

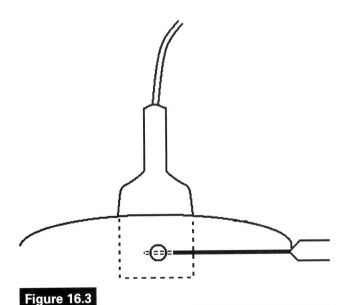

Figure 16.3

Schematic of a long-axis or horizontal approach that is used for core-needle biopsy with ultrasound guidance. The lesion is visualized in the center of the long axis of the transducer field, and the dermatotomy is made lateral to the edge of the transducer. This allows the needle to be placed horizontally, parallel to the chest wall, for a safer sampling when the needle is fired.

more control. For cysts, a 1-inch long, 21- to 25-gauge needle is used. For fine-needle aspiration biopsy, the smaller the needle, the better the sample, so a 25-gauge hypodermic needle is optimal. A vertical approach, as described by Fornage (19), may be used for needle placement for cyst aspiration or FNAB (Fig. 16.2). In this manner, the needle is placed the shortest distance from and directly into the mass. For this placement, the needle is placed at the midline of the long face of the transducer, and the needle is visualized once it is at the depth of the lesion. If a long axis or horizontal approach is used, the needle is placed at the short end of the transducer and is visualized in its entirety as it is advanced toward the lesion. The horizontal approach usually requires a longer needle to reach the lesion (Fig. 16.3).

For core-needle biopsy or vacuum-aspirated biopsy, a horizontal/oblique approach must be used. Because of the forward firing of the needle, it is imperative that an approach parallel to the pectoralis major muscle be used for safety (Fig. 16.4). Many of the core needles typically used for ultrasound-guided biopsy advance into the breast about 2 cm on firing. An angled approach could easily allow the needle to penetrate the chest wall. For core biopsy, the area is cleansed with antiseptic solution, and a sterile technique is used. The device is visualized in the scan plan. It can be very helpful to have the assistant hold the transducer so that the interventionalist can use both hands to control the needle and skin and to hold the biopsy gun. Lidocaine 1% is injected for local anesthesia, and a small dermatotomy is made. The location of the dermatotomy depends on the depth of the lesion. The deeper the lesion, the farther from the edge of the transducer is the dermatotomy made. If the dermatotomy is too close to

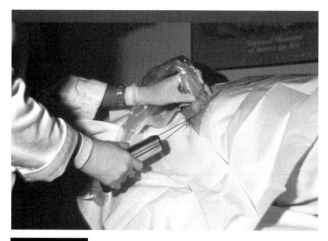

Figure 16.4

Ultrasound-guided core biopsy being performed with an automated core needle using a long-axis (horizontal) approach. The patient is turned to allow access to the lateral aspect of the breast and to allow room for the biopsy apparatus.

the edge of the transducer, the needle insertion will not be parallel to the chest wall.

Once the needle has been placed proximal to the lesion (pre-fire position), the patient is prepared for the first sample by reminding her that she will hear a loud sound. The gun is fired and the needle traverses the lesion (post-fire position) (Fig. 16.5). Vacuum-assisted probes (VAB) may also be used for ultrasound-guided biopsy (Fig. 16.6). Using VAB, the needle may be inserted through the lesion rather than fired, and then multiple samples are acquired utilizing suction. A clip may be placed under ultrasound guidance and is particularly important for very small lesions that may no longer be clearly evident on ultrasound after the biopsy. Some of the vacuum-assisted probes are designed for clip insertion through the probe. Also, clips loaded into a stiff introducer-type needle are excellent for direct clip placement following needle biopsy.

Ultrasound guided biopsy is an ideal method for the percutaneous biopsy of women with implants. The implant wall can be visualized as the procedure is performed. In the

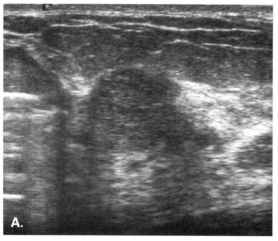

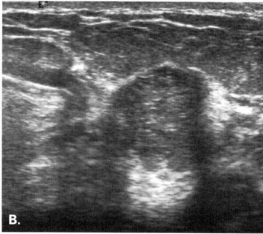

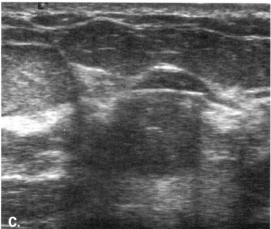

Figure 16.5

HISTORY: A 29-year-old with a new palpable right breast mass.

MAMMOGRAPHY: Sonography **(A)** demonstrates the lesion to be hypoechoic, slightly lobulated, and well-defined with no acoustic shadowing. All the features suggest that this is most likely a fibroadenoma. Vacuum-assisted biopsy was performed with ultrasound guidance. Pre-fire **(B)** and post-fire **(C)** sonographic images show that the needle has traversed the lesion. One pass was made.

HISTOPATHOLOGY: Fibroadenoma (concordant with imaging findings).

case of patients with implants, it is imperative that care be used in administering the local anesthesia and in the dermatotomy so that the implant is not punctured. The horizontal approach must be used for needle placement and tissue sampling. Automated core needles, rather than vacuum-assisted probes, are better suited for patients with very thin breast tissue over the implant (Fig. 16.7).

STEREOTACTIC BIOPSY

The advent of stereotaxis has greatly impacted the ease of accurate needle placement into small nonpalpable lesions and has allowed for a nonsurgical approach. Stereotactically guided needle biopsy can be performed for nodules as small as 3 mm. Stereotaxis can also be used for needle localizations and is particularly advantageous for the localization of a lesion seen clearly on only one view and superimposed over dense tissue on the orthogonal view. Stereotactic guidance with vacuum-assisted needles has become the standard or typical way of diagnosing suspicious microcalcifications.

Core biopsy can be performed with stereotactic, sonographic, or magnetic resonance imaging (MRI) guidance. Stereotactic biopsy units can be prone tables on which the breast is dependant through an aperture in the table, or upright units (20) that attach to the mammography equipment. When the patient is biopsied using an upright unit, she may sit up if the lesion is located in the superior aspect of the breast. However, if the lesion can be biopsied via a medial, lateral, or inferior approach, the patient lies on a stretcher in a decubitus position for the procedure (Fig. 16.8) (21,22).

The advantages of the upright unit are the ease in positioning the patient, the access to the posterior aspect of the breast, the comfort of the patient in not having to lie prone, the ability to use the room for general mammography as well as biopsy, and the interaction of the biopsy team with the patient. Advantages of the prone table unit are the access to the inferior aspect of the breast, the lack of patient visibility of the procedure, and the rarity of a vasovagal reaction.

The principle of stereotaxis is based on the movement of the x-ray tube relative to the breast at angles of a fixed degree of obliquity that allow for the precise calculation of the lesion location. The technique described here is based on the Siemen's Opdima stereotactic unit (Siemens Medical Solutions, Malvern, PA), but various stereotactic units are designed around similar basic principles and procedures. The breast is compressed and is not moved during the entire procedure. Two 15-degree oblique spot views of the lesion are made (stereotactic pair). The radiologist identifies the lesion on each image and confirms the reference point on the images. The reference point is a fixed point in the image receptor plate that is visible on the

images. Based on the position of the lesion target point versus the reference point, the X, Y, and Z coordinates of the lesion are calculated by the computer. The length of needle to be used must be chosen and entered into the computer.

At the stereotactic unit, the needle is then zeroed, thereby moving the needle guides into position at a $\Delta X = 0$, $\Delta Y = 0$, and $\Delta Z = 0$. This position indicates that the needle tip is over the lesion on the X and Y axes and that, when the gun is fired, the target point of the lesion will be at the level of the center of the needle's trough on the Z axis.

Following local anesthesia and a dermatotomy. the needle is placed through the guides. Repeat spot oblique views (a stereotactic pair) are made to confirm accurate needle placement. The needle position must be carefully analyzed on these pre-fire images, and these should show the needle tip at the leading edge of the lesion on both images (Fig. 16.9). If the needle is off position on the X, Y. or Z axis, its position must be adjusted based on the pre-fire images. If the needle is repositioned to any degree, a repeat stereotactic pair should be obtained. Examples of X, Y, Z, and complex errors are show in Figures 16.10 to 16.13, and methods to correct the errors are described.

Once the needle position is accurate, the sampling begins. With a vacuum-assisted probe or an automated core needle, the gun is fired. The needle is fired within the breast a distance specific for each particular needle and gun; most needles advance about 2 cm into the breast. Therefore, the thickness of the breast must be sufficient to accommodate this throw or stroke of the needle. Sampling begins by retrieving tissue cores at every 2 o'clock position with a vacuum-assisted probe. Typically two rotations are made, yielding 12 core samples. This circumferential sampling pattern is rapid and accurate.

If an automated core needle is used instead, the needle is oriented in position at ΔX, ΔY, and ΔZ at 0.0 mm. The gun is fired, and the first sample is retrieved by withdrawing the needle. The needle is replaced into the breast, and similar samples are obtained at ΔX at +2 or 3 mm, ΔX at −2 to 3 mm, ΔY at +2 to 3 mm, and ΔY at −2 to 3 mm (Fig. 16.14).

For the biopsy of calcifications, specimen radiography is performed to verify that the lesion has been correctly sampled (Fig. 16.15). This step is not necessary for noncalcified lesions. The vacuum probe is withdrawn 5 mm, and a clip is placed through the probe and deployed into the middle of the biopsy site. This change in the ΔZ of 5 mm is made because the clip tends to deploy forward at the end of the trough and will lie deep to the lesion once the compression is released. A final stereotactic pair is obtained to confirm that the clip has deployed, and the needle is withdrawn from the breast. Compression is applied to achieve hemostasis, the wound is cleansed, and Steri-Strips are applied to close the dermatotomy. An ice pack is placed over the breast for 20 to 30 minutes, and the wound is assessed for hemostasis before the patient is discharged.

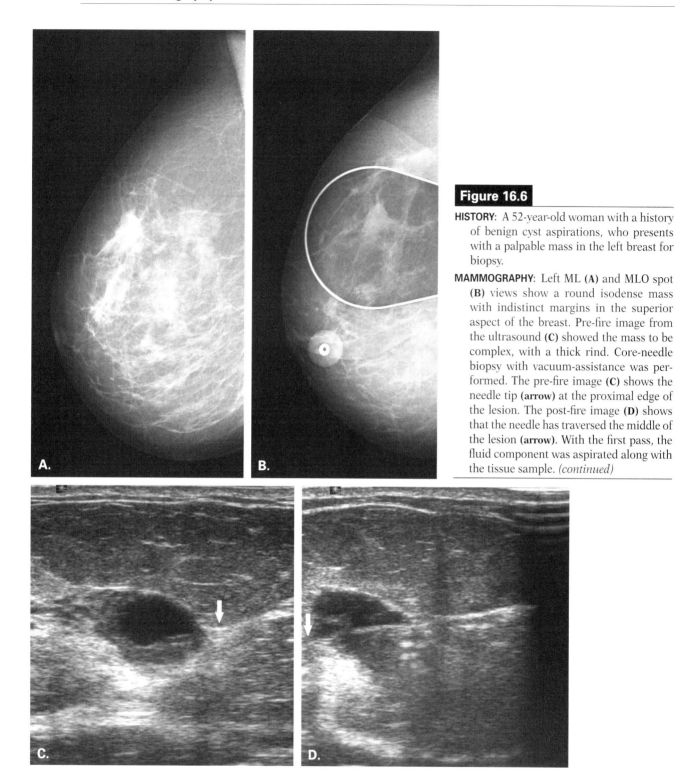

Figure 16.6

HISTORY: A 52-year-old woman with a history of benign cyst aspirations, who presents with a palpable mass in the left breast for biopsy.

MAMMOGRAPHY: Left ML (**A**) and MLO spot (**B**) views show a round isodense mass with indistinct margins in the superior aspect of the breast. Pre-fire image from the ultrasound (**C**) showed the mass to be complex, with a thick rind. Core-needle biopsy with vacuum-assistance was performed. The pre-fire image (**C**) shows the needle tip (**arrow**) at the proximal edge of the lesion. The post-fire image (**D**) shows that the needle has traversed the middle of the lesion (**arrow**). With the first pass, the fluid component was aspirated along with the tissue sample. *(continued)*

For aspiration procedures using stereotactic guidance, a coaxial system can be used to avoid multiple needle punctures. A 19- or 20-gauge outer cannula can be placed at the proximal edge of the lesion, and 22-gauge needles are passed through the cannula for aspiration.

Stereotactically guided fine-needle aspiration is of help for small well-defined masses that are new in comparison with prior examinations and that are not seen or are not definitely identified as cystic on ultrasound (Fig. 16.16). Fluid can be aspirated from these cysts under stereotactic guidance. Either pneumocystography or

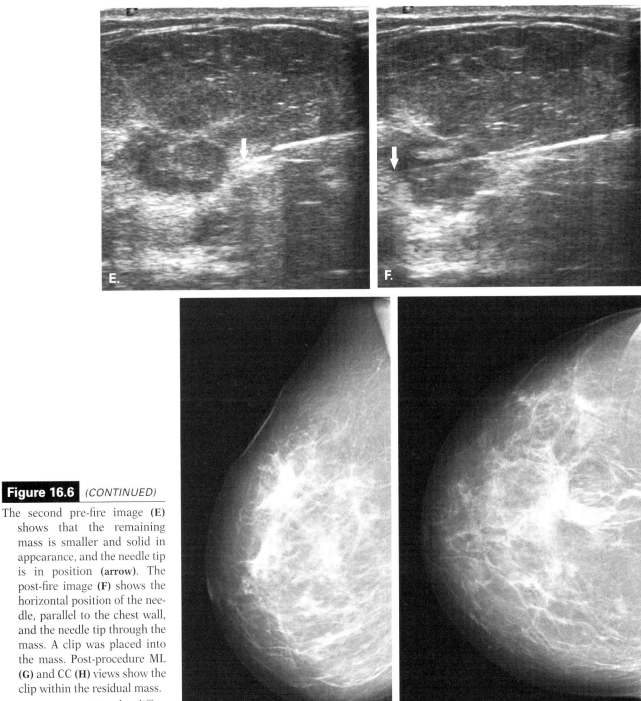

Figure 16.6 *(CONTINUED)*

The second pre-fire image **(E)** shows that the remaining mass is smaller and solid in appearance, and the needle tip is in position **(arrow)**. The post-fire image **(F)** shows the horizontal position of the needle, parallel to the chest wall, and the needle tip through the mass. A clip was placed into the mass. Post-procedure ML **(G)** and CC **(H)** views show the clip within the residual mass.

HISTOPATHOLOGY: Poorly differentiated invasive ductal carcinoma with papillary features.

follow-up mediolateral and craniocaudal views should be performed to confirm the disappearance of the nodule.

FINE-NEEDLE ASPIRATION BIOPSY

FNABs for palpable breast masses have been performed with success in lieu of open biopsy (23,24). For a ques-

tionably palpable lesion that cannot be satisfactorily aspirated by palpation only, or for a nonpalpable lesion, fine-needle aspiration can be performed under stereotactic or sonographic guidance. The following criteria are critical for fine-needle aspiration of nonpalpable lesions to be of value: (a) extremely accurate needle placement, (b) good techniques of aspiration and preparation of the smear, (c) experienced cytolopathologists

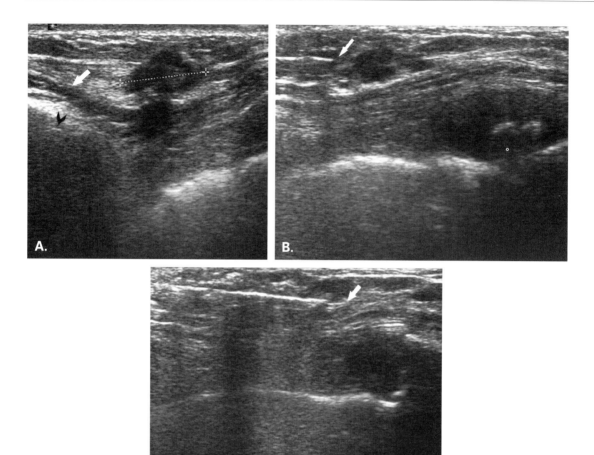

Figure 16.7

HISTORY: A 53-year-old woman with a history of breast implants who presents with an irregular mass identified on mammography in the right breast at 3 o'clock.

MAMMOGRAPHY: Right breast ultrasound **(A)** shows an irregular hypoechoic mass with angulated margins and some surrounding edema. The sonographic features are highly suggestive of malignancy. The breast parenchyma is very thin in this area. The pectoralis major muscle **(arrow)** is visualized, as well as the anterior edge of the subpectoral implant **(arrowhead)**.

Core-needle biopsy using an automated 14-gauge needle was performed. It is imperative that the needle be placed carefully and horizontally, keeping the needle and its trajectory parallel to the pectoralis major muscle and the chest wall. Pre-fire image **(B)** shows a proper needle position **(arrow)** proximal to the mass. Post-fire position **(C)** shows that the mass has been transversed **(arrow)** by the needle. Three core samples were obtained.

HISTOPATHOLOGY: Invasive ductal carcinoma.

for interpretation of the sample, and (d) accurate and consistent results for cytologic determination of benign and malignant lesions (25). The experience of the person performing the aspiration is reflected in the percentage of aspirates that have sufficient material for analysis (23,26).

Regardless of the mode of FNAB guidance, a 22- to 25-gauge needle is placed into the lesion, suction is applied, and the needle is moved back and forth within the lesion. The suction is released, the needle is withdrawn, and the aspirate is ejected from the needle onto the slides and is smeared and fixed. Multiple passes will increase the yield of cells for cytologic analysis. When mammographic guidance with a fenestrated plate was used for FNAB of nonpalpable breast lesions, Helvie et al. (27) found that only 46% of the aspirates

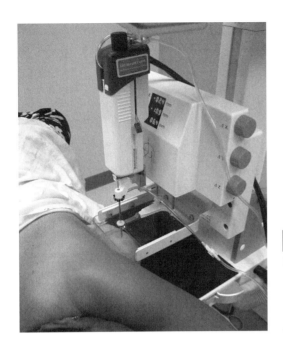

Figure 16.8

Patient is in position for stereotactic breast biopsy using an upright unit and a vacuum-assisted probe (Mammotome, Ethicon Endo-Surgery, Cincinnati OH). When the lesion is located in the upper aspect of the breast, a superior approach is used. For a lateral, medial, or inferior approach, the patient is placed in a decubitus position.

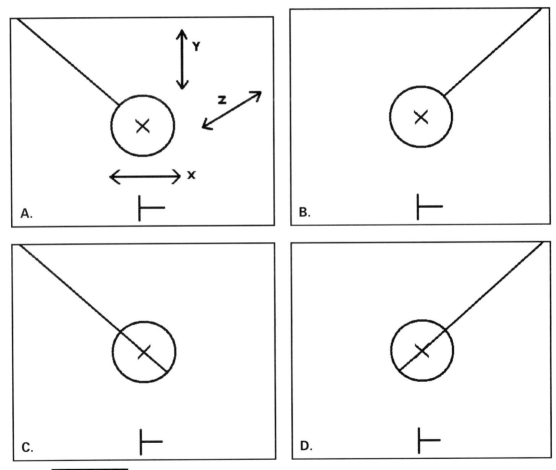

Figure 16.9

A, B: Accurate pre-fire needle position. The needle tip is at the leading edge of the lesion on both stereotactic images. The images must be analyzed together to understand where the needle tip is relative to the target point and where the needle tip will likely be once the gun is fired. The orientation of the X, Y, and Z axes are shown. **C, D:** Accurate post-fire needle position: After the gun has been fired, the needle has moved forward through the lesion, and the needle tip is traversing the target point on both images.

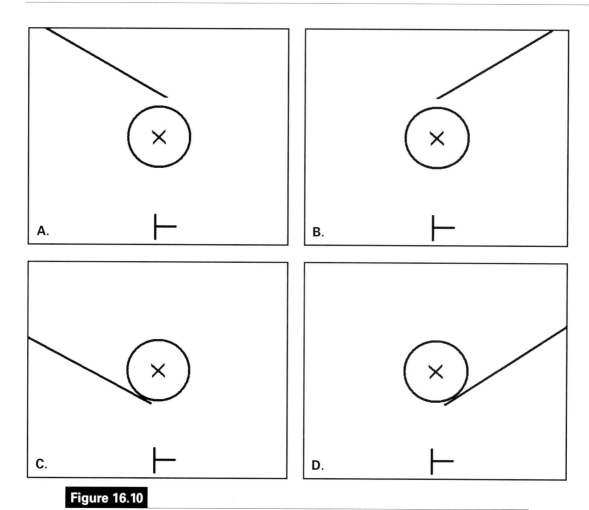

Figure 16.10

A, B: Y-axis error: The needle tip is above the target point on both images. If it is fired in this position, the lesion will be missed. This is the typical Y-axis error on the upright unit, because the patient has pulled back a bit and the lesion has moved back. The targeted point, therefore, lies anterior to the lesion on the stereotactic images. To correct this error, the ΔY is moved back (on the upright unit) or down (on the prone table). **C, D:** Y-axis error: The needle tip is below the target point on both views. This is the typical Y-axis error on the prone table, because the patient has pulled up a bit, moving the lesion above the needle tip. To correct this problem, the ΔY is moved up (on the prone table) or forward (on the upright unit).

of 215 lesions contained representative material. If an aspirate of a suspicious mammographic lesion is negative, core biopsy or open biopsy is necessary for accurate diagnosis.

Fine needle association biopsy under stereotactic guidance has been an option for the evaluation of nonpalpable solid lesions (28–38). Variable results from studies comparing cytology and histology for nonpalpable lesions have demonstrated a relatively high sensitivity and specificity for this procedure. For FNAB to be of value and to be cost effective, it is necessary that lesions called "malignant" be malignant and that no false positives occur. Otherwise, histologic confirmation would be

necessary prior to definitive treatment. Because of the small size of these lesions, the mixed nature of the aspirate (38), the necessity for highly accurate needle placement, and the technique for aspiration, the numbers of "insufficient for cytologic analysis" specimens during FNAB have ranged from 0% (31) to 36% (33), with most series reporting on insufficient sampling in approximately 20% of cases. In a review of 270 lesions that were biopsied using fine-needle aspiration techniques with either sonographic or stereotactic guidance, Ciatto et al. (39) found that the sensitivity was 88.5%, specificity was 94.6%, and inadequacy rate was 3.7% for malignant lesions and 22.9% for benign lesions when stereotactic

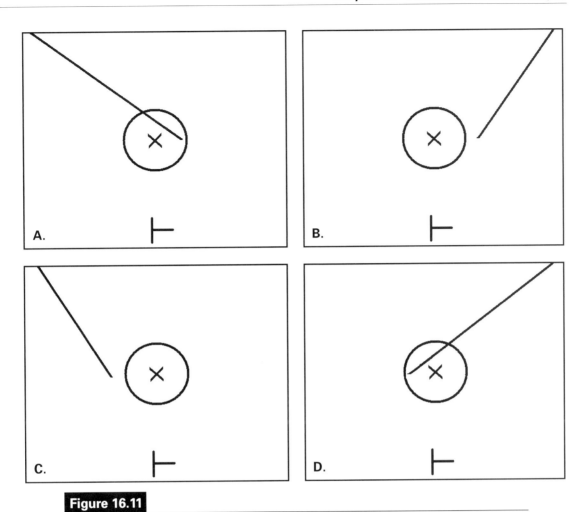

Figure 16.11

A, B: X-axis errors: The needle tip lies to the right of the lesion on both views. Although the needle appears to traverse the lesion on the **A** image, it is located far to the right of the lesion on the **B** view. If the needle is fired in this position, it will miss the lesion. To correct this problem the needle should be shifted to the left on the ΔX axis. **C, D:** X-axis error: The needle tip lies to the left of the lesion on both stereotactic images (an X-axis error). To correct this position, the ΔX is shifted to the right.

guidance was used. With sonography, the results were 96% sensitivity, 98.4% specificity, and 0% insufficient sampling for cancers, and 28.4% insufficient sampling for benign lesions. Stereotactic systems have allowed for improved sampling in comparison with the standard mammographic localization grid system (38).

The greatest advantage of FNAB is in the elimination of some open biopsies, but for this advantage to be present, it is critical that the radiologist and cytologist be highly experienced in the procedure. If any false-positive diagnoses should occur, then histologic confirmation prior to definitive therapy for "malignant" lesions would be necessary. Certainly, FNAB has a definite role in the evaluation of some benign lesions. Small equivocal masses that are

cysts can be aspirated with a high degree of accuracy and need not be subjected to open biopsy. Similarly, an option for lesions that are of low suspicion on mammography, such as "probable fibroadenomas," can be confirmed with cytologic analysis and followed mammographically rather than being resected.

CYST ASPIRATION

Cysts that are simple on ultrasound do not need to be aspirated unless they are markedly symptomatic (Fig. 16.16). A simple cyst is one that is anechoic, well-defined, with a thin wall and acoustic enhancement.

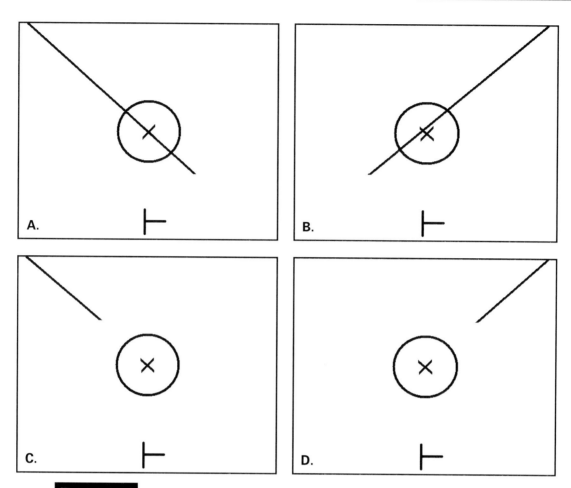

Figure 16.12

A, B: Z-axis error: In these images, the needle has traversed the image and is past the target point on both images. This indicates that the tip is deep to the lesion. This occurs in the following circumstances: (a) the gun has not been cocked, and the needle is inserted in the fired position, (b) the wrong needle length has been programmed into the unit, or (c) the ΔZ is not set to 0, but is set inferior to the target point. It can be very dangerous to fire the needle at this point. The needle can penetrate the opposite surface of the breast and hit the image receptor, breaking or bending it. **C, D:** Z-axis error: In these images, the needle is short of the target point on both images, indicating that the tip is shallow to where it should be. This problem occurs when the needle length has been incorrectly programmed into the computer, or when the ΔZ is set above the 0.00 mm.

Complicated cysts are those that may contain low-level echoes or lack enhancement (Fig. 16.17). These are typically aspirated when solitary, new, larger, or when associated with other lesions suspicious for malignancy in the same breast. Sometimes multiple simple cysts and complex cysts having a similar appearance are followed at a short interval rather than aspirating all that are not completely clear.

Cyst aspiration can be performed in various ways depending on how the mass is identified. A large palpable cyst may be aspirated by palpation alone. Cysts that are symptomatic and under pressure may be aspirated to relieve the symptoms, and this may be performed by palpation or with ultrasound guidance (Fig. 16.18). Ultrasound offers the ability to visualize the cyst and to verify that it is drained. Most often, cysts are aspirated using ultrasound guidance, which is how they are initially characterized. Either a short-axis approach (vertical) or a long-axis approach (horizontal) can be used, depending on the operator's skills and preferences. Particularly with the vertical approach, a 25-gauge hypodermic needle attached to a 20-cc syringe by a short piece of flexible tubing is ideal. A 1-inch needle is adequate in most cases unless the breast is very thick,

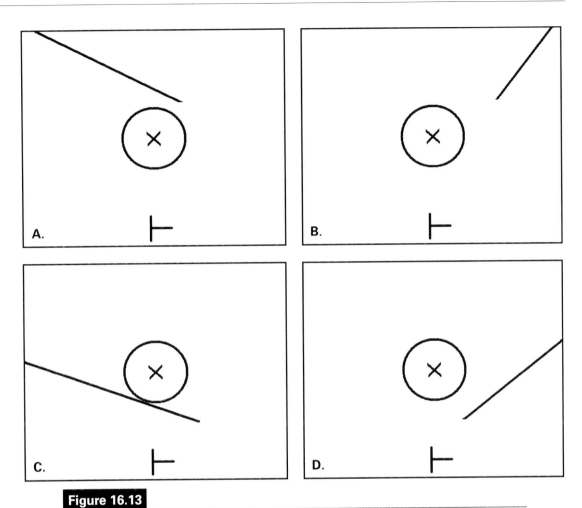

Figure 16.13

A, B: Complex errors: X and Y errors. X- and Y-axis error in which the needle tip lies to the right of and above the lesion. This is corrected by shifting the ΔX toward the left and the ΔY down or toward the chest wall (depending on the prone versus upright unit). **C, D:** X- and Y-axis errors in which the needle tip is to the right and below the lesion. This is corrected by shifting ΔX to the left and ΔY forward or up depending on the type of unit. *(continued)*

and the short needle length is safe and easy to handle. If the fluid is very thick, a larger gauge needle (21- or 22-guage) may be necessary. The smaller bore needles are easily visible on ultrasound.

Once the cyst is punctured and drained, a quick assessment of fluid type is needed before terminating the procedure. If the fluid appears bloody or very turbid, slides should be prepared and sent for cytologic analysis. In this situation, it is important to be able to identify the lesion later. in the event that atypia requiring excision is identified. Therefore, leaving a small amount of residual fluid is helpful. If the cyst completely collapsed and is no longer visible, placing a clip into the area may be helpful in the future, if excision is needed.

When cyst fluid is clear, straw-colored, or green, it is benign fluid and can be discarded. If the fluid is bloody or turbid, it should be sent for cytologic analysis. Usual cytologic findings that are benign and require no further evaluation are apocrine metaplasia, foamy macrophages, acellular fluid, and amorphous debris. Because the breast is a modified sweat gland, the epithelium is secretory or apocrine in nature.

PNEUMOCYSTOGRAPHY

The evaluation of a patient with a well-defined breast mass on mammography may include ultrasonography, needle aspiration, and occasionally pneumocystography. Pneumocystography can be performed if breast ultrasound is not available, if the sonographic findings are equivocal, or if the lesion is very small and not visible

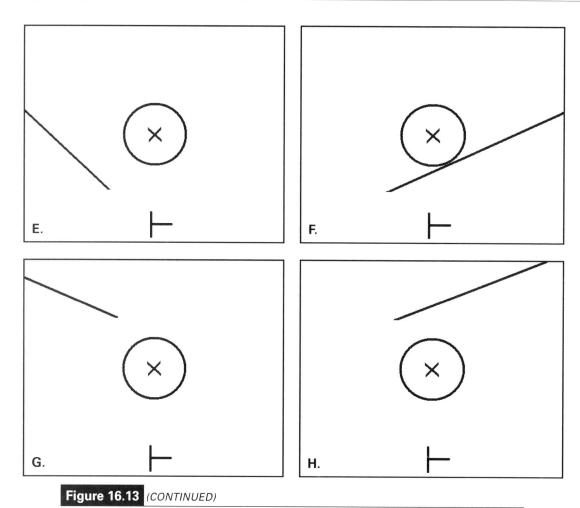

Figure 16.13 *(CONTINUED)*

E, F: X- and Y-axis error in which the needle tip is to the left and below (behind) the lesion. The correction is to shift the ΔX to the right and the ΔY up or forward prior to firing the gun. **G, H:** X- and Y-axis error in which the needle tip is to the left and above the lesion. The correction is to move the ΔX to the right and the ΔY down or back.

on ultrasound. Some studies (40) have shown a therapeutic value from breast cyst puncture and pneumocystography. Using pneumocystography, or air injection into the cyst cavity, an intracystic tumor can be identified. The incidence of intracystic carcinoma ranges from 0.2% (41) to 1.3% (42). Tabar et al. (40) identified 13 benign and 13 malignant tumors on a series of 434 pneumocystograms. The fluid aspirated from five to 13 cancers was not bloody, as is generally thought to be indicative of malignancy, and cytology performed in 11 of the cases was negative in eight (40). In a 1-year follow-up of 130 simple cysts diagnosed at pneumocystography, 88% did not refill after initial puncture, and 97% were definitively treated with pneumocystography after a repeat puncture. The presence of air within the cyst cavity may induce collapse and sclerosis of the wall (43).

Pneumocystography is a simple technique to perform and produces minimal discomfort to the patient. The aspiration of the cyst can be performed by palpating it, under ultrasound guidance (44), or under mammographic or stereotactic guidance. Palpable and nonpalpable cysts can be aspirated easily under mammographic guidance because the lesion can be fixed for puncture by compressing the breast. This technique is described as follows.

On viewing the initial mammogram, one determines the shortest distance from the lesion to the skin surface—medial, superior, or lateral. The localization compression plate is placed over the breast at the determined location, and an image is made. The patient remains in position with the breast compressed while the image is reviewed; the coordinates of the lesion are determined. A 20- to 22-gauge

(text continues on page 621)

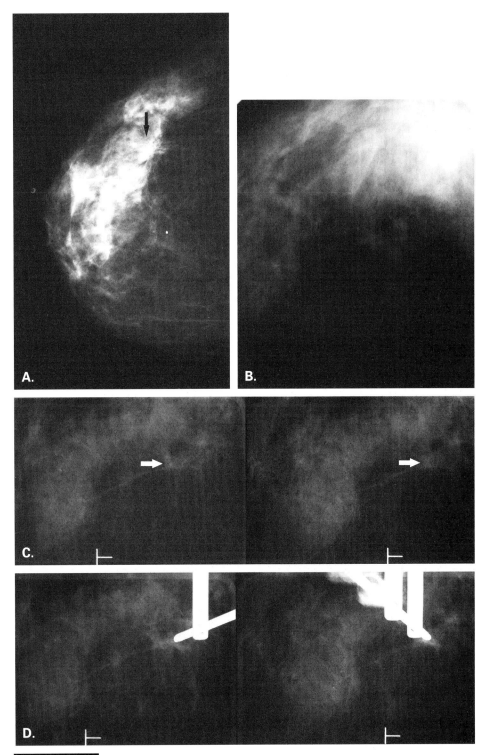

Figure 16.14

HISTORY: A 72-year-old woman for biopsy of a spiculated mass.

MAMMOGRAPHY: Preliminary left CC **(A)** and magnification CC spot **(B)** views show a small spiculated mass at the posterior edge of the parenchyma **(arrow)** laterally. A stereotactic pair **(C)** for targeting obtained with the aperture over the superior aspect of the breast shows the spiculated mass **(arrow)** on both images. The pre-fire set of stereotactic images **(D)** with the automated core needle in place shows the needle tip to lie just proximal to the center of the lesion on both images, which is a proper pre-fire position. Five core samples were obtained.

HISTOPATHOLOGY: Invasive ductal carcinoma.

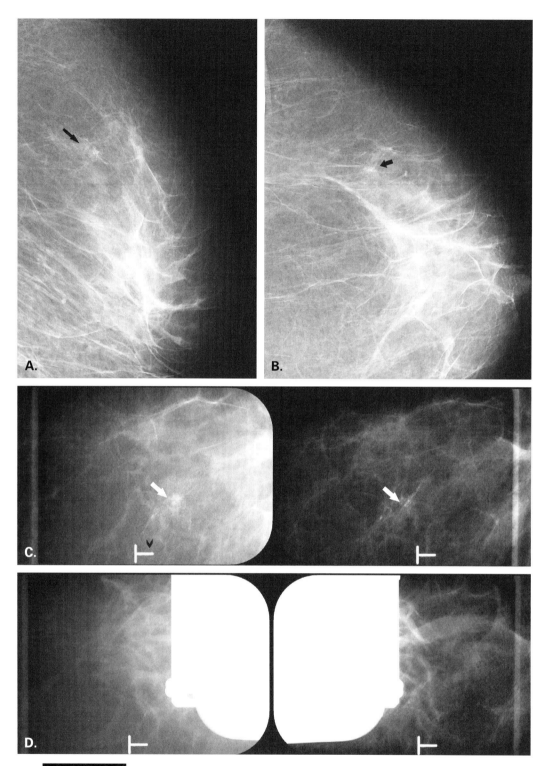

Figure 16.15

HISTORY: A 60-year-old woman with an abnormal screening mammogram, for additional evaluation.

MAMMOGRAPHY: Right magnification ML **(A)** and CC **(B)** views show scattered fibroglandular densities and clustered fine pleomorphic microcalcifications at 10 o'clock **(arrows)** that are suspicious for malignancy. Stereotactically guided vacuum-assisted biopsy was performed using an 11-gauge needle. Stereotactic pair **(C)** shows the microcalcifications **(arrow)** within the aperture, as well as the reference point in the unit **(arrowhead)**. After targeting the lesion, the needle has been positioned at $\Delta X = 0$, $\Delta Y = 0$, and $\Delta Z = 0$. In this position, the needle tip is at the leading edge of the abnormality on both views **(D)**. *(continued)*

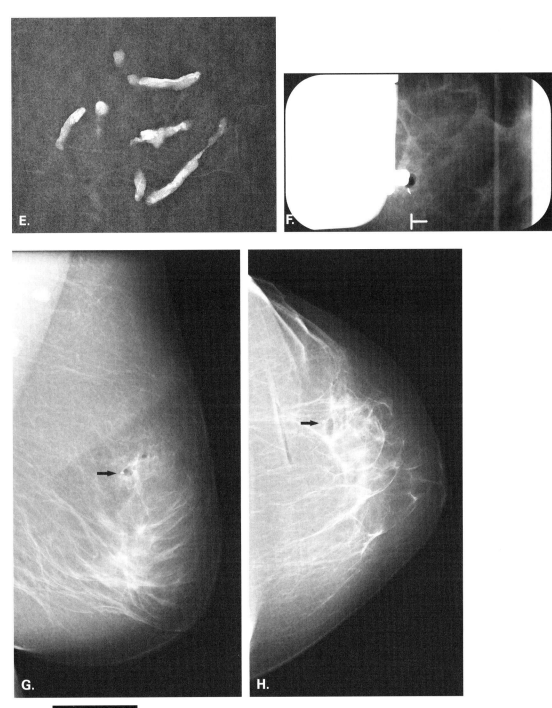

Figure 16.15 *(CONTINUED)*

Following sampling, the specimen radiograph **(E)** shows the calcifications to be included in the first cores. A clip was placed and a post-clip stereotactic image **(F)** shows that the calcifications have been removed, and the clip has been deployed. Post-clip mammography ML **(G)** and CC **(H)** views show the clip to be in accurate position **(arrows)** and that many of the calcifications have been removed. A small air pocket is present at the biopsy site.

HISTOPATHOLOGY: Ductal carcinoma in situ.

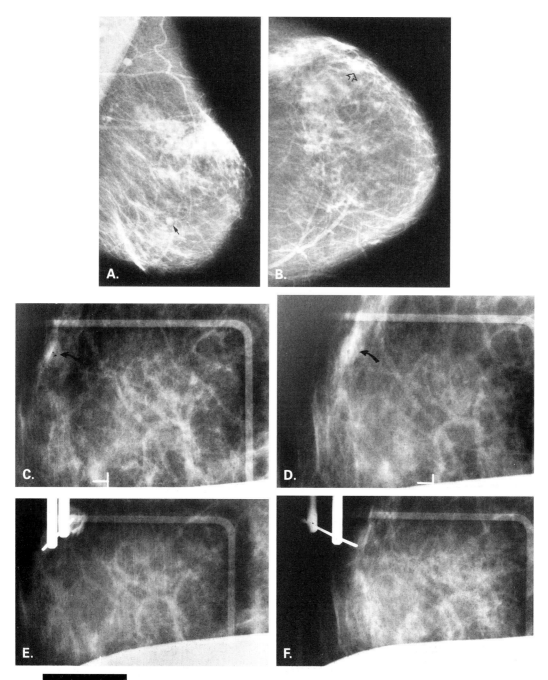

Figure 16.16

HISTORY: A 64-year-old G3, P2 woman with a positive family history of breast cancer, for screening.

MAMMOGRAPHY: Right MLO **(A)** and craniocaudal **(B)** preliminary stereotactic pair **(C** and **D)**, stereotactic pair with needle placement **(E** and **F)** from a stereotactically guided aspiration, and post-aspiration MLO **(G)** and craniocaudal **(H)** views. A relatively well-circumscribed 9-mm isodense mass nodule **(A** and **B)** is present in the right lower outer quadrant **(arrow)**. This nodule had developed since the previous study 3 years earlier. Ultrasound was performed and showed a small nodule to contain some internal echoes.

Stereotactically guided aspiration was performed to confirm that the new mammographic lesion was actually the small complicated cyst. Preliminary stereotactic pair **(C** and **D)** demonstrates the mass in the field and a dot marking the center **(arrow)** for targeting the coordinates of the lesion. Stereotactic pair views with the needle in place **(E** and **F)** show the needle within the nodule. Aspiration yielded 0.2 mL of clear fluid. *(continued)*

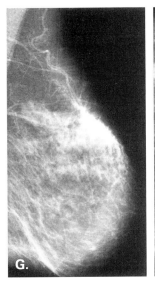
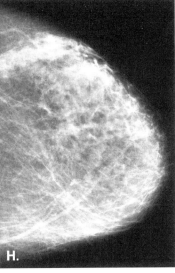

Figure 16.16 *(CONTINUED)*

Post-aspiration images MLO (**G**) and CC (**H**) demonstrate complete resolution of the nodule.

IMPRESSION: Simple cyst confirmed by stereotactically guided aspiration.

needle attached to a syringe is placed into the breast at this point and is slowly withdrawn while mild suction on the syringe is applied. When liquid is aspirated, the needle is held in place until aspiration is complete; the syringe is removed and replaced with a syringe containing a volume of room air, slightly less than the volume of fluid aspirated, and the air is injected into the cyst cavity (Fig. 16.19). If the fluid aspirated is bloody, it is sent for cytologic examination.

In mediolateral and craniocaudal projections, films are made immediately after injection of air. The walls of the cyst cavity should be thin and smooth (Fig. 16.20). Any intraluminal filling defect or focal irregularity of the wall is regarded with suspicion for an intracystic tumor. Benign intracystic papillomas and papillary carcinomas can be visualized in this way. If an intracystic abnormality is identified, excision of the lesion is indicated.

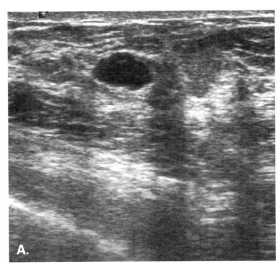
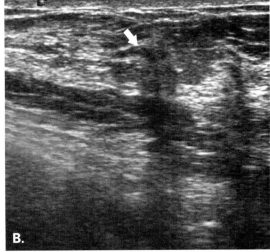

Figure 16.17

HISTORY: A 58-year-old woman with a history of complex cysts, for aspiration.

MAMMOGRAPHY: Right complicated cyst is seen on sonography, showing well-defined margins and low-level internal echoes. FNA was performed using a vertical approach and a 25-gauge needle. Post-aspiration image shows the cyst to have collapsed, and the needle tip is visible (**arrow**). Cloudy fluid was aspirated and sent for cytology.

CYTOLOGY: Scant amorphous debris.

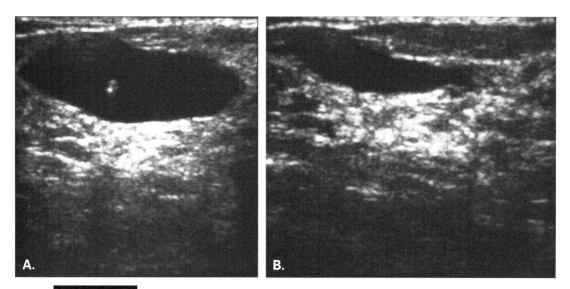

Figure 16.18

A symptomatic cyst is aspirated with ultrasound guidance, using a short-axis (vertical) approach. The needle tip is seen within the center of the cyst initially **(A)**. Clear fluid was aspirated, and the post-aspiration image **(B)** shows that the cyst has partially collapsed.

CORE BIOPSY

Core-needle biopsy can be performed using stereotactic, sonographic, or MRI guidance. Core-needle biopsy has evolved from the use of 18-gauge automated cutting needles to vacuum-assisted biopsy probes ranging from 14- to 8-gauge. With this evolution came the possibility of accurately diagnosing more types of mammographic abnormalities. One disadvantage of FNAB is the large number of nonspecific diagnoses, particularly for many benign lesions.

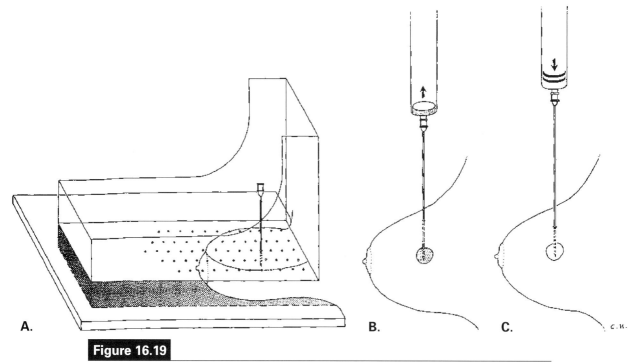

Figure 16.19

For pneumocystography under mammographic guidance, the needle is placed into the breast overlying the lesion to be aspirated **(A)**. The needle is slowly withdrawn into the lesion while aspiration is being performed **(B)** and, after aspiration is complete, air is injected **(C)**.

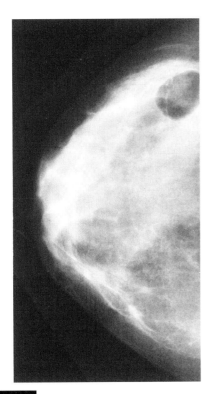

Figure 16.20

Left CC view from a pneumocystogram that was performed with mammographic guidance. The cyst has been drained and filled with air, showing a smooth, normal internal wall without filling defects.

With core-needle biopsy, specific histologies are obtainable from masses, focal asymmetries, and microcalcifications.

The size of the lesion no longer limits the ability to use core-needle biopsy, as it did initially. Mainero et al. (45)

found no significant relationship between lesion size and the ability to establish a specific diagnosis. In early series (46–49), before clips were available to mark the biopsy site, lesions less than 5 mm in size were not ideally biopsied percutaneously, since the entire mammographic lesion could be removed with the core needle. If the patient needed a subsequent excision, locating the original biopsy site was challenging and inaccurate. With the ability to deploy a clip, the biopsy of smaller lesions is feasible.

The diagnostic accuracy of a lesion biopsied using a core-needle technique is improved with an increase in the number of samples as well as increased experience in performing the procedure (50). Brenner et al. (50) found that more than 80% of the lesions (except for clustered microcalcifications) were diagnosed on the basis of two core samples; with five core samples, the accuracy was 98% for masses and 91% for calcifications (50). Liberman et al. (47) found that five cores taken with a 14-gauge automated needle yielded a diagnosis in 99% of masses but only 87% of calcifications.

Literature on the accuracy of needle biopsy has shown that the 14-gauge needle is superior to smaller needles for accuracy of diagnosis (51,52). The concept of the core needle is that it has an inner needle with a trough that pierces the tissue when the gun is fired. Instantaneously, the outer cutting cannula moves forward over the needle, transecting tissue that is contained in the trough. An example of the Bard (CR Bard, Cincinnati, OH) automated core needle is shown in Figure 16.21.

Another type of cutting needle, the Cassi (Sanarus Medical Inc., Pleasanton, CA), utilizes a freeze-stick concept (Fig. 16.22). The sharp inner stylet is advanced into the lesion, a quick freeze around the needle using CO_2 is

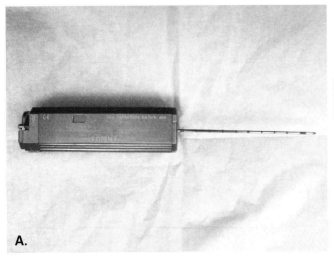

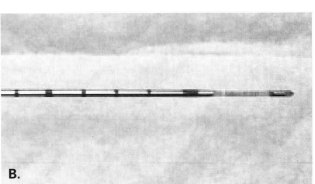

A.　　　　　　　　　　　　　　　　　　　　　**B.**

Figure 16.21

A: Automated core-needle and biopsy gun (Bard, CR Bard, Inc., Covington, GA). The 14-gauge needle is placed in the spring-loaded gun. **B:** The trough of the needle when open.

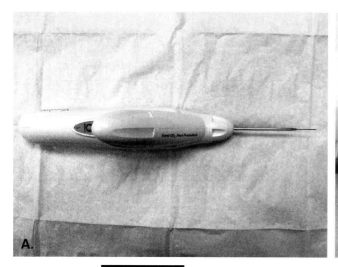
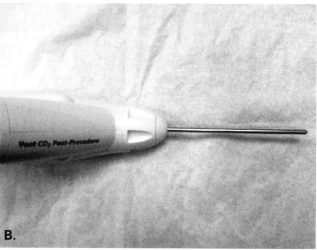

Figure 16.22

Freeze-stick device for breast biopsy (Cassi, Sanarus Medical, Inc., Pleasanton, CA). The tip is inserted under ultrasound guidance (A). CO_2 is expelled to freeze the tissue immediately around the needle, and the outer cannula fires forward (B).

applied to the hold the lesion, and the outer cutting cannula fires forward, severing the tissue around the stylet.

Vacuum-assisted probes were developed in the mid 1990s, the first being the Mammotome (Ethicon Endo-Surgery, Cincinnati, OH) (Fig. 16.23). This directional, vacuum-assisted device is fired into position so that its trough is in the middle of the lesion. The vacuum is then applied to pull the tissue into the trough of the needle and to transport it back up into the probe. The tissue is retrieved from a specimen chamber external to the breast; therefore, the probe stays in the breast while multiple

samples are acquired. The probe is rotated circumferentially as samples are acquired, thereby optimizing the volume of tissue acquired and the accuracy of the procedure. These probes range from 14 to 8 gauge in diameter.

In comparison with the automated 14-gauge core needles, the individual core specimen weights are much greater with the Mammotome. Burbank (53) reported mean specimen weights of 96 mg from the 11-gauge Mammotome probe versus 40 mg from the 14-gauge probe. Berg et al. (54) found the mean weights to be 17.7 mg from the automated 14-gauge core needle, 36.8 mg from the

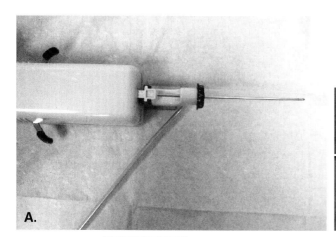
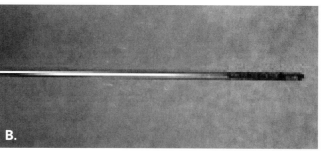

Figure 16.23

Vacuum-assisted biopsy probe (Mammotome, Ethicon Endo-Surgery, Cincinnati, OH. The open trough has small perforations within it that are used for applying suction and for draining fluid.

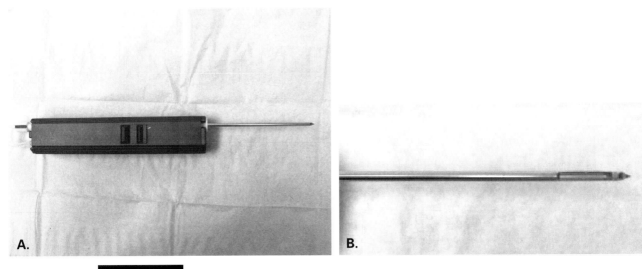

Vacuum-assisted, hand-held device (Vacora, CR Bard, Covington, GA). The 10-gauge needle is loaded in a gun that has a 30-cc syringe that provides suction for one sample (**A**). The needle is withdrawn, the sample collected, and the needle repositioned for additional samples. The open trough of the needle, which has a scalpel tip, is shown in **B**.

14-gauge directional vacuum-assisted probe, and 94.4 mg from the 11-gauge Mammotome probe.

Since the Mammotome was developed, several other vacuum-assisted probes are available. A vacuum-assisted probe that allows for only individual sampling is the Vacora (CR Bard, Inc., Covington, GA) (Fig. 16.24). This 10-gauge probe has a scalpel tip and is loaded into a gun that contains a 30-cc syringe that provides suction. One specimen is acquired, and the needle is removed from the breast; the specimen is retrieved and the needle must be repositioned for additional sampling. This type of needle is compatible with a coaxial cannula that facilitates repositioning the needle in the breast. The Vacora can be used with stereotactic or sonographic guidance.

Other directional, multisample probes are the EnCor (SenoRx Inc., Aliso Viejo, CA) and Suros (Suros Surgical Systems, Inc., Indianapolis, IN) types. In both cases, the system is closed, so that the individual specimens are not retrieved manually from the collection chamber, as they are with the Mammotome. Instead, the vacuum pulls the specimen back into a closed collection chamber that is dismounted from the unit at the termination of the procedure (Fig. 16.25).

Clip Placement

A clip is placed at the biopsy site to mark the area for future reference. If the lesion requires subsequent surgical excision, the clip marks the site for the needle localization. This is particularly important for small lesions, in which the entire mammographic abnormality may be removed by the core needle. A clip at a site of residual calcifications is also helpful on subsequent mammography to verify that the area had already been biopsied. In the case of larger cancers that might be treated first with neoadjuvant chemotherapy to reduce their size prior to surgery, the placement of a clip may be very important to document the location of the tumor (55). At times, the regression of the tumor is so great after the administration of the chemotherapy that the mass is no longer visible on mammography or ultrasound.

Clips may be deployed through vacuum-assisted probes, or they may be placed independently via an introducer. It is important to have a clear understanding of how the clip deploys so that it will be placed in an accurate position. With some types of clips that are inserted through the vacuum-assisted probes under stereotactic guidance, the probe must be withdrawn slightly so that the clip deploys in the middle of the biopsy cavity.

Clips do not necessarily deploy accurately, even though all the proper steps are followed. Rosen et al. (56) reported that 28% of clips were more than 1 cm from the target on at least one post-biopsy image. The migration of clips has occurred uncommonly, as documented on short- and long-term follow-up mammography (57–59). For these reasons, it is imperative that a post-procedure mammogram be obtained to verify the location of the clip relative to the biopsy site. This relationship should be described in the report. If any subsequent procedures are needed, the localization can be performed more accurately.

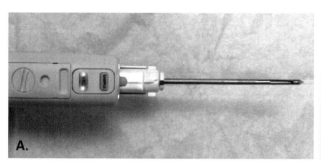
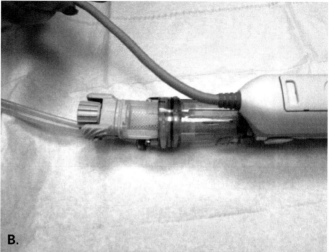

Figure 16.25

A vacuum-assisted system for ultrasound or stereotactic breast biopsy **(A)** (EnCor, SenoRx, Aliso Viejo, CA) has a closed system for specimen retrieval **(B)**.

Complications of Core Biopsy

Major complications of core-needle biopsy of the breast are rare. Infection can occur uncommonly and is managed with antibiotics. A clinically important hematoma has been described in less than 1% of patients in several series (46,60,61). The development of a large post-biopsy hematoma can present a clinical problem if the lesion is malignant and its visibility is obliterated by the fluid collection. This can result in a potential delay in surgery until the hematoma resorbs (62), if no clip has been placed to indicate the biopsy site.

An unusual complication of core biopsy is a milk fistula. This connection between the skin and the milk duct can occur if biopsy is performed in a lactating patient. Because of this, FNAB is performed first to attempt diagnosis in a lactating patient (63), and core biopsy is avoided.

Tumor cells can be displaced during core-needle biopsy. Actual seeding of the needle tract has only been reported once (64). Harter et al. (64) reported a case of seeding of the needle tract with mucinous carcinoma cells that were identified 2 weeks after a core biopsy performed with a 14-gauge core needle. Given the vast number of core biopsies that have been performed since then, this risk of seeding is exceedingly low.

A more commonly observed finding, however, is known as epithelial displacement, which can occur during core biopsy of the breast. Youngson et al. (65) described the presence of displaced epithelial fragments in the fibrous breast tissue or fat, adjacent to or within the tract of a core-needle biopsy. These epithelial fragments can mimic foci of invasion, but importantly, they are associated with the traumatic needle effect and, in these cases, no other true invasion is found elsewhere in the specimen. Epithelial cell displacement has been observed in benign lesions as well as malignancy, particularly in papillary ductal hyperplasia and papilloma (66). The viability of such displaced cells is not known.

Diaz et al. (67) studied of 352 cancer excisions in patients who had undergone core biopsy for diagnosis. The authors found that tumor cell displacement occurred in 32% of patients, and the incidence and amount of tumor cell displacement was inversely related to the interval between core biopsy and excision. Tumor cell displacement was observed in 37% of specimens previously biopsied with an automated gun versus 23% of specimens obtained via a vacuum-assisted needle. Tumor cell displacement was seen in 42% of patients who underwent excision in less than 15 days from the core biopsy, compared with only 15% of patients who underwent surgery more than 28 days from biopsy. This relation suggested than the displaced cells do not survive (67).

Pathologic Correlation

The performance of a successful core-needle biopsy is usually straightforward. The management of the results, however, can be challenging. A clear understanding before the procedure of what the anticipated results may be is extremely helpful when the pathology report arrives. This necessitates that a careful review of the imaging study is performed to characterize the lesion and to anticipate the outcome. The procedure is far from complete with the dictation of a report describing the procedure. The procedure is complete once the pathology report has been reviewed, correlated with the mammographic findings, the management recommendation is determined, and the patient and referring physician have been notified. The radiologist determines if the radiologic and pathologic findings are concordant and if surgical excision or re-biopsy are necessary (48,68).

Providing the pathologist with clinical information, the radiologic impression and whether calcifications are present is very helpful. The presence of calcifications should prompt the pathologist to search specifically for calcium to identify the area of interest within the various cores.

Calcification retrieval is imperative when the biopsy is performed for microcalcifications. Specimen radiography is performed during the procedure to confirm that calcifications have been removed (69). The 14-gauge Mammotome has been shown (70) to be superior to the 14-gauge automated needle in the ability to obtain calcifications on the specimen radiography (100% versus 91% respectively). Jackman et al. (71) reported calcification retrieval in 94% of 14-gauge automated core biopsies, 99% of 14-gauge directional vacuum-assisted biopsies, and >99% of 11-gauge vacuum-assisted biopsies. Liberman et al. (72) reported failure to remove calcifications in 5% of lesions; the lack of calcifications on specimen films was more likely in lesions <5 mm in size, for amorphous calcifications, and in cases where the probe was fired outside the breast (72).

If calcifications are not present on the specimen radiography, a review of the stereotactic images should be made to determine if the needle position is accurate. A repeat stereotactic pair may be helpful as well. Additional sampling is needed to try to obtain the calcifications.

If calcifications are present on specimen radiography, the case is completed and the tissue is sent to the laboratory. The pathologist must search the slides for calcifications to assure that the region of interest is included in his review. If no calcifications are identified initially, polarized light is used to try to identify calcium oxalate crystals, because calcium oxalate is not readily identifiable on hematoxylin and eosin staining. If no calcium is identified at this point, the tissue block is releveled, and more slides are prepared and stained. If, after the block is exhausted, no additional levels can be made, and no calcium is identified, the management of the case falls back to the radiologist and depends on the specimen radiography. When specimen radiography clearly shows the calcifications, and the review of the post-procedure mammogram shows that calcifications have been removed, the patient may be followed with mammography at 6 months. The lack of visualization of the calcium by the pathologist may have been the result of two problems: The microtome used for sectioning the tissue block can

hit a large calcification and pop it out of the tissue, or the calcification can float out of the tissue when it is stored in the formalin for an extended period prior to sectioning (73). An algorithm for the management of calcifications is shown in Figure 16.26.

When percutaneous biopsy yields a diagnosis of a high-risk lesion, surgical excision is performed. The presence of atypical ductal hyperplasia (ADH) should lead to surgical excision of the lesion (Fig. 16.27). Some controversy has arisen about lobular carcinoma in situ (LCIS), atypical lobular hyperplasia (ALH) radial scar, papillary lesions, and atypical columnar cell lesions, but most radiologists recommend excision of these. One of the reasons to excise a high-risk lesion is that the core biopsy may underestimate the disease, and therefore, excision of the remainder of the lesion may yield carcinoma. The other reason is to excise higher-risk tissue that has a greater potential to become malignant.

ADH is a proliferative lesion in the duct that has an appearance very similar to low grade ductal carcinoma in situ (DCIS). The distinction between ADH and DCIS may be determined in some cases by the number of ducts involved. A few ducts may be called ADH, but a more extensive lesion may be called DCIS. Therefore, in the cases of microcalcifications that are actually low-grade DCIS, acquiring a larger volume of tissue samples is important for a proper diagnosis. Underestimation rates for ADH vary with the type of needle used, ranging from 15% to 50% (74–81). With directional vacuum-assisted biopsy, the underestimation rate of ADH is less than it is with an automated core needle (74).

In a review of multiple series, Reynolds (75) found that of 630 ADH lesions, 37% were malignant on excision. Findings on excision were DCIS (76%) and invasive ductal carcinoma (24%). The automated 14-gauge core-needle biopsies were associated with an underestimation rate of 41% on average, whereas the vacuum-assisted 14- and 11-gauge probes are associated with cancer in 15% of cases. Jackman (76) reported an underestimation rate for ADH with automated core biopsy of 58%. Darling et al. (77) found the underestimation rate for ADH to be less with the 11-gauge vacuum probe than with the 14-gauge probe. Jackman et al. (78) reported an underestimation rate of DCIS to be 1.5 times more frequent when 10 or fewer specimens were obtained, than when more than 10 were taken.

When DCIS is found at stereotactic core-needle biopsy, approximately 20% to 25% of cases yield invasive carcinoma at surgical excision (82–84). Brem et al. (85) showed that the accuracy of diagnosis of invasive breast cancer was greater in lesions <30 mm. In lesions 30 mm or larger, the underestimation rate for DCIS was 43%. Like ADH, the 11-gauge probe improved the underestimation rate for DCIS, but 15% of the cases of DCIS were found by Won et al. (83) to be invasive at surgery.

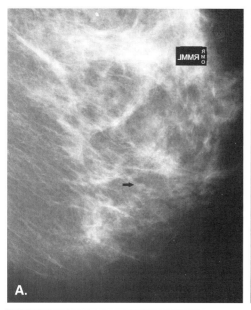

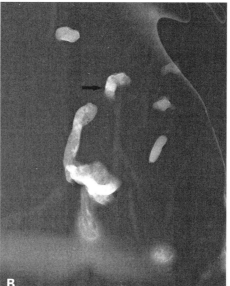

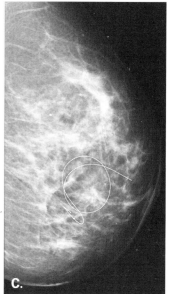

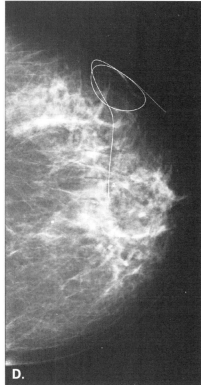

Figure 16.26

HISTORY: A 48-year-old woman recalled from screening for right breast microcalcifications.

MAMMOGRAPHY: Right magnification ML view **(A)** shows clustered amorphous microcalcifications in the inferior aspect of the breast **(arrow).** Stereotactic biopsy was performed with vacuum-assistance and 12 samples were acquired. Specimen radiography **(B)** showed the microcalcifications within the cores. Pathology showed atypical ductal hyperplasia and, because of this high-risk result, excision was recommended. Right ML **(C)** and CC **(D)** views from the needle localization show that the hookwire is in position at the clip placed during the biopsy procedure.

HISTOPATHOLOGY: Ductal carcinoma in situ, (initially called ADH on core biopsy).

Although the management of ALH or LCIS on percutaneous biopsy has been somewhat debatable, in a review of 35 patients with lobular neoplasia (LCIS or ALH), 17% were upgraded to DCIS or invasive cancer at excision (86). Based on this, the authors recommended surgical excision.

Radial scar is a proliferative lesion that may include ductal hyperplasia, atypical hyperplasia, or even DCIS. The rate of carcinoma found at radial-scar excision has

been reported to range from 0% to 40% (68). The risk of malignancy has been shown to be highest when the radial scar is associated with atypia.

Asymptomatic papillary lesions identified on core biopsy are also controversial (87–89). When atypia is present within a papilloma, the risk of malignancy is higher, and surgical excision is performed. Several series support the follow-up of patients with a core biopsy diagnosis of papilloma without atypia (89,90). A relationship also may

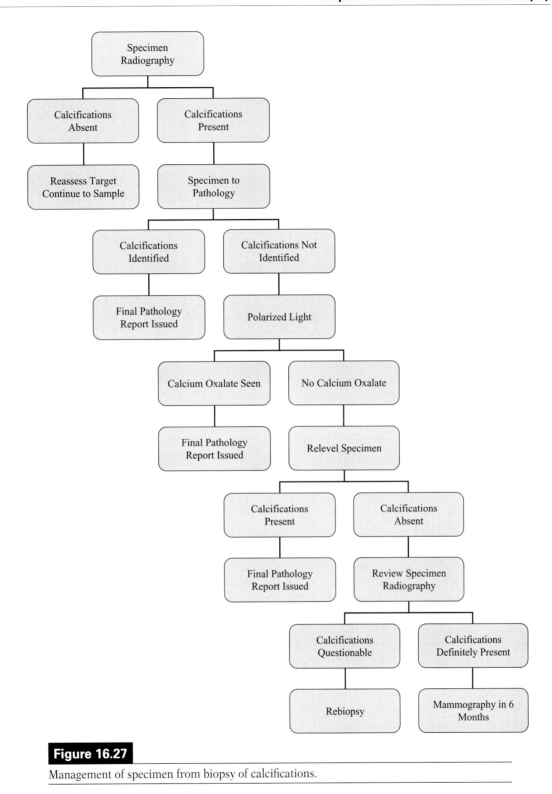

Figure 16.27

Management of specimen from biopsy of calcifications.

exist between sclerotic papillomas or micropapillomas and increased likelihood of malignancy on excision (89).

Columnar cell lesions include a wide variety of pathologic lesions characterized by columnar cells that line the terminal duct lobular unit. These etiologies range from columnar cell alternation of the lobules to DCIS with columnar cell features (68). When columnar cell change is associated with atypia, the management of this diagnosis on core biopsy is similar to that of atypical ductal hyperplasia—namely, excision (68).

Most often a fibroadenoma is clearly defined as such on core biopsy, and no further management is necessary.

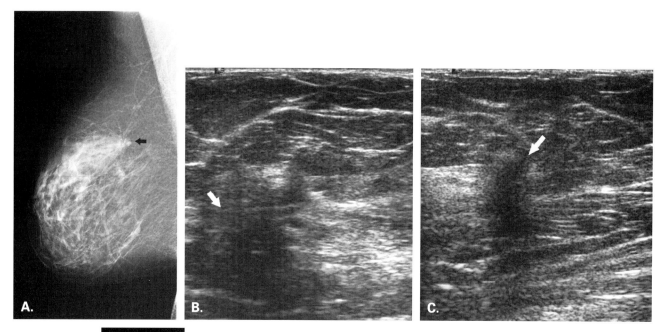

Figure 16.28

HISTORY: A 49-year-old for routine screening mammogram.

MAMMOGRAPHY: Left MLO **(A)** views show a small spiculated mass **(arrow)** in the left upper outer quadrant, highly suspicious for malignancy. The lesion was identified on ultrasound **(B)** **(arrow)**. Core biopsy was performed using an automated core 14-gauge needle **(C)**, showing the needle in position **(arrow)**. Pathology from the core biopsy showed fibrocystic change. Because the pathologic finding is not concordant with the mammographic finding, re-biopsy or excision was recommended.

HISTOPATHOLOGY: Invasive ductal carcinoma (initially benign on core biopsy and nonconcordant).

However, at times, a fibroadenoma can have a very cellular stroma that may raise the question or possibility of a phyllodes tumor. If this question is raised by the pathologist, excision of the entire lesion is performed.

An assessment for concordance determines if the lesion has been adequately sampled and diagnosed correctly. With FNAB, the negative cytologic aspiration in the face of a suspicious palpable mass prompts further tissue sampling, because the results are nonconcordant and the false-negative rate of FNAB is not insignificant. Percutaneous core biopsy has a greater degree of accuracy than FNAB, but it is not 100% accurate. Therefore, if the lesion is a BIRADS 5 mass or area of calcifications, for example, and the result is benign, one must consider carefully whether to follow the patient. Sclerosing adenosis can produce a small spiculated lesion that can be a concordant pathology. However, a spiculated mass that is called, for example, fibroadenoma or fibrocystic change, is not concordant (Fig. 16.28). Also, sufficiency of sampling must be considered. A dense mass should not yield "fat with scattered stromal elements" as the pathologic results.

The radiologist should also not hesitate to call the pathologist to discuss any concerns about the case. The anticipated malignant diagnosis that is not confirmed on the pathology report might prompt a conversation with the pathologist and a re-look at the slides prior to a re-biopsy. Sometimes additional leveling will reveal the lesion.

The correlation of the radiologic and pathologic findings is one of the key components of a successful percutaneous breast program. A careful selection of the type of procedure and skill in performing it contribute to the successful diagnosis of nonpalpable breast lesions.

REFERENCES

1. Bolmgren J, Jacobson B, Nordenstrom B. Stereotactic instrument for needle biopsy of the breast. *AJR Am J Roentgenol* 1997;129:121–125.
2. Gisvold JJ, Goellner JR, Grant CS, et al. Breast biopsy: a comparative study of stereotaxically guided core and excisional techniques. *AJR Am J Roentgenol* 1994;162:815–820.
3. Parker SH, Lovin JD, Jobe WE, et al. Stereotactic breast biopsy with a biopsy gun. *Radiology* 1990;176:741–747.
4. Elvecrog EL, Lechner MC, Nelson MT. Nonpalpable breast lesions: correlation of stereotaxic large-core needle biopsy and surgical biopsy results. *Radiology* 1993;188(2):453–455.

5. Parker SH, Lovin JD, Jobe WE, et al. Nonpalpable breast lesions: stereotactic automated large-core biopsies. *Radiology* 1991;180:403–407.

6. Liberman L, Gougoutas CA, Zakowski MF. Calcifications highly suggestive of malignancy: comparison of breast biopsy methods. *AJR Am J Roentgenol* 2001;177:165–172.

7. King TA, Cederbom GJ, Champaign JL, et al. A core breast biopsy diagnosis of invasive carcinoma allows for definitive surgical treatment planning. *Am J Surg* 1998;176:497–501.

8. Liberman L, LaTrenta LR, Dershaw DD, et al. Impact of core biopsy on the surgical management of impalpable breast cancer. *AJR Am J Roentgenol* 1997;168:495–499.

9. Jackman RJ, Mazoni FA, Finkelstein SI, Shepard MJ. Benefits of diagnosing nonpalpable breast cancer with stereotactic large-core needle biopsy: lower costs and fewer operations. *Radiology* 1996;201(p):311.

10. Rosenblatt R, Fineberg SA, Sparano JA. Stereotactic core needle biopsy of multiple sites in the breast: efficacy and effect on patient care. *Radiology* 1996;201:67–70.

11. Lee CH, Egglin TK, Philpotts L, et al. Cost-effectiveness of stereotactic core needle biopsy: analysis by means of mammographic findings. *Radiology* 1997;202:849–854.

12. Lindfors KK, Rosenquist CJ. Needle core biopsy guided with mammography: a study of cost-effectiveness. *Radiology* 1994;190:217–222.

13. Liberman L, Fahs MC, Dershaw DD, et al. Impact of stereotaxic core biopsy on cost of diagnosis. *Radiology* 1995;195:633–637.

14. Lind DS, Minter R, Steinbach B, et al. Stereotactic core biopsy reduces the re-excision rate and the cost of mammographically detected cancer. *Surg J Research* 1998;78:23–26.

15. Comstock CE. US-guided interventional procedures. In: Feig SA, ed. *Breast Imaging: Categorical in Diagnostic Radiologic*. Oak Brook, IL: RSNA; 2005:155–168.

16. Gordon PB, Goldenberg SL, Chan NHL. Solid breast lesions: diagnosis with US-guided fine-needle aspiration biopsy. *Radiology* 1993;189:573–580.

17. Parker SH, Jobe WE, Dennis MA, et al. US-guided automated large-core breast biopsy. *Radiology* 1993;187:507–511.

18. Simon JR, Kalbhen CL, Cooper RA, et al. Accuracy and complication rates of US-guided vacuum-assisted core breast biopsy: initial results. *Radiology* 2000;215:694–697.

19. Fornage BD, Coan JD, David CL. Ultrasound-guided needle biopsy of the breast and other interventional procedures. *Radiol Clin NA* 1992;30:167–185.

20. Caines JS, McPhee MD, Konok GP, et al. Stereotaxic needle core biopsy of breast lesions using a regular mammographic table with an adaptable stereotactic device. *AJR Am J Roentgenol* 1994;163:317–321.

21. Cousins JF, Wayland AD, Shaw de Paredes E. Stereotactic breast units: pros and cons. *Applied Radiol* 1998;27:8–14.

22. Welle GJ, Clark M, Loos S, et al. Stereotactic breast biopsy: recumbent biopsy using add-on upright equipment. *AJR Am J Roentgenol* 2000;175:59–63.

23. Wanebo HJ, Feldman PS, Wilhelm MC, et al. Fine needle aspiration cytology in lieu of open biopsy in management of primary breast cancer. *Ann Surg* 1984;199:569–579.

24. Palombini L, Fulciniti F, Vetrani A, et al. Fine needle aspiration biopsy of breast masses. *Cancer* 1988;61:2273–2277.

25. Kopans DB. Fine-needle aspiration of clinically occult breast lesions. *Radiology* 1989;170:313–314.

26. Lee KR, Foster RS, Papillo JL. Fine needle aspiration of the breast: importance of aspirator. *Acta Cytol* 1987;31:281–284.

27. Helvie MA, Baker DE, Adler DD, et al. Radiographically guided fine-needle aspiration of nonpalpable breast lesions. *Radiology* 1990;174:657–661.

28. Ciatto S, Del Turco MR, Bravetti P. Nonpalpable breast lesions: stereotaxis fine-needle aspiration cytology. *Radiology* 1989;173:57–59.

29. Dowlatshahi K, Gent HJ, Schmidt R, et al. Nonpalpable breast tumors: diagnosis with stereotaxis localization and fine-needle aspiration. *Radiology* 1989;170:427–433.

30. Masood S, Frykberg ER, McLellan GL, et al. Prospective evaluation of nonpalpable breast lesions. *Cancer* 1990;66:1480–1487.

31. Fajardo LL, Davis JR, Wiens JJ, Trego DC. Mammography-guided stereotactic fine-needle aspiration cytology of nonpalpable breast lesions: prospective comparison with surgical biopsy results. *AJR Am J Roentgenol* 1990;155:977–981.

32. Azavedo E, Svane G, Auer G. Stereotactic fine-needle biopsy in 2,594 mammographically detected nonpalpable lesions. *Lancet* 1989;1:1033–1035.

33. Lofgren M, Andersson I, Bondeson L, Lindholm K. X-ray guided fine-needle aspiration for the cytologic diagnosis of nonpalpable breast lesions. *Cancer* 1988;61:1032–1037.

34. Dent DM, Kirkpatrick AE, McGoogan E, et al. Stereotaxic localization and aspiration cytology of impalpable breast lesions. *Clin Radiol* 1989;40:380–382.

35. Evans WP, Cade SH. Needle localization and fine-needle aspiration biopsy of nonpalpable breast lesions with use of standard and stereotactic equipment. *Radiology* 1989;173:53–56.

36. Hann L, Ducatman BS, Wang HH, et al. Nonpalpable breast lesions: evaluation by means of fine-needle aspiration cytology. *Radiology* 1989;171:373–376.

37. Bibbo M, Scheiber M, Cajulis R, et al. Stereotaxic fine-needle aspiration cytology of clinically occult malignant and premalignant breast lesions. *Acta Cytol* 1988;32:193–201.

38. Lofgren M, Andersson I, Lindholm K. Stereotactic fine-needle aspiration for cytologic diagnosis of nonpalpable breast lesions. *AJR Am J Roentgenol* 1990;154:1191–1195.

39. Ciatto S, Catarzi S, Morrone, et al. Fine-needle aspiration cytology of nonpalpable breast lesions: US versus stereotaxic guidance. *Radiology* 1993;188:195–198.

40. Tabar L, Pentek Z, Dean PB. The diagnostic and therapeutic value of breast cyst puncture and pneumocystography. *Radiology* 1981;141:659–663.

41. Haagensen CD. *Disease of the Breast*. Philadelphia: WB Saunders, 1971.

42. Gatchell FG, Dockerty MB, Clagett OT. Intracystic carcinoma of the breast. *Surg Gynecol Obstet* 1958;106:347–352.

43. Hoeffken W, Hintzen C. Die diagnostik der mammazysten durch mammographie und pneumozystographie. *ROFO* 1970;112:9–18.

44. Fornage BD, Faroux MJ, Simatos A. Breast masses: ultrasound-guided fine-needle aspiration biopsy. *Radiology* 1987;162:409–414.

45. Mainiero MB, Philpotts LE, Lee CH, et al. Stereotaxic core needle biopsy breast microcalcifications: correlation of target accuracy and diagnosis with lesion size. *Radiology* 1996;198:665–669.

46. Sullivan DC. Needle core biopsy of mammographic lesions. *AJR Am J Roentgenol* 1994;162:601–608.

47. Liberman L, Dershaw DD, Rosen PP, et al. Stereotaxic 14-gauge breast biopsy: how many core biopsy specimens are needed? *Radiology* 1994;192:793–795.

48. Huynh PT, Shaw de Paredes E. Stereotactic large-gauge core biopsy of the breast: a review. *Radiologist* 1996;3(6):279–287.

49. Shaw de Paredes E, Langer TG, Cousins J. Interventional breast procedures. *Curr Prob Diag Radiol* 1998;27(5):133–184.

50. Brenner RJ, Fajardo L, Fisher PR, et al. Percutaneous core biopsy of the breast: effect of operator experience and number of samples on diagnostic accuracy. *AJR Am J Roentgenol* 1996;166:341–346.

51. Helbich TH, Rudas M, Haitek A, et al. Evaluation of needle size for breast biopsy: comparison of 14-, 16-, and 18-gauge biopsy needles. *AJR Am J Roentgenol* 1998;171:59–63.

52. Nath ME, Robinson TM, Tobon H, et al. Automated large-core needle biopsy of surgically removed breast lesions: comparison of samples obtained with 14-, 16-, and 18-gauge needles. *Radiology* 1995;197:739–742.

53. Burbank F. Stereotactic breast biopsy: comparison of 14- and 11- gauge Mammotome probe performance and complication rates. *Am Surg* 1997;63:988–995.

54. Berg WA, Krebs TL, Campassi C, et al. Evaluation of 14- and 11- gauge directional, vacuum-assisted biopsy probes and 14-gauge biopsy guns in a breast parenchymal model. *Radiology* 1997;205:203–208.

55. Reynolds HE, Lesnefsky MH, Jackson VP. Tumor marking before primary chemotherapy for breast cancer. *AJR Am J Roentgenol* 1999;173:919–920.

56. Rosen EL, Vo TT. Metallic clip displacement during stereotactic breast biopsy: retrospective analysis. *Radiology* 2001; 218:510–516.

57. Philpotts LE, Lee CH. Clip migration after 11-gauge vacuum-assisted stereotactic biopsy case report. *Radiology* 2002;222: 794–796.

58. Birdwell RL, Jackman RJ. Clip or marker migration 5-10 weeks after stereotactic 11-gauge vacuum-assisted breast biopsy: report of two cases. *Radiology* 2003;229:541–544.

59. Harris AT. Clip migration within 8 days of 11-gauge vacuum-assisted stereotactic breast biopsy: case report. *Radiology* 2003;228:525–554.

60. Parker SH, Burbank F, Jackman RJ, et al. Percutaneous large-core beast biopsy: a multi-institutional study. *Radiology* 1994;193:359–364.

61. Jackman RJ, Nowels LW, Shepard MJ, et al. Stereotaxic large-core needle biopsy of 450 nonpalpable breast lesions with surgical correlation in lesions with cancer or atypical hyperplasia. *Radiology* 1994;193:91–95.

62. Deutch BM, Schwartz MR, Fodera T, et al. Stereotactic core breast biopsy of a minimal carcinoma complicated by a large hematoma: a management dilemma. *Radiology* 1997;202: 431–433.

63. Schackmuth EM, Harlow CL, Norton LW. Milk fistula: a complication after core breast biopsy. *AJR Am J Roentgenol* 1993;161:961–962.

64. Harter LP, Curtis JS, Ponto G, et al. Malignant seeding of the needle track during stereotaxis core needle breast biopsy. *Radiology* 1992;185:713–714.

65. Youngson BJ, Liberman L, Rosen PP. Displacement of carcinomatous epithelium in surgical breast specimens following stereotaxic core biopsy. *Am J Clin Pathol* 1995;103: 598–602.

66. Youngson BJ, Cranor M, Rosen PP. Epithelial displacement in surgical breast specimens following needling procedures. *Am J Surg Pathol* 1994;18(9):896–903.

67. Diaz LK, Wiley EL, Venta LA. Are malignant cells displaced by large-gauge needle core biopsy of the breast? *AJR Am J Roentgenol* 1999;173:1303–1313.

68. Bassett LW, Apple SK, Hoyt AC. Breast core needle biopsy: imaging-pathology assessment of results In: Feig SA, ed. *Breast Imaging: Categorical in Diagnostic Radiologic*. Oak Brook, IL: RSNA; 2005:55–56.

69. Liberman L, Evans WP, Dershaw DD, et al. Radiography of microcalcifications in stereotaxic mammary core biopsy specimens. *Radiology* 1994;190:223–225.

70. Meyer JE, Smith DN, DiPiro PJ, et al. Stereotactic breast biopsy of clustered microcalcifications with a directional vacuum-assisted device. *Radiology* 1997;204:575–576.

71. Jackman RJ, Burbank FH, Parker SH, et al. Accuracy of sampling microcalcification by three stereotactic breast biopsy methods. *Radiology* 1997;205(p):325.

72. Liberman L, Smolkin JH, Dershaw DD, et al. Calcification retrieval at stereotactic, 11-gauge, directional, vacuum-assisted breast biopsy. *Radiology* 1998;208:251–260.

73. Moritz JD, Luftner-Nagel S, Westerhof JP. Microcalcifications in breast core biopsy specimens: disappearance at radiography after storage in formaldehyde. *Radiology* 1996;200:361–363.

74. Burbank F. Stereotactic breast biopsy of atypical ductal hyperplasia and ductal carcinoma is situ lesions: improved accuracy with directional, vacuum-assisted biopsy. *Radiology* 1997;202:843–847.

75. Reynolds HE. Core needle biopsy of challenging benign breast conditions: a comprehensive literature review. *AJR Am J Roentgenol* 2000;174:1245–1245.

76. Jackman RJ, Nowels KW, Rodriguez-Soto J, et al. Stereotactic, automated, large-core needle biopsy of nonpalpable breast lesions: false-negative and histologic underestimation rates after long-term follow-up. *Radiology* 1999;210:799–805.

77. Darling MLR, Smith DN, Lester SC, et al. Atypical ductal hyperplasia and ductal carcinoma in situ as revealed by large-core needle breast biopsy: results of surgical excision. *AJR Am J Roentgenol* 2000;175:1341–1346.

78. Jackman RJ, Burbank F, Parker SH, et al. Stereotactic breast biopsy of nonpalpable lesions: determinants of ductal carcinoma in situ underestimation rates. *Radiology* 2001;218: 497–502.

79. Philpotts LE, Lee CH, Horvath LJ, et al. Underestimation of breast cancer with 11-gauge vacuum suction biopsy. *AJR Am J Roentgenol* 2000;175:1047–1050.

80. Liberman L, Dershaw DD, Glassman JR, et al. Analysis of cancers not diagnosed at stereotactic core breast biopsy. *Radiology* 1997;203:151–157.

81. Brem RF, Behrndt VS, Sanow L, et al. Atypical ductal hyperplasia: histologic underestimation of carcinoma in tissue harvested from impalpable breast lesions using 11-gauge stereotactically guided directional vacuum-assisted biopsy. *AJR Am J Roentgenol* 1999;172:1405–1407.

82. Liberman L, Dershaw DD, Rosen PP, et al. Stereotaxic core biopsy of breast carcinoma: accuracy at predicting invasion. *Radiology* 1995;194:379–381.

83. Won B, Reynolds HE, Lazaridis CL, et al. Stereotactic biopsy ductal carcinoma in situ of the breast using an 11-gauge vacuum-assisted device: persistent underestimation of disease. *AJR Am J Roentgenol* 1999;173:227;229.

84. Lee CH, Carter D, Philpotts LE, et al. Ductal carcinoma in situ diagnosed with stereotactic core needle biopsy: can invasion be predicted? *Radiology* 2000;217:466–470.

85. Brem RF, Schoonjans JM, Goodman SN, et al. Nonpalpable breast cancer: percutaneous diagnosis with 11- and 8-gauge stereotactic vacuum-assisted biopsy devices. *Radiology* 2001; 219:793–796.

86. Foster MC, Helvie MA, Gregory NE, et al. Lobular carcinoma in situ or atypical lobular hyperplasia at core-needle biopsy: is excisional biopsy necessary? *Radiology* 2006;231(3):813–819.

87. Mercado CL, Hamele-Bena J, Singer C, et al. Papillary lesions of the breast: evaluation with stereotactic directional vacuum-assisted biopsy. *Radiology* 2001;221:650–655.

88. Philpotts LE, Shaheen NA, Jain KS, et al. Uncommon high-risk lesions of the breast diagnosed at stereotactic core-needle biopsy: clinical importance. *Radiology* 2000;216:831–837.

89. Sydnor MK, Shaw de Paredes E, Wilson JDH, et al. Underestimation of breast carcinoma in papillary lesions diagnosed on core needle biopsy. *Radiology*, in press.

90. Rosen EL, Bentley RC, Baker JA, Soo MS. Imaging guided core needle biopsy of papillary lesions of the breast. *AJR Am J Roentgenol* 2002;179(5):1185–1192.

Chapter 17

The Roles of Ultrasound and Magnetic Resonance Imaging in the Evaluation of the Breast

Imaging the breast has evolved from mammography alone to mammography with adjunctive modalities that primarily include ultrasound and magnetic resonance imaging (MRI). Until recent years, ultrasound and MRI have functioned as problem-solving tools and have been used to help to diagnose a mammographically and/or clinically detected abnormality. As these modalities have improved technologically and vast clinical experience has been acquired, so have their roles expanded from diagnostic tools to potential screening tools as well.

Ultrasound has many uses that relate to the evaluation of breast masses. Sonographic guidance is used frequently for the direction of percutaneous breast biopsies. MRI was initially used for the evaluation of implants, but it now has several roles that relate to the evaluation of carcinomas. With a dedicated breast coil and contrast enhancement, MRI has been of great value in identifying the extent of carcinoma and in helping to better plan patient management.

In this chapter, the discussion will not focus on the technical aspects of ultrasound or MRI. Instead, the focus will be on the roles of these ancillary modalities in complimenting mammography and the information that can be provided to enhance the clinical knowledge about the patient.

THE ROLE OF BREAST ULTRASOUND

The role of breast ultrasound has expanded considerably as the technique and resolution of the equipment have improved. With high-frequency linear array transducers and higher resolution, smaller lesions and greater detail are visualized. The initial primary role of ultrasound was the differentiation of solid versus cystic masses (1–4). Sonography is ideal for this role and is important in planning the management of the patient. The roles of ultrasound are shown in Table 17.1.

Of paramount importance in incorporating ultrasound in a breast-imaging program is the use of high-quality equipment and proper technique. High-frequency linear array transducers are typically used. Current transducers have frequency ranges of 15-18 MHz, 13-8 MHz, 12-5 MHz and 10-5 MHz (5). Setting the focal zone to the proper depth, at the level of the area of interest, optimizes the analysis of the lesion of interest. Setting the power and time-gain compensation at the proper level is extremely important so that the analysis of cystic versus solid masses is accurate. If the gain is set too low, a hypoechoic solid mass may be interpreted as anechoic and thought to be a cyst when in fact it is solid. Scanning may be performed in a longitudinal and transverse pattern or in a radial and antiradial orientation (5).

The ACR BI-RADS® Lexicon for Breast Imaging (6) also has descriptions for ultrasound reporting. In the BI-RADS® for ultrasound, the following are described: background echotexture, mass features, calcifications, special cases, and vascularity. Masses are described (6) according to their shape, orientation, margins, lesion boundary, echo pattern, posterior acoustic enhancement features, and

> **TABLE 17.1 The Roles of Ultrasound**

- Evaluation of the patient with a palpable mass
- Evaluation of the young or pregnant patient who is clinically symptomatic
- Evaluation of the patient with the mammographically identified round mass
- Implants evaluation for possible rupture
- Evaluation of suspicious areas of microcalcifications for an underlying mass
- Evaluation of focal areas of asymmetry
- Plan management of a solid mass
- Guidance for biopsy

effect on surrounding tissue. The background echotexture may be homogeneous-fat, homogeneous-fibroglandular, or heterogeneous.

Mass shapes may be oval, round, or irregular, and their orientation is parallel or not parallel to the chest wall. The margination of masses may be described as circumscribed or not circumscribed (indistinct, angular, microlobulated, or spiculated). The boundary of the lesion may be abrupt, or the mass may be surrounded by an echogenic halo. These findings parallel mammo-graphic findings in terms of the likelihood of benign versus malignant etiologies.

The echogenicity of masses may be described as anechoic, hyperechoic, hypoechoic, or isoechoic relative to the surrounding parenchyma, or they may be complex. Posterior acoustic features may be described as shadowing, enhancement, or no effect. Observation of the effect on surrounding tissue may include the following: ductal extension, changes in Cooper's ligaments, edema, architectural distortion, skin thickening, or skin retraction (6).

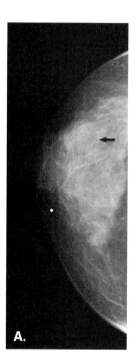
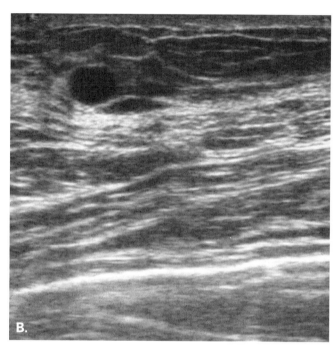
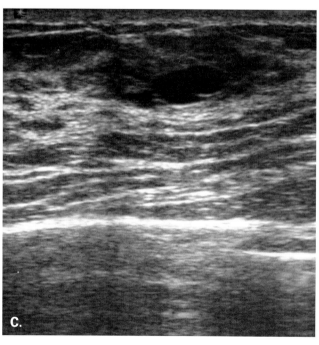

Figure 17.1

HISTORY: A 34-year-old woman with a small palpable mass in the left breast at 9 o'clock.

IMAGING: Left CC view **(A)** shows heterogeneously dense tissue and a BB marking a palpable lump. In addition, there is a vague rounded asymmetry located lateral to the nipple **(arrow)**. Ultrasound of these areas showed two simple cysts **(B,C)**. The cysts are anechoic, thin-walled, and very well defined, all of which are features of a simple cyst.

IMPRESSION: Simple cysts, BI-RADS® 2.

Assessment of Isodense Circumscribed Masses: Cystic Versus Solid

The diagnosis of a simple cyst with ultrasound is very accurate and has been reported to range from 96% to 100% (1–4,7). Careful scanning technique that includes proper gain, transducer frequency, and resolution of the equip-ment is necessary in order to achieve this highly reliable differentiation of solid versus cystic lesions. In addition, the criteria for a simple cyst must be adhered to in order to confirm that a lesion is clearly benign. The criteria for a simple cyst are as follows: smooth thin walls, no internal echoes (anechoic), and posterior acoustic enhancement (Figs. 17.1–17.3). With compound imaging where the scan

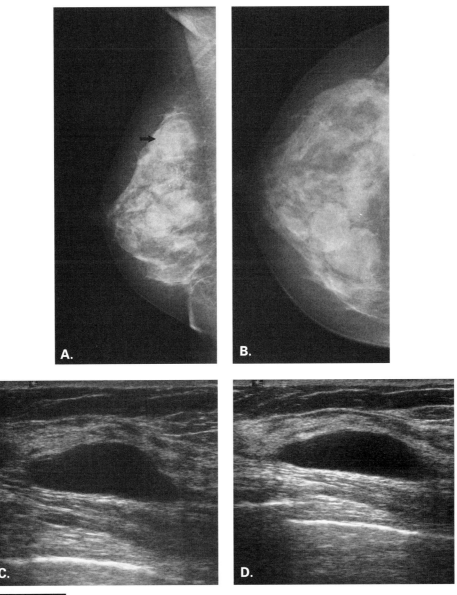

Figure 17.2

HISTORY: A 52-year-old woman who presents with left breast pain and a history of cysts in the past.

IMAGING: Left MLO (**A**) and CC (**B**) views show the breast to be heterogeneously dense. Multiple round circumscribed masses are present, all of which were stable, except for a 3-cm mass in the left axillary tail (**arrow**) that was new. Because of the interval change in the left axillary tail mass, ultrasound of this region was performed. Sonography at the 2 o'clock position (**C,D**) shows the mass to be very well defined, oval, and anechoic, with a thin wall and posterior acoustic enhancement. All these features meet the criteria for a simple cyst.

IMPRESSION: New mass left axillary tail, simple cyst, BI-RADS® 2.

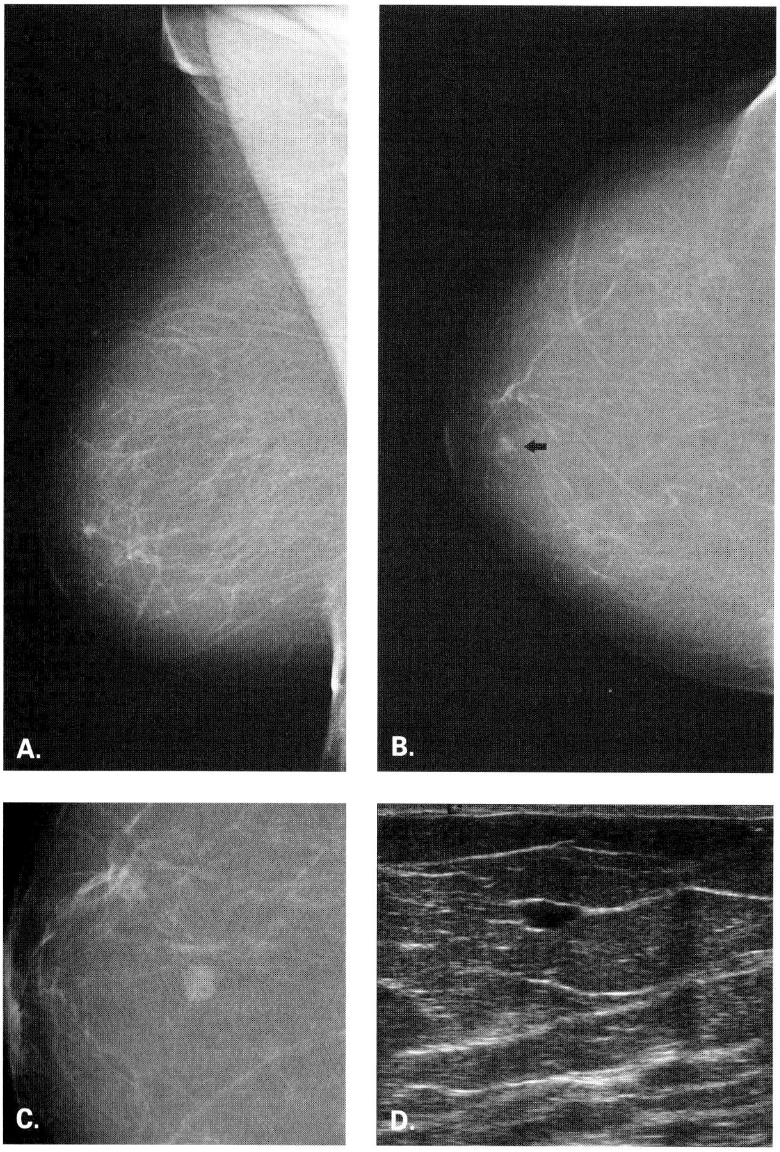

Figure 17.3

HISTORY: A 48-year-old woman for screening mammography.

IMAGING: Left MLO **(A)** and CC **(B)** views show the breast to be fatty replaced. There is a small, round, somewhat dense mass in the left subareolar area **(arrows)**. Spot compression CC view **(C)** shows the mass to be circumscribed, suggesting that it is most likely benign. The mass was larger in comparison with prior studies, and because of this interval change, ultrasound was performed. Left breast sonography **(D)** shows that the mass is very well defined and anechoic, with a thin wall, all features of a simple cyst.

IMPRESSION: Simple cyst, left breast, BI-RADS® 2.

plane is multidirectional, posterior acoustic enhancement may not be observed for some small cysts.

Importantly, the presence of acoustic enhancement behind a round or oval mass does not necessarily indicate that it is a cyst. Solid homogeneous masses, including breast cancers, may have acoustic enhancement as well. All the above-noted criteria must be met to call a mass a simple cyst. Thin septae may be present in a cyst and do not require biopsy. However, thick septae, a thick wall, or an intracystic solid component raises the concern for malignancy, and these findings do require tissue sampling (1,8).

Complicated cysts are those that contain low-level echoes. This may occur secondary to hemorrhage or inflammation or because the fluid is very thick (Fig. 17.4). Occasionally a very hypoechoic solid mass may have the appearance of a complicated cyst. Aspiration is usually performed when this finding is observed, especially if the mass is new, larger, or solitary. In a study of 150 cystic lesions, Berg et al. (9) found that none of the 38 complicated cysts that were aspirated proved to be malignant. Sebaceous cysts most often have the appearance of complicated cysts (Fig. 17.5), and because of their superficial location, their etiology is evident. Also, with sebaceous cysts, a thin track between the cyst and the skin surface is often visible.

Complex masses are those that contain both cystic and solid components. A thick rind around a cystic center, polypoid solid projections within a cystic mass, or a mass that has both fluid and solid components is complex. Such masses may represent necrotic tumors or intracystic benign or malignant tumors, but they also may represent several benign lesions. A cyst with marked inflammation or hemorrhage and clot may have this appearance. Similarly,

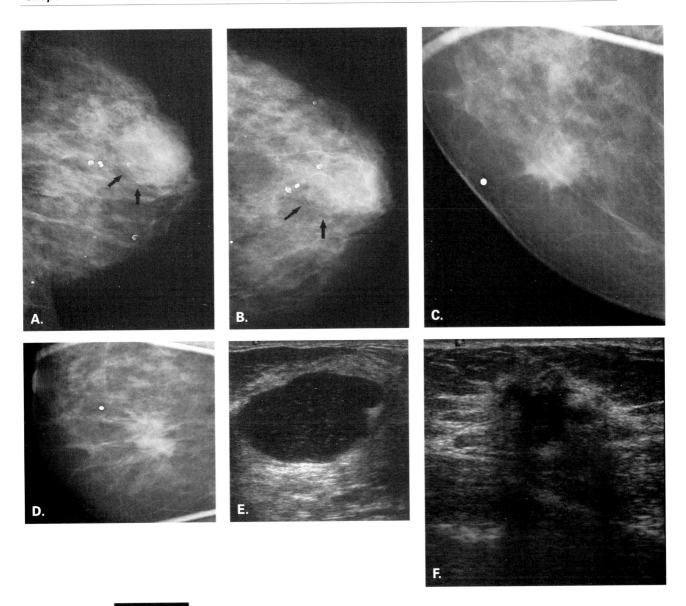

Figure 17.4

HISTORY: A 58-year-old woman with bilateral palpable masses.

IMAGING: Right ML **(A)** and CC **(B)** magnification views show dense parenchyma and scattered benign calcifications. There is a large round mass in the right subareolar area with a well-circumscribed margin and a fatty halo **(arrow)**, suggesting a benign etiology. In the left breast in the area of palpable concern, the spot compression CC **(C)** and ML **(D)** views show the palpable mass to be high density, irregular, with spiculated margins, and suspicious for malignancy. Right breast ultrasound **(E)** shows the round mass to be circumscribed and to contain low-level echoes suggesting a complicated cyst. The left breast ultrasound **(F)** shows the palpable mass to be irregular, hypoechoic, and shadowing and to have a branching ductal pattern in its periphery, highly suspicious for malignancy.

IMPRESSION: Right breast complicated cyst, left breast carcinoma.

HISTOPATHOLOGY: Right cyst aspiration showing benign-appearing green fluid. Left breast core biopsy showing invasive ductal carcinoma.

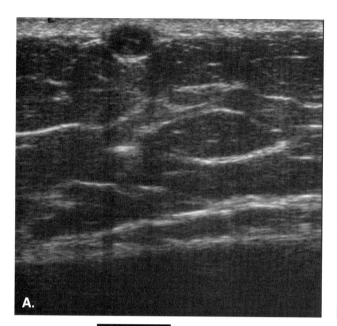

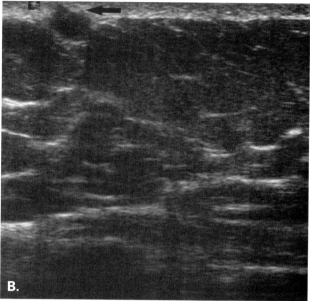

Figure 17.5

HISTORY: A 33-year-old woman with a small palpable mass in the left breast at 7 o'clock.

IMAGING: Mammography showed no abnormality to correspond with the palpable lesion. On ultrasound **(A,B)** the mass is complex, round, and located in the cutaneous area. The superficial fascial plane is not visible over the lesion, indicating that the mass is in the skin. A small track from the mass **(arrow)** is contiguous with the skin **(B)**.

IMPRESSION: Sebaceous cyst.

abscesses and hematomas usually appear as complex masses (Figs. 17.6 and 17.7). The management of a complex mass usually requires biopsy unless the finding is clearly a hematoma. Berg et al. (9) found that 7/23 complex masses with thick walls or thick septae and 4/18 lesions with an intracystic solid component proved to be malignant. Intracystic papillary carcinomas and necrotic high-grade malignancies may appear as complex masses on sonography (Figs. 17.8–17.10). Sampling of the solid portion of the mass is important, rather than aspiration of the fluid, so ultrasound has an important role in guiding the biopsy. Either percutaneous biopsy directed at the solid component of the mass or excision of the entire lesion is usually performed for diagnosis.

A solid mass on ultrasound is analyzed based on its contour, margination, orientation, and echogenicity. Although ultrasound cannot definitely diagnose a solid lesion as benign or malignant, there are criteria that are helpful in predicting a benign versus a malignant etiology. These features are based on the nature of benign masses, such as fibroadenomas, which are homogeneous lesions that have an encapsulated, very-well-defined margin (Figs. 17.11–17.14). Stavros et al. (10,11) described the criteria for solid benign versus malignant masses. The features of benign solid masses are listed in Table 17.2.

The sonographic features of fibroadenomas have been described in early papers (12,13) as hypoechoic, oval masses. Fibroadenomas are very well defined with a thin margin, and occasionally a pseudocapsule is evident. The lesions are usually elongated and wider than tall in orientation. Sometimes thin hyperechoic septae are seen with fibroadenomas. Most fibroadenomas have no effect on sound transmission, but some may enhance or shadow. When shadowing is identified, or when the orientation is not elongated or the borders are not well defined, biopsy is performed. A lesion that may have a similar appearance to a fibroadenoma is a phylloides tumor. On mammography, a large circumscribed mass is seen; on ultrasound, the mass is typically circumscribed and hypoechoic. The epithelial-lined clefts inside the mass may appear as small cystic spaces within the solid lesion on ultrasound (Fig. 17.15) (14).

> **TABLE 17.2 Ultrasound Features of Benign Solid Masses**

- Lack of any malignant features
- Intensely hyperechoic *or*
- Elliptical hypoechoic with a thin echogenic capsule
- Up to two or three gentle lobulations
- Posterior acoustic enhancement

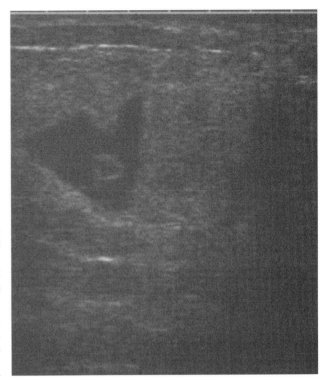

Figure 17.6

HISTORY: A 43-year-old patient with a history of trauma to the breast and a small palpable lump.

ULTRASOUND: Ultrasound of the lump demonstrates a complex mass, which has irregular margins extending along tissue planes. Within the mass is a solid-appearing component.

IMPRESSION: Complex mass consistent with organizing hematoma.

NOTE: Follow-up sonography in 1 to 3 months should be performed to confirm resolution of the hematoma and to verify that there is no residual mass.

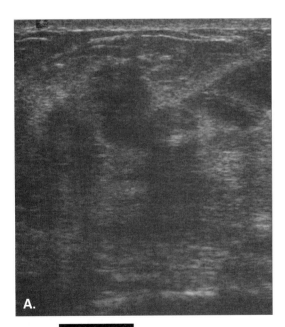

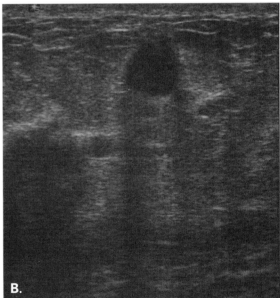

Figure 17.7

HISTORY: A 27-year-old woman with a tender palpable right breast mass. She had been treated with antibiotics and the mass had not resolved.

MAMMOGRAPHY: Right breast ultrasound over the lump shows it to be complex in appearance. Portions **(A)** of the mass are lobulated, of mixed echogenicity, and with some extensions into the tissue. Other portions appear more loculated and fluid filled **(B)**. There is surrounding hyperechoic edema. Mammography was performed and was noncontributory. The patient underwent vacuum-assisted biopsy of the area, and a large amount of purulent material was aspirated, along with the tissue specimen.

HISTOPATHOLOGY: Granulomatous inflammation.

NOTE: The patient underwent subsequent surgical drainage of the abscess and antibiotic therapy, and the area resolved.

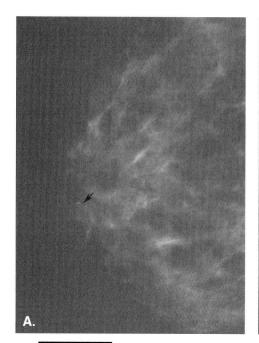
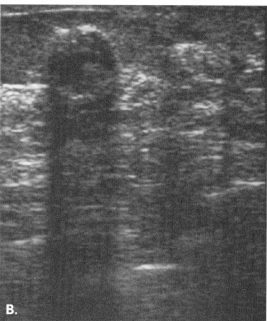

Figure 17.8

HISTORY: A 51-year-old woman with a palpable mass in the left breast at 6 o'clock.

IMAGING: Left ML view **(A)** shows a dense breast with benign eggshell calcification in the sub-areolar area **(arrow)**. The palpable mass is not seen on mammography. On ultrasound **(B)**, the palpable mass is observed and is complex, having a partially cystic component as well as an intracystic filling defect.

IMPRESSION: Intracystic lesion, papilloma versus carcinoma.

HISTOPATHOLOGY: Sclerotic intracystic papilloma.

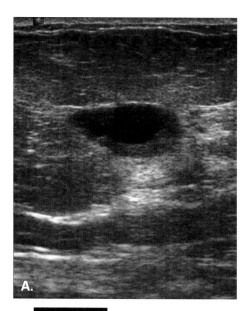
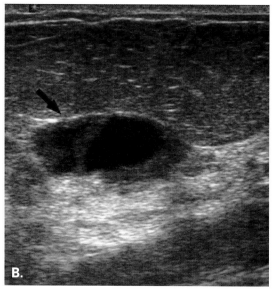

Figure 17.9

HISTORY: A 61-year-old woman with a history of a mass in the left breast, for further evaluation.

IMAGING: Left breast ultrasound **(A,B)** shows the palpable mass to be complex. The wall is thick and slightly irregular, and there is a cystic component as well. Parts of the mass appear more solid **(B, arrow)**, suggesting the presence of an intracystic mass. Alteratively, this could be a necrotic tumor or an abscess. Core needle biopsy with a vacuum probe was performed.

IMPRESSION: Complex mass, suspicious for carcinoma.

HISTOPATHOLOGY: Invasive ductal carcinoma with papillary features.

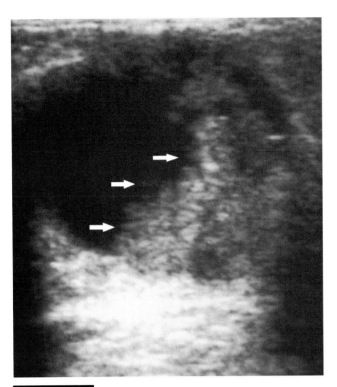

Figure 17.10

Ultrasound image of a palpable mass shows it to be complex. Portions are fluid filled, but the lateral wall is thickened with a solid component **(arrows)**. Excision showed intracystic papillary carcinoma. (Case courtesy of Dr. Christine Denison, Boston, MA.)

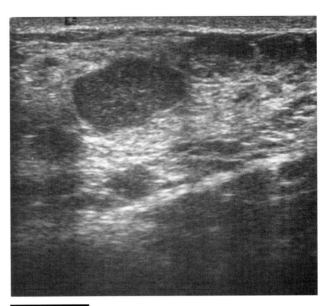

Figure 17.11

HISTORY: A 26-year-old woman with a new palpable breast mass.

IMAGING: Ultrasound shows the mass to be solid and to have benign features. It is well circumscribed, hypoechoic, and oval. There is a thin echogenic pseudocapsule surrounding the mass. Because the mass was new and palpable, it was biopsied.

IMPRESSION: Solid mass, likely a fibroadenoma.

HISTOPATHOLOGY: Fibroadenoma.

Lesions that are hyperechoic on ultrasound are typically those that contain fat. Hyperechoic masses include the following: fat necrosis (Figs. 17.16 and 17.17), lipomas, hamartomas, angiomas (Fig.17.18), and focal fibrosis. The appearance of fat necrosis ranges from anechoic masses to complex masses with mural nodules to solid masses of varying echogenicity (15). Lymph nodes also are hyperechoic in part, depending on the amount of fatty replacement. Normal nodes are elliptical and have a smooth cortex that is hypoechoic and a bright hyperechoic center that is the fatty hilum (16) (Fig. 17.19). Abnormal nodes have a thickened cortex and an indistinct margin, and they may have an increased anteroposterior (AP) diameter with obliteration of the fatty hilum (Fig. 17.20).

Based on the Stavros et al. (10) criteria, the likelihood of a solid mass with benign characteristics actually being benign is greater than 98%. Therefore, for a nonpalpable circumscribed mass on mammography that has benign sonographic features, early follow-up may be performed. However, for new palpable or enlarging solid masses, even with benign features, biopsy is usually performed for confirmation.

Malignancies tend to be more indistinct in margination and more firm, so their AP diameter is often greater than their transverse diameter. The features of malignant masses on ultrasound are listed in Table 17.3. Malignant masses may be markedly hypoechoic, irregular (17) shadowing lesions (Figs. 17.21–17.24). Because of the dense stromal reaction, the posterior acoustic shadowing with cancers may be intense. Some cancers have branching

▶ **TABLE 17.3 Sonographic Features of Malignant Solid Masses**

- Posterior acoustic shadowing
- Hypoechoic
- Irregular contour
- Taller-than-wide configuration
- Spiculation
- Angular or microlobulated margins
- Ductal extension, branching pattern
- Thick hyperechoic halo
- Increased vascularity
- Surrounding edema
- Microcalcifications

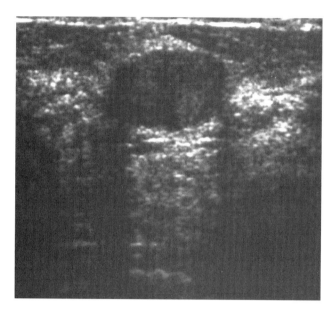

Figure 17.12

HISTORY: A 53-year-old woman with a palpable mass and a negative mammogram.

IMAGING: Single ultrasound image over the palpable mass shows it to be hypoechoic, oval, and well defined, features suggestive of a fibroadenoma. Because it was palpable, biopsy was performed.

HISTOPATHOLOGY: Fibroadenoma.

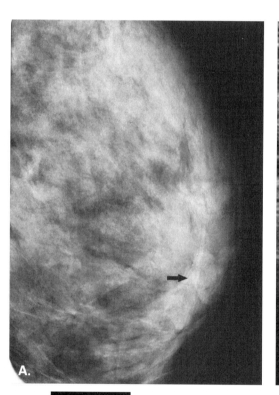

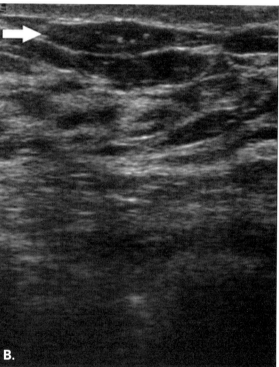

Figure 17.13

HISTORY: A 47-year-old woman recalled from screening mammography for right breast calcifications.

IMAGING: Right ML magnification view **(A)** shows a lobular mass that contains circumscribed margins in the subareolar area **(arrow)**. The mass has associated amorphous microcalcifications. Right breast ultrasound **(B)** shows the mass **(arrow)** to be oval, elongated, and well defined. There are some bright echoes within the lesion, likely related to the calcifications observed on mammography. Core needle biopsy was performed using ultrasound guidance.

HISTOPATHOLOGY: Fibroadenoma.

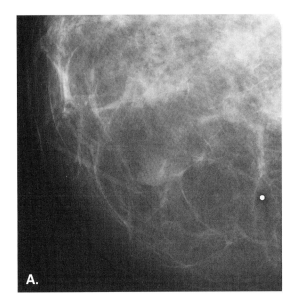

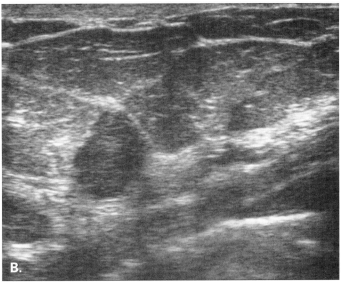

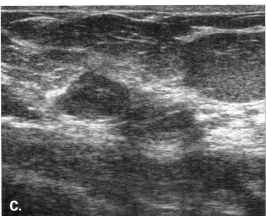

Figure 17.14

HISTORY: A 39-year-old woman recalled for a left breast mass found on screening mammography.

IMAGING: Left CC magnification view **(A)** shows a lobulated isodense mass located medially, having borders that are partially circumscribed and partially obscured. Because of this finding, ultrasound was performed. Sonography **(B,C)** reveals a hypoechoic, lobular mass that is partially defined. The lesion has multiple lobulations, and on some images, it has a slight indistinctness of the margins. Although this may represent a fibroadenoma, the sonographic features are not clearly benign. Biopsy was therefore performed.

HISTOPATHOLOGY: Fibroadenoma.

Figure 17.15

HISTORY: A 25-year-old woman with a new palpable right breast mass.

ULTRASOUND: Ultrasound of the palpable mass shows it to be oval, elongated, and smoothly marginated. The echo pattern is somewhat inhomogeneous. The shape of the mass suggests a fibroadenoma, particularly for a patient in this age group.

IMPRESSION: Solid mass, likely a fibroadenoma; recommend biopsy to confirm.

HISTOPATHOLOGY: Benign phylloides tumor.

NOTE: Phylloides tumors often have a heterogeneous echo pattern related to the cystic spaces within the stroma.

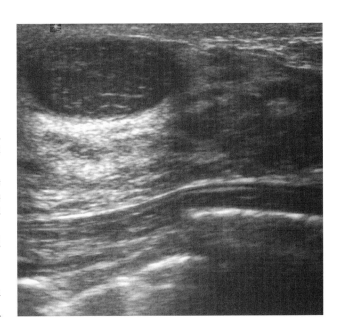

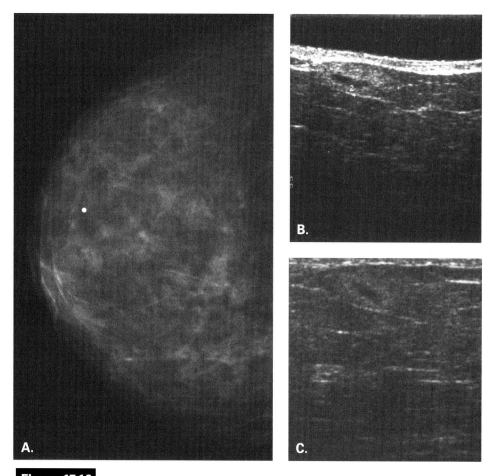

Figure 17.16

HISTORY: A 43-year-old woman with a small palpable mass in the left breast.

IMAGING: Left CC view **(A)** shows scattered fibroglandular tissue and a BB marking the palpable area of concern. No mammographic finding is present. *Ultrasound* **(B,C)** shows the palpable lesion to be heterogeneous in appearance. The periphery is hyperechoic, and the center is markedly hypoechoic and oriented obliquely toward the skin. The features are most suggestive of an area of resolving hematoma and fat necrosis. The patient had a vague history of recent trauma to this region. The area was followed in 4 weeks with ultrasound, and it resolved.

IMPRESSION: Fat necrosis, resolving hematoma.

linear extensions around their borders, which may indicate intraductal extension of tumor. Angular or microlobulated margins are also suspicious features for malignancy. A vertical orientation (taller than wide) is an ominous sign and has a high positive predictive value of being malignant (18,19). The highest positive predictive values for malignancy on the ultrasound of masses have been found to be the following findings: spiculation (87%), a thick hyperechoic halo (74%), and a taller-than-wide orientation (74%). The lowest predictive values of the malignant signs were associated with microlobulations and ductal extension (11).

Some cancers, particularly medullary or mucinous carcinomas, have a pushing edge and are homogeneous on ultrasound. These tumors may look round and smooth and be very hypoechoic, and because of the homogeneity of the mass, they may be associated with posterior acoustic enhancement. One must use great care in order not to misinterpret a medullary or a mucinous malignancy as a cyst. Also, some very-high-grade cancers or necrotic cancers may have this same appearance. Often in these cases, though, the orientation of the lesion is vertical rather than elongated or horizontal, as is seen in benign lesions.

A variety of benign conditions may have sonographic features that are indeterminate or frankly suspicious for malignancy. Prominent shadowing is associated with dense stromal areas that may be seen in scars, focal fibrosis, hyalinized fibroadenomas, and diabetic fibrous mastopathy (Fig. 17.25). Hypoechoic masses that are not completely circumscribed or that are inhomogeneous are

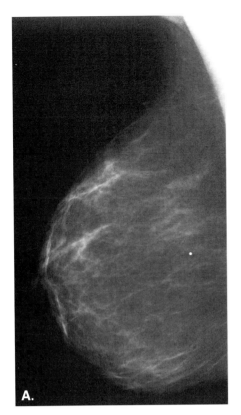

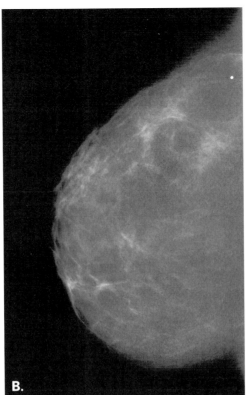

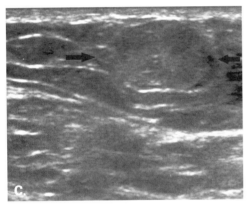

Figure 17.17

HISTORY: A 36-year-old woman with a new left breast palpable mass.

IMAGING: Left MLO **(A)** and CC **(B)** views with a BB over the palpable lump show a fatty-replaced breast, with no mammography abnormality. Sonographic image **(C)** of the palpable mass shows it to be well defined, hyperechoic, with areas of hypoechogenicity **(arrows)**. This lesion is located very superficially, a finding often seen in posttraumatic lesions. The findings are most suggestive of fat necrosis because of the negative mammogram and the sonographic findings.

IMPRESSION: Palpable mass, possible fat necrosis; recommend biopsy.

HISTOPATHOLOGY: Recent hemorrhage with fat necrosis.

seen in fibrocystic conditions at times. Radial scars (Fig. 17.26) and papillomas may also appear as solid masses that are not clearly benign.

An algorithm for the management of solid breast masses based on their sonographic features has been described by Stavros et al. (11). Based on this algorithm, one must first assess the lesion for any suspicious features. If a single suspicious feature is present, biopsy should be performed. If there are no suspicious features, one must search for benign characteristics. If there are no benign findings, classify the lesion as BI-RADS® 4A, suspicious, and perform a biopsy. If all the features are benign, the lesion is likely benign, and one can perform an early follow-up ultrasound.

Ultrasound in the Evaluation of the Palpable Mass

Breast ultrasound plays a critical role in the assessment of the patient with a palpable lump. For patients with a lump that is visible on mammography as a circumscribed mass, ultrasound differentiates cystic from solid etiologies. In the past, before percutaneous breast biopsy was widely used, a suspicious mass on mammography was not evaluated with ultrasound (4). However, both nonpalpable and palpable suspicious masses are often now imaged sonographically to determine if they are visible and if they can be biopsied with ultrasound guidance.

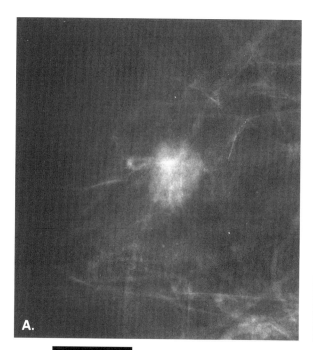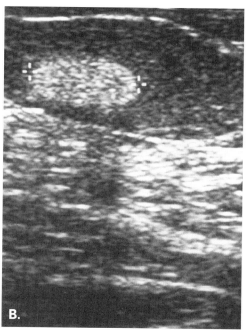

Figure 17.18

HISTORY: Postmenopausal patient recalled from screening mammography for a mass in the left breast.

MAMMOGRAPHY: Spot compression view **(A)** of the mass that was identified on screening shows the lesion to be isodense and to have microlobulated margins. The borders are somewhat suspicious for malignancy. Ultrasound **(B)** of the lesions shows it to be hyperechoic and oval and relatively well defined, suggesting most likely a benign etiology. Core needle biopsy was performed, based on the mammographic finding.

HISTOPATHOLOGY: Capillary angioma.

NOTE: Angiomas and other vascular lesions may be markedly hyperechoic on ultrasound.

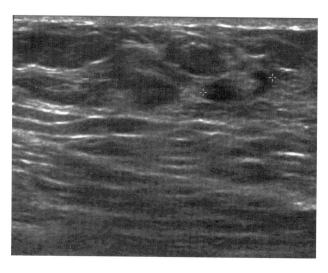

Figure 17.19

HISTORY: A 42-year-old woman with a small palpable breast mass in the upper outer quadrant.

IMAGING: Mammography was negative. Ultrasound of the mass shows an oval, hypoechoic circumscribed mass with a hyperechoic center consistent with the fatty hilum of a lymph node.

IMPRESSION: Intramammary node, BI-RADS® 2.

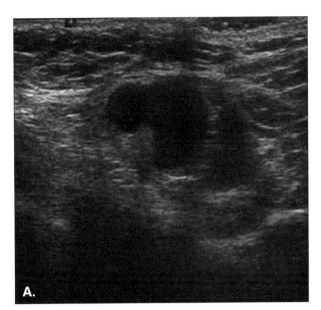 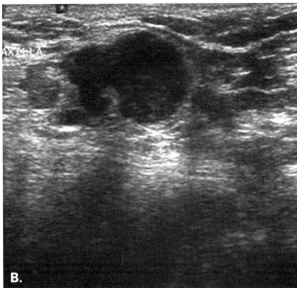

Figure 17.20

HISTORY: A 65-year-old woman with a history of left breast cancer treated with mastectomy, axillary node dissection, and chemotherapy 12 years ago. She now presents with a palpable mass in the left axilla.

ULTRASOUND: Sonography (**A,B**) of the left axilla shows a lobular mass that is taller than wide. The margins are partially circumscribed. The periphery of the mass is hypoechoic, and the center is hyperechoic, indicating that it is a lymph node. The size and contour of this node are abnormal. The widened nodular cortex of the node is suspicious for malignancy. Needle biopsy was performed using ultrasound guidance.

HISTOPATHOLOGY: Metastatic carcinoma consistent with primary breast cancer.

In the patient with a palpable mass and with vague, nonspecific mammographic findings or a negative mammogram, ultrasound is the next step in evaluation. Ultrasound may demonstrate a cancer or a benign mass that is not evident on mammography (Fig. 17.27). Various studies have shown the value of ultrasound in demonstrating palpable cancers that are mammographically occult (4,20–24).

In addition, a negative ultrasound is an important factor in determining the patient's management. A negative ultrasound and negative mammogram in the clinical situation of a palpable mass are associated with a risk of malignancy of <2%. Depending on the level of suspicion on clinical exam, clinical follow-up rather than biopsy may be performed when imaging is completely negative (25).

Ultrasound in Young or Pregnant Patients

In women younger than age thirty with a palpable mass, the most likely diagnosis is a fibroadenoma, with cysts and cancers being less likely. The workup of the patient is affected by the very low frequency of cancers is this age group and by the somewhat increased radiosensitivity of the breasts. Typically, mammography is not performed first, unless the patient is at high risk for breast cancer.

Most breast imagers (4,18,26,27) begin with ultrasound in the symptomatic young patient (Fig. 17.28). The exception to this is the very-high-risk patient (*BRCA1* or *BRCA2* carrier, history of treated Hodgkin disease, strong premenopausal family history, personal history of breast cancer). In the very-high-risk patient, bilateral mammography is performed first. A pitfall in this age group is the assumption that the patient has very dense breasts and that mammography is not helpful or will not detect cancer. Often in young women with breast cancer, a delay in diagnosis occurs for this reason (28).

In the usual-risk patient, ultrasound is performed to determine if the palpable mass is solid, cystic, or not seen. If the lesion is a cyst, no further workup is needed. If the lesion is solid and has the appearance of fibroadenoma, or if the lesion is clearly palpable but not seen on ultrasound, the next step is mammography. The mammographic examination may be limited to imaging the ipsilateral breast if the lesion does not have suspicious sonographic features. For a solid lesion that has any malignant features on ultrasound, bilateral mammography is usually performed. For new solid palpable masses, needle biopsy is typically performed for diagnosis, even if the lesion has an appearance suggestive of a fibroadenoma.

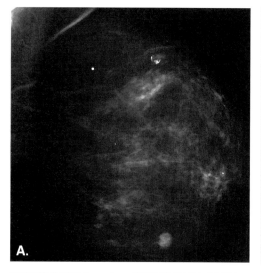

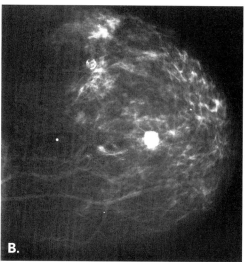

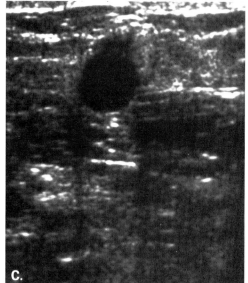

Figure 17.21

HISTORY: Screening mammogram on a 60-year-old woman.

IMAGING: Right MLO **(A)** and CC **(B)** views show heterogeneously dense tissue and scattered benign calcifications. At 6 o'clock, there is a dense, round, relatively circumscribed mass. Ultrasound **(C)** shows the mass to be markedly hypoechoic, round, and taller than wide. The anterior margin is slightly irregular and angulated. This mass should not be confused with a cyst because it is nearly anechoic. The worrisome features here are the vertical orientation and the indistinct anterior margin.

IMPRESSION: Markedly hypoechoic round mass, suspicious for carcinoma.

HISTOPATHOLOGY: Invasive ductal carcinoma.

In pregnant patients, ultrasound is also usually performed first. Limiting the radiation exposure is important, so depending on the ultrasound findings, mammography may be delayed until the second trimester of pregnancy. If, however, the sonographic finding has any aspects suspicious for malignancy, complete evaluation is needed without a delay. In pregnant patients, fibroadenomas, lactating adenomas, accessory breast tissue, galactoceles, and cancers occur. Because of the hormonal milieu, fibroadenomas may grow in these patients. Cancers also may grow more rapidly, so care must be taken not to delay the diagnosis of a suspicious mass.

In lactating patients, palpable masses are often abscesses or galactoceles; however, lactating adenomas, fibroadenomas, and cancers occur as well (Figs.17.29 and 17.30). Depending on the age and family history of the patient, ultrasound is often performed first. If ultrasound demonstrates a cyst, no further workup is necessary. For an apparent abscess, and depending on the

level of symptoms, treatment may be performed before mammography. For solid masses, mammography and further evaluation with biopsy are performed. For patients older than age 30, mammography is usually performed first.

Imaging of Asymmetries and Calcifications

Traditionally, focal asymmetries that are nonpalpable and identified on mammography have been managed based on their mammographic characteristics. For focal asymmetric densities or for questionable architectural distortion, ultrasound may be of value in trying to identify the presence of a mass. An ultrasound-detected mass within an area of mammographic asymmetry confirms that a true lesion is present and prompts biopsy (Figs. 17.31 and 17.32). In addition, sonographic guidance can be used to target the density, which sometimes can be difficult to target accurately with stereotaxis. When ultrasound is

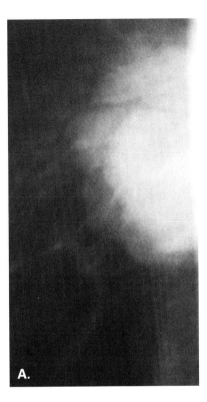

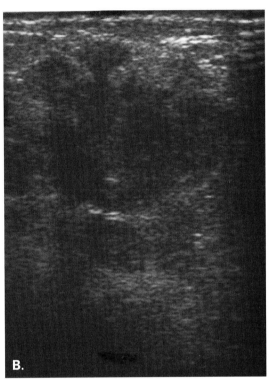

Figure 17.22

HISTORY: A 40-year-old woman with a palpable mass in the left breast inferiorly.

IMAGING: Left ML spot view **(A)** shows a high-density mass with microlobulated margins, highly suspicious for malignancy. On ultrasound **(B)**, the mass is of mixed echogenicity and has irregular margins with branching ductal extensions.

IMPRESSION: Highly suspicious for carcinoma.

HISTOPATHOLOGY: Infiltrating ductal carcinoma and DCIS, with one positive node.

A.

B.

negative for a mass, the asymmetry must be managed based on its mammographic characteristics.

Microcalcifications may occasionally be seen on high-resolution ultrasound but most often are not visible. Therefore, sonography is not used to evaluate the etiology of microcalcifications. However, performing breast ultrasound is most helpful in planning interventions and management in one circumstance. When microcalcifications having a suspicious appearance for ductal carcinoma in situ (DCIS) are present, particularly when the area is larger than a cluster, ultrasound is a helpful adjunct to mammography (Fig. 17.33).

The most likely diagnosis for BI-RADS® 5 microcalcifications is DCIS. If needle biopsy is performed and demonstrates DCIS, lumpectomy without an assessment of the axilla is performed. If final pathology on the excision shows invasive carcinoma also, the axillary nodes are then sampled in a second surgery. The preoperative identification of invasive carcinoma is important in surgical planning in that lumpectomy with axillary node sampling is performed as one procedure. Ultrasound may demonstrate a solid mass within a region of calcifications, and this finding suggests the presence of an invasive cancer. Therefore, percutaneous ultrasound-guided biopsy of the mass is most helpful in treatment planning.

Screening Ultrasound

The role of ultrasound in the detection of clinically occult breast cancer remains uncertain. Early literature using a water path scanner (20,29) found that screening ultra-

sound was not an acceptable substitute for mammography to detect breast cancer. Small nonpalpable breast cancers were not adequately identified with ultrasound.

With significant improvements in the ultrasound technology and with better resolution, greater detail is available, and small cancers are identifiable. Since 1995, several studies (30–35) have evaluated the value of screening ultrasound, primarily in women with dense parenchyma on mammography. The prevalence of cancers detected by ultrasound alone in these series ranged from 0.27% to 0.9%, and the mean tumor size ranged from 9.0 to 11.0 mm (36).

In an analysis of the 42,838 screening ultrasound examinations reported in six series, Feig (36) calculated a positive predictive value in biopsies performed based on a suspicious ultrasound examination of 11.4%. This is less than the literature shows for mammographically detected lesions but is certainly not an insignificant number. In one of the largest series, Kolb et al. (32) found 246 cancers on screening ultrasounds of 11,130 asymptomatic women with dense breasts and negative mammography. The authors found that mammographic sensitivity declined with increasing breast density and that screening ultrasound increased the detection of small early-stage breast cancers.

In addition to a true screening ultrasound in the patient with negative mammography, ultrasound may be performed to assess the extent of carcinoma by searching for other mammographically occult cancers (Fig. 17.34). Full breast ultrasound imaging has been shown to be useful in identifying other mammographically and clinically occult foci of tumor in the patient with a known breast cancer in the ipsilateral breast (37). Although MRI is more

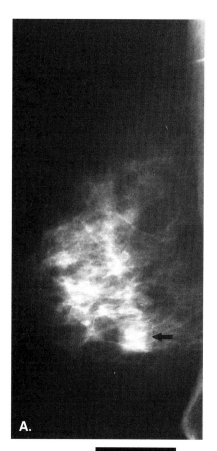
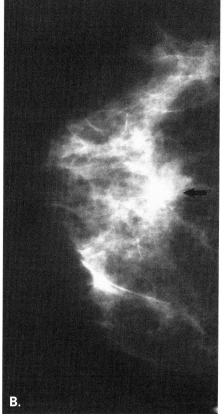
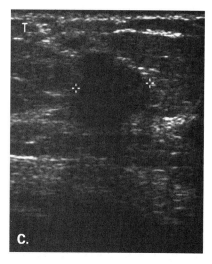

Figure 17.23

HISTORY: Premenopausal woman with a palpable mass in the left breast at 6 o'clock.

MAMMOGRAPHY: Left MLO (**A**) and CC (**B**) views show heterogeneously dense tissue. There is an irregular mass with indistinct margins located inferiorly (**arrow**). Ultrasound (**C**) shows the mass to be microlobulated, markedly hypoechoic, and taller than wide. This mass has very suspicious features on sonography, and it should not be confused with a cyst because it is so hypoechoic.

IMPRESSION: Highly suspicious for carcinoma.

HISTOPATHOLOGY: Invasive lobular carcinoma.

---

frequently used in this role, ultrasound may be helpful initially or as a second-look procedure. The cost of ultrasound is less than that of MRI, and if multicentric disease is identified, the clinical plan for breast is not changed by adding MRI. If MRI detects a mammographically occult lesion that is not clinically apparent and that is suspicious for multifocal or multicentric carcinoma, biopsy is necessary. With knowledge of the location and size of the lesion, a second-look ultrasound may identify the abnormality, which can then be biopsied more easily with ultrasound guidance. LaTrenta et al. (38) found an ultrasound correlate for 23% of suspicious lesions identified on MRI.

Occasionally, mammographically occult cancers are identified incidentally. When an ultrasound is performed as a diagnostic test to evaluate a particular lesion or lesions, scanning adjacent tissue or the rest of the breast may lead to the observation of an abnormality that is sus-

picious. If such a lesion is identified, further evaluation is needed, because a mammographically occult carcinoma certainly may be present (Fig. 17.35).

Implant Imaging

The imaging of patients with augmented breasts with silicone prostheses may include ultrasound to search for rupture. The specificity for ultrasound in the identification of implant rupture has been reported to range from 55% to 79%, and sensitivity is 59% to 85% (18,39–41). Both intracapsular rupture and extracapsular rupture can be identified on ultrasound, whereas mammography does not show intracapsular rupture. MRI is also of great value in the assessment of implants for rupture.

The normal implant has an anechoic appearance on ultrasound. A prominent reverberation artifact is visible

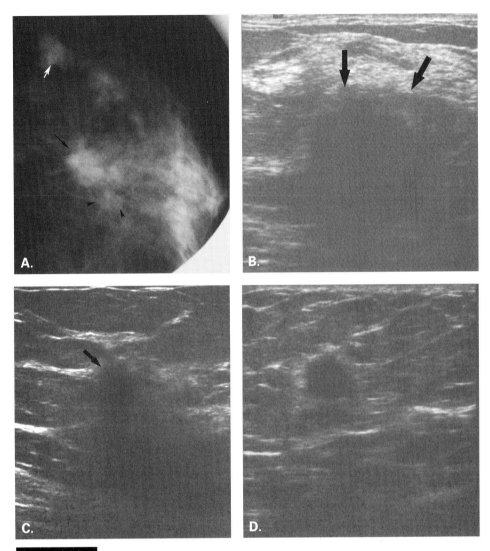

Figure 17.24

HISTORY: A 41-year-old patient with a palpable mass in the 12 o'clock position of the right breast.

IMAGING: Right CC view **(A)** shows a large, dense spiculated mass centrally **(arrow)**. Adjacent to this mass is a smaller spiculated lesion **(arrowhead)**, and there is a dense lobular mass in the lateral aspect of the breast. Sonography of the right breast **(B)** shows a large dense mass **(arrows)** centrally that is producing very prominent shadowing, corresponding to the palpable mass noted on mammography. Adjacent to this lesion is a small irregular mass **(arrow)** with very prominent central shadowing **(C)**. The lateral lesion **(D)** is more rounded and slightly indistinct in margination. The internal echo texture is homogeneous and hypoechoic. Each of these lesions has different sonographic features of malignancy.

HISTOPATHOLOGY: Multicentric invasive ductal carcinoma.

in the anterior aspect of the implant. Radial folds are often visible as linear bands connecting to the implant wall. Setting the focal zone and depth to an appropriate level to image through the implant and the use of a lower frequency transducer at times is necessary for adequate visualization and assessment of the prosthesis.

When an intracapsular rupture occurs, the implant wall is broken, but the silicone remains contained within the fibrous capsule that the body forms around the implant. In this situation, the broken wall of the implant is floating within the silicone. The wall structure is visible on ultrasound as multiple parallel linear echoes in a stair-step pattern. These correspond to the so-called linguine sign on MRI. Diffuse internal echoes may also be seen in the case of intracapsular rupture.

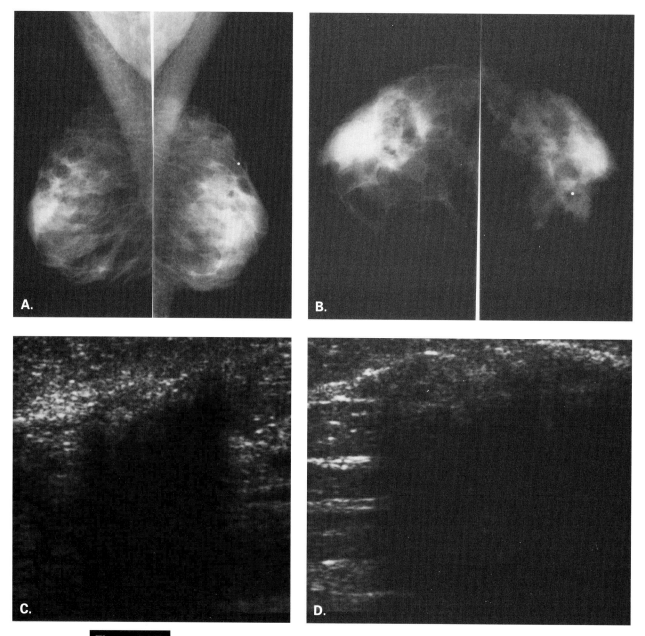

Figure 17.25

HISTORY: A 34-year-old insulin-dependent diabetic woman with a palpable right breast mass. Clinical exam showed firm tissue in the right periareolar area.

IMAGING: Bilateral MLO **(A)** and CC **(B)** views show dense parenchyma bilaterally, with no focal abnormality. A BB marks the palpable abnormality on the right. On the right breast ultrasound **(C)**, very dense acoustic shadowing is seen, suspicious for carcinoma. Sonography of the left breast **(D)** shows a similar pattern.

IMPRESSION: Dense shadowing bilaterally, likely diabetic fibrous mastopathy.

HISTOPATHOLOGY: Fibrous mastopathy.

When the rupture extends beyond the fibrous capsule, an extracapsular rupture is present. This may be evident on mammography as droplets of silicone beyond the apparent implant lumen. On ultrasound, "silicone cysts" may be evident as small, hypoechoic nodules beyond the confines of the prosthesis. With the intense tissue reaction to the silicone, a characteristic feature is seen on ultrasound: the snowstorm appearance (42–44) (Figs. 17.36 and 17.37), which is echogenic noise or shadowing related to the tissue's reaction to silicone.

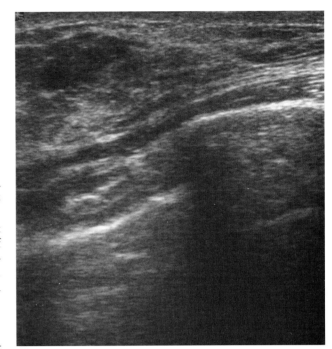

Figure 17.26

HISTORY: A 48-year-old woman with a palpable mass in the right breast.

IMAGING: Mammography showed dense breast tissue and did not reveal the mass. On ultrasound, the lesion is hypoechoic and of mixed echogenicity; the shape of the mass is lobular, its borders are partially defined, and its orientation is elongated. These findings suggest a fibrocystic etiology, but carcinoma can not be excluded.

IMPRESSION: Solid mass, BI-RADS® 4; recommend biopsy.

HISTOPATHOLOGY: Radial scar.

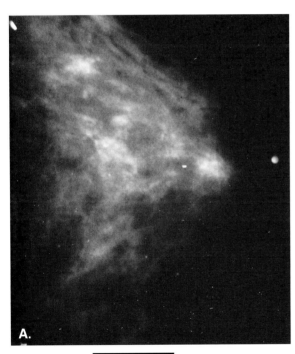

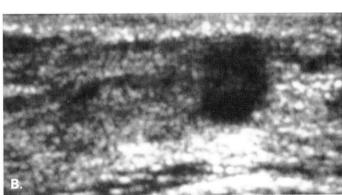

Figure 17.27

HISTORY: A 58-year-old woman with a history of left mastectomy. She reports a new palpable right subareolar mass.

IMAGING: Right CC view **(A)** shows heterogeneously dense tissue with vague increased density in the subareolar region. Ultrasound **(B)** was performed to evaluate the palpable mass. Sonography shows the lesion to be taller than wide, indistinct and hypoechoic with acoustic enhancement. The orientation and borders of the lesion are suspicious for malignancy.

HISTOPATHOLOGY: Invasive ductal carcinoma.

NOTE: Sonography of a palpable mass should be performed if mammography is negative or equivocal. Particularly when the parenchyma is dense, a noncalcified lesion may be obscured on mammography.

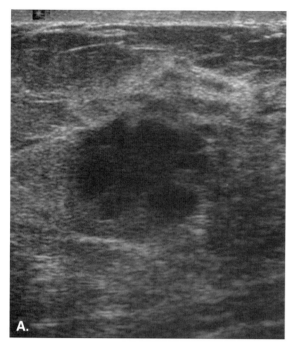
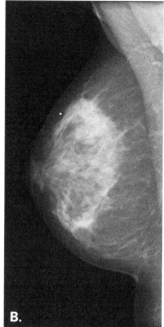
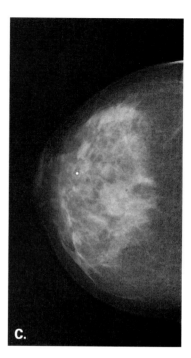

Figure 17.28

HISTORY: A 25-year-old woman with a 3-day history of a tender firm mass in the left breast. She had been gardening on the day of onset of the mass but she had not noticed any injury.

IMAGING: Left ultrasound was performed first because of the age of the patient. Sonography of the palpable mass **(A)** shows it to be round, slightly indistinct, and heterogeneous in echo pattern. The differential includes carcinoma versus an inflamed cyst versus abscess versus hematoma. Left mammography was performed before biopsy. Left MLO **(B)** and CC **(C)** views show the breast tissue to be dense, compatible with the patient's age. A BB marks the palpable mass at 12 o'clock, which is lobular, isodense, and obscured. Vacuum-assisted core needle biopsy was performed using ultrasound guidance. Purulent material was retrieved along with the core tissue sample.

HISTOPATHOLOGY: Acute and chronic mastitis with granulation tissue.

NOTE: The abscess was drained via the vacuum-assisted biopsy probe and resolved with antibiotic therapy.

Breast Interventions

Ultrasound has played an extremely important role in guiding breast interventions (45). With sonographic guidance, needle localization, cyst aspiration, fine-needle aspiration biopsy, core biopsy, and vacuum-assisted biopsy can be performed (46–48). The technology has evolved and the needles and devices have been developed to offer a variety of choices for tissue diagnosis.

Advantages of ultrasound for percutaneous biopsy are many. The lack of radiation, the ease of positioning the patient, and patient comfort (49) are evident to the patient as advantages. The equipment is multiuse and not strictly used for biopsy. The cost of equipment is less than stereotactic equipment, and the cost of the procedure is less (50). The accuracy of tissue sampling is great, and the ability to observe the needle trajectory as the sample is acquired in real time is important in assessing an adequate and accurate sample. The ability to visualize the

lesion and rapidly aspirate or sample it leads ultrasound guidance to be the procedure of choice for many interventionists.

THE ROLE OF MAGNETIC RESONANCE IMAGING OF THE BREAST

The clinical roles of breast MRI include the following:

- Neoadjuvant chemotherapy: assessment of response
- Determination of extent of disease in a patient with invasive carcinoma
- Search for an occult malignancy with a positive axillary node
- Assessment of postoperative patient with breast reconstruction and possible recurrent malignancy
- Assessment of possible chest wall invasion of primary breast cancer

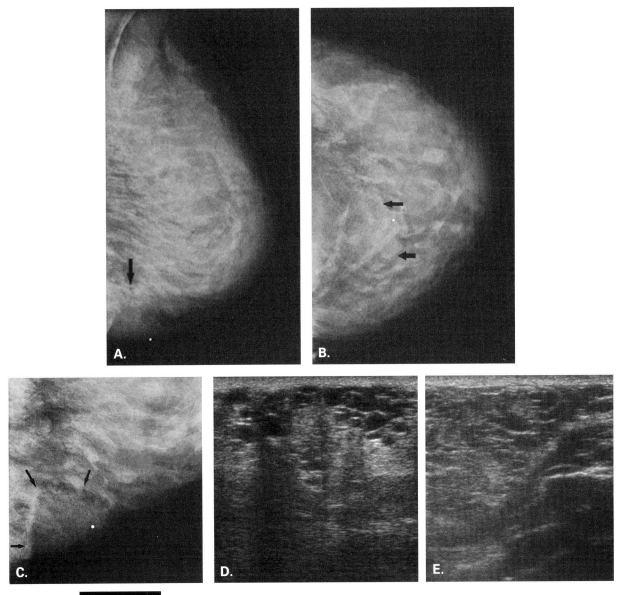

Figure 17.29

HISTORY: A 32-year-old woman with no family history of breast cancer who is 2 months postpartum and who presents with a firm right breast mass.

MAMMOGRAPHY: Right ML **(A)**, CC **(B)** and spot ML **(C)** views show the breast to be extremely dense, compatible with a lactating state. There is a focal area of increased density having a very glandular appearance **(arrows)** corresponding to the palpable mass at 5 o'clock. Clinical examination demonstrated a very firm, glandular region in the right inner-lower quadrant. The patient reported that she had always had this fullness, but it had become more masslike since her delivery. Ultrasound **(D,E)** showed multiple dilated ducts that extend up to the skin line throughout the palpable region. No solid mass was identified.

IMPRESSION: Accessory breast, stimulated by breastfeeding.

NOTE: The accessory breast that does not have a communication to the skin can become quite engorged during lactation.

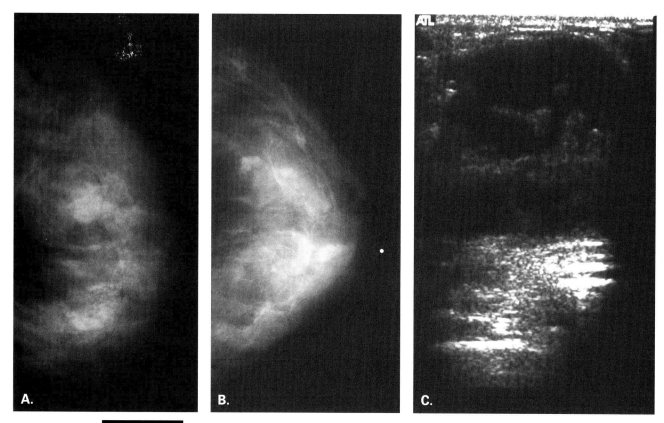

Figure 17.30

HISTORY: A 33-year-old lactating patient with a red, tender right breast.

MAMMOGRAPHY: Right ML **(A)** and CC **(B)** views show extremely dense tissue compatible with a lactating state. The area marked by the BB as palpable is generally more dense, but no definite finding is identified otherwise. On ultrasound **(C)**, there is a complex mass in the subareolar area corresponding to the lump. This mass appears to have some thick internal septations and is partially fluid filled. The edges are somewhat indistinct. Given the history and physical findings, this most likely represents an abscess. The patient was treated with drainage and antibiotics, and the abscess resolved.

IMPRESSION: Abscess in a lactating breast.

- Assessment of the contralateral breast in patients with primary breast cancer
- Assessment of postlumpectomy patient for residual disease
- Assessment of abnormal ductal lavage with negative mammography and ultrasound
- Search for cancer in a patient with silicone augmentation
- Assessment for implant rupture

These clinical recommendations were defined by the Interventional Working Group on Breast MRI in 2004 (51).

The technique for MRI imaging for tumor assessment includes the use of a breast coil and a 1.5T magnet, and dynamic imaging with injection of gadolinium DTPA. High resolution with an in-plane resolution of 1 mm or less and a slice resolution of 2 mm or less are recommended (51). A challenge for breast MRI is to achieve a high temporal res-

olution in conjunction with a high spatial resolution. The temporal resolution is needed in order to be able to scan rapidly and repetitively, and to assess for neovascularity, patterns of enhancement, and the washout of contrast. Biopsy capability is necessary so that when MRI-detected suspicious lesions are identified and are not visible on mammography or ultrasound, MRI-guided needle localization (52,53) or core biopsy can be performed (54,55).

Magnetic Resonance Imaging of Augmented Breasts

Early work with breast MRI was primarily for the evaluation of implant rupture. MRI has been shown (56–59) to be the most effective modality for the diagnosis of rupture. Silicone has a unique MRI frequency and a long T_1 and T_2 relaxation time. On T_2-weighted images, silicone has a

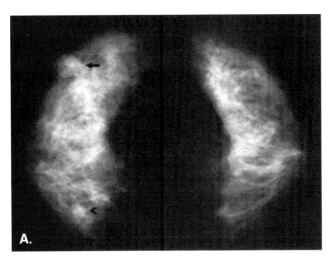

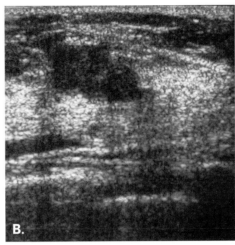

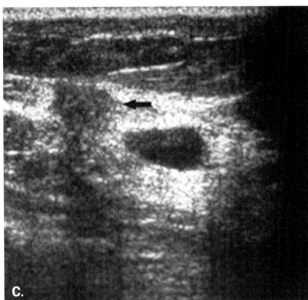

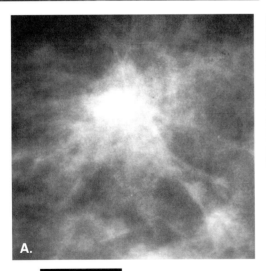

Figure 17.31

HISTORY: A 41-year-old woman for screening mammography.

MAMMOGRAPHY: Bilateral CC views **(A)** show heterogeneously dense tissue. In the lateral aspect of the left breast, there is a lobulated, relatively circumscribed mass **(arrow)**. When comparing the breasts as mirror images, an area of architectural distortion is also noted, superimposed over the dense tissue in the left breast medially **(arrowhead)**. Ultrasound **(B)** of the lateral mass shows it to be hypoechoic and lobulated with features most compatible with a fibroadenoma. Sonography of the medial aspect of the breast **(C)** shows two masses: a complex cyst as well as a small solid mass that is associated with dense shadowing **(arrow)**.

IMPRESSION: Three masses likely representing a cancer, a fibroadenoma, and a complicated cyst.

HISTOPATHOLOGY: Fibroadenoma (lateral mass), invasive ductal carcinoma (medial mass).

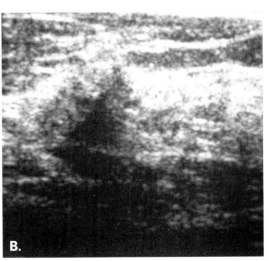

Figure 17.32

Spot compression view **(A)** performed for an area of asymmetry shows a small dense area of distortion centrally. Ultrasound **(B)** is helpful in this situation in confirming the presence of an irregular mass, suspicious for carcinoma. Also, sonographic guidance is an ideal method for directing percutaneous breast biopsy.

HISTOPATHOLOGY: Invasive lobular carcinoma.

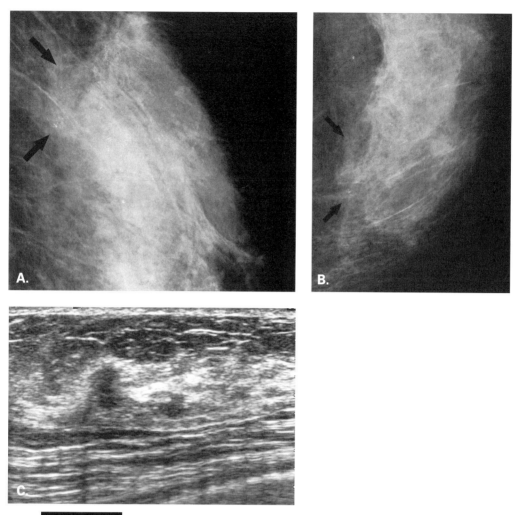

Figure 17.33

HISTORY: A 47-year-old woman who had been followed for 2 years for microcalcifications in the right breast and who now presents for a second opinion.

IMAGING: Right ML magnification **(A)** and CC magnification **(B)** views show fine pleomorphic microcalcifications in a regional distribution in the upper inner aspect of the breast **(arrows)**. These are highly suspicious for malignancy and do not meet the criteria for a probably benign lesion. Ultrasound was performed to search for an underlying mass. On ultrasound **(C)** of the area of microcalcifications, a mass is identified. The lesion is taller than wide, hypoechoic, and somewhat irregular, all features that are highly suspicious for malignancy. The presence of the mass raises the likelihood of an invasive component. Core needle biopsy of the mass was performed under sonographic guidance.

IMPRESSION: Highly suspicious for malignancy.

HISTOPATHOLOGY: Invasive ductal carcinoma, DCIS.

signal intensity greater than fat and less than water. The wall of the implant, composed of silicone polymer, is of lower signal intensity than the silicone gel contents (59).

The normal single-lumen implant has an oval shape and uniform signal intensity. Radial folds may be seen and represent infolding of the silicone wall or shell. These are linear invaginations that are of low signal and attach to the wall. Radial folds are a normal finding and do not indi-

cate signs of rupture. Typically, radial folds have a sharp angulation with the fibrous capsule that helps to differentiate them from an intracapsular rupture, which is oriented parallel to the capsule (60).

In patients with an intracapsular rupture, the silicone shell is broken, and the silicone has extravasated into the space within the fibrous capsule. In these patients, the silicone shell is floating within the silicone and has the

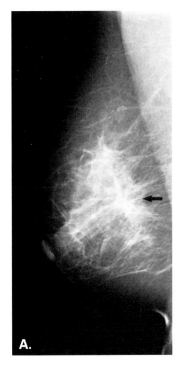

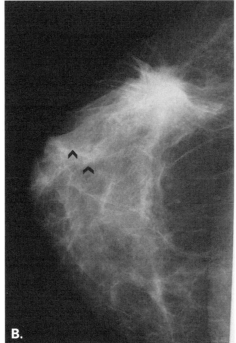

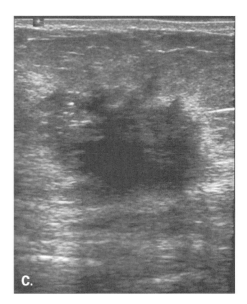

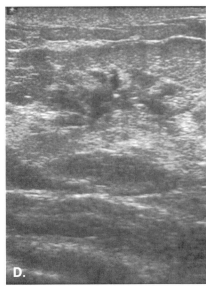

Figure 17.34

HISTORY: A 42-year-old woman with a palpable mass in the left breast at 3 o'clock posteriorly.

MAMMOGRAPHY: Left MLO (**A**) and CC (**B**) magnification views show a high-density spiculated mass with associated fine linear microcalcifications (**arrow**) that are highly suspicious for malignancy. This corresponded to the palpable mass. No other suspicious mass was noted on mammography, but the calcifications do extend in a ductal distribution from the mass anteriorly (**B, arrowheads**). Left breast ultrasound was performed to evaluate the palpable mass and the remainder of the breast. The palpable mass (**C**) is microlobulated, shadowing, hypoechoic, and taller than wide. The borders are indistinct, and there is some surrounding hyperechogenicity, compatible with edema, all of which are malignant features. In the subareolar area (**D**), a second solid irregular lesion that has indistinct margins and is also hypoechoic is seen. This lesion is also highly suspicious for malignancy.

IMPRESSION: Multifocal carcinoma.

HISTOPATHOLOGY: Invasive ductal carcinoma with DCIS at both sites.

appearance of the linguine sign within the silicone. The low signal wall appears to float within the silicone gel (Figs. 17.38 and 17.39).

With extracapsular rupture, the silicone extends outside the capsule into the breast tissue and the axilla. Droplets of silicone are visible on MRI beyond the confines of the fibrous shell that is around the silicone (Fig. 17.40). Reported sensitivity and specificity of breast MRI for rupture have been retrospectively reported to be 94% and 97%, respectively (59). The most reliable signs of rupture are the linguine sign (59) and free silicone in the extracapsular area (59).

Problem-solving Magnetic Resonance Imaging

MRI is performed to assess the breast for malignancy in several important clinical situations. The technical considerations for tumor assessment include the following requirements: use of a breast coil, contrast administration, subtraction or fat suppression or both, T_1- and T_2-weighted sequences, scan thickness of no more than 3 mm, image acquisition time to allow for repeated scans through the same area in 60 to 90 seconds, and the ability to calculate time-intensity curves.

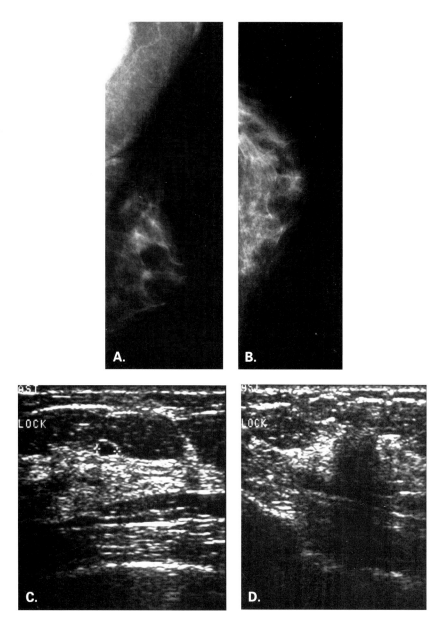

Figure 17.35

HISTORY: A 38-year-old patient who presents with a small palpable mass in the right upper-outer quadrant.

MAMMOGRAPHY: Right MLO **(A)** and CC **(B)** views showed dense parenchyma and no dominant mass. Ultrasound **(C)** was performed and showed a small cyst that corresponded to the palpable finding. More inferiorly in the same breast in an area that was not palpable, ultrasound **(D)** demonstrated an irregular solid mass with dense shadowing, highly suspicious for carcinoma.

IMPRESSION: Right cyst that is palpable; right suspicious solid mass, an incidental finding.

HISTOPATHOLOGY: Invasive lobular carcinoma.

NOTE: Occasionally screening ultrasound or ultrasound of the remainder of the breast that is being evaluated for a specific finding will reveal a mammographically and clinically occult carcinoma. If a suspicious sonographic finding is observed, biopsy using ultrasound guidance is performed.

Because of the tumor neovascularity and angiogenesis, the contrast rapidly flows into the area of the tumor. With arteriovenous shunting, there is a rapid washout of contrast. Because of this phenomenon, tumors tend to enhance rapidly and intensely compared with benign lesions. Because of the vascular characteristics of malignancy, the contrast also rapidly washes out (61). Therefore, rapid image acquisitions are necessary to observe this phenomenon, and the scans are typically performed over about 8 minutes to observe the enhancement and washout of lesions. Time-intensity curves may be calculated over enhancing regions of interest. Malignancies usually exhibit the cancer curve (62), reflecting the rapid peak at 90 seconds to 2 minutes and then immediate washout. Benign lesions tend to continually enhance or to plateau. The sensitivity of breast MRI for detection of invasive breast cancer is high, ranging from 88% to 99%, but the specificity is lower

(28%–80%) (63–68). Even in cases of DCIS, early contrast enhancement has been demonstrated, and tumor angiogenesis has been found in the stroma in these cases (69).

The pattern of enhancement and shape of masses on MRI suggest their possible etiologies. On T_2-weighted images, certain benign lesions are high in signal, particularly cysts, lymph nodes, and myomatous fibroadenomas (70). The vast majority of breast cancers are not high in signal on T_2-weighted images, although occasionally necrotic tumors or mucinous carcinomas (71) may be bright on T_2. The shape of lesions on MRI can be described as round, oval, lobulated, or irregular; the margins are smooth, irregular, or spiculated (70); and these findings parallel the mammographic findings.

Patterns of enhancement are homogeneous or heterogeneous. Findings that are suspicious for malignancy include heterogeneous enhancement, rim enhancement, enhancing

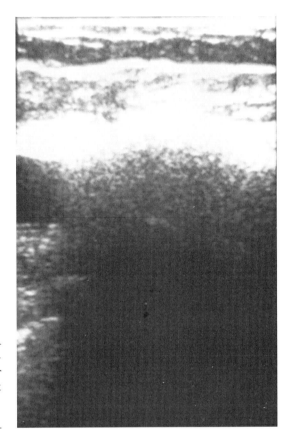

Figure 17.36

HISTORY: Patient with a history of silicone implants with a question of rupture.

IMAGING: Ultrasound over the left axillary tail shows signs of extracapsular rupture. There is an echogenic focus anterior to the edge of the implant with associated dense acoustic shadowing, the snowstorm appearance.

IMPRESSION: Extracapsular silicone implant rupture.

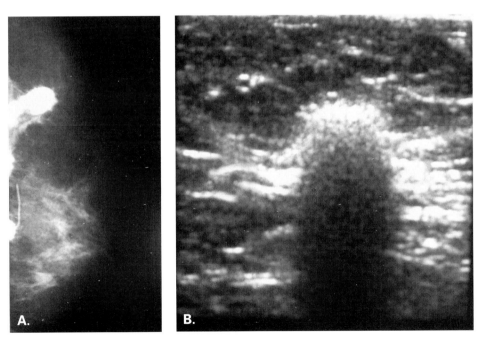

Figure 17.37

HISTORY: Postmenopausal patient with newly diagnosed lymphoma and a palpable right breast mass. She had a history of removal of silicone implants for rupture years ago.

IMAGING: Right exaggerated CC lateral view **(A)** show a hyperdense indistinct mass laterally, extending along the chest wall. The density is much greater than that of breast parenchyma, suggesting the possibility of free silicone rather than a breast mass. Ultrasound **(B)** shows the mass to be associated with very echogenic shadowing, consistent with free silicone.

IMPRESSION: Free silicone granulomas.

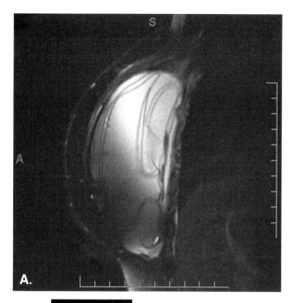

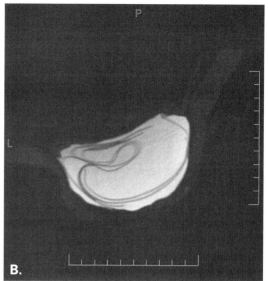

Figure 17.38

HISTORY: Patient with a history of silicone implants with a question of rupture.

IMAGING: Sagittal **(A)** and axial **(B)** T$_2$-weighted MRI images. Within the silicone is a serpiginous structure that is not connected to the wall. The silicone conforms to the shape of an implant, and there is no extension beyond this shape. The structure within the silicone represents the broken implant wall that is floating within the silicone. The fibrous capsule around the implant is intact and is containing the silicone.

IMPRESSION: Intracapsular rupture of the silicone implant (linguine sign). (Case courtesy of Dr. Deanne Lane, Houston, TX.)

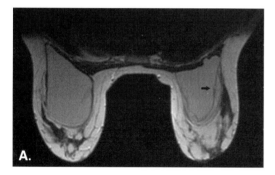

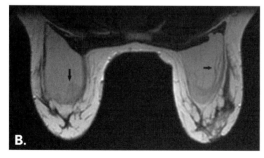

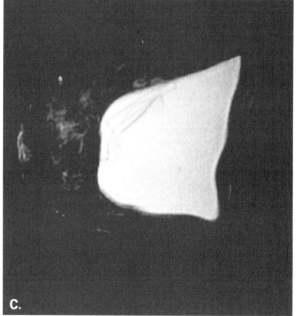

Figure 17.39

HISTORY: Patient with a history of augmentation with silicone implants, with a question of rupture.

MAMMOGRAPHY: Bilateral axial T$_2$-weighted MRI images **(A,B)** show low signal serpiginous structures **(arrows)** within the silicone. A sagittal inversion recovery image of the right breast **(C)** also shows the linguine sign, which represents the broken implant wall floating within the silicone. The silicone is contained by the fibrous capsule that formed around the implant, so this is not an extracapsular rupture.

IMPRESSION: Bilateral intracapsular ruptures of silicone prostheses. (Case courtesy of Dr. Neeti Goel, Harrisburg, PA.)

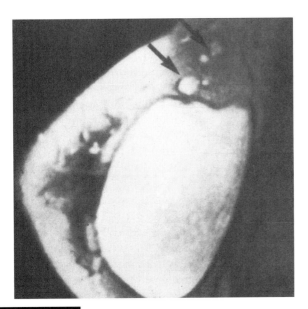

septations, or central enhancement (70). Liberman et al. (72) found that MRI features with the highest positive predictive value of malignancy were a spiculated margin (80% cancers), rim enhancement (40% cancers), and an irregular shape (38% cancers). Dark internal septations are characteristic of fibroadenomas. Inflamed cysts and fat necrosis may show thin rims of enhancement. Nonmass patterns of enhancement may be linear or segmental, which suggest a ductal orientation, and are worrisome for DCIS. Regional or diffuse enhancement patterns are more often benign, but it is important to look for symmetry when this finding is observed. When linear or segmental enhancement has a clumped or irregular pattern, it is particularly suspicious for DCIS (70) (Fig. 17.41). Orel et al. (73) described MRI findings of DCIS and found that 77% of cases showed ductal enhancement and regional enhancement or a peripherally enhancing mass.

Figure 17.40

HISTORY: Patient with a history of silicone implants and a question of rupture.

IMAGING: Sagittal MRI image of the left breast shows the implant to be slightly irregular in contour. There are multiple rounded "masses" **(arrows)** extending toward the axillary tail having the same signal intensity as the silicone. The findings are typical of extracapsular rupture.

IMPRESSION: Extracapsular rupture of a silicone implant. (Case courtesy of Dr. Patricia Abbitt, Gainesville, FL.)

Magnetic Resonance Imaging for the Assessment of Local Extent of Carcinoma

As more and more women undergo breast conservation therapy, it is critical that careful preoperative assessment of the patient be performed to assure that she is a good candidate for this treatment. MRI is particularly helpful for assessing the size, number, and location of breast cancers. MRI has been demonstrated to more accurately assess tumor size than mammography (74–78). Weinstein et al. (79) found that MRI imaging showed more extensive tumor

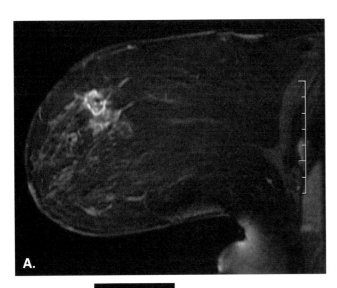

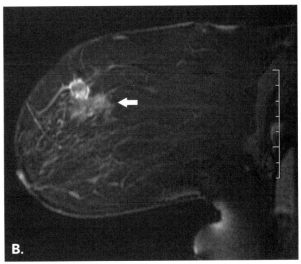

Figure 17.41

MRI study on a patient who had recently undergone a core biopsy for DCIS in the right breast. Subtraction T_1-weighted postcontrast images show an enhancing lesion in the upper aspect of the breast **(A,B)**. Within this area of enhancement is a central susceptibility artifact from the clip that was deployed during the biopsy. A moderate amount of clumped enhancement surrounds the biopsy site, consistent with residual tumor **(arrow)**.

HISTOPATHOLOGY: DCIS. (Case courtesy of Dr. Neeti Goel, Harrisburg, PA.)

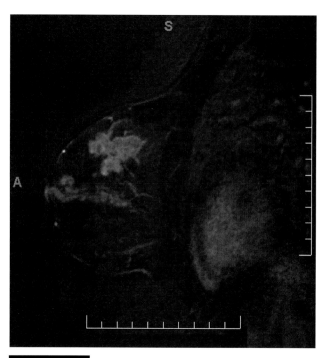

Figure 17.42

HISTORY: Patient with biopsy-proven cancer in the left upper-outer quadrant, for assessment of extent of disease.

IMAGING: T_1-weighted sequence postcontrast, subtraction sagittal image shows a large rim-enhancing irregular mass in the upper aspect of the breast, corresponding to the cancer. Extending anterior to the mass is clumped linear enhancement that is suggestive of intraductal extension of tumor. In addition, there is a separate area of linear enhancement in the subareolar region, likely representing another focus of DCIS. Biopsy of this region was performed as well.

HISTOPATHOLOGY: Invasive ductal carcinoma, DCIS, multicentric. (Case courtesy of Dr. Deanne Lane, Houston, TX.)

than conventional imaging and affected the clinical management in 50% of patients with invasive lobular carcinoma.

Additional foci of tumor representing either multifocal or multicentric disease may be demonstrated on MRI, when only the index lesion is evident on mammography (80–82) (Figs. 17.42 and 17.43). In the patient with multicentric carcinoma, mastectomy is indicated, so the preoperative diagnosis of multiple cancers greatly affects patient management. Orel et al. (83) found that as a result of the increased sensitivity of MRI compared with mammography, clinical staging and treatment were altered in 11% of patients with breast cancer.

Boetes et al. (75)—in a study of 60 women with 61 cancers that were evaluated with mammography, ultrasound, and MRI before mastectomy—found that MRI was the most accurate method to assess the size and number of malignancies. Liberman et al. (84) found additional sites of ipsilateral cancer with MRI in 27% of women with percutaneous proven breast cancer. The yield was highest in

women with family history of breast cancer or an infiltrating lobular histology.

In a study of 67 patients with dense breasts and cancers, MRI depicted 100% of the multifocal or multicentric cancers (20 patients), whereas mammography found 35% and ultrasound depicted 31% of the additional malignancies (85). In a study comparing mammography, ultrasound, and MRI in patients with known breast cancers, Berg et al. (86) found that mammography had a sensitivity of 100% for additional foci in fatty breasts, but the sensitivity was 45% in dense breasts. The sensitivity of mammography for the detection of invasive ductal carcinoma was 89%; invasive lobular carcinoma, 34%; and DCIS, 55%. MRI sensitivities for the same lesions were 95%, 96%, and 89%, respectively (86). Sardanelli et al. (87) also found MRI to be significantly more sensitive than mammography in the detection of multiple malignant foci in dense breasts, but there was not a significant difference in fatty breasts.

The depiction of additional foci in the same breast or the contralateral breast should prompt biopsy before any change in the definitive treatment plan (Fig. 17.44). Because of the limited specificity of MRI, additional enhancing lesions may represent other foci of cancers, but in most cases, they are benign. Liberman (88) found that biopsies performed because of MRI-depicted contralateral lesions were benign in 80% of patients. Contralateral cancers have been identified on MRI in 2% to 9% of cases (89,90). Therefore, histologic sampling of additional findings on preoperative breast MRI should be performed before treatment decision making is affected (91).

Postoperative MRI assessment of the patient with newly diagnosed breast cancer may also yield important information that affects the final surgical management and treatment. Normal finding after lumpectomy is a seroma, which has a smooth, thin rim of enhancement. Positive surgical margins might suggest the presence of residual disease and prompt imaging with MRI. The observation of linear clumped enhancement around the lumpectomy site suggests the presence of residual DCIS. MRI can confirm the presence of residual carcinoma as well as possible other foci elsewhere in the breast. Orel et al. (80) evaluated MRI for the assessment of residual tumor and found that MRI had a positive predictive value of 82% and a negative predictive value of 61% for assessment of residual tumor.

Assessment of Recurrent Carcinoma

In the early postoperative period, the lumpectomy site may be visible on subtraction images as having thin rim-like enhancement. This pattern of enhancement may persist until 18 months after surgery. From this point on, enhancement at the lumpectomy site should be viewed with suspicion for malignancy.

In patients who have been treated with breast conservation therapy, the sensitivity of mammography for the

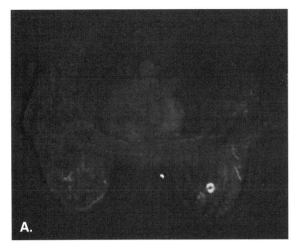

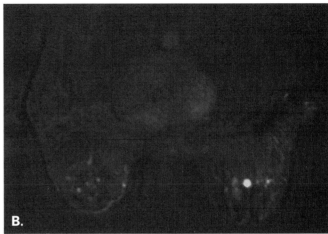

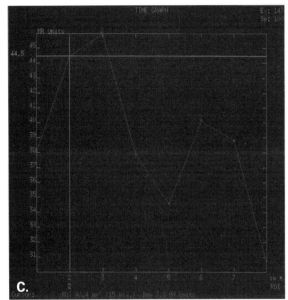

Figure 17.43

HISTORY: A 44-year-old woman with a strong family history of breast cancer and with newly diagnosed breast cancer, for assessment of extent of disease.

MRI: T_1-weighted subtraction postcontrast images show a rim-enhancing mass in the right breast **(A,B)**. Adjacent to this lesion is some clumped enhancement suggestive of the possibility of intraductal extension. Multiple small enhancing foci were seen in the opposite breast. A time-intensity curve **(C)** over the larger mass shows the typical cancer curve of rapid wash in and rapid wash out of contrast.

IMPRESSION: Possible intraductal extension of tumor.

HISTOPATHOLOGY: Invasive ductal carcinoma, DCIS.

detection of local possible recurrence has been reported to be 55% to 70% (92,93). MRI is useful, particularly after the first 18 months, to detect local recurrence (94,95). In the first 12 months after treatment, fat necrosis at the lumpectomy site is associated with poorly defined enhancement patterns that may be confused with tumor.

Findings on mammography that might suggest the possibility of recurrence are an increase in size or density of the scar or an increase in skin thickness. Because of the overall edema of the breast and the difficulty in compressing some irradiated breasts, these findings may be subtle. With recurrence, MRI demonstrates enhancement at the region of the scar or elsewhere in the breast (Fig. 17.45) and may show diffuse skin enhancement when an inflammatory recurrence is present.

Neoadjuvant Chemotherapy

In patients with locally advanced breast cancer or in patients with large tumors relative to the breast size,

neoadjuvant chemotherapy may be given to reduce the tumor burden before surgery. In patients with large tumors (>5 cm), the use of neoadjuvant chemotherapy has been shown to reduce the need for mastectomies and to increase the rate of lumpectomies by 175% (96).

In addition to trying to reduce the tumor burden with neoadjuvant chemotherapy, one may be able to determine potential outcome. Those tumors that show a marked response to neoadjuvant therapy may be those with an overall better outcome (91). The lack of response to the chemotherapy usually prompts surgery rather than completing the preoperative chemotherapy regimen.

MRI has been found to be better than mammography and ultrasound in the assessment of the size of tumor (91). However, overestimates of residual tumor by MRI range from 6% to 52% (97,98), and underestimates range from 10% to 23% (97,98). Underestimation of disease has been found to be greater in invasive lobular carcinoma and has been reported to occur in 78% of cases (99).

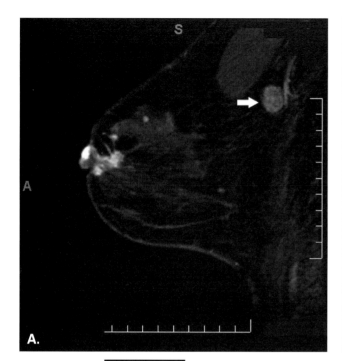

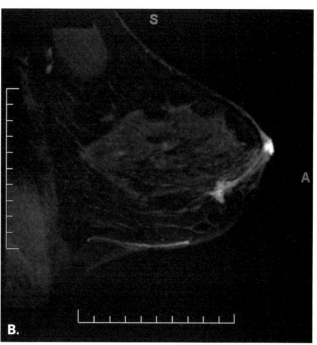

Figure 17.44

HISTORY: Patient with biopsy-proven left breast cancer, referred to assess for extent of disease.

MAMMOGRAPHY: Left **(A)** and right **(B)** sagittal subtraction postcontrast imaging. There is a lobular enhancing mass that has heterogeneous enhancement located in the left subareolar area **(A)**. This lesion is highly suspicious for malignancy, and this corresponded to the biopsied cancer. Multiple small enhancing foci are noted in the same breast. An enlarged enhancing node is also noted in the inferior axillary region **(arrow)** on the left, suspicious for metastatic involvement with tumor. On the right **(B)**, there is linear, ductal enhancement in the subareolar area, extending back toward a small lobulated enhancing mass in the inferior pole of the breast.

IMPRESSION: Multicentric carcinoma left breast with positive axillary adenopathy; DCIS and invasive cancer right breast.

HISTOPATHOLOGY: Left invasive ductal carcinoma, multicentric; mucinous carcinoma, right breast. (Case courtesy of Dr. Deanne Lane, Houston, TX.)

The Positive Axillary Node

The vast majority of patients who have metastatic breast cancer in the ipsilateral axillary nodes have a clinical or mammographic presentation of the cancer within the breast. Occasionally, though, the primary cancer may be clinically and mammographically occult, yet the patient presents with an enlarged axillary node that is positive for adenocarcinoma on biopsy. MRI can be valuable in these circumstances in identifying the primary breast cancer.

The treatment of patients with a positive node and no primary cancer identified in the breast has been controversial, yet in most cases, mastectomy has been performed. With MRI detection of the primary cancer, the patient may be able to undergo breast conservation therapy. In addition, the histology and the cellular features of the tumor are important to treatment planning (74,100). Obdeijn et al. (101) studied the role of MRI in 31 women

with metastatic carcinoma in axillary nodes from an unknown primary site and with negative mammography and physical exam. MRI revealed the primary breast cancer in 40% of the patients who had no prior history of malignancy.

Other Clinical Situations

MRI plays a role in several other clinically and mammographically equivocal situations. In patients with suspicious nipple discharge and negative imaging, MRI may identify the source of the discharge. A papilloma may be identified as an intermediate signal-intensity mass within a dilated duct on T_2-weighted images and is a homogeneously enhancing mass after contrast (74). Small peripheral papillomas are round enhancing masses, and DCIS is often seen as linear or clumped enhancement. Orel et al. (102) suggested the role of MRI imaging to identify benign

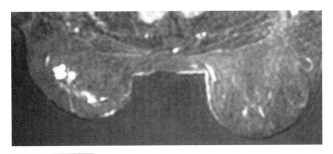

Figure 17.45

HISTORY: A 52-year-old patient with a history of left breast cancer treated with lumpectomy and radiotherapy 7 years previously. She reports increased heaviness of the treated breast.

IMAGING: Mammography showed postoperative changes with questionable increase in skin thickness on the left. MRI was performed and shows signs of recurrence on the subtraction postcontrast T_1-weighted axial image. There are three enhancing lobular masses in the left breast, suspicious for recurrence. The lesions were identified on ultrasound. Biopsy was performed using ultrasound guidance.

IMPRESSION: Enhancing masses in the treated breast, most suggestive of recurrent carcinoma.

HISTOPATHOLOGY: Invasive lobular carcinoma, multicentric, recurrent.

and malignant causes of discharge and to potentially serve as an alternative to galactography.

Ductal lavage is sometimes performed in high-risk women to search for atypical cells. This procedure involves flushing fluid into the ducts and collecting the expressed fluid for cytologic analysis. In patients with positive or suspicious ductal lavage findings and negative imaging, MRI may be used to search for a potential malignancy (51).

Equivocal mammographic findings, such as focal asymmetries that do not have an associated clinical or sonographic finding, may occasionally be evaluated with MRI. In these situations, a negative MRI may prompt follow-up rather than biopsy for a density that is of low suspicion, whereas a positive MRI leads to biopsy (74).

THE ROLE OF MAGNETIC RESONANCE IMAGING IN SCREENING FOR BREAST CANCER

The limitations of screening mammography are greater in women with dense parenchyma that may obscure underlying noncalcified masses. Younger women tend to have denser breasts, but this is not necessarily so. Breast density depends on a number of factors, including body habitus, weight, and parity, as well as parenchymal factors. The risk of breast cancer is less in younger women, and the risk of the disease increases with age.

Young women who are at high risk of developing breast cancer or those women who are at higher risk and who have dense breasts are those who may potentially benefit most from screening MRI. MRI has a high sensitivity for the detection of invasive cancers greater than 3 mm in size, and parenchymal density does not limit its sensitivity. Therefore, if screening MRI is to be used, the populations it may best serve are those women who are at high risk for breast cancer and those with dense parenchyma. Several small studies have reported on screening MRI-detected breast cancers in high-risk women (103–106). Morris et al. (103) found 14/367 high-risk women (4%) to have MRI-detected, mammographically occult breast cancers. Kriege et al. (107) from the Netherlands reported on screening 1,909 high-risk women who had proven genetic mutations or positive family history. Clinical examination, mammography, ultrasound, and MRI were used to screen the women, and 45 cancers were found, 22 of which were seen on MRI only.

A number of potential problems exist with MRI screening, including the following (108): the ability to tolerate the procedure or be a candidate for MRI, contrast reaction, cost of the procedure, high number of false positives, determination of protocols for "probably benign" MRI-detected lesions, and accessibility to a breast MRI facility. The potential for MRI to detect cancers in certain select populations is great.

Because of many of the above cited disadvantages, screening MRI will not likely be a replacement for mammography or a generally used study. MRI, like ultrasound, plays an important role in the comprehensive evaluation of women with breast abnormalities, many of which are detected on mammography. The gold standard for early detection of breast cancer and the tool proven to reduce mortality for this disease remains mammography.

REFERENCES

1. Hilton SW, Leopold GR, Olson LK, et al. Real-time breast sonography: application in 300 consecutive patients. *AJR Am J Roentgenol* 1986;147:479–486.
2. Bassett LW, Kimme-Smith C. Breast sonography. *AJR Am J Roentgenol* 1991;156:449–455.
3. Sickles EA, Filly RA, Callen PW. Benign breast lesions: ultrasound detection and diagnosis. *Radiology* 1984;151:467–470.
4. Jackson VP. Present and future role of ultrasound in breast imaging. *In: Radiological Society of North America Categorical Course in Physics* Hous AG and Yaffe MJ eds. Radiological Society of North America. Oak Brook, IL. 1993;241–247.
5. Mendelson EB. Breast US: performance, anatomy, pitfalls, and BI-RADS®. *Breast Imaging: RSNA Categorical Course in Diagnostic Radiology* Feig SA ed. Radiological Society of North America. Oak Brook, IL. 2005;107–113.
6. American College of Radiology. *Breast Imaging and Data System (BIRADS)*. Reston, VA: ACR, 2003.
7. Jellins J, Kossoff G, Reeve TS. Detection and classification of liquid-filled masses in the breast by gray scale echography. *Radiology* 1977;125:205–212.

8. Reuter K, D'Orsi CJ, Reale F. Intracystic carcinoma of the breast: the role of ultrasonography. *Radiology* 1984;153: 233–234.

9. Berg WA, Campassi CI, Ioffe OB. Cystic lesions of the breast: sonographic-pathologic correlation. *Radiology* 2003; 227:183–191.

10. Stavros AT, Thickman D, Rapp CL, et al. Solid breast nodules: use of sonography to distinguish between benign and malignant lesions. *Radiology* 1995;196(1):123–134.

11. Stavros AT, Rapp CL, Kaske TI, et al. Hard and soft sonographic findings of malignancy. In: *Breast Imaging: RSNA Categorical Course in Diagnostic Radiology*, ed. Feig SA, Radiological Society of North America, Oak Brook, IL. 2005;125–142.

12. Cole-Beuglet C, Soriano RZ, Kurtz AB, et al. Fibroadenoma of the breast: sonomammography correlated with pathology in 122 patients. *AJR Am J Roentgenol* 1983;140:369–375.

13. Fornage BD, Lorigan JG, Andry E. Fibroadenoma of the breast: sonographic appearance. *Radiology* 1989;172: 671–675.

14. Buchberger W, Strasser K, Heim K, et al. Phylloides tumor: findings on mammography, sonography and aspiration cytology in 10 cases. *AJR Am J Roentgenol* 1991;157: 715–719.

15. Soo MS, Kornguth PJ, Hertzberg BS. Fat necrosis in the breast: sonographic features. *Radiology* 1998;206:261–269.

16. Gordon PB, Gilks B. Sonographic appearance of normal intramammary lymph nodes. *J Ultrasound Med* 1988;7: 545–548.

17. Cole-Beuglet C, Soriano RZ, Kurtz AB, et al. Ultrasound analysis of 104 primary breast carcinomas classified according to histopathologic type. *Radiology* 1983;147: 191–196.

18. Gordon PB. US for problem solving in breast imaging: tricks of the trade. In: *A Categorical Course in Breast Imaging* ed by Kopons DB and Mendelson EB. Radiological Society of North America. Oak Brook, IL. 1995;121–131.

19. Harris KM, Ilkhanipour ZS, Ganott MA. Vertically oriented solid breast mass: a predictor of malignancy at sonography [abstract]. *Radiology* 1992;185(P):112(abst).

20. Sickles EA, Filly RA, Callen PW. Breast cancer detection with sonography and mammography: comparison using state-of-the-art equipment. *AJR Am J Roentgenol* 1983;140: 843–845.

21. Egan RL, Egan KL. Automated water-path full-breast sonography: correlation with histology in 176 solid lesions. *AJR Am J Roentgenol* 1984;143:499–507.

22. Bassett LW, Kimme-Smith C, Sutherland LK, et al. Automated and hand-held breast US: effect on patient management. *Radiology* 1987;165:103–108.

23. Kopans DB, Meyer JE, Lindfors KK. Whole-breast US imaging: four-year follow-up. *Radiology* 1985;157:505–507.

24. Croll J, Kotevich J, Tabrett M. The diagnosis of benign disease and the exclusion of malignancy in patients with breast symptoms. *Semin Ultrasound* 1982;3:38–50.

25. Soo MS, Rosen EL, Baker, JA, et al. Negative predictive value of sonography with mammography in patients with palpable breast lesions. *AJR Am J Roentgenol* 2001;177:1167–1170.

26. Harris VJ, Jackson VP. Indications for breast imaging in women under age 35 years. *Radiology* 1989;172:445–448.

27. Bassett LW, Ysrael M, Gold RH, et al. Usefulness of mammography and sonography in women less than 35 years of age. *Radiology* 1991;180:831–835.

28. Shaw de Paredes E, Marstellar LP, Eden BV. Breast cancers in women 35 years of age and younger: mammographic findings. *Radiology* 1990;177:117–119.

29. Kimme-Smith C, Bassett LW, Gold RH. High frequency breast ultrasound: hand-held versus automated units: examination for palpable mass versus screening. *J Ultrasound Med* 1988;7:77–81.

30. Buchberger W, Niehoff A, Obrist A, et al. Clinically and mammographically occult breast lesions: detection and classification with high-resolution sonography. *Semin Ultrasound CT MR* 2000;21:325–336.

31. Kaplan SS. Clinical utility of bilateral whole-breast US in the evaluation of women with dense breast tissue. *Radiology* 2001;221:641–649.

32. Kolb TM, Lichy J, Newhouse JH. Comparison of the performance of screening mammography, physical examination, and breast US and evaluation of factors that influence them: an analysis of 27,825 patient evaluations. *Radiology* 2002;225:165–175.

33. Leconte I, Feger C. Galant C, et al. Mammography and subsequent whole-breast sonography of nonpalpable breast cancers: the importance of radiologic breast density. *AJR Am J Roentgenol* 2003;180:1675–1679.

34. Crystal P, Strano S, Shcharynski S, et al. Using sonography to screen women with mammographically dense breasts. *AJR Am J Roentgenol* 2003;181:177–182.

35. Gordon PB, Goldenberg SL. Malignant breast masses detected only by ultrasound: a retrospective review. *Cancer* 1995;76:626–630.

36. Feig SA. Current status of screening US. *Breast Imaging: RSNA Categorical Course in Diagnostic Radiology* ed. Feig SA, Radiological Society of North America. Oak Brook, IL. 2005;143–154.

37. Berg WA, Gilbreath PL. Multicentric or multifocal cancer: whole breast US in preoperative evaluation. *Radiology* 2000;214(1):59–66.

38. LaTrenta LR, Menell JH, Morris EA, et al. Breast lesions detected with MR imaging: utility and histopathologic importance of identification with US. *Radiology* 2003;227: 856–861.

39. Everson LI, Parantainen H, Detlie T, et al. Diagnosis of breast implant rupture: imaging findings and relative efficacies of imaging techniques. *AJR Am J Roentgenol* 1994; 163:57–60.

40. Berg WA, Caskey CI, Kuhlman JE, et al. Comparative evaluation of MR imaging and US in determining breast implant failure [abstract]. *Radiology* 1994;193(P):318(abst).

41. Herzog PM, Exner K, Holtermueller KH, et al. Detection with US of implant rupture and siliconomas [abstract]. *Radiology* 1993;189(P):155(abst).

42. Rosculet KA, Ideda DM, Forrest ME, et al. Ruptured gel-filled silicone breast implants: sonographic findings in 19 cases. *AJR Am J Roentgenol* 1992;159:711–716.

43. Barlow RE, Torees WE, Sones PJ, et al. Sonographic demonstration of migrating silicone. *AJR Am J Roentgenol* 1980;135:170–171.

44. Palmon LU, Forshager MC, Everson LI, et al. US of ruptured breast implants: sensitivity of snowstorm appearance [abstract]. *Radiology* 1994;193(P):177(abst).

45. Comstock CE. US-guided interventional procedures. *Breast Imaging RSNA Categorical Course in Diagnostic Radiology* ed by Feig SA. Radiological Society of North America. Oak Brook, IL. 2005;155–168.

46. Staren ED, O'Neill TP. Ultrasound-guided needle biopsy of the breast. *Surgery* 1999;126:629–634; discussion 634–635.

47. Rubin E, Mennemeyer ST, Desmond RA, et al. Reducing the cost of diagnosis of breast carcinoma: impact of ultrasound and imaging-guided biopsies on a clinical breast practice. *Cancer* 2001;91:324–332.

48. Parker SH, Jobe WE, Dennis MA, et al. US-guided automated large-core breast biopsy. *Radiology* 1993;187:507–511.

49. Mainiero MB, Gareen IF, Bird CE, et al. Preferential use of sonographically guided biopsy to minimize patient discomfort and procedure time in a percutaneous image-guided breast biopsy program. *J Ultrasound Med* 2002;21:1221–1226.

50. Liberman L, Feng TL, Dershaw DD, et al. US-guided core breast biopsy: use and cost-effectiveness. *Radiology* 1998;208:717–723.

51. Harms SE, Rabinovitch R, Julian TB, et al. Report of the working groups on breast MRI: report of the breast cancer staging group. *Breast J* 2004;10(2):S3–S8.

52. Orel SG, Schnall MD, Newman RW, et al. MR imaging-guided localization and biopsy of breast lesions: initial experience. *Radiology* 1994;193:97–102.

53. Heywang-Kobrunner SH, Huynh AT, Viehweg P, et al. Prototype breast coil for MR-guided needle localization. *J Comput Assist Tomogr* 1994;18(6):876–881.

54. Kuhl CK, Morakkabati N, Leutner CC, et al. MR imaging-guided large-core (14-gauge) needle biopsy of small lesions visible at breast MR imaging alone. *Radiology* 2001;220: 31–39.

55. Fischer U, Vossherich R, Keating D, et al. MR-guided biopsy of suspect breast lesions with a simple stereotaxic add-on device for surface coils. *Radiology* 1994;192:272–273.

56. Gorczyca DP, Schneider E, DeBruhl ND, et al. Silicone breast implant rupture: comparison between three-point Dixon and fast spin-echo MR imaging. *AJR Am J Roentgenol* 1994;162:305–310.

57. Gorczyca DP, DeBruhl ND, Ahn CY, et al. Silicone breast implant ruptures in an animal model: comparison of mammography, MR imaging, US, and CT. *Radiology* 1994;190: 227–232

58. Gorczyca DP, Sinha S, Ahn CY, et al. Silicone breast implants in vivo: MR imaging. *Radiology* 1992;185:407–410.

59. Gorczyca DP. Magnetic resonance imaging of the augmented breast and breast tumors. *Breast J* 1996;2(1): 18–22.

60. Soo MS, Kornguth PJ, Walsh R, et al. Complex radial folds versus subtle signs of intracapsular rupture of breast implants: MR findings with surgical correlation. AJR *Am J Roentgenol* 1996;166:1421–1427.

61. Kinkel K, Helbich TH, Esserman LJ, et al. Dynamic high-spatial-resolution MR imaging of suspicious breast lesions: diagnostic criteria and interobserver variability. *AJR Am J Roentgenol* 2000;175:35–43.

62. Kuhl CK, Mielcareck P, Klaschik S, et al. Dynamic breast MR imaging: are signal intensity time course data useful for differential diagnosis of enhancing lesions? *Radiology* 1999;211:101–110.

63. Harms SE, Flaming DP, Hesley KL, et al. Fat-suppressed three-dimensional MR imaging of the breast. *RadioGraphics* 1993;13(2):247–267.

64. Kaiser WA, Zeitler E. MR imaging of the breast: fast imaging sequences with and without Gd-DTPA. *Radiology* 1989;170:681–686.

65. Harms SE, Flaming DP, Hesley KL, et al. MR imaging of the breast with rotating delivery of excitation off resonance: clinical experience with pathologic correlation. *Radiology* 1993;186:493–501.

66. Heywang-Kobrunner SH. Contrast-enhanced magnetic resonance imaging of the breast. *Invest Radiol* 1994;29:94–104.

67. Kaiser WA, Zeitler E. MR imaging of the breast: fast imaging sequences with and without Gd-DTPA. *Radiology* 1989;170:681–686.

68. Orel S, Schnall MD, LiVolsi VA, et al. Suspicious breast lesions: MR imaging with radiologic-pathologic correlation. *Radiology* 1994;190:485–493.

69. Gilles R, Zafrani B, Guinebretiere JM, et al. Ductal carcinoma in situ: MR imaging-histopathologic correlation. *Radiology* 1995;196:415–419.

70. Morris EA. Breast MR imaging: performance, reporting with BI-RADS®, and pitfalls in interpretation. *Breast Imaging: RSNA Categorical Course in Diagnostic Radiology*, ed. Feig SA, Radiological Society of North America, Oak Brook, IL. 2005;175–184.

71. Kawashima M, Tamaki Y, Nonaka T, et al. MR imaging of mucous carcinoma of the breast. *AJR Am J Roentgenol* 2002;179:179–183.

72. Liberman L, Morris EA, Joo-Young Lee M, et al. Breast lesions detected on MR imaging: features and positive predictive value. *AJR Am J Roentgenol* 2002;179:171–178.

73. Orel SG, Mendonca MH, Reynolds C, et al. MR imaging of ductal carcinoma in situ. *Radiology* 1997;202:413–420.

74. Newstead GM. Problem-solving MR Imaging of the breast. *Breast Imaging: RSNA Categorical Course in Diagnostic Radiology*, ed. Feig SA, Radiological Society of North America, Oak Brook, IL. 2005;191–198.

75. Boetes C, Mus RD, Holland R, et al. Breast tumors: comparative accuracy of MR imaging relative to mammography and US for demonstrating extent. *Radiology* 1995;197(3): 743–747.

76. Davis PL, Staiger MJ, Harris KB, et al. Breast cancer measurements with magnetic resonance imaging, ultrasonography, and mammography. *Breast Cancer Res Treat* 1996;37:1–9.

77. Yang WT, Lam WW, Cheung H, et al. Sonographic, magnetic resonance imaging and mammographic assessments of preoperative size of breast cancer. *J Ultrasound Med* 1997;16:791–797.

78. Gribbestad IS, Nilsen G, Fjosne H, et al. Contrast-enhanced magnetic resonance imaging of the breast. *Acta Oncol* 1992;31(8):833–842.

79. Weinstein SP, Orel SG, Heller R, et al. MR imaging of the breast in patients with invasive lobular carcinoma. *AJR Am J Roentgenol* 2001;176:399–406.

80. Orel SG, Reynolds C, Schnall MD, et al. Breast carcinoma: MR imaging before re-excisional biopsy. *Radiology* 1997; 205:429–436.

81. Esserman L, Hylton N, Yassa L, et al. Utility of magnetic resonance imaging in the management of breast cancer: evidence for improved preoperative staging. *J Clin Oncol* 1999;17:110–119.

82. Drew PJ, Chatterjee S, Turnbull LW, et al. Dynamic contrast enhanced magnetic resonance imaging of the breast is superior to triple assessment for the preoperative detection of multifocal breast cancer. *Ann Surg Oncol* 1999;6:599–603.

83. Orel SG, Schnall MD, Powell CM, et al. Staging of suspected breast cancer: effect of MR imaging and MR-guided biopsy. *Radiology* 1995;196:115–122.

84. Liberman L, Morris EA, Dershaw DD, et al. MR imaging of the ipsilateral breast in women with percutaneously proven breast cancer. *AJR Am J Roentgenol* 2003;180:901–910.

85. Van Goethem M, Schelfout K, Dijckmans L, et al. MR mammography in the pre-operative staging of breast cancer in patients with dense breast tissue: comparison with mammography and ultrasound. *Eur Radiol* 2004;14(5):809–816.

86. Berg WA, Gutierrez L, NessAiver MS, et al. Diagnostic accuracy of mammography, clinical examination, US, and MR imaging in preoperative assessment of breast cancer. *Radiology* 2004;233(3):830–849.

87. Sardanelli F, Giuseppetti GM, Panizza P, et al. Sensitivity of MRI versus mammography for detecting foci of multifocal, multicentric breast cancer in fatty and dense breasts using the whole-breast pathologic examination as a gold standard. *AJR Am J Roentgenol* 2004;183:1149–1157.

88. Liberman L. Assessment of extent of disease using magnetic resonance imaging. In Morris EA, Liberman L, eds. *Breast MRI: Diagnosis and Intervention*. New York: Springer, 2005: 200–213.

89. Hungness ES, Safa M, Shaughnessy EA, et al. Bilateral synchronous breast cancer: mode of detection and comparison of histologic features between the 2 breasts. *Surgery* 2000; 128:702–707.

90. Rieber A, Merkle E, Bohm W, et al. MRI of histologically confirmed mammary carcinoma: clinical relevance of diagnostic procedures for detection of multifocal or contralateral secondary carcinoma. *J Comput Assist Tomogr* 1997;21: 773–779.

91. Birdwell RL, Smith DN. MR imaging use in breast cancer staging and the assessment of treatment. *Breast Imaging: RSNA Categorical Course in Diagnostic Radiology*, ed. Feig SA, Radiological Society of North America, Oak Brook, IL. 2005;199–207.

92. Orel SG, Troupin RH, Patterson EA, et al. Breast cancer recurrence after lumpectomy and irradiation: role of mammography in detection. *Radiology* 1992;183(1):201–206.

93. Berenberg AL, Jochelson MS, Harris JR. Mammographic detection of recurrent cancer in the irradiated breast. *AJR Am J Roentgenol* 1987;148:39–43.

94. Dao TH, Rahmouni A, Campana F, et al. Tumor recurrence versus fibrosis in the irradiated breast: differentiation with dynamic gadolinium-enhanced MR imaging. *Radiology* 1993;187:751–755.

95. Lewis-Jones HG, Whitehouse GH, Leinster SJ. The role of MRI in the assessment of local recurrence breast carcinoma. *Clin Radiol* 1991;43:197–204.

96. Fisher ER, Anderson S, Tan-Chiu E, et al. Fifteen year prognostic discriminates for invasive breast carcinoma. *Cancer* 2001;91:1679–1687.

97. Yeh E, Slanetz P, Kopans DB, et al. Prospective comparison of mammography, sonography, and MRI in patients undergoing neoadjuvant chemotherapy for palpable breast cancer. *AJR Am J Roentgenol* 2005;184:868–877.

98. Rosen EL, Blackwell KL, Baker JA, et al. Accuracy of MRI in the detection of residual breast cancer after neoadjuvant chemotherapy. *AJR Am J Roentgenol* 2003;181:1275–1282.

99. Rieber A, Brambs HJ, Gabelmann A, et al. Breast MRI for monitoring response of primary breast cancer to neoadjuvant chemotherapy. *Eur Radiol* 2002;12:1711–1719.

100. Chen C, Orel SG, Harris E, et al. Outcome after treatment of patients with mammographically occult, magnetic resonance imaging-detected breast cancer presenting with axillary adenopathy. *Clin Breast Cancer* 2004;5:72–77.

101. Obdeijn IMA, Brouwers-Kuyper EMJ, Tilanus-Linthorst MMA, et al. MR imaging-guided sonography followed by fine-needle aspiration cytology in occult carcinoma of the breast. *AJR Am J Roentgenol* 2000;174:1079–1084.

102. Orel SG, Dougherty CS, Reynolds C, et al. MR imaging in patients with nipple discharge: initial experience. *Radiology* 2000;216:248–254.

103. Morris EA, Liberman L, Ballon DJ, et al. MRI of occult breast carcinoma in a high-risk population. *AJR Am J Roentgenol* 2003;181:619–626.

104. Kuhl CK, Schmutzler RK, Leutner CC, et al. Breast MR imaging screening in 192 women proved or suspected to be carriers of a breast cancer susceptibility gene: preliminary results. *Radiology* 2000;215:267–279.

105. Tilanus-Linthorst MM, Obdeijn IM, Bartels KC, et al. First experiences in screening women at high risk for breast cancer with MR imaging. *Breast Cancer Res Treat* 2000;63:53–60.

106. Stoutjesdijk MJ, Boetes C, Jager GJ, et al. Magnetic resonance imaging and mammography in women with a hereditary risk of breast cancer. *J Natl Cancer Inst* 2001;93:1095–1102.

107. Kriege M, Brekelmans CT, Boetes C, et al. Efficacy of MRI and mammography for breast-cancer screening in women with a familial or genetic predisposition. *N Engl J Med* 2004;351:427–437.

108. Lee CH. Current status of MR imaging screening for breast cancer, in *Breast Imaging: RSNA Categorical Course in Diagnostic Radiology*, ed. Feig SA, Radiological Society of North America, Oak Brook, IL. 2005;209–216.

Page numbers followed by "*f*" refer to figures; page numbers followed by "*t*" refer to tables.